Diagnosis and Management of Primary Bone Tumors

Won-Jong Bahk

Diagnosis and Management of Primary Bone Tumors

Volume 1

Springer

Won-Jong Bahk
Department of Orthopaedic Surgery
Cheju Halla General Hospital
Jeju-si, Korea (Republic of)

ISBN 978-981-96-3483-5 ISBN 978-981-96-3484-2 (eBook)
https://doi.org/10.1007/978-981-96-3484-2

This Springer imprint is published by the registered company Springer Nature Singapore Pte Ltd.
The registered company address is: 152 Beach Road, #21-01/04 Gateway East, Singapore 189721, Singapore

Preface

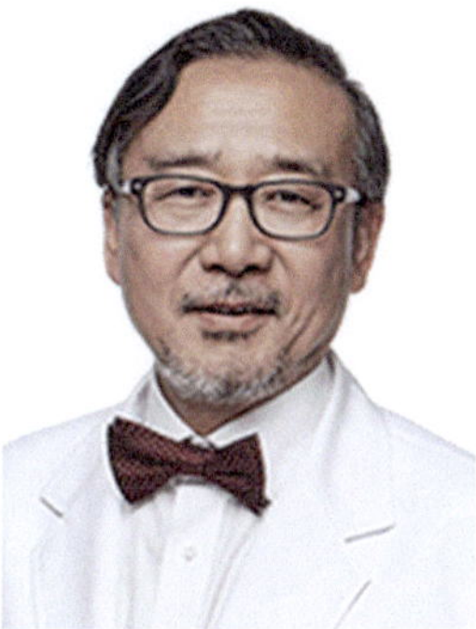

Fundamentally, there are diverse subtypes of bone tumors, either benign or malignant lesions, depending on the tissue components originated and location of the bone including intramedullary cavity, cortex or periosteum. As is well known, each subtype presents protean radiologic manifestations and variable pathologic findings in each case and even in the same cases depending on the phases of tumors. The other unique factors such as inadequate samples by poor biopsy technique, tissues obtained from reactive zone, and callus tissue by unrecognized stress or fatigue fracture which is not existed in tumors of other organs can make a diagnosis of bone tumors more confusing and difficulty. Thus, the emphasis throughout the books is on an integrated team approach to diagnosis and management highlighting the important role of clinical, radiologic, and pathologic correlation, so-called "diagnostic triangle," for reducing the possibility of diagnostic error and avoiding inadequate under- or over-treatment. In addition, microscopic findings of callus tissue are precisely described based on the weekly age of the tissue and the importance of the histologic recognition of it for correct diagnosis. Appearances on the full range of imaging studies including plain radiographs, CT scan, MRI, bone scans, SPECT CT as well as PET/CT scan are illustrated in addition to the pathologic findings in as many cases as possible. Attention is also drawn to the role of long-term follow-up radiographs ensuring if the diagnosis with management is reasonable for all physicians.

Jeju-si, Korea (Republic of) Won-Jong Bahk

Acknowledgments

First of all, I would like to express the deepest appreciation from the bottom of my heart to Professor Emeritus Joseph M. Mirra and Young-Whee Bahk for giving me a special inspiration of these Books. I also would like to acknowledge Professor Emeritus Yong-Koo Kang, Professors Yang-Guk Chung (The Catholic University of Korea) and Whan-Sung Cho (Seoul National University) as well as Sungtaek-Jung (Chunnam National University), Jung-Il Kim (Busan National University), Jong-Hoon Park (Korea University), "Young-Hoon" Kim, Min-Wuk Joo, Jae-Young Lee, Yong-Suk Lee (The Catholic University of Korea), Sung-Wook Seo, Se-Jun Park (Samsung Medical Center) for their courtesy of cases. Many thanks are due to Kyung-Jin Seo (Professor of Department of Hospital Pathology, Uijeongbu St. Mary's Hospital) for his expertise photographic work of microscopic features, and Woo-Jin Chang (Librarian of the Catholic University of Korea) for his expertise bibliographic work. I have to appreciate Clinical Assistant Professor Ji Hoon Bahk (The Catholic University of Korea) for his effort to arrange the numerous references and citation. Finally, I would like to pay a special and hearty tribute to my wife Kyeong-Hee Lee, my son Ji Hoon Bahk, daughter-in-law Jueun Kwak, and my lovely grandson Yu Joon Bahk for everything we have always shared hand-in-hand to make comfortable and stable my family during all these prolong perspiring, endeavoring, and inspiring years.

Contents

Part I

General Considerations

1 General Considerations

1.1 Introduction

The term *tumor* originated from the Latin word *tumere* meaning to swell, which refers to a new growth of certain tissues in which the multiplication of cells is uncontrolled and progressive, and also called *a neoplasm* [1]. The word *tumor* is defined as those neoplastic conditions and tumor-like lesions that mimic or may be mistaken for a true neoplasm [2]. Bone tumors are traditionally classified as benign (noncancerous) or malignant (cancerous). *Benign bone tumors* lack the properties of spreading to local structures or to distant parts of the body, which tend to grow slowly with distinct borders and have a favorable chance for recovery. However, *malignant bone tumors* have a property of local invasiveness with cortical destruction and soft tissue extension as well as spreading and metastasis to other organs via the bloodstream or the lymphatics with less chance of recovery and survival. Bone tumors are also classified as *primary bone tumor* which arises in bone or from bone-derived cells and tissues and *secondary bone tumor* which first starts in another part of the body and metastasize to the skeleton, mainly through the vascular or sometimes lymphatic system. The latter secondary is also called a *metastatic bone cancer* which is the same type of cancer as the original primary cancer. For example, cancer cells may spread from the primary cancer of the lung to the bone, producing a new secondary cancer. The cancer cells in the bone are identical to those in the lung. Another different type of *second cancer* can newly occur as a late effect of the first cancer or its treatment, or it may be unrelated to the first cancer. More recently, *Double or multiple primary cancers* or *subsequent neoplasm* has been diagnosed in the same individual with increasing incidence. As the population of cancer survivors from their first cancer diagnosis has increased and continues to age, the incidence of *second cancers* has risen dramatically from 9% of all cancer diagnoses in 1975–1979 to 19% in 2005–2009 [3]. The risk of development varies substantially depending on the age of the patients, the type of initial primary cancer, and its management, including chemotherapy, radiotherapy, and bone marrow transplantation, prevalence of second cancer risk factors, lifestyle and environment, genetic susceptibility to second cancer etiology, and exposure to other cancer risk factors. Precancerous conditions include benign tumors or lesions with abnormal cells, which are associated with a risk of developing into cancer, so-called *malignant change or transformation*. Higher risk precursors for malignant transformation include Ollier's disease and Maffucci's syndrome, familial retinoblastoma syndrome, or Rothmund Thompson syndrome. Moderate risk groups include multiple osteochondromas, Paget's disease, and radiation osteitis. Lower risk can be associated with bone infarction, long-term chronic osteomyelitis (OM), prosthetic implants, osteogenesis

W.-J. Bahk, *Diagnosis and Management of Primary Bone Tumors*,
https://doi.org/10.1007/978-981-96-3484-2_1

imperfecta, or some benign bone tumors such as fibrous dysplasia (FD), giant cell tumor (GCT), osteoblastoma (OB), and chondroblastoma (CB) [4]. Correct diagnosis of bone tumors has been well known to be difficult to make for a variety of reasons, including the many tumor subtypes, the protean radiologic manifestations, and variable pathologic findings depending on the phases of the tumor, the presence of reactive host bone changes, overlapping findings between benign and malignant tumors, and issues relating to adequacy of biopsy. The aims of these books (Volume 1 & 2) are to offer the best guidance in negotiating these potential difficulties for a correct diagnosis of bone tumors by a clinical-radiologic-pathologic correlation and to provide adequate options for management and outcomes for each tumor. Early in 1958, Jaffe [5] emphasized the *diagnostic triangle* of the cooperative approach by the orthopedic surgeon, radiologist, and pathologist to reach a rational diagnosis, and the concept is still valuable in diagnosis of bone tumors (Fig. 1.1a). They should share their points of view on a bone lesion, including clinical factors such as patient age, location in a particular bone or part of a bone, solitary or multiple lesions, and other preexisting conditions for a rational diagnosis as well as radiologic and pathologic findings. For a simple example, a differential diagnosis of osteofibrous dysplasia from FD cannot be attained only with a microscopic finding of irregular, curvilinear trabeculae of woven bone with osteoblastic rimming and intervening bland spindle cells in some cases. However, it is easily distinguished by adding only one radiograph with an *eccentric cortex-based* lesion exclusively in the tibia and/or fibula with an open growth plate indicating a young child (Fig. 1.1b). Conversely, a diagnosis of fibrous dysplasia can also be easily made by radiographic findings of a *concentric intramedullary* lesion with a "ground-glass" density in the midshaft of other long bones (Fig. 1.1c). Even such an approach cannot avoid all diagnostic errors, but it can certainly make them fewer and less glaring. The recent advent of molecular diagnostic techniques has expanded this diagram into a *diagnostic quadrangle* to reduce diagnostic errors [6], but the technique is not covered in this edition of the books (Vol. 1 & 2). These books provide a comprehensive conventional guide to the radiologic and pathologic diagnosis, biopsy technique, as well as clinical outcomes and radiologic follow-up results after conservative or surgical management in primary benign and malignant bone tumors. In addition, histologic findings of callus tissue caused by fatigue or stress fracture and even pathologic fracture that

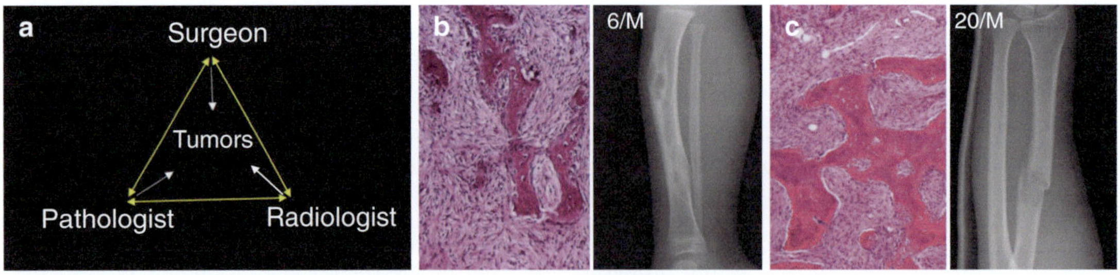

Fig. 1.1 Diagnostic triangle. (**a**) Early in 1958, a cooperative approach by surgeons, radiologists, and pathologists was already emphasized by Jaffe to share their points of view on a bone lesion for a rational diagnosis. *Simple examples*: (**b**) A differential diagnosis of OFD from FD cannot be assured only by a microscopic finding of irregular, curvilinear trabeculae of woven bone with exuberant osteoblastic rimming and intervening bland spindle cells (Left). However, a diagnosis of OFD is easily made by adding only a single radiograph which shows multiple eccentric cortex-based bubbly lesions of tibia diaphysis with open growth plates indicating a young growing child (Right). (**c**) A microscopic finding of irregular, curvilinear trabeculae of woven bone is also seen with prominent osteoblastic rimming simulating OFD (Left). However, a diagnosis of FD is easily made by an additional radiographic finding of a concentric radiolucent lesion and minimally displaced fracture with *"ground-glass"* density in the midshaft of the radius, and a closed growth plate, indicating an adult (Right)

can make a diagnosis more complicated will be presented by the age of the callus to reduce the wrong diagnosis in its own chapter. The emphasis throughout the books is on an integrated team approach to diagnosis and management, highlighting the important role of clinical, radiologic, and pathologic correlation in reducing the possibility of diagnostic error and avoiding undertreatment or overtreatment. Appearances on the full range of imaging studies are illustrated, including plain radiographs, CT scans, MRI, bone scans, and SPECT CT as well as PET/CT scans. Attention is also drawn to the role of long-term follow-up radiographs, ensuring if the diagnosis with management is reasonable. The incidence, favorite ages, and locations described of each tumor are based on the published data mainly from several major centers such as Mayo Clinic, Rizzoli Institution, or Massachusetts General Hospital, as well as published books edited by Campanacci M, Unni KK, Mirra JM, Czerniak B, or others. Survival rates of primary malignant bone tumors are based on the recent analysis of the National Cancer Institute Surveillance, Epidemiology, and End Results (SEER) program as well as of Mayo Clinic, Rizzoli Institution, MD Anderson Cancer Center group, and others.

1.2 Bone Tumors

Bone is a compact type of hardened connective tissue surrounded by periosteum, muscles, and soft tissue, which consists of a variety of components, including bone and cartilage cells, membranes, neurovascular structures, extracellular mineralized matrix, and central bone marrow. Therefore, there are diverse subtypes of benign and malignant bone tumors depending on the tissue components originated and the location of the bone, including intramedullary cavity, cortex, or periosteum. Each subtype may exhibit protean radiologic manifestations and variable pathologic findings depending on the phases of tumors. The other unique factors, such as inadequate samples by poor biopsy technique and callus tissue by unrecognized stress or fatigue fracture, which does not exist in tumors of other organs, can make a diagnosis of bone tumors more confusing and difficult. Thus, an expert team should be composed of orthopedic surgeon, radiologist, pathologist, radiation, and medical oncologist for a correct diagnosis and adequate management of the broad spectrum of bone tumors.

1. *Incidence*

Primary bone tumors are rare compared to tumors occurring in other organs, and most are benign in nature. However, malignant bone tumors account for a significant proportion of cancers occurring in childhood and adolescence. The true incidence of benign bone tumors is unknown because most of the patients are asymptomatic and do not seek medical attention. Many of them are discovered incidentally on imaging studies for other reasons and remain undiagnosed. The most common benign bone tumors are osteochondroma (OC), enchondroma (EC), and osteoid osteoma (OO) [2, 7]. The solitary osteochondroma affects probably as many as 1–2% of the population, and fibrous cortical defect can be seen in as many as 5–10% of children on radiographic studies. OC, EC, and OO were reported to represent 8.5%, 3.0%, and 2.8% of primary biopsy-analyzed bone tumors, respectively [2]. As for soft tissue tumors, benign conditions of bone are 100 times more frequent than malignant primary bone tumors [7]. The incidence of primary bone sarcoma is much less. Primary bone sarcomas account for only about 0.2% of all malignancies [6–8]. Bone sarcomas occur at a rate that is approximately one-tenth that of soft tissue sarcomas when compared to that of the closely related group of soft tissue sarcomas [9]. According to the Sarcoma Foundation of America, sarcoma accounts for about 1% of adult cancers and 15–20% of childhood cancers diagnosed in the United States [10]. The incidence specifically regarding bone sarcomas is considered one-fifth to one-sixth of all sarcomas, with an incidence of about 1 new case/100,000 inhabitants/year [7]. However, malignant bone tumors are outnumbered by metastases from carcinoma or hematologic malignancies, including myeloma. The most frequently diagnosed subtypes of primary malignant bone tumors are osteosarcoma (OSA), chondrosarcoma (CSA), and Ewing sarcoma (ESA), followed by chordoma [7, 11], which represent about 36%, 27%, 14%, and 8% of all bone sarcomas, respectively [6]. OSA and ESA develop mainly in children and young adults, whereas CSA is usually found in middle aged and older adults. Although the most common cancers causing death are carcinomas arising from the lung, stomach, colorectum, pancreas, prostate, and breast, primary malignant bone tumors rank as as the third leading cause of death in patients with cancer younger than 20 years despite the very low incidence. Survival rates for bone sarcoma depend on many factors, including age, location, histologic grade, stage, feasibility to surgical resection, and response to chemotherapy or radiotherapy of bone sarcoma. According to 2022 estimates for sarcomas in the United States by Sarcoma Foundation of America [10], 5-year survival rate for primary bone sarcoma was up to 87% when the cancer was diagnosed at the localized stage, 83% if it spread to surrounding tissues or organs and/or the regional lymph nodes, and 55% when the cancer had spread to distant parts of the body (metastatic disease).

2. *Favorite ages and locations* (Tables 1.1 and 1.2)

Typically, there are predilections for certain ages and locations of specific bone tumors, which allow a significant reduction in the diagnostic spectrums. The majority of benign bone tumors or lesions including nonossifying fibroma (NOF), simple bone cyst (SBC), aneurysmal bone cyst (ABC), chondroblastoma (CB), osteoid osteoma (OO), osteoblastoma (OB), osteofibrous dysplasia (OFD), Langerhans cell histiocytosis (LCH), and chondromyxoid fibroma (CMF) usually occur during growing period in the first two decades of life. There is no significant gender predilection with any clinical significance in most cases. Among locally aggressive benign bone tumors, GCT occurs mostly in skeletally mature patients between 20 and 40 years of age after epiphyseal closure, while CB typically occurs in younger patients between 10 and 20 years of age before epiphyseal closure. Typically, the age-specific incidence rates of primary bone sarcomas show a bimodal distribution with a first peak occurring in the first and second decades during the growing period and a second peak in adult patients in the fifth to seventh decades of life [6, 12]. Of the malignant bone tumors, the most common histologic subtypes occurring in the first two decades of life include ESA and OSA. Other rare cases such as neuroblastoma, retinoblastoma, rhabdomyosarcoma, and leukemia occur also in that young age. On the contrary, CSA, secondary OSA, chordoma, myeloma, undifferentiated pleomorphic sarcoma (UPS), and fibrosarcoma (FSA) usually occur after the fifth decade. Metastatic cancer to bone, secondary sarcoma in preexisting benign bone tumors, or after irradiation often develop in older

Table 1.1 Favorite ages of specific bone tumors

< 10 years	Rare—Nonossifying fibroma, osteofibrous dysplasia, Langerhans' cell histiocytosis, neuroblastoma, retinoblastoma, leukemia, rhabdomyosarcoma
10–20 years	Most tumors—Enchondroma, osteochondroma, osteoid osteoma, chondroblastoma, chondromyxoid fibroma, simple bone cyst, aneurysmal bone cyst, osteosarcoma, Ewing sarcoma
20–40 years	Giant cell tumor
40–50 years	Chondrosarcoma, lymphoma, fibrosarcoma
> 50 years	Myeloma, metastasis

Table 1.2 Favorite locations of specific bone tumors

Epiphysis	Giant cell tumor, chondroblastoma, clear cell chondrosarcoma
Metaphysis	Nonossifying fibroma, fibrous dysplasia, chondromyxoid fibroma, osteochondroma, enchondroma, simple bone cyst, aneurysmal bone cyst, osteoblastoma, osteosarcoma, chondrosarcoma
Diaphysis	Langerhans' cell histiocytosis, osteoid osteoma, enchondroma, osteofibrous dysplasia, Ewing's sarcoma, chondrosarcoma, adamantinoma
Arch spine	Aneurysmal bone cyst, osteoid osteoma, osteoblastoma
Body spine	Hemangioma, giant cell rumor, osteosarcoma

patients between sixth and eighth decades of life. In addition, most bone tumors occur in favorite locations of predilection for certain bones, which provide a valuable clue or strong suggestion for a certain diagnosis in combination with favorite ages. Most primary bone tumors, including OC, EC, NOF, SBC, ABC, CMF, FD, and OSA, affect the metaphysis or meta-diaphysis if long bone is involved. However, ESA, CSA, OO, or LCH occurs mostly in the diaphysis. GCT, CB, or clear cell CSA occur most favorably in the epiphysis and extends frequently to the metaphysis. If GCT purely affects the metaphysis or diaphysis rather than epiphysis, serum level of calcium, phosphate, and parathyroid hormone (PTH) should be checked to exclude "brown tumor" in primary hyperparathyroidism which almost always occurs in the metaphysis or diaphysis. A heavily ossified mass pasted on the intact posterior cortex of the distal femur is a strong indication of parosteal OSA, and thus biopsy is not necessary for a histologic confirmation. Almost exclusively, adamantinoma and OFD affect the cortex of the diaphysis of the tibial and/or fibula. CSA exhibits a predilection for the meta-diaphysis of the femur and humerus, as well as flat bones such as pelvis, ribs, scapula, and sternum, but rarely short tubular bones of hands and feet or spines. EC most often most often involves the short tubular bones of the hands and feet accounting for over half of the cases, followed by meta-diaphysis of the distal femur, proximal humerus and fibula, and distal tibia. It is uncommon in truncal bones such as pelvis, rib, and scapula. In the spine, ABC, OO, or OB involves more commonly in the posterior element including transverse or spinous process and pedicle. In contrast, hemangioma, GCT, or OSA usually affects anterior elements such as the body. Chordoma is almost exclusively located in the axial skeleton from the base of the skull to the coccyx. About 80–90% of cases occur in the sacro-coccygeal and spheno-occipital regions, and the remaining cases arise in the mobile cervical and lumbar spine. The thoracic spine is rarely affected. In the sacrum, chordoma usually involves caudal sacrum below S3, while other tumors such as GCT, CSA, or OSA frequently occur at higher sacral levels.

3. *Clinical information*

1) Clinical history and symptoms

Most bone tumors have a predilection for a specific age group. Thus, age of the patients is one of the important clinical information when assessing a bone tumor. The characteristics of the pain and its duration are other valuable information particularly when they are correlated with radiologic and histologic findings. For example, a differentiation of cellular EC from Grade 1 CSA has been well known to be extremely difficult by histologic findings alone. However, clinical information of symptoms is valuable to increase the probability of a correct diagnosis. Most patients with EC are asymptomatic and fortuitously discovered during image studies including plain radiographs or MRI for other reasons or bone scan and PET/CT scan as a part of staging workup in cancer patients (refer Figs. 1.3, 1.4, and 1.5 in Enchondroma chapter). A history of asymptomatic and incidentally found lesion provides a greater chance of EC rather than CSA. When pain exists, it may occur immediately after mild injury by slip or fall and strenuous physical activities in about half of patients with EC. The remaining half of patients have more vague and milder pain of longer duration, which is more ominous to interpret because longstanding, vague pain is also typical of grade 1 CSA [13]. The most important key is to evaluate the nature of the pain whether it directly originates from the lesion in the bone or from the other reasons. In many patients, the pain is localized in the shoulder joint not directly referred to the upper arm with bony lesion. When findings of rotator cuff tear, microfracture, capsular injury, or unrelated arthritic change on MRI, it would be the cause of the shoulder pain and indicates more likely a diagnosis of EC (refer Fig. 5 in Enchondroma chapter). However, the vague pain localized in the upper arm rather than the shoulder joint which seems to be directly referable to the bony lesion suggests more likely a diagnosis of low-grade CSA. Localized swelling or palpable hard mass or limitation of joint motion may rarely be associated.

2) Pertinent past history and family history

A positive familial history is very rare in bone tumors with two rare exceptions being hereditary multiple osteochondromatosis and neurofibromatosis.

3) Physical examination

If presnet, the palpable mass is usually stony hard with or without localized tenderness. The adjacent joint can be swollen with joint effusion, and the range of the joint motion can be limited due to pain or mechanical blocking. *Café au lait* pigmentations that have irregular borders resembling "the coast of Maine" are observed in polyostotic FD. In contrast, the skin pigmentations in neurofibromatosis and Jaffe-Campanacci syndrome (multiple NOF with extraskeletal abnormalities) show regular borders resembling "the coast of California." Careful physical examination is necessary to find the hidden spots in the axillary fossa and gluteal folds. Sexual precocity in young girls associated with various endocrinopathies or exophthalmos can be detected during physical examination in some cases of polyostotic FD.

4) Laboratory Data

The laboratory data are usually nonspecific in bone tumors. However, blood chemistry shows an elevated serum level of certain substances which can be of diagnostic value. Alkaline phosphatase level is increased in any condition with tremendous osteoblastic activity as in OSA, fracture callus, osteoblastic metastasis from prostate carcinoma, and Paget's disease. It will return to normal level in a few days after surgical removal of OSA, and a re-elevation of the alkaline phosphatase level is an ominous sign suggesting a probable local recurrence or metastasis. Neutrophils and erythrocytes sedimentation rate (ESR) can be elevated in some cases of ESA or LCH. Laboratory findings including anemia, hypercalcemia, reverse A/G ratio (low albumin and high globulin), proteinuria, and Bence-Jones proteinuria are associated with plasma cell myeloma (PCM). In addition, serum and urine immunoelectrophoresis (IEP) or immunofixation electrophoresis (IFE) can identify abonormal myeloma protein.

4. *Characteristics of imaging modalities*

A. *Plain radiographs*

Plain radiograph is an essential and indispensable tool in the diagnosis of bone tumors. Bone is a compact type of hardened connective tissue consisting of variuos types of bone and cartilage cells, hematopoietic marrow cells periosteal cells, fibroblasts, fat cells, nerve cells, vascular cells, smooth muscle cells, notochordal cells, or histiocytes, and various types of extracellular mineralized matrix. Therefore, protean radiologic manifestations are observed in the diverse subtypes of bone tumors depending on their aggressiveness and phases even in the same entity, and they may be nonspecific and difficult to diagnose. In addition, bone destruction cannot be detected on conventional radiographs until the host is destroyed to a certain degree. In its earliest stage, tumors arising in the medullary cavity may spread invisibly through the intertrabecular spaces, and a large amount of cancellous bone should be destructed before the loss will be seen on conventional radiographs which require longer periods of time to be detected [14]. However, almost all primary bone tumors penetrate the cortex at a rather early stage and may be seen more easily on radiographs due to the greater contrast density between osteolytic area and intact bone compared to the cancellous bone. This is more likely in the long bones where the cortex is usually thicker, and the fairly uniform density of the overlying soft tissues is not likely to obscure the pattern of destruction. However, the thinness of the cortex and confusing shadows of overlying gas often obscure the pattern of destruction in the spongy bones such as the spine and pelvis [15]. In the earlier 1950s, Ardran [16] reported up to 30% of postmortem vertebral body thickness could escape detection on radiographs, and Lachman [17] described that 30% of overall bone density was necessary to be destroyed before any alteration could be detected. A decade later, Clain [18] described that approximately 10% of the patients with metastatic cancer had normal X-rays when first seen, and they complained of pain for some time before the radiographs showed vertebral deposits. He also found that certain sites of bone metastasis (notably vertebra) showed a higher incidence of negative radiographic findings than other sites at the first investigation. Edelstyn and colleagues [19] reported the defects were detected on lateral radiograph only when 50–75% of the cancellous bone thickness was removed, and greater deficit was necessary on anteroposterior view in an experimental study on human lumbar vertebrae with conical holes of gradually increased size in the center of the cancellous body as being a reasonable approximation to a naturally occurring metastasis. The figure was approximately twice as great as Ardran's that of 30%. Thus, alternative more sensitive methods such as bone scan, SPECT/CT imaging, CT scan, MRI, or PET/CT scan should be obviously necessary for early detection of changes of bone structure in bone tumors. The most important first step of radiologic interpretation is to get the age of the patient and the location of the tumor, which can narrow the scope of differential diagnosis. A systemic approach to radiographic interpretation should include evaluating the following factors [20].

1. *Number of the lesion; solitary/multiple*

   The number of bone lesions is important because primary malignant bone tumors rarely present multifocal lesions, but metastatic cancers or hematologic malignancies affect multiple bones more frequently. Benign bone tumors are also usually solitary, but multiple lesions are more common in cases of EC, OC, FD, NOF, LCH, or brown tumors of hyperparathyroidism. Bone scan is useful to detect multiple bony lesions but cannot provide information regarding types of pathologic processes.

2. *Location of the lesion within the bone* (Table 1.2)

   The location of the lesion within a certain bone is a very important determination for diagnosis and subclassification of bone tumors. A preferential location for each tumor includes long bone or flat bone, axial or appendicular skeleton as mentioned in the Introduction. The location of the lesion in a long bone is typified by its longitudinal involvement (epiphysis, metaphysis, diaphysis), which allows narrowing the diagnostic spectrum. An apophysis of long bone (a growth center not contributing to bone growth) is the equivalent of an epiphysis. It is also categorized by its transverse location (medulla, cortex, periosteum) that subclassifies the tumor into intramedullary, intracortical, or periosteal to parosteal (juxtacortical) tumors. This subclassification can be useful for a decision of surgical margin and provide a prognostic implication.

3. *Patterns of bone destruction by Lodwick* (Figs. 1.2, 1.3, and 1.4)

   The radiographic patterns of destruction, host bone response pattern to the lesion, and margin of the lesion are the most important factors to determine the growth rate and the degree of aggressiveness of the tumor. The destruction pattern usually correlates to pathologic indolence or aggressiveness. The transition zone between the host bone and the tumor presents range from a well-defined to an ill-defined infiltrative margin. A lesion with sharp margin with a narrow transitional zone is regarded as nonaggressive benign tumor particularly when surrounded by a thin rim of reactive sclerosis. This pattern suggests a slow growth of the tumor to provide sufficient time to make the reactive sclerosis by the host bone. In contrast, an ill-defined lesion with a wide transition zone suggesting rapid growth indicates locally aggressive benign or malignant bone tumors. Three basic patterns of *geographic*, *moth-eaten*, and *permeative* destruction in bone tumors have been described by Lodwick [15, 21] (Fig. 1.2). Biological aggressiveness increases with faster growth speed from geographic via moth-eaten to permeated destruction (Fig. 1.3).

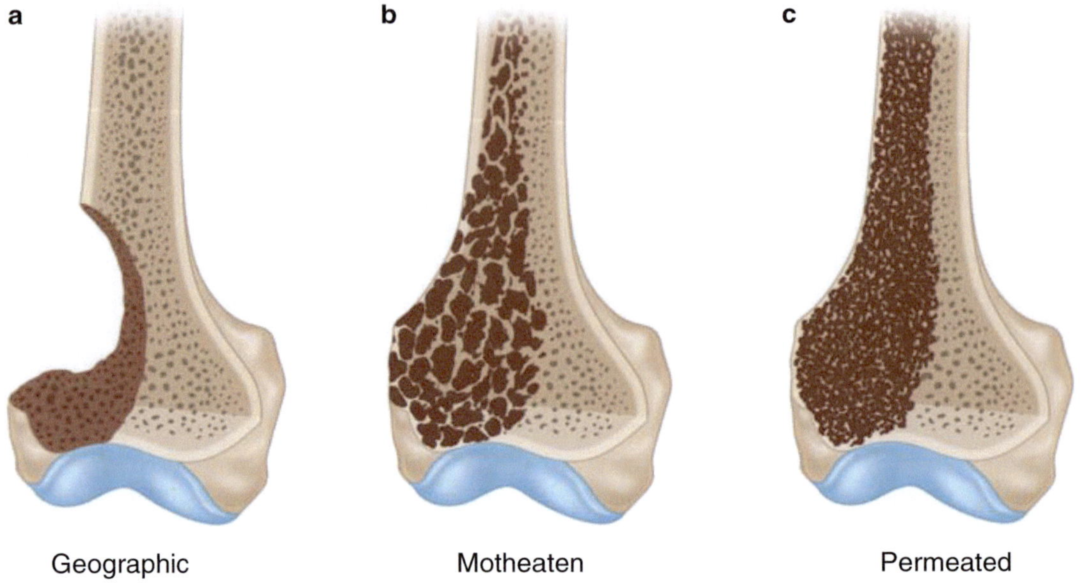

Fig. 1.2 Patterns of bone destruction by Lodwick. (**a**) Grade I: *"Geographic"* bone destruction typified by a large, uniformly destroyed area implies the slowest growth rate with a well-defined margin which is indicative of the least aggressive benign bone tumors. (**b**) Grade II: *"Moth-eaten"* bone destruction is typified by multiple small holes of irregular sizes, which are usually confluent and imply moderately aggressive growth that is seen in the geographic pattern. (**c**) Grade III: *"Permeated"* bone destruction is characterized by innumerable, uniformly tiny holes in the cortical bone with indistinct margins of bone destruction implying the most rapid rate of growth. The cortex may appear intact with greatly diminished density because of multiple penetrating holes. Biological aggressiveness increases from type geographic via moth-eaten to permeated destruction

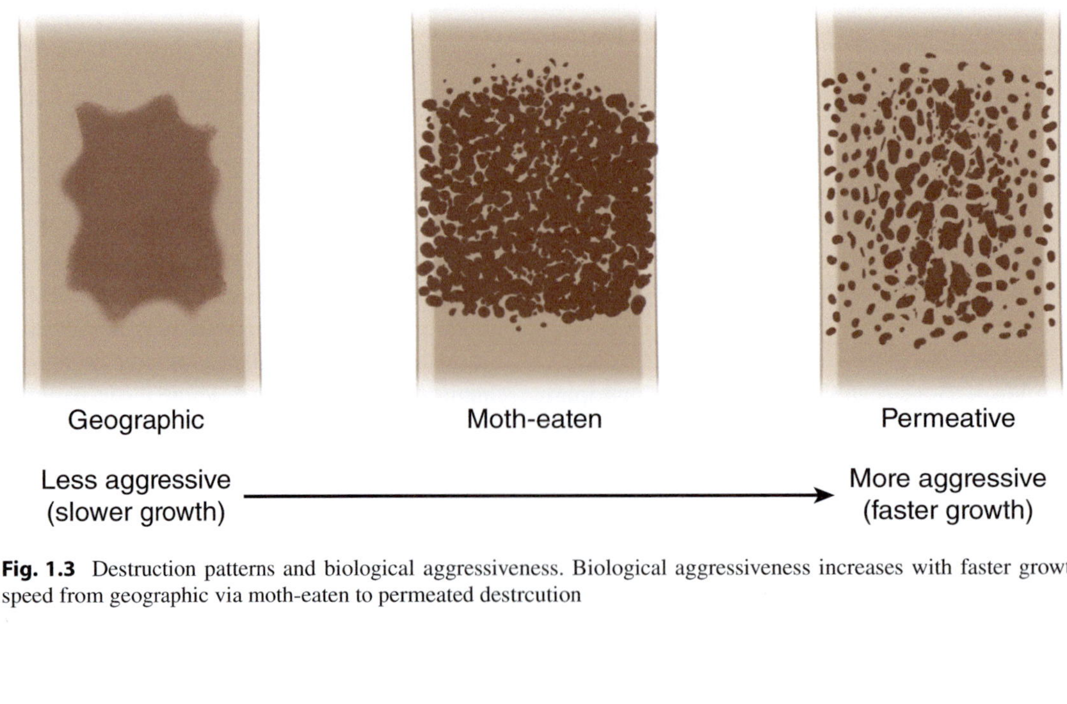

Fig. 1.3 Destruction patterns and biological aggressiveness. Biological aggressiveness increases with faster growth speed from geographic via moth-eaten to permeated destrcution

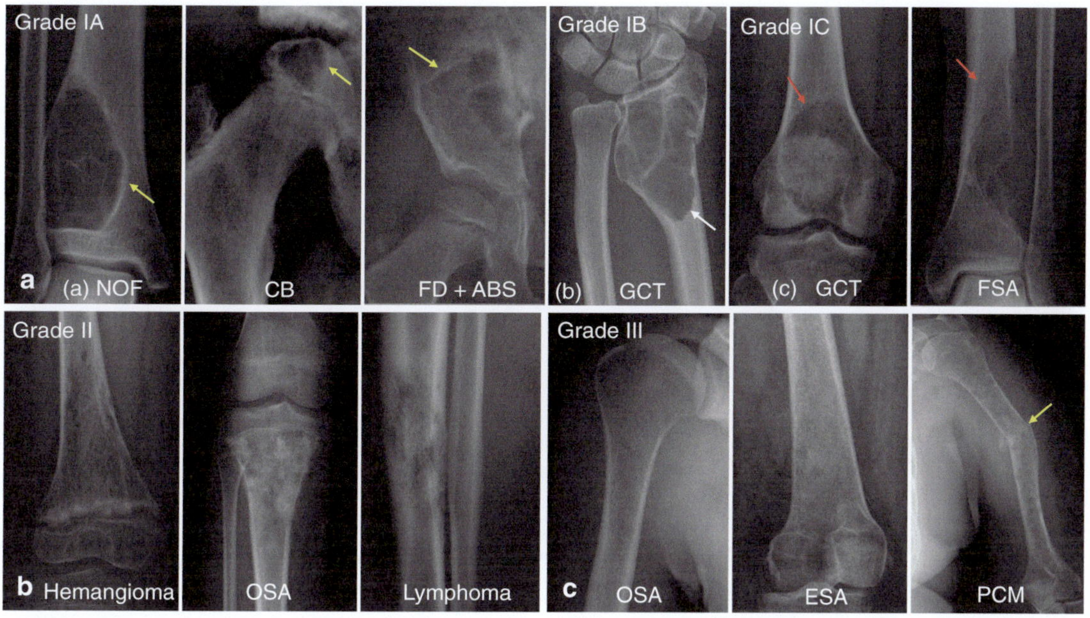

Fig. 1.4 Examples of each bone destruction pattern. (**a**) Grade I (*geographic destruction*) is subdivided into Grade: IA, IB, and IC, depending on the presence or absence of reactive changes. (a) Grade IA is geographic lesions with sclerotic margin as seen in NOF, CB, and FD (yellow arrows). (b) Grade IB is still sharply edged geographic lesions but no discernible sclerotic margins as seen in GCT (white arrow). (c) Grade IC is geographic lesions with a wider zone of transition or ill-defined margin as seen in GCT and FSA (red arrows). (**b**) Grade II (*moth-eaten destruction pattern*) is characterized by multiple small holes of irregular sizes (2–5 mm) with coalescence of each other, which is apparently due to more aggressive or rapid tumor growth. Hemangioma, OSA, and lymphoma present this pattern. (**c**) Grade III (*permeated destruction*) is typified by innumerable, uniformly tiny holes (less than 1 mm) in the cortical bone, which can be too tiny to be perceived with preserved cortical architecture in certain cases. OSA, ESA, and PCM present this pattern. Note pathologic fracture is associated with a markedly thinned cortex, but preserved cortical architecture in the case of PCM (yellow arrow)

1. *Grade I geographic destruction* (Fig. 1.4a):

   This pattern is characterized by one or more large, well-defined, uniformly destroyed areas with sharply defined margins which can be regular, scalloped, or ragged. The transition zone between destroyed bone and intact bone is narrow and sharp suggesting a relatively slow growth rate. More indolent tumors tend to be well defined by a narrow transition zone with a rim of reactive sclerosis. Most benign or some low-grade malignant bone tumors can exhibit this pattern. Geographic destruction can be further divided into three subtypes of IA, IB, and IC, based on the presence of reactive changes including sclerotic rim and expansion of cortex. *Subtype IA* is a geographic lesion with sclerotic margin which can be seen in SBA, NOF, EC, CMF, CB, FD, and some GCT. *Subtype IB* is a well-defined geographic lesion, but no sclerotic rim as seen in most GCT. *Subtype IC* is a locally infiltrative geographic lesion with an ill-defined margin, which can be observed in GCT, aggressive form of EC, CB, desmoplastic fibroma (DF), low-grade FSA, or CSA. The relative biological aggressiveness increases from subtypes A to C.

2. *Grade II moth-eaten destruction* (Fig. 1.4b)

   This pattern is characterized by multiple small holes of irregular sizes (2–5 mm) with a tendency to coalesce, which are apparently due to more aggressive or rapid tumor growth than the geographic pattern. The cortex is greatly weakened by the multiple confluent holes which completely penetrate the cortex, often producing a pathological fracture. The margin of each hole is poorly defined. Mostly, this pattern can be seen in malignant tumors including OSA, CSA, FSA, myeloma, lymphoma, or metastatic cancer, among others. However, some benign lesions or tumors such as OM, hemangioma, LCH, or some GCT may present this pattern. In addition, acute disuse osteoporosis occurring in the distal area to the tumor due to severe pain or limitation of joint motion may also give rise to a spotty moth-eaten pattern simulating a malignant tumor. It is, however, quite different from the uniform pattern of osteoporosis in bed-ridden, debilitated, or elderly people.

3. *Grade III permeated destruction* (Fig. 1.4c):

   This type is typified by innumerable, uniformly tiny holes (less than 1 mm) in the cortical bone, which can be occasionally too tiny to be perceived. The transitional zone is wider and more ill-defined, and the cortex usually seems to be fuzzy or indistinct. Since the number and size of the holes gradually diminish from the maximum zone of destruction to the point where no destruction at all can be observed, the actual border of the lesion is hard to define. The very rapid growth and highly infiltrative nature of the tumors do not allow time for the geographic destruction of bone and rim of reactive bone formation that can be seen in the more slowly growing tumors. The tiny holes are the enlarged Haversian systems by tumor enzyme and/or osteoclastic activity due to very rapid spread of infections or some malignant bone tumors [20]. Although an ill-defined segmental loss of bone density is observed, the cortex outline may often appear intact despite the numerous penetrating tiny holes which may be too small to be perceived and allow to form a large soft tissue mass without significant cortical destruction, particularly in hematologic malignancies. Only a few benign lesions or tumors including OM or LCH can exhibit this pattern of destruction. Malignant tumors most frequently associated with this pattern are OSA, metastatic cancers, or hematologic cancers such as myeloma, lymphoma, and leukemia. Any combination of three types can be seen in a single lesion, indicating a change from the slow-growing nature of the lesion toward a more aggressive pattern and malignant change or even dedifferentiation.

4. *Responses of bone to tumor* (Fig. 1.5).

   (a) Rim of host bone sclerosis (Fig. 1.5a)

   A complete rim of surrounding reactive sclerosis indicates a high probability of benignancy (a). However, it is also rarely present in slow-growing, low-grade bone sarcoma, and thus it is not pathognomonic for benign tumors (b). Loss of completeness of the rim may indicate a regression of old benign lesion (c), or even a malignant transformation of preexisting benign lesion (d).

   (b) Bent bone

   Normal bones cannot bend or expand because they are mineralized hard structures. However, the bone may appear *bent* by the healing of repeated fractures and remodeling in some conditions such as rickets, fibrous dysplasia, and Paget's disease.

   (c) "Expanded" or "ballooned" bone (Fig. 1.5b).

   If the tumor grows slowly enough, the periosteum can lay down a reactive new bone which becomes a new cortex and blends imperceptibly into the adjacent host cortex appearing *expanded* to *balloon-shaped* bone. The *expansion* without cortical perforation is usually a sign of benignancy, particularly when it is regular and symmetric. However, it can be observed rarely in low-grade malignant bone tumors or slow-spreading metastases from renal and thyroid carcinoma.

   (d) "Eccentric expansion" or "bubbling out" of bone (Fig. 1.5c).

   The tumor can eccentrically bulge out from the host bone surrounded by a thin rim of periosteal new bone mostly in benign bone tumors such as CMF or ABC, but also rarely in low-grade sarcoma. The periosteal surrounding rim is equivalent to the intramedullary rim of sclerotic new bone, which also indicates a slow growth of the tumor.

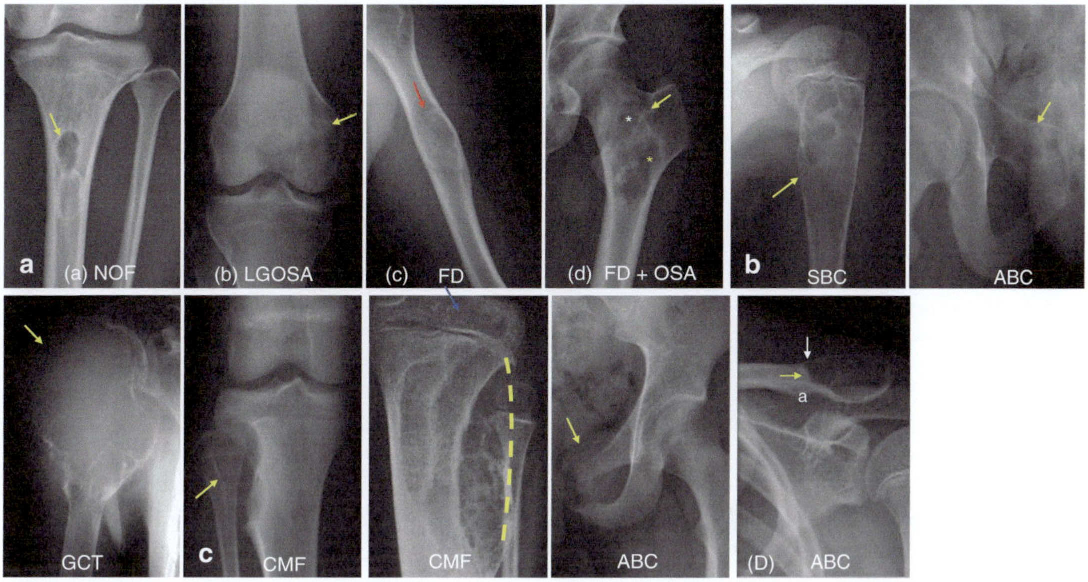

Fig. 1.5 Host bone responses to tumors (**a**) (a) A complete rim of reactive sclerosis usually indicates high probability of benignancy as in NOF. (b) However, it may also rarely be present in slow-growing sarcoma such as low-grade OSA, and thus it is not always pathognomonic for a benign tumor. (c) The absence of completeness or haziness of the rim with *"ground glass"* density may indicate a regression or ancient FD (red arrow). (d) The incomplete sclerotic rim (yellow arrow) surrounding the lesion of *"ground-glass"* density (white asterisk) and ill-defined osteolytic lesion (yellow asterisk) may suggest a malignant transformation of preexisting FD. (**b**) The "expansion" without cortical perforation is usually a sign to benignancy, particularly when it is regular and symmetric. SBC, ABC, and GCT expand the underlying host bones (arrows). (**c**) The tumor can eccentrically bulge out from the host bone with a thin rim of periosteal new bone, so-called *bubbling-out,* mostly in benign bone tumors but rarely, in low-grade sarcoma. A thin periosteal surrounding rim is equivalent to the intramedullary rim of sclerotic new bone, which also indicates slow growth of benign tumors. CMF and ABC present this pattern of host response (yellow arrows and dotted line). (**d**) A thin reactive shell of periosteal new bone (white arrow) encircles the expanded lesion in a *"balloon-like"* fashion. The Codman's triangle (a) fuses with the thin reactive rim appearing as a *"finger-in-the-balloon"* appearance with the distal calvicle shaft protruding into the expanded area (yellow arrow) and supported by a buttress of preiosteal reaction

(e) "Finger-in-the-balloon" appearance (Fig. 1.5d).

A thin reactive shell of periosteal new bone can be extended from the Codman's triangle area fusing together and beginning to encircle the lesion in a *balloon-like* fashion. With the shaft end of long bone protruding into the expanded area with the buttress of periosteal reaction, the overall contour becomes a *finger-in-the-balloon* appearance, which is most frequently seen in ABC although not a pathognomonic sign. It can rarely be observed in other types of cystic lesions (Fig. 1.1a in Brown tumor of hyperparathyroidism chapter).

5. *Soft tissue mass formation* (Fig. 1.6).

Malignant bone tumors can markedly destroy the cortex and extend into the surrounding soft tissue to form a naked mass without shell or rim of periosteal new bone (Fig. 1.6a). Such a naked soft tissue mass is a strong indication of high-grade malignant bone tumor. However, locally aggressive benign tumors including GCT or ABC in its early rapid-growing phase can also make the naked soft tissue mass (Fig. 1.6b).

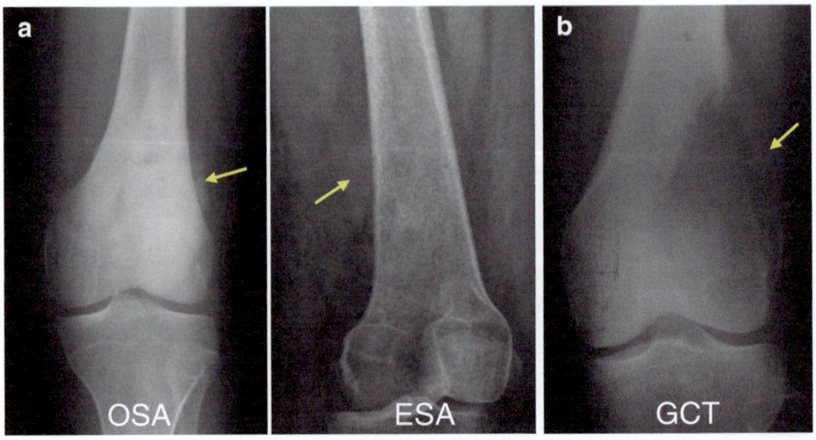

Fig. 1.6 Naked soft tissue mass. (**a**) A naked soft tissue mass without shell or rim of periosteal new bone can be made through the destructed cortex (arrows), which strongly indicates a high-grade bone sarcoma such as OSA and ESA. (**b**) However, GCT may also present a soft tissue mass during its early, radipldy growing phase (arrow)

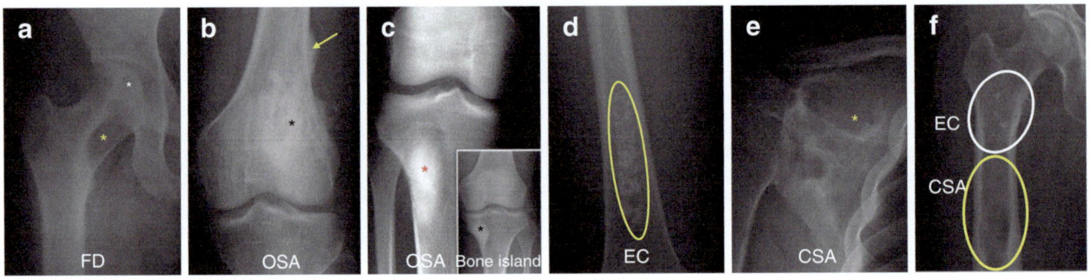

Fig. 1.7 Intralesional densities. (**a**) A characteristic *"ground-glass"* density asterisks is seen in FD. (**b**) *"Fluffy"* to *"cloud-like"* density (asterisk) with a naked soft tissue mass (arrow) and metaphyseal location strongly suggest OSA. (**c**) *"Ivory-like"* or sclerosing density (asterisk) is seen in the osteoblastic variant of OSA. A similar density is also observed in giant bone island (inset). To distinguish both entities, a biopsy is necessary. (**d**) *"Stippled"* or *"rings and arcs"* foci of mineralization are typically observed with an irregularly defined oblong radiolucent lesion within an imaginary line (dotted circle) in EC. (**e**) *"Windblown"* and spotty densities within the large expansile radiolucent lesion (asterisk) are seen in CSA. (**f**) An osteolytic lesion with endosteal deep scalloping and cortical thickening (yellow circle) is observed adjacent to neighboring area with *"stippled"* foci of mineralization consistent with preexisting EC (white circle), suggesting secondary central CSA

6. *Intralesional densities* (Figs. 1.7 and 1.8).

   (a) "Ground glass" density

   This type of density reflects numerous small woven bone trabeculae which is highly indicative of FD. The density is variable depending on the amount of woven bone formation and its state of mineralization. If the woven bones are more prominent, the lesion appears closer to *ground-glass* density, but if those are sparser as in old or ancient lesions, the lesion appears more radiolucent (Fig. 1.7a). Rarely, low-grade OSA may exhibit a similar density mimicking FD, and it is also very difficult to distinguish them even by histologic examination.

   (b) "Fluffy" to "Cloud-like" density

   Tumor-producing osteoid-to-bone matrices usually appear as *fluffy* to *cloud-like* or amorphous if they are immature woven bones. When such density is associated with ill-defined destruction affecting the metaphysis of long bone with naked soft tissue mass and Codman's triangle, particularly in children or adolescents younger than 20 years of age, it is virtually pathognomonic for OSA (Figs. 1.7b and 1.8). Rarely, stress or fatigue fracture callus may produce "fluffy" density simulating OSA, and it must be distinguished by histologic examination.

(c) *"Ivory-like" density*

One large uniformed area of *ivory-like* density, being equivalent to the normal cortex, can be seen when when the matrix is heavily mineralized tumor bone which is excessive to the proportion of tumor cells, so-called sclerosing OSA. However, the identical density can be seen in a huge bone island (Fig. 1.7c and 1.8).

(d) *"Stippled", "Flocculant", "Popcorn-like" to "Rings and arcs" calcification*

These densities indicate EC or preexisting foci of EC in secondary CSA. The particular *ring and arc-like* appearance reflects a histologic finding of the peripheral plates of reactive host lamellar bone encasing the small cartilage nodules, so-called *lamellar bone encasement*. The spotty or stippled round densities suggest foci of endochondral ossification or dystrophic calcification on microscopic examination (Figs. 1.7d and 1.8).

(e) "Windblown" densification

This kind of density along with spotty densities may represent prominent reactive woven bone or dystrophic calcification in the growing cartilage nodules, often representing CSA (Fig. 1.7e). If the affected bone is expanded associated with internal windblown density and radiolucnet area having spotty densification in neighboring areas, secondary CSA from preexisting EC should be suspected (Fig. 1.7f).

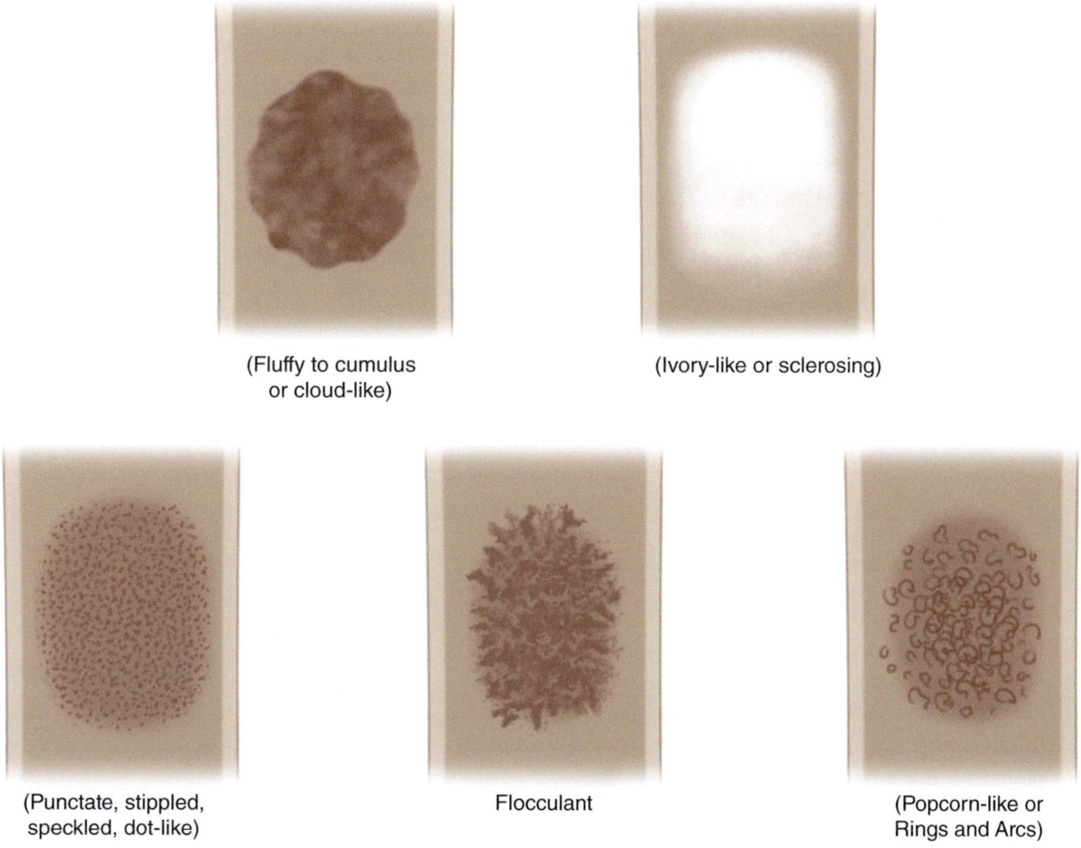

Fig. 1.8 A schema of variable intralesional densities

7. *Periosteal reaction* (Fig. 1.9)

The periosteum is an unstable sensitive structure having the feasibility to respond to injury stimulation or pressure from the enlarging tumor by new bone deposition. The degree and pattern of periosteal reaction can vary depending on the rate of growth or local aggressiveness. Slow-growing benign tumors usually make a continuous periosteal reaction on the cortical surface and provoke a solid buttress at the peripheries under the periosteum. However, rapidly growing malignant bone tumors destructing the cortex tend to produce a discontinuous periosteal reaction.

(a) Triangular cuff (*"Codman's triangle"*)

A rapidly expanding tumor mass can destroy the cortex and elevate the periosteum with a triangular cuff of reactive periosteal bone at the edge of the tumors. The apex of the triangle represents the most periphery of the irritated periosteum (Fig. 1.9a). It is most frequently seen in malignant bone tumors and occasionally in rapidly growing benign lesions such as ABC or OM.

(b) Multiple lamellate, parallel periosteal lines (*"Onion-skinning"*)

The periosteal new bone may unusually deposit in a multiple lamellate pattern paralleling the cortical surface, so-called *onion skinning*, which is most commonly seen in OM, ESA (Fig. 1.9b), or rare cases of OSA involving the diaphysis. However, it can be seen in rapidly growing benign bone tumors such as LCH (Fig. 1.9b). The multiple lamellated periosteal reaction is basically attributable to cyclic tumor growth.

(c) Perpendicular or spiculate periosteal lines (*"sunburst"* appearance)

The periosteum is attached to the cortex by perpendicularly oriented Sharpey's fibers. Rapid and continuous periosteal lifting and stretching by the tumor irritate the periosteum to lay down reactive new bone along the Sharpey's fibers to make the perpendicular lines, so-called *spiculate* or *sunburst* (Fig. 1.9c). This pattern of periosteal reaction can be seen often in ESA, intramedullary or periosteal OSA, and some metastatic cancers.

(d) Thick dense periosteal reaction

The periosteal reaction can be very thick and dense in irritative benign lesions including OO, OM, or trauma (Fig. 1.9d).

B. *Radionuclide bone scan*

Bone scan using technetium-99 m-labeled diphosphonate radioisotope is highly valuable for evaluation of musculoskeletal abnormalities because it is exquisitely sensitive in detecting biopathology and is uniquely able to assess metabolic and physiological profiles of diseased bones

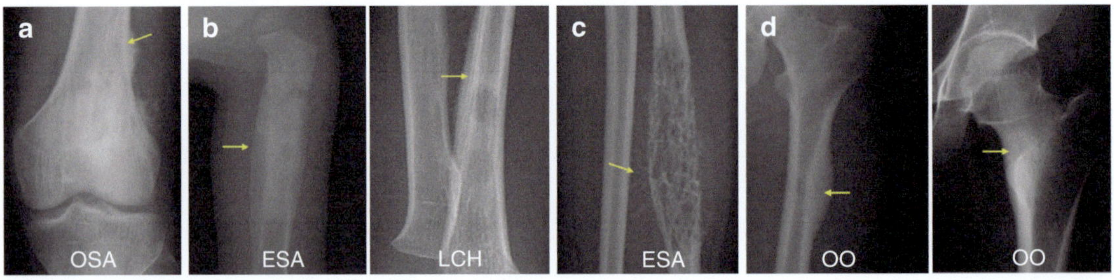

Fig. 1.9 Periosteal reaction (arrows). (**a**) Triangular cuff ("Codman's triangle") is typically seen in OSA. (**b**) Multiple lamellated, parallel periosteal lines ("Onion-skinning") are characteristically observed in ESA and LCH. (**c**) Typically, perpendicular periosteal lines (*"sunburst"* appearance) are seen in ESA. (**d**) Thick dense periosteal reaction is typically seen in OO, in which a nidus is buried

and joints as well as even adjacent soft tissue structures [22]. The early uptake of the radionuclide occurs in the area with richer blood supply, and late uptake occurs in the area of osteogenesis where calcium salt crystals are formed. The process of active osteogenesis such as bone tumors, reactive new bone formation, soft tissue tumors adjacent to the bone, OM, fracture, and degenerative or inflammatory process presents a vividly hot uptake of the isotope. Radionuclide bone scan is not specific, but it plays several roles in evaluation of the bone lesions; (1) It provides information on active or stable to quiescent status of the lesion, which may offer an indication for surgical management (2) It plays an excellent role in screening the entire skeleton with a single examination for multifocal benign bone tumors such as OCs, ECs, NOFs, or LCHs as well as multifocal metastatic cancers (3) Some conditions that are not clearly depicted on anatomic images such as tiny nidus of OO or small metastatic deposition can be detected on bone scan (4) It provides the extent of the tumor and detect *skip metastases* defined as synchronous smaller foci of tumor occurring in the same bone anatomically separated from the primary lesion or on the opposing side of a joint [23]. (5) Finally, it may play a role as an indicator of the response to neoadjuvant chemotherapy and is useful in serial monitoring of local recurrence or bone metastasis after management. Pinhole bone scan (PBC) can provide more unique and decisive information in making a specific diagnosis of bone and joint lesions [24]. Gamma correction of PBC image is a more recently developed process that can efficiently extract specific signs from bland amorphous uptake of the radioisotope on naive unprocessed pinhole bone image [25, 26]. In occult fracture, the mechanism making the fracture stand out more clearly is the subtraction of the lower tracer uptake in edema, hyperemia, hemorrhage, and reactive inflammation. The same principle can apply to the depiction of nidi and fibro-vascular zones in OO by presenting a pathognomonic *hotter spot within hot area* sign [27] (refer Fig. 2B in OO chapter). PBC with gamma correction is readily accessible, easily performed, widely available, as well as economical.

C. *CT scan*

Plain radiograph provides only a two-dimensional image of a more complicated three-dimensional anatomic structure of bone, but a CT scan imparts an additional axial image without complicated overlapping structures. In addition, it can offer to a greater extent the contrast between fat, muscle, bone, and bone marrow space. CT scan can exhibit specific patterns in some bone tumors. For example, *polka-dot* sign on axial views and *corduroy* or *jail bar* sign on sagittal and coronal images are pathognomonic for vertebral hemangioma. It may provide better declination of soft tissue mass, thin rim of sclerosis around the soft tissue extension, tumors invisible on plain radiograph, calcific matrices, thickness of cartilage cap, extension of the tumor into the joint, separation of periosteal or parosteal tumor from medullary tumor, and patterns of ossification. CT scan is superior to MRI in the evaluation of ossification or mineralization, and it is widely used to detect distant metastases to the lung and other intra-abdominal organs.

D. *Magnetic resonance imaging (MRI)*

MRI can offer three-dimensional cuts in coronal, sagittal, and axial plane. It provides a better declination of both bone and soft tissue and is very sensitive to detect even early alterations of fatty bone marrow. In general, MRI is better than CT in demonstrating the extent of tumor in bone marrow and soft tissues. Bony or marrow lesions are often not visible on plain radiographs, particularly in their early phase, and are subtle even on CT scans. MRI is better than CT for showing normal marrow, while CT scan is better than MRI for revealing normal cortex. The general superiority of MRI is due to two main factors [28]. Firstly, MRI is able to show a high-contrast difference of signal intensity (SI) between soft-tissue structures which is of about equal density on CT. Secondly, MRI permits direct coronal and sagittal images which are particularly valuable in evaluating the longitudinal extent of the lesion in the medullary canal. The extent is critical in planning the resection level in limb-salvage operation or amputation. MRI is of greatest value in the evaluation of the conditions of cartilage, growth plate, muscle, neurovascular bundles, fat, fluid or blood, hemosiderin component, and adjacent soft tissues. It is also prominently valuable in the analysis of the tumor response to radiotherapy or chemotherapy, restaging after neoadjuvant chemotherapy, and post-therapeutic follow-up for local recurrence. *Skip metastases* localized to the marrow, which are not evident on plain radiographs or CT scans can also be detected on MRI. Contrast-enhanced MRI can depict the most vascularized or necrotic areas of the tumor, thereby helping avoid inadequate sampling during biopsy [29].

E. *18F-FDG PET/CT scan*

Numerous primary bone tumors are encountered on PET/CT, and many are FDG-avid. The FDG avidity of several benign tumors may be as high as, or even higher, than that of the malignant tumors. A predictable spectrum of the uptake is not always applicable, particularly when comparing tumors of different histologic groups. For example, GCTs have been reported to be more avid than grouped CSAs [30–32]. In a study of 202 pathologically proven primary bone tumors, the authors found significantly higher FDG uptake in sarcomas than in latent or active benign lesions but no significant difference between the FDG uptake of high-grade malignancies and benign aggressive lesions [30]. However, another study found a trend toward higher uptake in benign aggressive lesions than the malignancies [32]. In general, the uptake is more avid in locally aggressive lesions, and significantly more active in malignant tumors than benign lesions [30–34]. However, the degree of FDG uptake does not necessarily reflect malignant potential in bone tumors. After the diagnosis of certain primary malignant bone tumors, PET/CT is useful for whole-body staging, the evaluation of neoadjuvant chemotherapeutic response, and detection of local recurrence or distant metastasis during follow-up after management.

5. *Microscopic examination of cells and matrices*

   The skeleton is histologically composed of a variety of types of cells originally derived from embryonal mesenchyme, which can produce variable matrices respectively. Thus, there are diverse subtypes of benign and malignant bone tumors and variable pathologic findings depending on the phases of each tumor or even the same tumor [2]. In addition, callus tissue by fatigue or stress fracture and pathologic fracture in the preexisting bone tumors can make a diagnosis more confusing particularly when the callus is very young and unripe. The time of the fracture event may be important to play a crucial role in distinguishing the reparative process of callus from an underlying benign or malignant bone tumors. Callus passes through varying phases of maturation, and each phase presents distinct histologic findings according to the age of the lesion changing on a weekly basis during the first two months, at least [35].

A. *The variety cells within the bones developing primary bone tumors*

   (a) *Osteoblasts and chondroblasts*

   Osteoblasts and chondroblasts reside within bone, and each of them produces a distinct matrix: osteoblasts generate "*bony matrix*" of osteoid, woven, and lamellar bone, while chondroblasts form "*cartilaginous matrix*" of chondroid, hyaline, elastic, or myxoid cartilage. Both may also contribute "*fibrous tissue*" formation. They can produce intermediate mixtures of matrices such as chondro-osteoid, fibro-chondroid, or fibro-chondro-osteoid. These cells can develop bone-forming tumors such as OO, OB, or OSA and cartilage-forming tumors such as OC, EC, CMF, or CSA.

   (b) *Fibroblasts*

   The ordinary spindle-like cells are also present within the bone, which may produce fibrous tissue, collagen matrix, or even osseous matrix. Mirra (2) suggested most spindle cells are more closely related to osteoblast precursor cells and referred to the cells as *fiber-osteoblasts*. These cells produce fibrous tissue and osseous matrix which are typically seen in FD, low-grade OSA, or even fracture callus. They can also develop FSA and DF of bone.

(c) *Periosteal cells*

The periosteal cells form the fibrous layer of the periosteum surrounding the bone under normal conditions. However, they can produce bone or cartilage matrix by various stimuli, including injury, fracture, infection, tumors, or other conditions. These cells can develop parosteal or periosteal OSA/CSA.

(d) *Bone marrow hematopoietic cells*

Bone marrow is the soft and flexible sponge-like tissue of primary hematopoiesis and is found in the cavities of cancellous bones and the medullary cavity of the long bones. There are two major types of red marrow (hematopoietic with abundant blood cells) and yellow marrow (predominantly filled with fat cells and stem cells that can become cartilage, fat, or bone cells). Bone marrow is richly innervated by nerves and is highly vascularized tissue. Tumors such as PCM, lymphoma, or leukemia can rarely develop directly from the red marrow tissues or more frequently from such blood cancers. Other tumors can arise from the lipocytes, nerves, or vessels within the bone. In addition, a special type of histiocytes, so-called Langerhans cells, can abnormally proliferate to develop LCH.

(e) *Lipocytes*

These cells can often give rise to intraosseous lipoma or very rarely, liposarcoma liposarcoma.

(f) *Nerve cells*

Most bones contain naked nerve fibers lacking the myelinated sheath of Schwann cells. However, myelinated nerves pass through foramina only in the skull and mandible. Therefore, primary neurofibroma and Schwannoma can be extremely rare in the long bones if ever.

(g) *Vascular cells*

Endothelial cells of blood vessels within the bone may give rise to vascular tumors such as hemangioma, epithelioid hemangioendothelioma, or angiosarcoma.

(h) *Smooth muscle cells*

These cells are present in the wall of blood vessels of the bone, which develop extremely rarely primary leiomyoma or leiomyosarcoma of bone.

(i) *Notochordal cells*

These cells may appear within the vertebrae or base of the skulls in the form of rest, which can develop benign notochordal cell tumors or malignant chordoma.

(j) *Histiocytes*

These cells may also be found in the bone, and give rise to benign fibrous histiocytoma or UPS.

(k) *Epithelial cells*

Rarely, the epithelial cells may be a part of intraosseous elements. These cells in the form of epidermal rest can be incorporated into bones formed by endochondral ossification in close apposition to the skin and give rise to the OFD or adamantinoma exclusively located in the tibia and/or fibula.

B. *Associated callus of unrecognized fracture*

It is very important to accurately indentify and interpret callus tissue to distinguish fracture callus due to clinically unrecognized fatigue or stress, particularly in the early phase, from a preexisting benign or malignant bone tumor. The *fracture callus* presents variable sequences of healing events, beginning with an exclusive growth of primitive mesenchymal cells which can be easily mistaken for a certain type of malignant bone tumor. And it goes through the phase of a primitive chondro-osteoid matrix, which may still make a misdiagnosis of OSA, particularly before the advent of prominent osteoblastic rimming. However, the callus would not be mistaken for sarcoma anymore in the next phase of prominent osteoblastic rimming with injured vessels. Finally, the process would terminate with completely normal lamellar bone and bone marrow by remodeling. It will take 2–3 months to be remodeled with chronologic phases of maturation on a week-to-week basis during the early months [35]. The process of approximately estimated aging of the callus will be discussed more precisely, based on pathologic findings of the samples obtained during fracture treatment at each phase in Fracture Callus chapter.

C. *Hematoxylin and Eosin (H&E) stain*

This stain is one of the principal tissue stains used in histologic examination and gold standard in histologic diagnosis, but often nonspecific. The specimens obtained from biopsy or surgical procedure are adequately decalcified in 5% or 10% nitric acid for varying hours depending on the hardness of the specimens prior to processing and embedding in paraffin wax. Sections of decalcified, formalin-fixed, paraffin-embedded bone specimens are cut. The prepared sections are stained with standard H&E stain. When adequately decalcified, the base nature of hematoxylin stains the nuclei of cells *purplish blue* or *dark purple* and the acidic nature of eosin stains the extracellular matrix and cytoplasm *pinkish*. Other structures can take on different shades, hues, and combinations of these colors.

D. *Pleomorphism and anaplasia*

Pleomorphism is defined as alterations in the size and shape of nuclei and cytoplasm of cells, which should not be automatically considered as cancerous because benign lesions may exhibit such pleomorphism. Extremely rarely, certain benign bone tumors may present bizarre or pleomorphic features simulating cytologic anaplasia. However, they absolutely lack abnormal mitosis and are called *pseudoanaplastic* or *pseudomalignant* tumors. Such findings can be seen in the lesions managed by irradiation or embolization. A diagnostic guideline for *pseudoanaplastic* tumors of bone was suggested as follows [36]. Firstly, mitotic figures should not be present or extremely scarce, and if present, should be typical, but neve atypical. Rare cases may contain a few typical mitoses, but far fewer than would be expected for their bizarre, highly anaplastic-looking appearance. Careful attention should be paid to distinguish true mitoses and karyorrhectic pseudomitoses. Special immunohistochemical stains for cellular proliferation, such as Ki-67, can be useful. Because the majority of the lesions with significant cytological aberrations are true sarcomas, a repeat biopsy is recommanded if the first biopsy samples seem to be inadequate. Secondly, the clinical and radiographic features should be within a range of the benign lesion being considered to be *pseudoanaplastic*. Such lesions are typically small to moderate, growth is absent to imperceptible, or it may be found incidentally to some other process. Finally, the clinical behavior of the lesion should be benign without any evidence of aggressiveness with soft tissue mass formation, local recurrence, and regional or distant metastases. Out of over 4000 cases of bone tumors retrieved from the personal database of Mirra JM, only 15 (0.35%) met these criteria [35]. By Dorland's [1] definition, *anaplasia* is a loss of differentiation of cells and their orientation to one another and to their axial framework and blood vessels, which is also called undifferentiation. Clinically, it shows uncontrolled, ceaseless, life-threatening growth often with single or multiple distant metastases. Microscopically, *anaplasia* presents an increased nuclear/cytoplasm (N/C) ratio, open and prominent chromatin with abnormal clumping, enlarged single or multiple nucleoli, abnormal mitoses, or hyperchromatism with significant deep-blue color of the nuclei beyond the normal range.

E. *Matrices produced by tumor cells*

Bone tissue consists of collagen, proteoglycan, crystals of calcium and phosphate (known as hydroxyapatite), and related cells of osteoblasts and osteocytes. The tumor cells also produce osseous and cartilaginous matrix, fibrous tissue, and collagen matrix.

(a) Collagen

Collagen produced by spindle fibroblasts is the main structural protein in the extracellular matrix and imparts tensile strength to bones. Collagen presents longitudinally or wavy spindled bundles which can be easily observed by polarized light. NOF, DF, and FSA produce typically prominent collagen fibers without any other matrices.

(b) Fibrin

Fibrin is a fibrous, nonglobular protein involved in the clotting of blood. Thus, it is usually evident in areas of hemorrhage. There are no visible fibers in it under polarized light.

(c) Osteoid

Osteoid is an unmineralized, organic portion of the bone matrix that forms prior to the maturation of bone tissue. It is produced by osteoblasts and is homogeneously stained pink. Identification of osteoid is very important for the differentiation of OSA, CSA, FSA, DF, and others because fibrin, collagen, and chondroid can be deposited in similar patterns and are also stained pink. The process of bone formation begins by secreting the osteoid of fibrous protein called collagen. The osteoid consists mostly of fibers (type I collagen) and ground substance (chondroitin sulfate and osteocalcin). Then, the osteoid becomes mineralized by hydroxyapatite to get the bone hardness. Osteoblasts are alkaline phosphatase positive. The lesions rich in osteoid or bone matrix include callus, OO, OB, FD, OFD, and OSA.

(d) Woven bone

Woven bone is characterized by a random, more disoriented, deposition of collagen fibers in criss-cross or woven pattern. It is temporary structure that is normally replaced by stronger, more organized structure of lamellar bone. In phylogeny, woven bone is preceded lamellar bone and is sometimes referred to as "*primitive (woven) bone*". This type of bone tissue is primarily found during embryonic development and fracture healing, but can be also found in any pathologic condition in which new bone formation occurs, such as benign or maignant osteogenic bone tumors, osteomyelitis, and Paget's disease.

(e) Lamellar bone

Lamellar bone is a mature and stronger type of bone tissue, characterized by a well-organized collagen fibers arranged in lamellae, with parallel orientation within each sheet and alternating perpendicular orientation between adjacent sheets. This pattern of deposition is particularly well observed by polarized light. This peculiar alternative pattern of layering gives much greater strength to the bone. Besides the normal process, this type of bone can be found in reparative process, including myositis ossificans and facture callus. Although low-grade of parosteal OSA may produce thin streamer of lamellar pattern of bone (Refer Chapter 10 Parosteal Osteosarcoma), moderate and high grade OSA never produce lamellar type of bone.

(f) Chondroid

Chondroid is a primitive form of cartilage, which is rich in collagen and devoid of proteoglycan. Thus, it is tinctorially identical to osteoid, except that it is produced by cartilagenous tumors, such as CB, CMF, or some mesenchymal CSA. If the color is blue to purple, the matrix is cartilage rather than chondroid, reflecting its rich proteoglycan contents. Chondroid is usually deposited in masses with a more rounded border, and less fibrillar than osteoid. In addition, there are usually characteristic peri-lacunar chondrocyte-like spaces within the matrix when compared to osteoid. Chondroid or cartilage matrix can be deposited in chondroma, CB, CMF, CSA, and chondrogenic OSA. When a pathologist condsidered chondroid to be blue or purple rather than pink in color, a red-stained matirx can be misinterpreted as osteoid, and the lesion may be mistaken for an osteogenic tumor.

F. *Immunohistochemistry (IHC)*

IHC is a widely used ancillary testing method using anatomical, immunological, and biochemical techniques to image discrete tumor cells in tissues.

IHC is a process of selectively identifying antigens in certain cells of tissue section by using the principal antibodies which bind to the specific antigens in examined biological tissues [37]. It is a useful tool to provide diagnostically valuable information on the histogenesis and differentiation of cells and is routinely used to detect the presence of specific protein markers that can assist with more accurate differential diagnoses in doubtful cases. IHC stains specific for protein markers of each tumor cell have evolved to complement the H&E stains which are nonspecific and other special stain techniques. The common antigens for bone and soft tissue tumors are summarized as follows. *Vimentin* is common for most mesenchymal cell tumors; *desmin* for skeletal and smooth muscle tumors; *actin* for skeletal and smooth muscle tumors as well as tumors with myofibroblastic differentiation such as nodular fasciitis, DF, FSA or UPS; *cytokeratin* for epithelial tumors such as chordoma and adamantinoma; *epithelial membrane antigen (EMA)* for nerve sheath tumors; CD 68 and alpha-1-antitrypsin for fibro-histiocytic tumors; *myoglobin* for skeletal muscle; factor VIII and CD31 for vascular tumor; *S100 protein* for nerves sheath tumors, chondroblastic tumors, chordoma, lipoblastic tumor, LCH, rhabdomyoma; *CD34* for vascular tumors and benign nerve sheath tumors; *MIC2 gene product (CD99)* for ESA; and *CD45* (common leukocyte antigen) for lymphoma.

G. *Special stains*

Although the majority of bone tumors and tumor-like conditions can be accurately diagnosed with a simple H&E stain technique, some cases should be frequently supplemented with special stains as well as IHC. *Periodic Acid-Schiff (PSA) stain* is principally used for the demonstration of intracytoplasmic glycogen in ESA and clear cell CSA. It is necessary to distinguish ESA from neuroblastoma or lymphoma which is usually negative for PAS. *Reticulin stain* represents fine fibrillary material deposited in the intercellular matrix with an exquisite honeycomb pattern of reticulin fibers encompassing the individual chondroblasts in CB. *Trichrome stain* is frequently used to demonstrate the presence of extracellular substances of connective tissue such as collagen. It is rarely used in the diagnosis of bone tumors, but it is frequently used for histomorphometric evaluation of mineralized versus nonmineralized osteoids in metabolic bone diseases [6]. *Congo red stain* is useful for amyloid examination with non-polarized and polarized light. Amyloid appears as a reddish deposit under nonpolarized light and green birefringence under polarized light (refer to Fig. 1L, 2E in Amyloidosis chapter).

6. *Grading and staging*

   (a) *Grading systems*

   Variable histologic grading for malignant bone tumors has been proposed in an attempt to predict the behavior on the basis of histological findings because bone tumors vary widely in their clinical and biologic behavior. An exact grading in malignant bone tumors can provide guidelines for adequate surgical management with or without adjuvant therapy and predict the prognosis. However, the clinical significance can be limited by the interobserver variability because of the subjective interpretation of the histologic findings. Early in 1920, Broder's four-tier grading system was introduced in 537 cases of squamous epitheliomas of the lip, which has been widely adopted since then. *Grade I* is a well-differentiated tumor in which 75–100% of cells are differentiated, *Grade II* is a moderately differentiated tumor in which 50–75% of cells are differentiated, *Grade III* is a poorly differentiated tumor in which 25–50% of cells are differentiated, and *Grade IV* is an anaplastic tumor in which less than 25% of cells are differentiated [38]. This grading system was applied to skin cancer in 1921, then gastro-urinary tract cancer in 1922, and head and neck cancer in 1925. Later in 1939, it was also applied for soft tissue FSA [39]. Since the designation, several sarcoma grading systems have been developed based on two-, three-, or four-tier concepts, but none of these systems is precise. The four-tier system usually has no admittedly objective differences between the two lowest grades. The three-tier system has a problem in the intermediate grade, which may behave as a fully malignant tumor capable of metastasis or as a locally aggressive tumor only. In general, grading systems include the status of differentiation, degree of atypia, and mitotic activity including abnormal mitoses. More recently, the Mayo Clinic group proposed a grading of bone sarcoma based on a combination of histologic diagnosis and Broder's grading system, which assesses cellularity and degree of cytologic features of anaplasia [40, 41]. Although the necrosis and mitotic figures are more common in higher-grade malignant bone tumors, the degree of necrosis and mitotic numbers are not used as criteria for grading. There are also two-, three-, or four-tier grading systems for malignant bone tumors. The four-tier system has the disadvantage of minimal differences between each grade with admittedly subjective interpretation. The histological grade, 1 through 3, is useful to determine the prognosis and to decide whether adjuvant therapy is necessary in many sarcoma cases. Grade 1 shows minimal or subtle anaplasia, which is difficult to differentiate from benign tumors. Grade 2 shows a moderate degree of anaplasia, which can be recognized as malignant from cytologic findings alone. However, some benign conditions including early callus or ABC may exhibit the overlapped histologic findings of striking cellularity, plumpness, and mitoses. Grade 3 shows severe anaplasia with strikingly bizarre cytologic pleomorphism, including gigantic cells having huge nuclei and frequent atypical mitoses [2]. The three-tier system has also a problem with the intermediate grade 2, which cannot predict if the tumor has a capability metastasis or a local aggressiveness only. Therefore, there is no generally accepted grading system for bone sarcomas to date. Thus, the World Health Organization (WHO) endorses the use of a two-tier system designating bone tumors as low grade (grades 1 and 2 in a four-tier system) or high grade (grades 3 and 4 in a four-tier system) [4]. However, the two-tier system also has a drawback that it is not always possible to classify the tumor as definitively low or high grade [6]. Grading of malignant bone tumors is an important part of staging for chemotherapy and surgical treatment as well as prediction of prognosis.

(b) *Staging systems*

Staging systems have been developed to predict prognosis and to decide the surgical margin and adjuvant chemotherapy or radiotherapy depending on various prognostic factors by several authors. A staging system for bone tumors aims (1) to evaluate the significant prognostic factors of risk of local recurrence and distant metastases, (2) to serve as a useful guide in the selection of an appropriate surgical procedure, and (3) to provide guidelines for adjunctive therapies as well [42]. There are separate staging systems for benign (stages 1, 2, 3) and malignant bone tumors (stages I, II, III) in Enneking's surgical staging system [43].

(i) *Benign bone tumors*

The staging system for benign bone tumors consists of three categories of stage 1 (inactive or latent), stage 2 (active), and stage 3 (aggressive) lesions based on radiographic characteristics of the tumor.

1. Stage 1. *Inactive* benign lesions are usually asymptomatic and often discovered incidentally on radiographs for other reasons. On radiographs, they are typically well-defined by a varying degree of cortex-like sclerotic reactive bone without deformation or expansion of the host bone. They may slowly grow and attain a large size, but eventually reach a steady state where they do not grow anymore. The histologic characteristics include low cell-to-matrix ratio, matured well-differentiated matrices, benign cytologic features, encapsulation by mature fibrous tissue or cortical bone, and little or no reactive mesenchymal proliferation, inflammatory infiltrate, or neo-angiogenesis about the lesion.
2. Stage 2. *Active* benign lesions are usually discovered due to discomfort or mild pain, pathologic fracture, or mechanical dysfunction. Radiographically, they usually have irregularly well-defined margin. The inner aspect is often irregular or corrugated, giving a septate appearance. Expansion, bulging, or deformation of the overlying cortex is frequently observed. They grow steadily and continue to enlarge during follow-up observation. The

histologic characteristics include a relatively balanced cell-to-matrix ratio with homogenous distribution of the matrix, well-differentiated matrices, benign cytologic findings, intact capsule of mature fibrous tissue, and/or cancellous bone. In addition, there can be a narrow zone of mesenchymal, inflammatory, and vascular reactive tissue between the capsule and the surrounding normal tissue as well as resorption of preexisting bone by osteoclasts rather than by neoplastic cells as a mechanism of expansion.

3. Stage 3. *Aggressive* benign lesions are usually discovered because of discomfort, pain, growing mass or pathologic fracture. The radiographic features include a ragged permeative interface with indistinct margin, cortical scalloping or destruction, periosteal reaction such as Codman's triangles, and even soft tissue mass formation. Histologic features are high cell-to-matrix ratio, differentiated matrices of varying degrees of maturity, and predominantly benign cytologic characteristics without equivalent anaplasia or pleomorphism. However, there can be frequent hyperchromatic and plump nuclei, occasional typical mitoses but never atypical ones, or vascular invasion within the lesion. In addition, finger-like projections of the tumor extend through the gaps in the (pseudo)capsule and grow into the surrounding reactive zone. Despite the benign cytologic characteristics, the invasive behavior of these lesions is more like that of a low-grade malignancy occasionally with pulmonary implantation [42].

(ii) *Malignant bone tumors*

Based on plain radiograph, CT scan, MRI, bone scintigraphy, and PET/CT scan as well as histological evaluation, several authors have proposed the staging system to subclassify malignant bone tumors according to prognostic factors such as tumor size, localization, compartmental extension, histologic grade, and the presence or absence of metastasis. However, two staging systems, the TNM staging system and Enneking's surgical staging system, are mostly used for musculoskeletal malignant tumors.

1. *TNM staging system* with three parameters of primary tumor (T), regional lymph node (N), and metastasis (M) was designed by the American Joint Committee on Cancer (AJCC) and adopted by the International Union Against Cancer (UICC), which is used to assess any intramedullary malignant tumors, but not for juxtacortical surface sarcomas and hematopoietic malignancies such as multiple myeloma and lymphoma [44, 45]. Histological confirmation of the tumors with histological subtype and grade should be obtained. (T) stands for the primary tumor. Tx is designated for tumors which cannot be assessed, and T0 for no evidence of primary tumor. T1 represents a tumor confined within the cortex, and T2 extends to the adjacent soft tissue beyond the cortex through the breakage. Size 8 cm in the greatest dimension is the cut-off point between T1 and T2. Discontinuous tumors from the primary tumor site, *skip lesion*, are defined as T3. (N) stands for regional lymph nodes. Nx designates the lymph nodes that cannot be assessed. N0 represents no detectable lymph node metastases and N1 for the presence of metastases. (M) stands for distant metastasis. M0 represents the absence of detectable distant metastases, and M1 for the presence of distant metastases. The tumors are histologically classified into two major categories of low (Grades 1 and 2) and high (Grades 3 and 4) according to their histologic grade. The TNM classification, grading, and

Table 1.3 TNM classification of bone sarcomas [44, 45]

T—Primary Tumor
TX Primary tumor cannot be assessed
T0 No evidence of primary tumor
T1 Tumor 8 cm or less in greatest dimension
T2 Tumor more than 8 cm in greatest dimension
T3 Discontinuous tumors in the primary bone site
N—Regional Lymph Nodes
NX Regional lymph nodes cannot be assessed
N0 No regional lymph node metastasis
N1 Regional lymph node metastasis
M—Distant Metastasis
M0 No distant metastasis
M1 Distant metastasis
M1a Lung
M1b Other distant sites

Table 1.4 TMN staging grouping [44, 45]

Stage	Tumor (T)	Lymph node (N)	Metastasis (M)	Grade
IA	T1	N0	M0	Low
IB	T2	N0	M0	Low
IIA	T1	N0	M0	High
IIB	T2	N0	M0	High
III	T3	N0	M0	Any grade
IVA	Any T	N0	M1a	Any grade
IVB	Any T	N1	Any M	Any grade

staging system are summarized in Tables 1.3 and 1.4.

2. *Enneking's staging system* is based on the biologic aggressiveness and local extent of disease based on the compartmentalization concept of bone and soft tissue [42, 43], which was adopted by the Musculoskeletal Tumor Society (MSTS) for orthopedic surgeons to decide options of surgical management. It is based on the biologic and clinical aggressiveness and local extent of the disease. The local aggressiveness is based on histologic grading and specific histologic types, and the extent of the lesion is based on the localization of the compartment concept of bone and soft tissue. The staging system considers the surgical or histologic grade (G; G1, G2), surgical site or anatomic extent (T; T1, T2), and absence or presence of metastasis (M; M0, M1). Low-grade G1 (Broder's I or II) is a locally aggressive tumor with a lower probability of metastases such as GCT, low-grade medullary or parosteal OSA, clear cell CSA, secondary CSA, FSA, Kaposi's sarcoma, hemangioendothelioma, adamantinoma, and chordoma. High-grade G2 (Broder's III and IV) is an aggressive tumor with higher metastatic potential including high-grade conventional OSA, radiation sarcoma, Paget's sarcoma, ESA, grade 3 CSA, FSA, malignant GCT, UPS, or angiosarcoma. When a tumor is confined within a bone medullary cavity, it is considered an intra-compartmental tumor (T1), and extending beyond the cortex into adjacent soft tissue, joint, or another bone is considered an extra-compartmental tumor (T2) (Table 1.5). The presence or absence of metastases is the third major factor related to both prognosis and surgical planning. Malignant tumor cells spread to the lung most commonly through the hematogenous route, and regional metastasis to lymph nodes can occur less commonly. Those metastatic lesions implicate the same ominous prognostic significance with little chance for prolonged survival. Based on these parameters, Enneking developed the Surgical Staging System in which a malignant bone tumor is divided into three stages in articulation with surgical treatment. *Stage I* is of low histologic grade and *stage II* is of high grade. *Stage III* is any kind of tumor with metastases. The stages are subdivided into A and B based on the compartmentalization of the lesion. When the tumor is confined to the bone, it is considered stage A, and if the tumor also involves the soft tissue beyond the cortex, it is considered stage B. Thus, low-grade tumors are subclassified into stages IA and IB, and high-grade tumors into stages IIA and IIB depending on the anatomic extent of the neoplasm (Table 1.6).

Table 1.5 Definitions of anatomic extent in the Musculoskeletal Tumor Society Staging System [42, 43]

Intra-compartmental	Extra-compartmental
Intra-articular	Soft tissue extension
Superficial to deep fascia	Deep fascial extension
Paraosseous	Intraosseous or extrafascial extension
Intrafascial compartment	Extrafascial compartment

7. *Biopsy* (Fig. 1.10)
Biopsy is a procedure to obtain tumor tissue for confirmatory histologic analysis, and the procedure should avoid post-biopsy morbidity, minimize potential tumor spread, and

Table 1.6 Enneking surgical staging system for malignant bone tumors [43]

Stage	Grade	Site	Metastasis
IA	Low	Intra-compartmental	None
IB	Low	Extra-compartmental	None
IIA	High	Intra-compartmental	None
IIB	High	Extra-compartmental	None
III	Any	Any	Regional or distant

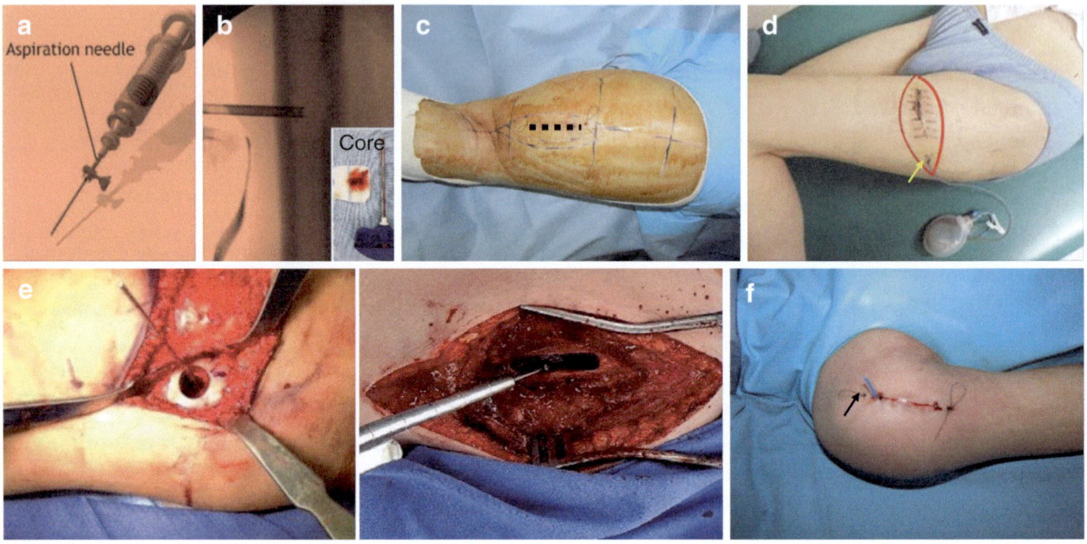

Fig. 1.10 Types and principles of biopsy. (**a**) Fine needle aspiration (FNA) biopsy. (**b**) Trocar biopsy under C-arm image intensifier control. (**c**) A small longitudinal surgical incision (black dotted line) allows for easy extension of the incision for subsequent surgery. (**d**) However, a larger transverse incision wound is extremely difficult to excise and makes a huge defect particularly when drain is exited far from the incision line as in this case (arrow). This case is an extreme examination of soft tissue sarcoma. (**e**) If a hole is necessary to be made in the bone, it should be rounded (Left) or ovoid or oblong with rounded ends, which is an example of a window created for cocurrent frozen biopsy and extended curettage (Right) to avoid stress concentration preventing a subsequent fracture. (**f**) The drain should be inserted in line with the biopsy incision to allow the drain scar to be easily incorporated into a subsequent surgical incision (arrow)

should not delay or alter future treatments. It is not indicated for asymptomatic latent bone lesions or symptomatic active bone lesions which appear entirely benign on imaging studies. Some bone tumors such as OO, OC, or parosteal OSA with a typical radiographic appearance can be primarily resected without a biopsy. For other bone tumors, microscopic examination of formalin-fixed decalcified tumor tissue obtained from biopsy which is routinely embedded in paraffin and stained with H&E is fundamental to make a correct diagnosis in correlation with clinical and radiologic findings (diagnostic triangle). Most bone lesions can be accurately diagnosed with this simple staining technique, but special stains to identify various cell components and extracellular matrices or IHC with immunologic detection of individual molecules using specific antibodies for a differential diagnosis can also be necessary. In addition, cytometry and histomorphology techniques may be recruited to quantify the subjective microscopic findings of cellular features and tissue architecture. More recently, transmission electron microscopy with a sophisticated resolution level has been introduced to understand the pathogenesis of bone tumors, but it is usually not used practically. The simple routine stain and special techniques can collaborate with each other and provide a more precise diagnosis. Biopsy should be performed after completion of all image studies including plain radiograph, CT scan, MRI, bone scan, SPECT/CT imaging, as well as PET/CT scan to avoid alterations of the natural findings by biopsy-induced hemorrhage, edema, or inflammatory changes. A properly and timely performed biopsy is the critical step in a multimodality approach. Biopsy should be considered as a first step in the surgical procedure and planned as carefully as the definitive surgical procedure. There are two principal types of biopsy: *closed biopsy* such as fine needle aspiration (FNA) or trocar biopsy and *open incision biopsy*. Any kind of biopsy track and all tissue exposed during biopsy are considered to be contaminated by tumor cells, which should be completely removed during future surgical resection. The importance of careful planning and adequate performance of a biopsy cannot be overemphasized because a poorly performed biopsy often fails to allow proper diagnosis, negatively affects survival, compromises the ability to perform limb-preserving surgery, and ultimately necessitates an unnecessary amputation [46]. Thus, biopsy is of paramount importance and should be done by an expert orthopedic oncologist who will perform subsequent surgical management.

A. *Closed biopsy*

Closed biopsy is a simple, rapid, and minimally invasive procedure by various transcutaneous instruments, which reduces the risk of tumor contamination, infection, or fracture. However, it may produce complications such as bleeding or hematoma, neurovascular injury by blind technique, and infection with a lower risk [47]. Closed biopsy techniques have been more widely used under the guidance of various imaging techniques such as C-arm image intensifier, CT scan, or sometimes MRI. However, it may be extremely difficult or even impossible to diagnose diverse and complex bone tumors on the basis of a small amount of material obtained by closed biopsy techniques in some cases. For example, the variants of OSA with focal minimal osteoid production such as chondroblastic, fibroblastic, telangiectatic, small-cell, and giant-cell rich types require incision biopsy to obtain adequate and enough specimens rather than needle or trocar biopsy. Thus, the closed biopsy technique would not be routinely recommended for every bone tumor, particularly if there is no experienced team.

(a) FNA biopsy (Fig. 1.10a)

Early in 1931, Coley et al. [48] introduced a diagnosis of bone lesions by needle biopsy. However, the procedure was not realized until 1970 when it was simplified by Lalli [49] who used image-intensified fluoroscopy. FNA provides only fluid and cytologic (cellular) specimens and is not routinely used for bone sarcoma. FNA biopsy can be basically suitable for osteolytic bone lesions particularly with cortical thinning or breakage forming soft tissue mass. It is less traumatic with a minimal chance of contamination, safe, cost-effective, well-tolerated by the patients, and preserves most of the tissue without complications. However, the main drawback of FNA is the high incidence of false negatives, and it does not permit the evaluation of tissue architecture. In addition, the obtained samples are always inadequate for ancillary, ICH, cytogenetic, or molecular studies. It usually requires an experienced team approach for clinical, radiographic, and pathologic correlation because of the small amount of tumor tissue. If the diagnosis rendered is very unusual for the age or location of the entity or if the diagnosis does not fit the clinical and radiographic findings, then open biopsy should be considered [50]. The overall diagnostic accuracy rates of FNA have been reported with a wide range from 60% to 100% depending on experience, selection bias, needle passes/attempts, inadequate or insufficient samples, and histologic verification at follow-up [51–54]. By Mayo Clinic's experience with FNA done during a period from 1993 to 2003, the number of nondiagnostic biopsies has disappointingly not diminished with increasing experience. By FNA biopsy, "nondiagnostic" biopsy was most common (39%), followed by metastatic cancer. Myeloma, lymphoma, and OSA were the most frequent primary bone tumors diagnosed [55]. Rarely, local recurrences of sarcoma have been reported in closed needle biopsy tracts [54, 56, 57]. The trajectory of the needle is important because the tract can harbor malignant cells. Trans-compartmental approach should be avoided whenever possible. In addition, the trajectory of the needle should be given strong consideration to be included in future wide resection with the primary site on this subject.

(b) Trocar, core-needle, or tru-cut biopsy (Fig. 1.10b)

Trocar biopsy has evolved to obtain larger-sized cores of tumor tissue as an alternative to FNA, which improves accuracy of diagnosis with a lower false negative rate. It is particularly useful in easy cases where histologic confirmation is certainly sure even with a small amount of biopsy specimen in correlation with the clinical-imaging findings. It is a safe and fast technique for obtaining a more adequate amount of sample to provide both cytologic and stromal elements of the lesion. It is also useful in deep locations including hip joint, pelvis, sacrum, and vertebra but can produce hematoma or neurovascular injury by blind technique with potential contamination of the tissue plane. In a series of 270 biopsies, high accuracy of the trocar biopsy has been reported with an overall accuracy rate of 91% and failure rate of 9%. The authors did not find specific contraindications with regard to the kind of lesion, and the site of the lesion did not influence the rate of success, except for the pelvis [58]. More recent studies have reported similar diagnostic accuracy for core-needle biopsy compared to open biopsy [47, 59–62]. A closed biopsy can be acceptable for (1) confirmation of metastatic disease, (2) diagnosis of SBC, (3) screening for OM to differentiate from bone tumors, (4) histologic confirmation of a typical clinic-radiologic presentation of sarcoma, and (5) confirmation of local recurrence [2]. However, trocar biopsy is not adequate for diagnosis of some tumors. For example, incision biopsy is required to obtain more extensive and adequate samples for a correct diagnosis of various OSAs of chondroblastic, fibroblastic, telangiectatic, small-cell, and giant-cell rich subtypes, which usually produce only focal minimal osteoid. If osteoid is not discovered in an inadequate small sample, they can be easily mistaken for CSA, FSA, small round cell tumor, or malignant GCT (refer Histologic findings in Osteosarcoma chapter).

B. *Open incision biopsy*

Open incision biopsy has been considered the gold standard in bone and soft tissue tumors for a long time, with an accuracy of 94–99%. However, it can bring a higher chance of complications than a closed biopsy, including hematoma, tumor spread, and wound problems that may interfere with future treatments. In an analysis of 597 patients who underwent a biopsy for bone and soft tissue sarcomas, only about 60% of the 85 needle biopsies led to the correct diagnosis as compared with 76% of the 512 incisional biopsies [63]. The authors reported the rate of major errors in diagnosis was 14%, the rate of complications was 16%, and unnecessary amputation was performed in about 3% of these patients. Errors, complications, and changes in clinical course were two to 12 times greater when the biopsy was done in a referring institution instead of in a treatment center. More recently, an increasing number of studies suggest similar diagnostic accuracy with a lower risk of complications for percutaneous techniques compared to open biopsy [47, 51, 53, 58–61]. Incision biopsy is more often indicated for difficult cases which that require extensive samples for detailed histological analysis, including IHC, special stains, cytometry or histomorphology technique, and even electron microscopy.

Principles of incision biopsy If a tourniquet is used, the limb should be elevated before inflation without exsanguination by compression to prevent squeezing the tumor cells into the systemic circulation. A small longitudinal incision should be carefully placed to access the tumor without contamination of critical structures, which easily allows for extension of the incision for a future definitive surgery (Fig. 1.10c). However, a biopsy wound by large transverse incision can make adequate wide excision more difficult and produce a huge defect even with tumor contamination in later surgery (Fig. 1.10d). The approach should be made directly to the lesion through a single compartment rather than contaminating an intermuscular plane by muscle dissection, and major neurovascular structures should be avoided. Samples should be taken from the periphery of the tumor due to the frequent presence of central necrosis, and they can be obtained from the soft tissue mass if exists. If a hole is necessary to be made in the host bone, it should be round to oval or oblong with rounded ends to avoid stress concentration preventing a subsequent fracture (Fig. 1.10e). In cadaver femora study, Clark et al. [64] revealed that an oblong hole with rounded ends afforded the greatest residual strength and found that increased width of the hole caused a significant reduction in strength but increased length did not. They concluded the hole should have very rounded, smooth ends. If the defect needs to be enlarged to get enough specimens, an increase in its length is less detrimental to bone strength than an increase in its width. The hole must be plugged with bone cement to minimize hematoma formation and spillage of tumor cells through the hole. During biopsy, a frozen section should be sent to ensure that the sample is adequate and enough for additional histologic analysis. With meticulous hemostasis after deflation of tourniquet, bring the drain out of the skin in line with biopsy incision to allow the drain track is easily included in a future surgical incision for wide resection (Fig. 1.10f). Skeletal sarcomas were reported to recur after resection and prosthetic reconstruction at open biopsy sites with a much higher rate (38%) when the biopsy scar was not excised than when the scar is excised (7%) [65].

8. Principles of surgical management
   A. *Surgical margins* (Fig. 1.11)

   Surgical margins are the quality and quantity of the tissues surrounding the tumor after its surgical removal [66]. In 1980, Enneking and colleagues advocated an evaluation system for surgical margins of four types, *intralesional*, *marginal*, *wide*, and *radical margin*,

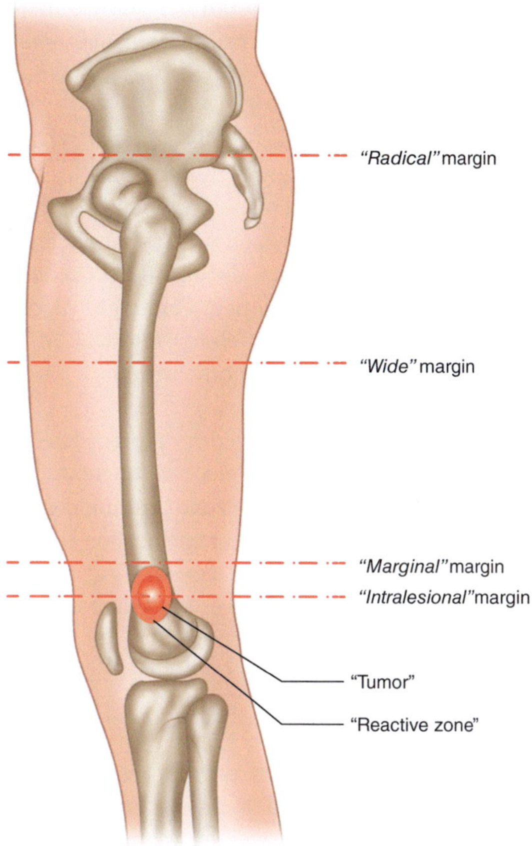

Fig. 1.11 Surgical margin by Enneking. Enneking et al. advocated surgical margins of four types including intralesional, marginal, wide, and radical margin based on the relationship of the surgical margin to the *"tumor"* and its pseudo-capsular *"reactive zone"* [42]. (**1**) *"Intralesional"* margin is accomplished by a procedure of tumor removal throughout the lesion, which allows severe contamination of all the exposed tissues during the procedure. (**2**) *"Marginal"* margin is achieved by a procedure of tumor removal in one piece throughout the (pseudo)capsule or reactive zone surrounding the tumor. (**3**) *"Wide"* margin is obtained by a procedure in which the lesion, its (pseudo) capsule and/or reactive zone, and a surrounding cuff of normal tissue are taken as a single block. The procedure is intra-compartmental en-bloc resection with normal tissue cuff and may leave the *"skip"* lesions. (**4**) *"Radical"* margin is achieved by a procedure in which the lesion, (pseudo)capsule, reactive zone, and the entire muscles or bone involved are removed as one block. The procedure is extra-compartmental en-bloc resection with the entire anatomic compartment of origin bounded by its natural barriers resulting in no residual tumor.

based on the relationship of the surgical margin to the *tumor* and its pseudo-capsular *reactive zone* [42].

(a) Intralesional margin

This margin is accomplished by a procedure of tumor removal through the lesion. Macroscopic or microscopic tumor is left at the margins of the wound with contamination of all exposed tissues during the procedure such as incisional biopsy, curettage, piecemeal debulking, or subtotal removal of a tumor to be managed by other means.

(b) Marginal margin

This margin is achieved by a procedure of tumor removal in one piece throughout the pseudocapsule or reactive zone surrounding the tumor. Marginal excision or enucleation is usually performed for benign tumors. If performed in malignant tumors, the procedure leaves microscopic disease at the margin of the wound producing a local recurrence in most cases.

(c) Wide margin

This margin can be obtained by a procedure in which the lesion, its pseudocapsule and/or reactive zone, as well as the surrounding cuff of normal tissue are taken out as a single block. The procedure is intra-compartmental en-bloc resection with normal tissue cuff but may leave the "skip" lesions if present.

(d) Radical margin

This margin is achieved by a procedure in which the lesion, pseudocapsule, reactive zone, and the entire muscles or bone involved are removed as one block. Longitudinally, the plane of dissection goes through or beyond the joint proximally and distally to the bone involved and through the tendinous origin and insertion of involved muscles. Transversely, the dissection passes beyond the major fascia septa of the involved soft tissue compartments or beyond the periosteum of intraosseous lesions. The procedure is extra-compartmental en-bloc resection with the entire anatomic compartment of origin bounded by its natural barriers resulting in no residual tumor.

B. *Surgical options according to the tumor stage*

Benign Bone Tumors

(a) Benign stage 1 (inactive) tumor

When the lesion is asymptomatic, periodic observation is enough to watch if the lesion grows or changes. Intralesional curettage can be necessary if it is painful.

(b) Benign stage 2 (active) tumor

Intralesional removal with or without local adjuvant treatment is indicated.

(c) Benign stage 3 (aggressive) tumor

Extended curettage using high-speed burr with or without local adjuvant therapy or even wide resection with reconstruction for recurrent cases can be indicated.

Malignant Bone Tumors

(a) Malignant stage IA

Extended curettage using high-speed burr with local adjuvants or wide resection with reconstruction is necessary.

(b) Malignant stage IB

Wide resection with reconstruction is indicated.

(c) Malignant stage IIA

Wide resection with reconstruction is indicated occasionally with chemotherapy or radiotherapy.

(d) Malignant stage IIB

C. Wide resection or even radical excision with reconstruction by various methods is indicated usually with chemotherapy or radiotherapy. Amputation may be necessary in some cases such as severely contaminated lesions, poor bone stalk or inadequate soft tissue coverage for reconstruction after resection, repeated local recurrence, uncontrollable infection, or useless limb.

1. Curettage and filling of the defect (Fig. 1.12).
   A. Simple curettage

   Most benign bone tumors (stage 1 or 2) except locally aggressive tumors (stage 3) are treated adequately by simple curettage without local adjuvants. Curettage is done through the cortical window of varying size according to the lesion size. The size of the window needs to be at least as large as the lesion itself so as not to leave residual tumor on the undersurface of the near cortex (Fig. 1.12a).

   B. Extended curettage

   Locally aggressive benign bone (stage 3) tumors including ABC, GCT, CB, OB, or CMF and even low-grade malignant tumors such as grade 1 CSA are generally treated by extended curettage using high-speed burr, often with local adjuvant therapy such as liquid nitrogen, alcohol, phenol, hydrogen peroxide, thermal electrocauterization, argon beam, plasma coagulation, and iodine to extend destruction of any microscopic tumor cells remaining within the tumoral cavity (Fig. 1.12b–d). However, these agents may produce side effects such as wound healing problems, nerve injury, tendon rupture, bleeding, infection, pathological fracture, and/or skin and soft tissue necrosis. Concerns regarding the efficacy and associated morbidity by the adjuvants have been raised, and the superiority of a single adjuvant has not been documented [67]. Early in 1968, Marcove and colleagues [68] introduced cryosurgery into orthopedic oncology for the treatment of aggressive bone tumors by direct pouring of liquid nitrogen into the cavity made by curettage. Repeated freezing and thawing are performed in three cycles at a temperature of at least minus 60 °C, especially in more aggressive cases where most extensive necrosis is desired. Three cycles of freezing-thawing resulted in tumor cell death up to 2 cm from the inner cavity margin [69]. Cryosurgery appeared to be an effective method of avoiding limb ablation and controlling the painful lesions in primary locally aggressive benign or low-grade malignant bone tumors, and even in metastatic carcinomas [68–71]. Adequate exposure, meticulous curettage and burring, soft-tissue mobilization and protection, and routine use of internal fixation with PMMA for reconstruction are essential to improve outcome and to reduce the incidence of fracture and infection [72]. Argon beam coagulation is gaining popularity as an adjuvant therapy in orthopedic surgery due to the ease, precision, and confined nature of the argon beam coagulator directly delivering electrical current to the bone defect through an inert argon gas beam. It results in desiccation, coagulation, and shrinkage of the remained tumor cells without possible complications such as chemical burn and necrosis which can be produced by phenol and liquid nitrogen [73, 74]. More recently, a closed cryoablation device using metal probes through which argon and helium gasses are delivered into the tumor cavity for freezing and thawing was developed [75]. The authors reported a low rate of local recurrence (3.4%) without skin necrosis, infection, neurapraxia, or thromboembolic complication as well as a low incidence of perioperative fractures (3.4%). Phenol can coagulate all proteinaceous substances to produce tumor cell necrosis and is highly corrosive to cause chemical burns on direct contact. Thus, careful technique such as using cotton-tipped cautery or gauze packing over the borders of the tumor cavity is mandatory. Then, the cavity is washed with saline solution lavage or neutralized with alcohol after several minutes. However, its poor tissue penetration limits the resultant tumor necrosis to superficial cell layers [76–79].

   C. Options of filling the bone defect followed by curettage

   The cavitary defect of host bone followed by curettage can be filled with various substances including graft bone, demineralized

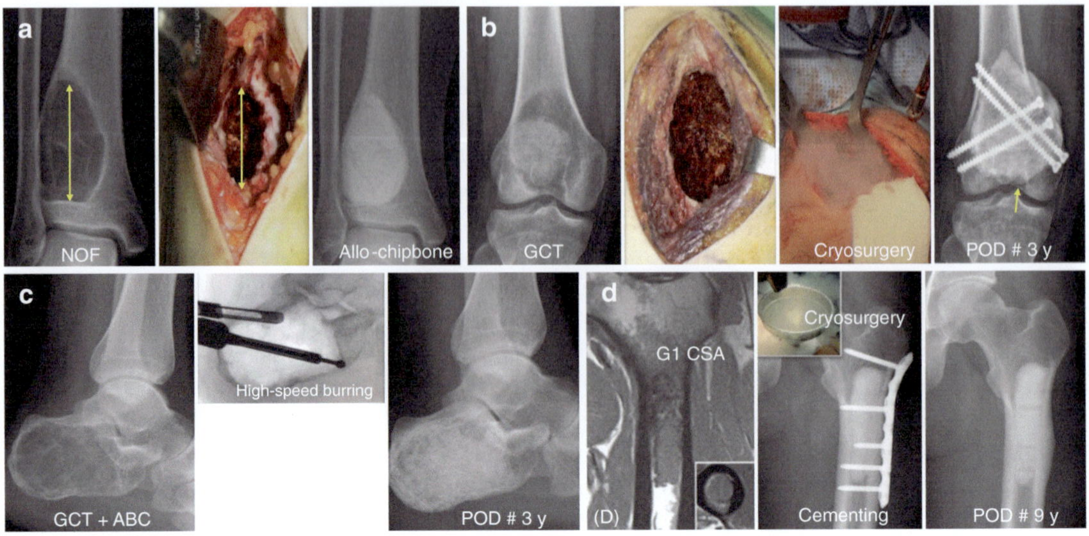

Fig. 1.12 Curettage. (**a**) *Simple curettage:* A large NOF is simply curetted without adjuvant therapy, and the large defect is impacted with allogenic chip bone. Most benign bone tumors except locally aggressive tumors (stage 3) can be treated adequately by such simple curettage. The size of the window needs to be at least as large as the lesion itself (double-headed arrows) so as not to leave residual tumor on the undersurface of the cortex. (**a**) *Extended curettage* using high-speed burr: Locally aggressive benign tumors including GCT (**b**), GCT with secondary ABC, (**c**) and low-grade CSA (**d**) are managed by an extended curettage with or wihtout cryosurgery. Follow-up radiographs in each case show no evidence of local recurrence. The early degenerative change of the joint is prevented by using subchondral autogenous bone graft of 1–2 cm thickness before cementing on a follow-up radiograph at 3 years after surgery (yellow arrow in **b**)

bone matrix (DBM), polymethylmethacrylate (PMMA) bone cement, and synthetic bone substitutes such as calcium sulfate and calcium phosphate composite often in combination with autogenous bone, bone marrow aspirates, or demineralized matrix.

(a) Autogenous bone graft

It may provide all three essential elements of osteogenic, osteoinductive, and osteoconductive properties according to the type of autogenous bone graft, which provides the most rapid and reliable bone regeneration along with the final bonding between host bone and grafting material, so-called *osteointegration*. However, it may be complicated with unnecessary morbidity such as residual pain, infection, neurovascular injury, and cosmetic disadvantages at the harvest site. In addition, the amount of graft bone is limited and may not be enough for large cavities particulate in small children or elderly patients with severe osteoporosis. The osteogenic property is best provided by fresh cancellous autograft containing viable donor osteocytes, or their precursor cells which directly promote primary bone formation. Osteoinduction refers to the ability of the graft to recruit pluripotent mesenchymal stem cells differentiating into bone-forming cells. Osteoconduction refers to the scaffolding, which provides an environment for new bone apposition by capillary ingrowth and recruitment of osteoprogenitor cells. The common donor sites include the iliac crest, proximal and distal end of tibia, distal radius, and greater trochanter of the femur, rib, or fibula. Autogenous cortical bone graft provides osteoconductive property with minimal osteoinductive and osteogenic properties, which is best suitable for structural defects for which immediate mechanical stability is required for healing. Cancellous bone graft is the most commonly used source of autogenous graft, providing all of the osteoinductive, osteoconductive, and osteogenic properties. Cortico-cancellous bone grafts can provide the advantages of both cortical and cancellous bone with immediate structural stability and osteoconductive property from the cortical bone as well as osteogenic and osteoinductive properties from the cancellous bone. Free vascularized grafts can be harvested as cortico-cancellous type with a vascular pedicle which offer the most predictable incorporation and are indicated for large bone defects [80]. Vascularized grafts are traditionally harvested from the iliac crest with its deep circumflex iliac artery, fibula with branches of the peroneal artery, distal end of the radius with the supraretinacular artery, or ribs with the posterior intercostal artery. Early in 1907, Ryall [81] reported the first case of iatrogenic tumor transplantation, being ipsilateral total chest wall contamination from a single scalpel used during mastectomy. Years later in 1913, Mayo [82] documented a traumatic dissemination of cancer during a surgical procedure for malignant disease. He realized the possibility of spontaneous ontogenous grafting of carcinoma especially at points of contact, which may be induced by surgical manipulations. Subsequently, Saphir [83] reported the presence of viable tumor cells on the scalpel used for the biopsy of breast cancer, and Brandes et al. [84] described the cancer transplantation via a surgeon's gleoves, which was contaminated with malignant cells during biopsy. Years later, iatrogenic implantation of GCT at the bone graft harvest site of iliac crest from the original site of proximal tibia was first reported by Joynt and Ortved [85]. More recently, iatrogenic seeding cases have been reported at the bone graft harvest site probably due to contamination by tumor cells from the primary lesion of bone in GCT or much more commonly, in malignant lesions [86–91]. Therefore, autogenous bone should be carefully harvested using a different set of instruments, gloves, and drapes to prevent possible contamination of the donor site by tumor cells from the primary bone lesions.

(b) Allogenous bone graft (Fig. 1.12a, c)

This type of graft bone is readily available in enough quantities without any further operative morbidity, although it has only osteoconductive profile. The current increasing availability has made it possible to manufacture various customized types, such as dowels, strips, chips, or even long cortical grafts. Allograft can be used in the fresh frozen or freeze-dried forms, and cortical or cancellous grafts. A theoretically possible risk of disease transmission can be intercepted by the use of freeze-dried cancellous allograft. However, the manufacturing procedure can significantly weaken the biologic and mechanical properties initially present in the bone tissue.

(c) Demineralized bone matrix (DBM)

DBM is produced by decalcification of cortical bone followed by process to reduce the potential for infection and immunogenic reaction by the host. It is an osteoconductive and osteoinductive commercial biomaterial. DBM retains the trabecular collagenous structure of the original tissue and can serve as a biologic osteoconductive scaffold. Bone demineralization process does not eliminate all potent osteogenic agents, which are now more bioavailable despite the loss of structural strength. Many DBMs retain proteinaceous components such as growth factors which are known to be potent osteogenic agents. DBM has been validated as a versatile bone biomaterial with more osteoinductive potential than standard mineralized allograft in orthopedic repair.

(d) Synthetic substitutes (Tricalcium phosphate-ceramic and hydroxyapatite).

They have only osteoconductive potential but are readily available. They are usually used in combination with autogenous bone graft, bone marrow aspirates, or DBM, which can be effective to fill relatively large defects.

(e) Polymethylmethacrylate (PMMA) Bone Cement (Fig. 1.12b, d)

PMMA cement is useful to fill large cavitary defects in addition to its use as an adjuvant. It provides immediate stability to allow early ambulation and rehabilitation and reduces the risk of pathologic fracture with easy detection of local recurrence by radiolucency between the cement and host bone. Although the cement produces heat during polymerization, the heat is not effectively delivered to the deeply seated tumors. In a rabbit model, a 1- to 2-mm rim of thermal necrosis was reported after filling a bone cavity with PMMA [92]. In a dog model, bone marrow cells were necrotized at 60 °C but not below 5 °C. The authors measured the maximum temperature which never exceeded 46 °C under surgical conditions [93]. The heat developed during polymerization was sharply decreased between the center of the PMMA block and its interface with the adjacent bone [92, 93]. Other authors also suggested that the polymerization heat alone has no necrotizing effect, although hot toxic chemicals during polymerization may inhibit bone blood perfusion and remodeling [94, 95]. However, the heat may lead to early cartilage degeneration of the adjacent joint, and thus subchondral autogenous bone graft of 1–2 cm thickness before cementing is necessary to protect the articular cartilage by forming a barrier between the cement and the articular cartilage [96–98] (Fig. 1.12b). More recently, cement with ferromagnetic compounds was developed to generate heat by hysteresis loss under an alternate magnetic field in a rabbit tibia model, which may be applicable for the hyperthermic treatment of bone tumors [99]. Similar studies aiming to develop an optimized composition of magnetic bone cement area which would be sufficient to kill tumor cells are still going [100–102].

2. *Wide resection and reconstruction (Limb-salvage surgery)* (Figs. 1.13, 1.14, and 1.15).

The primary goal in surgery of bone sarcomas is the complete removal of tumor by local resection with adequate margin or amputation. Progressive advances in diagnostic imaging, chemotherapy, radiation therapy, and surgical techniques for resection, sometimes using navigation systems and reconstruction, allow limb salvage surgery rather than amputation to be a reasonable option in most patients with malignant bone tumors. However, limb salvage surgery cannot be allowed in rare cases with neurovascular involvement, significantly displaced pathologic fracture, or severe contamination due to local recurrence or wrongly performed biopsy. Four basic concerns are addressed for limb-sparing procedures instead of amputation (1). The survival rate should not be worse when compared to that after amputation (2). The morbidity or complications need to be low and not delay the subsequent chemotherapy or radiotherapy (3). Better function of the salvaged limb should be expected when compared to the function after amputation (4). There should be psychosocial benefits for patients who undergo limb-salvage surgery instead of amputation [103]. There have been no randomized, controlled trials comparing the outcomes of limb-preserving surgery with amputation due to the inability to randomize treatment and the subjective nature of important outcome measures. However, retrospective studies reported no difference between both strategies in terms of the disease-free interval or total survival [103, 104]. Some authors have even reported a significant survival benefit limb-preserving surgery over amputation [105, 106].

A. *En bloc resection with adequate wide margin*

The surgeon should dissect and cut cautiously to avoid hemorrhage and reactive tissue or scar tissue by previous biopsy in normal tissue for prevention of contamination during the entire surgery. The incision should include the tract of closed biopsy or all scars including stitch marks from the previous incision biopsy in a wide wedge (Fig. 1.13b). The subcutaneous and underlying fascia should be excised more widely including hemorrhage area or reactive tissues. The muscles can be resected subtotally or totally on both sides of the scar tract. Peritumoral intra-

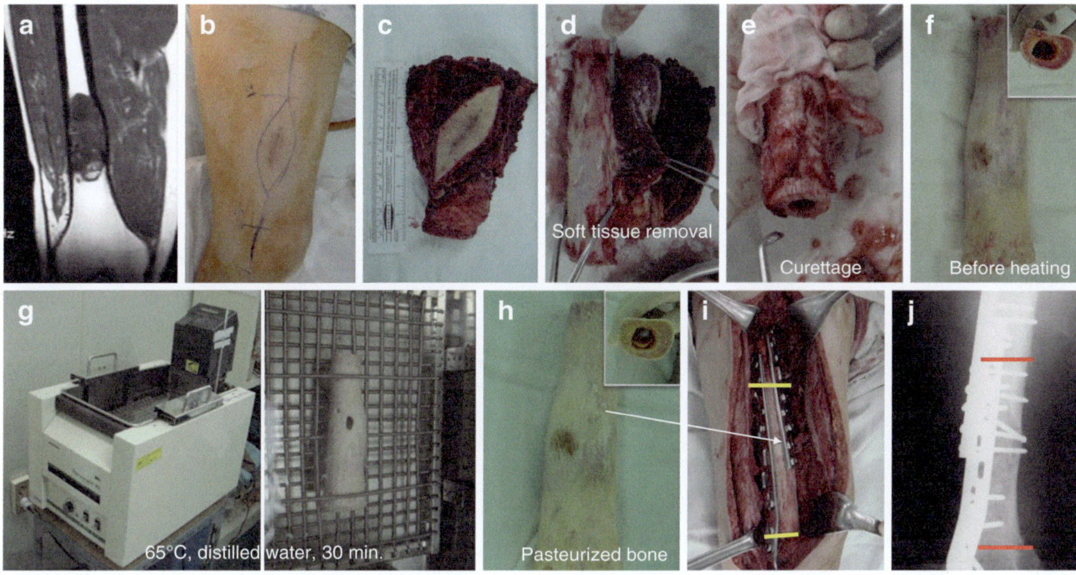

Fig. 1.13 Pasteurization procedure. (**a**) MRI shows a malignant bone tumor involving the diaphysis of distal femur. (**b**) A skin incision, including the previous biopsy scar with stich marks, is made. (**c**) The procedure includes en-bloc resection with wide margin including the whole tumor with a part of normal bone, bony lesion, and surrounding cuff of normal tissue. (**d**) The resected specimen is cleaned up by removal of surrounding soft tissues including periosteum and muscles. (**e**) The bone marrow and tumor cells are thoroughly curetted. (**f**) The fully cleaned bone specimen before heat treatment is shown with focal areas of blood tinged. The medullary bone remains red in color (inset). (**g**) The specimen is sterilized by pasteurization at a low temperature of 60–65 °C for 30 minutes. (**h**) The Pasteurized bone no longer shows blood-tinged areas on the cortical surface and red-clored meduallry bone (inset). (**i**) The sterilized bone is perfectly repositioned (between yellow lines) and rigidly fixed using dual plates. (**j**) Postoperative radiograph notes perfect match in size and shape (between red lines) and alignment

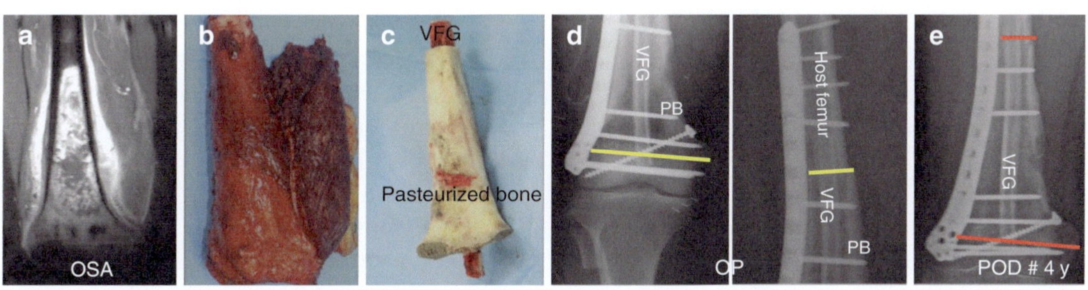

Fig. 1.14 Pasteurized bone augmented by VFG. (**a**) MRI shows a malignant bone tumor involving the meta-diaphysis of distal femur. (**b**) A specimen by En-bloc resection with wide margin including a part of the host bone with whole tumor, surrounding normal muscle, and all contaminated areas from the previous incision biopsy. (**c**) After pasteurization, VFG is inserted into the pasteurized bone (PB) to reinforce mechanical strength and to promote union between the PB and the host bone junction. (**d**) Immediate postoperative radiograph reveals a good repositioning of the PB (between yellow lines). (**e**) Follow-up radiograph at 4 years after surgery reveals good union of the PB (between red lines) with no evidence of local recurrence

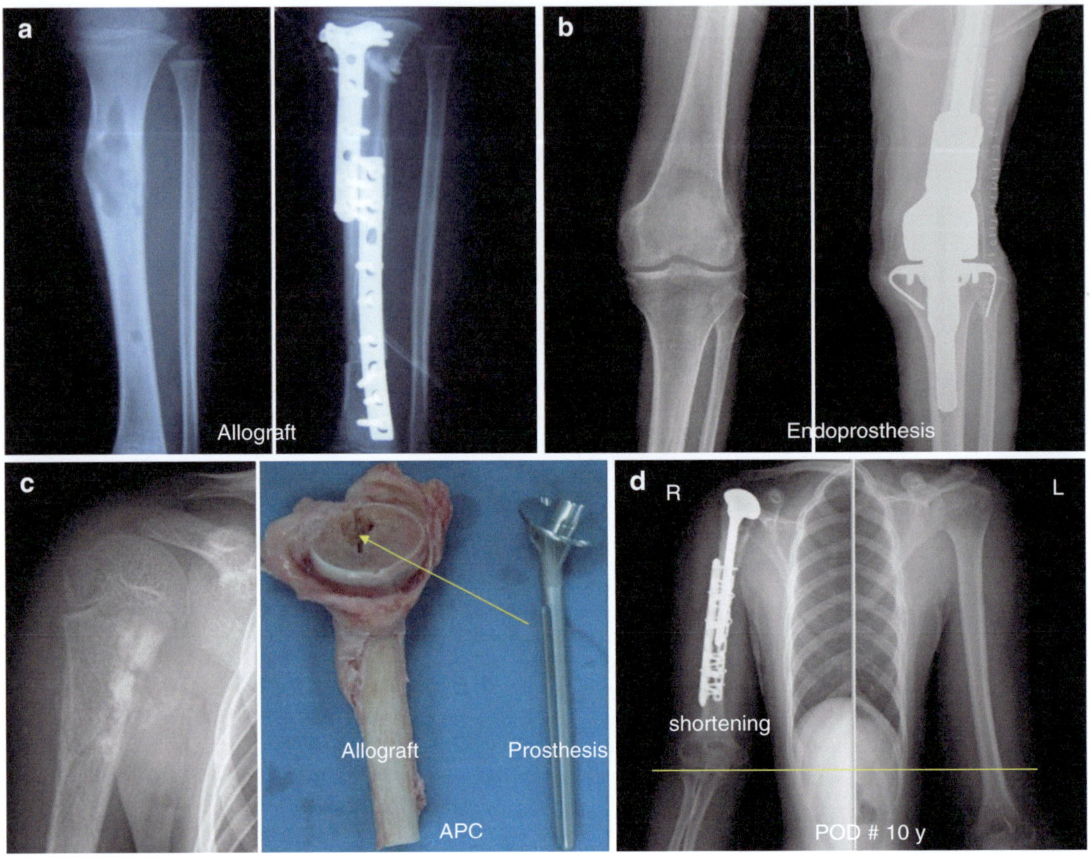

Fig. 1.15 Reconstruction by various methods. (**a**) Allograft, (**b**) endoprosthesis, and (**c**) allo-prosthesis composite (APC) are used for reconstruction. (**d**) Follow-up radiograph at 10 years after reconstruction with APC notes a significant shortening of the right upper arm. However, the patient is very active and doing well without physical dysfunction and psychological problems

or extra-compartmental hematoma may be formed by previous biopsy or pathologic fracture. The intra-compartmental hematoma can be removed by including the compartment in the resection procedure, but an extra-compartmental hematoma around the major neurovascular structure may require amputation. With gentle dissection, the major neurovascular bundles should be separated from the tumor by a layer of normal tissue if possible. However, the major vessels with adhesion to the rumor must be resected en-bloc, and artery should be repaired with bypass surgery. As previously mentioned, Enneking et al. advocated four surgical margins including intralesional, marginal, wide, and radical based on the relationship of the surgical margin to the neoplasm and its pseudo-capsular reactive zone [42], which have been popularly used. However, there is a drawback with a wide range of definitions of the wide margin and severe dysfunction after a radical margin. Thus, the modified system for surgical margins was accepted by the Japanese Orthopedic Association years later. A surgical margin in the modified system is based on the distance of the margin from the tumor's reactive zone and classified into four categories: intralesional, marginal, adequate or inadequate wide, and curative margin [107]. A curative wide margin (curative margin) passes through the region outside the reactive zone at a distance of more than 5 cm from the tumor-reactive zone. A wide margin passes through outside the reactive zone with more than 1–4 cm of normal tissue cuff but is not enough to be curative, which is further classified into two subtypes including adequate and inadequate wide margin. An adequate wide margin is a margin that is 2 cm or more from the reactive zone, and an inadequate wide margin is a margin that is 1 cm outside the reactive zone. Marginal margin passes through the reactive zone. Intralesional margin passes inside the tumorous parenchyma. The *reactive zone* is in this system strictly defined as a discolored area around a tumor observed by gross inspection, which consists of hemorrhagic tissue, scar tissue, degenerated muscle, edema, or the tumor (pseudo)capsule. The *Barrier* refers to any tissue that has resistance against tumor invasion, including fascia, joint capsule, tendon, tendon sheath, periosteum, vascular sheath, cartilage, pleura, peritoneum, and epineurium. A thin fascia is considered to be the equivalent of 2 cm of normal tissue, a thick fascia is 3 cm, and a joint cartilage is 5 cm [108]. Later, Kawaguchi et al. analyzed this system in 837 patients with musculoskeletal sarcoma, and they determined the safety margins in various situations. If preoperative chemotherapy is not done or is ineffective in high-grade sarcoma, a margin greater than 3-cm wide is necessary. A 2-cm wide margin is permissible if the preoperative modality is effective. However, a curative margin is required for recurrent tumors whether low-grade or high-grade. For low-grade sarcoma, an adequate wide margin is also essential but a limited wide margin with partial marginal margins may be acceptable if barriers exist [109].

B. *Options for reconstruction of the defect*

Generally, reconstructions followed by wide resection have much higher rates of complication than those of standard total joint arthroplasties because of the large defect by extensive bone and soft tissue loss in addition to the compromising effects by irradiation and chemotherapy. In addition, these reconstructions are often done in young patients who grow rapidly and are extremely active. Muscle transfer to gain adequate motor function or soft tissue coverage, including local or free flaps for wound closure to prevent subsequent infection is often necessary after reconstruction. The options for reconstructions including biologic, nonbiologic, and combined methods are summarized in Table 1.7.

I. Biologic reconstruction

Biologic reconstruction can be achieved by autogenous bone, including fibula graft, recycled autograft, or distraction osteogenesis as well as allogenic bone graft from a bone bank.

(a) Autograft: (non)vascularized fibular graft and recycled bone
    (i) Fibular graft: non-vascularized and vascularized fibula graft

A nonvascularized fibula graft (NFG) has been a gold standard for biological reconstructions for large bone defects for various reasons including trauma or resection for tumor treatment or others during many decades because of its remodeling capacity at the donor site, simpler operative technique, less expensive, and shorter operative time [110, 111]. Occasionally, NFG is still a useful alternative to vascularized fibula graft (VFG), especially where there is a good cover with soft tissue and good blood supply. Krieg and Hefti [110] reported a good long-term result with an increased diameter of the graft in 70% and a relatively low rate of donor site complication (16%). Fatigue fracture occurred in seven cases (23%) but only two cases needed treatment. Nowadays, VFG has been more frequently used for reconstructions for larger defect because of the limited biologic activity and higher risk of resorption of NFG. Early in 1975, Taylor et al. [112] reported the first successful distant transfer of a composite fibular graft by

Table 1.7 Options for reconstruction followed by resection

Biologic	Autograft—VFG, autoclave, pasteurization, irradiation Distraction osteogenesis Allograft
Nonbiologic	Tumor prosthesis
Combined	Allograft prosthesis composite (APC)

microvascular anastomoses. Years later in 1981, Weiland [113] reported its first use after resection of bone tumors. VFG is necessary to reconstruct bony defects more than 6 cm or defects occasionally with poorly vascularized tissue. However, NFG does not provide either the stability of a hypertrophied graft or biologic stimulus for healing in these situations. VFG unite more rapidly with the host bone and is more resistant to infection than NFG by virtue of their inherent vascularity. VFG are particularly useful to restore a large diaphyseal defect due to their shape and mechanical properties [113].

(ii) Recycled autograft: autoclaving, irradiating and freezing, pasteurization (Fig. 1.13).

It has been widely used for reconstruction when bone banks for allograft are not readily available particularly in Korea and Japan due to a lack of wide acceptance of bone donation, primarily because of the cultural and religious backgrounds. Therefore, recycled autogenous host bone grafting processed by extracorporeal procedures including heat [114–117], irradiation [118, 119], or freezing [120, 121] has been widely used as an alternative to allograft. Of these, pasteurization with low-temperature saline can kill the tumor cells while preserving bone morphogenic protein (BMP). The procedure includes en-bloc resection with wide margin of a part of the host normal bone, soft tissue, or muscle as well as biopsy scar with stitch marks. Then, the resected specimen is cleaned up by removal of surrounding soft tissues including periosteum and muscles followed by a thorough curettage of tumor cells and bone marrow. The prepared bone is sterilized by pasteurization at a low temperature of 60–65 °C for 30 minutes. The pasteurized bone is accurately repositioned and rigidly fixed with dual plates (Fig. 1.13). In a rabbit model, irradiation and pasteurization produced a more favorable outcome in terms of bone union based on radiographic and histological evaluations. Pasteurization had the best overall outcomes with the preservation of osteocytes and bone marrow cellularity [122]. It can be an acceptable temporary spacer in terms of histological regeneration in retrieved grafts [115]. This approach has several benefits, including elimination of host immunological response and disease transmission, ease of anatomical reinsertion with a perfect size and shape match, biologic healing, and low cost. Most importantly, the risk of local recurrence seemed to be low because there were no viable tumor cells on the resected tumor bones which were treated with the different methods of sterilization such as pasteurization, boiling, autoclaving, and irradiation in a rabbit model [123]. However, they are mechanically weak and brittle depending on the sterilization process used, which may contribute to delayed union or nonunion, fracture of the processed bone, and degeneration or destruction of the articular cartilage. Therefore, VFG may be necessary to reinforce mechanical strength and to promote the union (Fig. 1.14). Additionally, the recycled bone does not allow an adequate evaluation of chemotherapy effects and postoperative margin.

(iii) Distraction osteogenesis

Bone lengthening by the Ilizarov technique using an external fixator is another biological approach to repair large segmental bone defects. It has been widely used for the management of nonunion, leg-length discrepancy, deformity, OM, and traumatic bone defects as well as for large defects followed by bone tumor resection [124–127]. Despite the advantages of ability to restore all defects of any diameter and length as well as permission of early weight bearing and joint motion, there is a limited number of studies about the reconstruction of bony defects following en-bloc resection for bone tumors due to long treatment period, risk of pin tract infection, delayed ossification or maturation, functional limitations by wrongly placed K-wires traversing muscles, and pain caused by loosening of K-wires [126, 128, 129].

(b) Allografts (Fig. 1.15a)

Frozen allografts have been used longer than any other options in Western countries where they are readily available. They are favored by some surgeons for their potential for longevity by their function as a biologic reconstruction to allow host-to-allograft incorporation. In addition, osteoarticular allografts can allow preserving the joint which is not affected by the tumor and provide the ability of soft tissue or peri-articular ligament reconstruction. There is also no donor-site morbidity as well. However, they have a high rate of complications such as infection, fracture, joint instability, delayed or nonunion, articular degeneration or collapse, and failure of ligament or tendon attachments requiring additional surgeries in many cases. The allograft can be reinforced by VFG for promoting union and prevention of graft fracture in some cases (Fig. 1.14). Resorption of the graft or leg length discrepancy can be associated. Sizing mismatch may also exist even in a large bone bank. Immunologic complications and risk of disease transmission possibly exist but are generally out of concern. In comparing different types, intercalary allografts have better clinical outcomes than osteoarticular allografts, allograft prosthetic composites, and allografts used for arthrodesis [130, 131].

II. Non-biologic reconstruction: Modular endoprostheses (Fig. 1.15b)

Currently available endoprosthetic systems provide lightweight, strong, inert profiles for skeletal reconstruction by great improvements in implant materials with increased durability. Prosthetic reconstruction carries a lower risk of deep infection than allografts, and nonunion is not a concern. They avoid the risk of disease transmission and immune responses that may exist in allograft reconstruction. In addition, most endoprostheses are modular to allow incremental lengthening of the limb in growing children. Endoprosthetic reconstruction can provide immediate stability allowing early rehabilitation with early joint motion and immediate weight bearing particularly when performed with bone cement. However, they also carry early complications with the extensive nature in most musculoskeletal oncology procedures including wound problems such as necrosis or dehiscence, superficial or deep infection, thrombo-embolic conditions, neurapraxia, and joint instability. They are also associated with late complications such as infection, aseptic loosening, polyethylene wear or dissociation of modular components, joint or prosthetic insatiability, or fatigue fracture if the patients are cured of disease, which can be successfully treated with revision surgery. However, late infection remains the most serious complication in consideration of insufficient attachment of soft tissues to the metallic components. The survival rate of endoprostheses, complications, and functional outcomes may vary depending on the anatomic site, type of prosthesis, and fixation technique including cementing.

III. Combined biologic and non-biologic tools: Allograft-Prosthesis Composite (Fig. 1.15a).

Allograft-endoprosthesis composite (APC) was introduced to overcome the complications of megaprosthesis. It is made of a revision-type prosthesis cemented into an allograft which allows biologic fixation with the remaining soft tissue sleeve (Fig. 1.15c). By using APC, the advantages of both modular implant arthroplasty and osteoarticular allograft can be obtained, and the disadvantages encountered when either reconstruction is used alone are diminished. Compared to other techniques, APC has many advantages including restoration of bone stock, customization with conventional implant components, durable and stable articulation with joint stability by soft tissue attachment of tendons and ligaments, avoidance of cartilage degradation, and preservation of the medullary canal of the host bone. However, drawbacks such as infection, delayed- or nonunion at the graft-host junction, allograft resorption, or periprosthetic fracture can exist. When performed in a growing child, length discrepancy is also expected. But the patient may be tolerable without further surgery if the upper extremity is involved (Fig. 1.15d). A prolonged period of protected weight bearing is required to allow for graft incorporation. Therefore, APC is best suited for revision settings with inadequate length of remaining bone stock to secure the tumor prosthetic stem as well as in those with benign aggressive tumors or low-grade sarcomas, who do not need chemotherapy.

3. *Amputation*

Amputation or disarticulation may be indicated in rare cases with severe neurovascular involvement, significantly displaced fracture, or widespread contamination due to local recurrence or inadequately done biopsy. Various problems such as infection, wound dehiscence, chronic painful limb, phantom limb pain, and appositional bone overgrowth requiring revision surgery can be also complicated. Harris and his colleagues [132] compared the long-term function by an extensive questionnaire and the psychological effects based on questionnaire responses and reviews regarding amputation, arthrodesis, and arthroplasty for tumors around the knee. The study suggested the patients with an amputation were very active, and they were the least worried about damaging the affected limb. However, they had difficulty walking on steep, rough, or slippery surfaces. The authors did not find any difference in psychological and physical function among patients who were treated with different types of surgery. There has been no study regarding a difference between amputation and limb salvage in terms of psychologic outcome or quality of life in long-term survivors of sarcoma. Therefore, surgeons should provide full and objective information on advantages and disadvantages in terms of functional and cosmetic expectations as well as the potential complications of each procedure to the patients and families for making a final decision in light of long-term goals and lifestyle consideration.

4. *Consideration for pediatric patients*

In pediatric patients with skeletal immaturity who have a varying degree of remaining growth potential, limb-preservation surgery is challenging in maintaining equal limb length throughout the child's growth. Future longitudinal and radial growth of the remaining limb is expected to lead to limb length discrepancy (LLD) that may severely limit the limb and joint function, especially in the lower limb. However, some patients are very active and may not worry about damaging the affected limb in upper extremities without any psychological problems and physical dysfunction. A varying degree of LLD can be managed by several options such as amputation with external prosthesis, rotationplasty, arthrodesis, epiphysiodesis, distraction osteogenesis, or expandable tumor prosthesis depending on the patient's age with remaining growth potential and desire. Limb preservation is almost impossible for children under 5 years of age, leaving amputation as the only reasonable option for most cases. It is possible in patients between 5 and 14 years if LLD is managed by distraction osteogenesis using an Ilizarov technique or expandable endoprosthesis. A standard nonexpandable tumor endoprosthesis is usually preferable for patients older than 14 years of age with near completion of growth. Lengthening of 1–2 cm can be obtained during the initial procedure in patients with near maturity. The limb length discrepancy may be minimized by epiphysiodesis of the contralateral limb. Current development of expandable prostheses allows for avoiding procedures such as amputation or rotationplasty with the decreased risk of infection and gradual lengthening without repeated invasive procedures. However, the total lengthening still remains small with high failure rate related to implant breakage, stem loosening, and limited durability even with third-generation noninvasive prostheses, which necessitate reoperations leading to poor functional outcomes and patient satisfaction [133–136]. A systemic review of 292 patients from the literatures between 1997 and 2017 reported that the overall complication and revision rate was 43% with an increase to 59% in 5–10 years' follow-up, and 89% in over 10 years' follow-up. The authors reported minimally invasive model had lower complication rates than noninvasive prostheses, particularly mechanical complications, mainly because of increased rates of lengthening and device failure in the noninvasive models. Patients with distal femur tumor averaged 4.4 lengthening procedures achieving a mean length gain of 43 mm [137]. Although expandable prostheses are not the final answer to

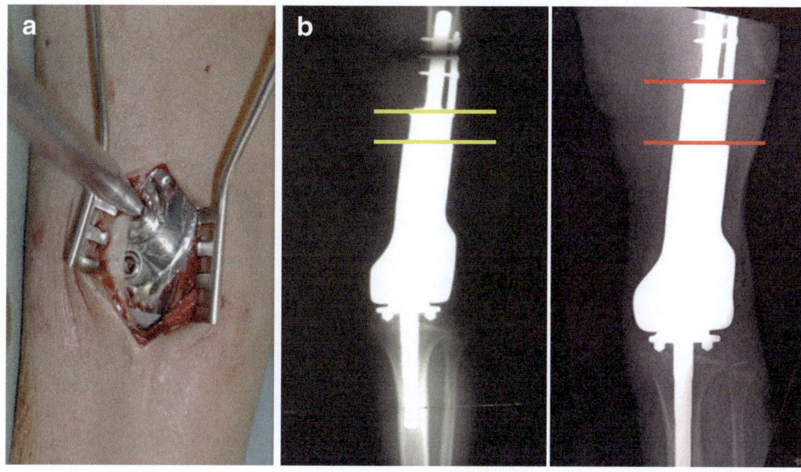

Fig. 1.16 Expandable prosthesis in growing young patients. (**a**) Leg length discrepancy is corrected by a minimally invasive procedure through a small incision. (**b**) With a single minimally invasive procedure, the tumor prosthesis is lengthened by 12 mm (between lines)

the treatment of bone sarcomas in growing pediatric patients due to the frequent high rate of complications, it may still be an appropriate temporary option until the patient's full maturity [138]. The leg length discrepancy can be corrected by minimally invasive procedure (Fig. 1.16) or electromagnetic coil.

References

1. Newman Dorland WA, Dorland's illustrated medical dictionary. 32nd ed. Philadelphia: Elsevier, Saunders; 2012. p.1985.
2. Mirra JM, Picci P. General considerations. In: Mirra JM, editor. Bone tumors: clinical, radiologic, and pathologic correlations. 2nd ed. Philadelphia: Lea & Febiger; 1989. p. 13–34.
3. Morton LM, Onel K, Curtis RE, Hungate EA, Armstrong GT. The rising incidence of second cancers: patterns of occurrence and identification of risk factors for children and adults. Am Soc Clin Oncol Educ Book. 2014;34(1):e57–67.
4. Flanagen AM, Blay JY, Bovée JVMG, Bredella MA, Cool P, Nielsen GP, Yoshida A. Bone tumors: introduction. In: WHO Classification of Tumours Editorial Board, editor. Soft tissue and bone tumours. 5th ed. Lyon: International Agency for Research on Cancer; 2020. p.340–344.
5. Jaffe HL. Introduction. In: Jaffe HL, editor. Tumors and tumorous conditions of the bones and joints. Phildelphia: Lea & Febiger; 1958. p. 14.
6. Czerniak B. General considerations. In: Dorfman HD, Czerniak B, editors. Dorfman and Czerniak's bone tumors (eBook). 2nd ed. Elsevier; 2016. p. 1–56.
7. Picci P. Epidemiology of bone lesions. In: Picci P, Manfrini M, Donati DM, Gambarotti M, Righi A, Vanel D, Dei Tos AP, editors. Diagnosis of musculoskeletal tumors and tumor-like conditions. Cham: Springer; 2020. p. 3–9.
8. SEER Cancer Statistics Factsheets: bone and joint cancer. National Cancer Institute, Bethesda. 2016. http://seer.cancer.gov/statfacts/html/bones.html. Accessed 15 Feb 2023.
9. Toro JR, Travis LB, Wu HJ, Fletcher CD, Devesa SS. Incpatterns of soft tissue sarcomas, regardless of primary site, in the Surveillance, Epidemiology and End Results program, 1978-2001: an analysis of 26,758 cases. Int J Cancer. 2006;119:2922–30.
10. 2022 Estimates for sarcomas in the United States. Sarcoma Foundation of America, Washington, DC. 2022. https://www.curesarcoma.org/wp-content/uploads/Sarcoma-Statistics-2022.pdf. Accessed 15 Feb 2023.
11. Dorfman HD, Czerniak B. Bone cancers. Cancer. 1995;75(S1):203–10.
12. Franchi A. Epidemiology and classification of bone tumors. Clin Cases Miner Bone Metab. 2012;9(2):92–5.
13. Mirra JM, Eckardt JJ. Enchondroma versus chondrosarcoma. In: Mirra JM, editor. Bone tumors: clinical, radiologic, and pathologic correlations. 2nd ed. Philadelphia: Lea & Febiger; 1989. p. 476–535.
14. Lodwick GS. The radiological diagnosis of metastatic cancer in bone. In: Tumors of Bone and Soft Tissue. Proceedings of a Conference at the University of Texas, M. D. Anderson hospital and Tumor Institute. Chicago: Year Book Medical Publishers; 1965. p. 253–268.
15. Lodwick GS. A systematic approach to the roentgen diagnosis of bone tumors. In: Tumors of Bone and Soft Tissue. Proceedings of a Conference at the University of Texas, M. D. Anderson hospital and Tumor Institute. Chicago: Year Book Medical Publishers; 1965. p. 49–68.

16. Ardran G. Bone destruction not demonstrable by radiography. Br J Radiol. 1951;24(278):107–9.
17. Lachman E. Osteoporosis. The potentialities and limitations of its roentgenographic diagnosis. Am J Roentgenol. 1955;74:714–5.
18. Clain A. Secondary malignant disease of bone. Br J Cancer. 1965;19(1):15–29.
19. Edelstyn G, Gillespie P, Grebbell F. The radiological demonstration of osseous metastases. Experimental observations. Clin Radiol. 1967;18(2):158–62.
20. Mirra JM. Basics of clinicoradiologic interpretation. In: Mirra JM, editor. Bone tumors: clinical, radiologic, and pathologic correlations. 2nd ed. Philadelphia: Lea & Febiger; 1989. p. 55–103.
21. Lodwick GS. Editor solitary malignant tumors of bone: the application of predictor variables in diagnosis. Semin Roentgenol. 1966;1(3):293–313.
22. Bahk YW. Introduction and fundamentals of pinhole scintigraphy. In: Bahk YW, editor. Combined Scintigraphic and radiographic diagnosis of bone and joint diseases. Berlin Heidelberg New York: Springer-Verlag; 1994. p. 1–12.
23. Enneking W, Kagan A. “Skip” metastases in osteosarcoma. Cancer. 1975;36(6):2192–205.
24. Bahk YW, Kim OH, Chung SK. Pinhole collimator scintigraphy in differential diagnosis of metastasis, fracture, and infections of the spine. J Nucl Med. 1987;28(4):447–51.
25. Bahk YW, Jeon HS, Kim JM, Park JM, Chung Y-A, Kim EE, et al. Novel use of gamma correction for precise 99m Tc-HDP pinhole bone scan diagnosis and classification of knee occult fractures. Skeletal Radiol. 2010;39(8):807–13.
26. Bahk YW, Kim SH, Chung YA, Bahk WJ, Park JM, Kang YM, et al. Depiction of nidi and fibrovascular zones of osteoid osteomas using gamma-correction Tc-99m HDP pinhole bone scan and conventional radiograph, and correlation with CT, MRI, and PVC phantom imaging. Nucl Med Mol Imaging. 2011;45(1):21–9.
27. Bahk YW. Osteoid osteoma. In: Bahk YW, editor. Combined scintigraphic and radiographic diagnosis of bone and joint diseases: including gamma correction interpretation. 5th ed. eBook: Springer; 2017. p. 452–3.
28. Zimmer W, Berquist T, McLeod R, Sim F, Pritchard D, Shives T, et al. Bone tumors: magnetic resonance imaging versus computed tomography. Radiology. 1985;155(3):709–18.
29. Ojala R, Sequeiros RB, Klemola R, Vahala E, Jyrkinen L, Tervonen O. MR-guided bone biopsy: preliminary report of a new guiding method. J Magn Reson Imaging. 2002;15(1):82–6.
30. Schulte M, Brecht-Krauss D, Heymer B, Guhlmann A, Hartwig E, Sarkar MR, et al. Grading of tumors and tumorlike lesions of bone: evaluation by FDG PET. J Nucl Med. 2000;41(10):1695–701.
31. Aoki J, Watanabe H, Shinozaki T, Takagishi K, Ishijima H, Oya N, et al. FDG PET of primary benign and malignant bone tumors: standardized uptake value in 52 lesions. Radiology. 2001;219(3):774–7.
32. Costelloe CM, Chuang HH, Chasen BA, Pan T, Fox PS, Bassett RL, et al. Bone windows for distinguishing malignant from benign primary bone tumors on FDG PET/CT. J Cancer. 2013;4(7):524–30.
33. Tian R, Su M, Tian Y, Li F, Li L, Kuang A, et al. Dual-time point PET/CT with F-18 FDG for the differentiation of malignant and benign bone lesions. Skeletal Radiol. 2009;38:451–8.
34. Dimitrakopoulou-Strauss A, Strauss LG, Heichel T, Wu H, Burger C, Bernd L, et al. The role of quantitative 18F-FDG PET studies for the differentiation of malignant and benign bone lesions. J Nucl Med. 2002;43(4):510–8.
35. Mirra JM. Benign lesions: callus and stress fracture. In: Mirra JM, editor. Bone tumors: clinical, radiologic, and pathologic correlations. 2nd ed. Philadelphia: Lea & Febiger; 1989. p. 155–74.
36. Bahk WJ, Mirra JM. Pseudoanaplastic tumors of bone. Skeletal Radiol. 2004;33(11):641–8.
37. Ramos-Vara J, Miller M. When tissue antigens and antibodies get along: revisiting the technical aspects of immunohistochemistry—the red, brown, and blue technique. Vet Pathol. 2014;51(1):42–87.
38. Broders AC. Squamous-cell epithelioma of the lip: a study of five hundred and thirty-seven cases. JAMA J Am Med Assoc. 1920;74(10):656–64.
39. Broders AC, Hargrave R, Meyerding HW. Pathological features of soft tissue fibrosarcoma with special reference to the grading of its malignancy. Surg Gynecol Obstet. 1939;69:267–80.
40. Inwards CY, Unni KK. Classification and grading of bone sarcomas. Hematol Oncol Clin North Am. 1995;9(3):545–70.
41. Unni K, Dahlin D, editors. Grading of bone tumors. Semin Diagn Pathol. 1984;1(3):165–72.
42. Enneking WF, Spanier SS, Goodman MA. A system for the surgical staging of musculoskeletal sarcoma. Clin Orthop Relat Res. 1980;153:106–20.
43. Enneking WF. A system of staging musculoskeletal neoplasms. Clin Orthop Relat Res. 1986;204:9–24.
44. Edge SB, Byrd DR, Compton CC, Fritz AG, Greene FL, Trotti A. Bone (primary malignant lymphoma and multiple myeloma are not included.). In: Edge SB, Byrd DR, Compton CC, Fritz AG, Greene FL, Trotti A, editors. AJCC Cancer Staging Manual, 7th ed. New York: Springer-Verlag; 2010; p. 281–7.
45. Bovée JVMG, Flanagen AM, Lazar AJ, Nielsen GP, Yoshida A. TMN staging of tumors of bone. In: WHO Classification of Tumours Editorial Board, editor. Soft Tissue and Bone Tumours. 5th ed. Lyon: International Agenchy for Research on Cancer; 2020. p. 339.
46. Bickels J, Jelinek JS, Shmookler BM, Neff RS, Malawer MM. Biopsy of musculoskeletal tumors: current concepts. Clin Orthop Relat Res. 1999;368:212–9.

47. Le HB, Lee ST, Munk PL, editors. Image-guided musculoskeletal biopsies. Semin Intervent Radiol; 2010: © Thieme Medical Publishers.
48. Coley BL, Sharp GS, Ellis EB. Diagnosis of bone tumors by aspiration. Am J Surg. 1931;13(2):215–24.
49. Lalli A. Roentgen-guided aspiration biopsies of skeletal lesions. Can Assoc Radiol J. 1970;21(2):71–3.
50. Vetrani A, Fulciniti F, Boschi R, Marino G, Zeppa P, Troncone G, et al. Fine needle aspiration biopsy diagnosis of giant-cell tumor of bone. An experience with nine cases. Acta Cytol. 1990;34(6):863–7.
51. El-Khoury G, Terepka R, Mickelson M, Rainville K, Zaleski M. Fine-needle aspiration biopsy of bone. J Bone Joint Surg. 1983;65(4):522–5.
52. Layfield L, Glasgow B, Anders K, Mirra J. Fine needle aspiration cytology of primary bone lesions. Acta Cytol. 1987;31(2):177–84.
53. Palombini L, Marino D, Vetrani A, Fulciniti F. Fine-needle aspiration biopsy in primary malignant and metastatic bone tumors. Appl Pathol. 1983;1:76–81.
54. Schwartz HS, Spengler DM. Needle tract recurrences after closed biopsy for sarcoma: three cases and review of the literature. Ann Surg Oncol. 1997;4:228–36.
55. Unni KK, Inwards Y. Introduction and scope of study. In: Dahlin's bone tumors: general aspects and data on 10,165 cases. Philadelphia: Lippincott Williams & Wilkins; 2010. p. 1–8.
56. Ayala A, Raymond A, Ro J, Carrasco C, Fanning C, Murray J. Needle biopsy of primary bone lesions. MD Anderson experience. Pathol Annu. 1989;24:219–51.
57. Davies N, Livesley P, Cannon S. Recurrence of an osteosarcoma in a needle biopsy track. J Bone Joint Surg Br. 1993;75(6):977–8.
58. Van der Bijl A, Taminiau A, Hermans J, Beerman H, Hogendoorn P. Accuracy of the Jamshidi trocar biopsy in the diagnosis of bone tumors. Clin Orthop Relat Res. 1997;334:233–43.
59. Adams SC, Potter BK, Pitcher DJ, Temple HT. Office-based core needle biopsy of bone and soft tissue malignancies: an accurate alternative to open biopsy with infrequent complications. Clin Orthop Relat Res. 2010;468:2774–80.
60. Pohlig F, Kirchhoff C, Lenze U, Schauwecker J, Burgkart R, Rechl H, et al. Percutaneous core needle biopsy versus open biopsy in diagnostics of bone and soft tissue sarcoma: a retrospective study. Eur J Med Res. 2012;17(1):1–5.
61. Rimondi E, Staals EL, Errani C, Bianchi G, Casadei R, Alberghini M, et al. Percutaneous CT-guided biopsy of the spine: results of 430 biopsies. Eur Spine J. 2008;17:975–81.
62. Sung KS, Seo SW, Shon MS. The diagnostic value of needle biopsy for musculoskeletal lesions. Int Orthop. 2009;33:1701–6.
63. Mankin HJ, Mankin CJ, Simon MA. The hazards of the biopsy, revisited. For the members of the Musculoskeletal Tumor Society. J Bone Joint Surg. 1996;78(5):656–63.
64. Clark C, Morgan C, Sonstegard DA, Matthews LS. The effect of biopsy-hole shape and size on bone strength. J Bone Joint Surg. 1977;59(2):213–7.
65. Cannon SR, Dyson PHP. Relationship of the site of open biopsy of malignant bone tumors to local recurrence following resection and prosthetic replacement. Proc J Bone Joint Surg Br. 1987;69:492.
66. Campanacci M. Introduction. In: Campanacci M, editor. Bone and soft tissue tumors. Wien: Springer-Verlag; 1999. p. 1–70.
67. Bickels J, Campanacci DA. Local adjuvant substances following curettage of bone tumors. J Bone Joint Surg. 2020;102(2):164–74.
68. Marcove RC, Miller TR, Cahan W. The treatment of primary and metastaticbone tumors by repetitive freezing. Ann N Y Acad Sci. 1968;44(5):532–44.
69. Marcove RC, Weis LD, Vaghaiwalla MR, Pearson R, Huvos AG. Cryosurgery in the treatment of giant cell tumors of bone. A report of 52 consecutive cases. Cancer. 1978;41(3):957–69.
70. Marcove RC, Miller TR. The treatment of primary and metastatic localized bone tumors by cryosurgery. Surg Clin North Am. 1969;49(2):421–30.
71. Marcove R. The management of bone tumors. Clin Bull Mem Sloan-Kettering Cancer Cent. 1971;1:7–10.
72. Bickels J, Meller I, Shmookler BM, Malawer MM. The role and biology of cryosurgery in the treatment of bone tumors: a review. Acta Orthop Scand. 1999;70(3):308–15.
73. Cummings JE, Smith RA, Heck RK. Argon beam coagulation as adjuvant treatment after curettage of aneurysmal bone cysts: a preliminary study. Clin Orthop Relat Res. 2010;468:231–7.
74. Lewis VO, Wei A, Mendoza T, Primus F, Peabody T, Simon MA. Argon beam coagulation as an adjuvant for local control of giant cell tumor. Clin Orthop Relat Res. 2007;454:192–7.
75. Bickels J, Kollender Y, Merimsky O, Isaakov J, Petyan-Brand R, Meller I. Closed argon-based cryoablation of bone tumours. J Bone Joint Surg Br. 2004;86(5):714–8.
76. Lack W, Lang S, Brand G. Necrotizing effect of phenol on normal tissues and on tumors: a study on postoperative and cadaver specimens. Acta Orthop Scand. 1994;65(3):351–4.
77. Mittag F, Leichtle C, Kieckbusch I, Wolburg H, Rudert M, Kluba T, et al. Cytotoxic effect and tissue penetration of phenol for adjuvant treatment of giant cell tumours. Oncol Lett. 2013;5(5):1595–8.
78. Nithyananth M, Priscilla AJ, Boopalan P, Titus V, Lee VN. Time required for effective action of phenol against giant cell tumour cells. J Orthop Surg. 2014;22(1):104–7.
79. Yun Y, Kim N, Han D, Kang E. An investigation of bone necrosis and healing after cryosurgery, phenol cautery or packing with bone cement of defects in the dog femur. Int Orthop. 1993;17:176–83.

80. Khan SN, Cammisa FP Jr, Sandhu HS, Diwan AD, Girardi FP, Lane JM. The biology of bone grafting. J Am Acad Orthop Surg. 2005;13(1):77–86.
81. Ryall C. Cancer infection and cancer recurrence: a danger to avoid in cancer operations. Lancet. 1907;170(4393):1311–6.
82. Mayo WJ. Grafting and traumatic dissemination of carcinoma in the course of operations for malignant disease. JAMA J Am Med Assoc. 1913;60(7):512–3.
83. Saphir O. The transfer of tumor cells by the surgical knife. Surg Gynecol Obstet. 1954;63:775–6.
84. Brandes WW, White W, Sutton J. Accidental transplantation of cancer in the operating room; with a case report. Obstet Gynecol. 1946;82:212–4.
85. Joynt G, Ortved W. The accidental operative transplantation of benign giant cell tumor. Ann Surg. 1948;127(6):1232–9.
86. Cole G Jr, Sindelar WF. Iatrogenic transplantation of osteosarcoma. South Med J. 1995;88(4):485–8.
87. Yip K, Lin J, Kumta S. A pelvic osteosarcoma with metastasis to the donor site of the bone graft: a case report. Int Orthop. 1997;20:389–91.
88. Dias RG, Abudu A, Carter SR, Grimer RJ, Tillman RM. Tumour transfer to bone graft donor site: a case report and review of the literature of the mechanism of seeding. Sarcoma. 2000;4(1–2):57–9.
89. Ferguson PC, Sommerville S, Grimer RJ. Possible metastasis of osteosarcoma to a remote biopsy site: a case report. Clin Orthop Relat Res. 2004;424:216–20.
90. Ofluoglu O, Donthineni R. Case report: iatrogenic seeding of a giant cell tumor of the patella to the proximal tibia. Clin Orthop Relat Res. 2007;465:260–4.
91. Gulia A, Puri A, Salunke A, Desai S, Jambhekar N. Iatrogenic implantation of giant cell tumor at bone graft donor site and clinical recommendations to prevent "a rare avoidable complication". Eur J Orthop Surg Traumatol. 2013;23:715–8.
92. Feith R. Side-effects of acrylic cement implanted into bone: a histological, (micro) angiographic, fluorescence-microscopic and autoradiographic study in the rabbit femur. Acta Orthop Scand. 1975;46(sup161):1–136.
93. Wilkins RM, Okada Y, Sim FH, Chao EYS, Gorgki J. Methylmethacrylate replacement of subchondral bone: a biomechanical and morphologic analysis. In: Enneking WF, editor. Limb-sparing surgery in musculoskeletal oncology. New York: Churchill Livingstone; 1987. p. 179–85.
94. Malawer M, Marks M, McChesney D, Piasio M, Gunther S, Schmookler B. The effect of cryosurgery and polymethylmethacrylate in dogs with experimental bone defects comparable to tumor defects. Clin Orthop Relat Res. 1988;226:299–310.
95. Stürup J, Nimb L, Kramhøft M, Jensen JS. Effects of polymerization heat and monomers from acrylic cement on canine bone. Acta Orthop Scand. 1994;65(1):20–3.
96. Benevenia J, Rivero SM, Moore J, Ippolito JA, Siegerman DA, Beebe KS, et al. Supplemental bone grafting in giant cell tumor of the extremity reduces nononcologic complications. Clin Orthop Relat Res. 2017;475:776–83.
97. Campanacci M. Curettage of giant cell tumor of bone. Reconstruction with subchondral grafts and cement. Chir Organi Mov. 1990;75:212–3.
98. van der Heijden L, van de Sande MA, Heineken AC, Fiocco M, Nelissen RG, Dijkstra PS. Mid-term outcome after curettage with polymethylmethacrylate for giant cell tumor around the knee: higher risk of radiographic osteoarthritis? J Bone Joint Surg. 2013;95(21):e159.
99. Takegami K, Sano T, Wakabayashi H, Sonoda J, Yamazaki T, Morita S, et al. New ferromagnetic bone cement for local hyperthermia. J Biomed Mater Res. 1998;43(2):210–4.
100. Kubota M, Yokoi T, Ogawa T, Saito S, Furuya M, Yokota K, et al. In-vitro heat-generating and apatite-forming abilities of PMMA bone cement containing TiO2 and Fe3O4. Ceram Int. 2021;47(9):12292–9.
101. Miola M, Laviano F, Gerbaldo R, Bruno M, Lombardi A, Cochis A, et al. Composite bone cements for hyperthermia: modeling and characterization of magnetic, calorimetric and in vitro heating properties. Ceram Int. 2017;43(6):4831–40.
102. Ruskin EI, Coomar PP, Sikder P, Bhaduri SB. Magnetic calcium phosphate cement for hyperthermia treatment of bone tumors. Materials. 2020;13(16):3501.
103. Simon M, Aschliman M, Thomas N, Mankin H. Limb-salvage treatment versus amputation for osteosarcoma of the distal end of the femur. J Bone Joint Surg Am. 1986;68(9):1331–7.
104. Rougraff BT, Simon MA, Kneisl JS, Greenberg DB, Mankin HJ. Limb salvage compared with amputation for osteosarcoma of the distal end of the femur. A long-term oncological, functional, and quality-of-life study. J Bone Joint Surg Am. 1994;76(5):649–56.
105. Evans DR, Lazarides AL, Visgauss JD, Somarelli JA, Blazer DG, Brigman BE, et al. Limb salvage versus amputation in patients with osteosarcoma of the extremities: an update in the modern era using the National Cancer Database. BMC Cancer. 2020;20:1–11.
106. Papakonstantinou E, Stamatopoulos A, Athanasiadis DI, Kenanidis E, Potoupnis M, Haidich A-B, et al. Limb-salvage surgery offers better five-year survival rate than amputation in patients with limb osteosarcoma treated with neoadjuvant chemotherapy. A systematic review and meta-analysis. J Bone Oncol. 2020;25:100319.
107. Japanese Orthopaedic Association Musculoskeletal Tumor Committee. Evaluation method of surgical margin for musculoskeletal sarcoma. 1st ed. Tokyo: Kanehara; 1989. p. 3–22.
108. Kawaguchi N, Matumoto S, Manabe J. New method of evaluating the surgical margin and safety margin for musculoskeletal sarcoma, analysed on the basis of 457 surgical cases. J Cancer Res Clin Oncol. 1995;121:555–63.

109. Kawaguchi N, Ahmed AR, Matsumoto S, Manabe J, Matsushita Y. The concept of curative margin in surgery for bone and soft tissue sarcoma. Clin Orthop Relat Res. 2004;419:165–72.
110. Krieg AH, Hefti F. Reconstruction with non-vascularised fibular grafts after resection of bone tumours. J Bone Joint Surg Br. 2007;89(2):215–21.
111. Agarwal A, Kumar A. Fibula regeneration following non-vascularized graft harvest in children. Int Orthop. 2016:1–7.
112. Taylor GI, Miller GD, Ham FJ. The free vascularised bone graft: a clinical extension of microvascular techniques. Plast Reconstr Surg. 1975;55:533–44.
113. Weiland AJ. Vascularized free bone transplants. J Bone Joint Surg Am. 1981;63-A:166–9.
114. Khattak MJ, Umer M, Umar M. Autoclaved tumor bone for reconstruction: an alternative in developing countries. Clin Orthop Relat Res. 2006;447:138–44.
115. Bahk WJ, Kang HG, Park SY, Cho HS, Cho Y, Seo KJ. Histological findings of regeneration in retrieved pasteurized bone grafts. J Orthop Sci. 2019;24(4):737–41.
116. Ehara S, Nishida J, Shiraishi H, Tamakawa Y. Pasteurized intercalary autogenous bone graft: radiographic and scintigraphic features. Skeletal Radiol. 2000;29:335–9.
117. Manabe J, Ahmed AR, Kawaguchi N, Matsumoto S, Kuroda H. Pasteurized autologous bone graft in surgery for bone and soft tissue sarcoma. Clin Orthop Relat Res. 2004;419:258–66.
118. Lietman SA, Tomford WW, Gebhardt MC, Springfield DS, Mankin HJ. Complications of irradiated allografts in orthopaedic tumor surgery. Clin Orthop Relat Res. 2000;375:214–7.
119. Chen Z, Chen Z, Zhang G. Fibula grafting for treatment of aggressive benign bone tumor and malignant bone tumor of extremities. Chin Med J. 1997;110(02):125–8.
120. Tsuchiya H, Wan S, Sakayama K, Yamamoto N, Nishida H, Tomita K. Reconstruction using an autograft containing tumour treated by liquid nitrogen. J Bone Joint Surg Br. 2005;87(2):218–25.
121. Yamamoto N, Tsuchiya H, Tomita K. Effects of liquid nitrogen treatment on the proliferation of osteosarcoma and the biomechanical properties of normal bone. J Orthop Sci. 2003;8:374–80.
122. Yasin NF, Ajit Singh V, Saad M, Omar E. Which is the best method of sterilization for recycled bone autograft in limb salvage surgery: a radiological, biomechanical and histopathological study in rabbit. BMC Cancer. 2015;15(1):1–11.
123. Singh VA, Nagalingam J, Saad M, Pailoor J. Which is the best method of sterilization of tumour bone for reimplantation? A biomechanical and histopathological study. Biomed Eng Online. 2010;9(1):1–15.
124. Canadell J, San-Julian M, Cara J, Forriol F. External fixation in tumour pathology. Int Orthop. 1998;22:126–30.
125. Erler K, Yildiz C, Baykal B, Atesalp AS, Ozdemir MT, Basbozkurt M. Reconstruction of defects following bone tumor resections by distraction osteogenesis. Arch Orthop Trauma Surg. 2005;125:177–83.
126. Kapukaya A, Suba¸ si M, Kandiya E, Özate¸ s M, Yilmaz F. Limb reconstruction with the callus distraction method after bone tumor resection. Arch Orthop Trauma Surg. 2000;120:215–8.
127. Millett P, Lane J, Paletta G Jr. Limb salvage using distraction osteogenesis. Am J Orthop. 2000;29(8):628–32.
128. Green SA. Complications of pin and wire external fixation. Instr Course Lect. 1990;39:219–28.
129. Ilizarov GA. Clinical application of the tension-stress effect for limb lengthening. Clin Orthop Relat Res. 1990;250:8–26.
130. Mankin HJ, Gebhardt MC, Jennings LC, Springfield DS, Tomford WW. Long-term results of allograft replacement in the management of bone tumors. Clin Orthop Relat Res. 1996;324:86–97.
131. Ortiz-Cruz E, Gebhardt MC, Jennings LC, Springfield DS, Mankin HJ. The results of transplantation of intercalary allografts after resection of tumors. A long-term follow-up study. J Bone Joint Surg. 1997;79(1):97–106.
132. Harris IE, Leff A, Gitelis S, Simon M. Function after amputation, arthrodesis, or arthroplasty for tumors about the knee. J Bone Joint Surg. 1990;72(10):1477–85.
133. Eckardt JJ, Kabo JM, Kelley CM, Ward WG Sr, Asavamongkolkul A, Wirganowicz PZ, et al. Expandable endoprosthesis reconstruction in skeletally immature patients with tumors. Clin Orthop Relat Res. 2000;373:51–61.
134. Ruggieri P, Mavrogenis AF, Pala E, Romantini M, Manfrini M, Mercuri M. Outcome of expandable prostheses in children. J Pediatr Orthop. 2013;33(3):244–53.
135. Staals EL, Colangeli M, Ali N, Casanova JM, Donati DM, Manfrini M. Are complications associated with the Repiphysis® expandable distal femoral prosthesis acceptable for its continued use? Clin Orthop Relat Res. 2015;473:3003–13.
136. DiCaprio MR, Friedlaender GE. Malignant bone tumors: limb sparing versus amputation. J Am Acad Orthop Surg. 2003;11(1):25–37.
137. Portney DA, Bi AS, Christian RA, Butler BA, Peabody TD. Outcomes of expandable prostheses for primary bone malignancies in skeletally immature patients: a systematic review and pooled data analysis. J Pediatr Orthop. 2020;40(6):e487–e97.
138. Saghieh S, Abboud MR, Muwakkit SA, Saab R, Rao B, Haidar R. Seven-year experience of using Repiphysis® expandable prosthesis in children with bone tumors. Pediatr Blood Cancer. 2010;55(3):457–63.

Part II

Bone-Forming (Osteoblastic) Tumors and Lesions

Fracture Callus

2

Most pathologic fractures associated with bone tumors present with a clear history of minor or trivial trauma and a previous clinical history of underlying lesions. However, diagnostic problems would be met in the bone tumor with a fracture through a previously unknown bony lesion which is not easily detectible due to concealed lesion by the spiral or oblique fracture on radiograph, and in unrecognized stress or fatigue fracture without a history of memorable trauma. A complete comprehensive understanding of remarkable microscopic sequences of fracture repair is essential for a correct diagnosis of bone tumors with unrecognized concealed fractures because the histologic findings include exclusive growth of primitive mesenchymal cells in the beginning and primitive chondro-osteoid matrix without osteoblastic rimming in the next phase, both of which can be easily misinterpreted as sarcoma. However, the absolute criterion for malignancy including mitotic figures and frank pleomorphism are never seen in fracture callus. Several histologic features useful for differentiation of fracture callus from osteosarcoma (OSA) have been described. Fracture callus exhibits a typical zonal architecture with areas of immature cartilage merging with woven bone and myofibroblasts, whereas OSA tends to be more diffuse. Maturing woven bone in fractures forms trabeculae with prominent rimming, which connect together and produce variable-sized circles. In contrast, OSA produces a more lace-like pattern of woven bone embedding individual tumor cells and lacks well-formed trabeculae. Lastly, the space between woven bone trabeculae consists of a mixture of vascular and reactive fibroblastic cells in maturing fracture, whereas there is largely a matrix in the stroma of OSA [1]. The repair process after general fracture goes through four stages including formation of hematoma at the fracture ends, formation of a fibrocartilaginous callus, formation of a bony callus, and remodeling with addition of compact bone, which make histologic features vary greatly with time. The chronologic stages can be considerably overlapped [2]. *(A) Hematoma formation* (days 1 to 5): The hematoma immediately following the fracture releases pro-inflammatory cytokines such as tumor necrosis factor-alpha (TNF-α), bone morphogenetic proteins (BMPs), interleukins, and platelet-derived growth factors (PDGF), which recruit macrophages, monocytes, and lymphocytes to remove damaged, necrotic tissue. *(B) Fibrocartilaginous callus formation* (days 5 to 11): The VEGF initiates angiogenesis and recruits local fibroblasts and capillaries to form granulation tissue or pro-callus. The cytokines also recruit further primitive mesenchymal cells and differentiate pluripotential cells into immature fibroblasts, osteoblasts, and chondroblasts which lay down collagen-rich fibrocartilaginous and osteoid matrices mimicking fibrosarcoma, chondrosarcoma, or OSA. *(C) Bony callus formation* (days 11 to 28): The cartilaginous callus begins

W.-J. Bahk, *Diagnosis and Management of Primary Bone Tumors*,
https://doi.org/10.1007/978-981-96-3484-2_2

to undergo enchondral ossification. The cartilaginous callus is resorbed and begins to calcify by further differentiation of chondroblasts, chondroclasts, as well as osteoblasts and osteoclasts with RANK-L expression. A hard, calcified callus of immature bone forms at the end of the stage. *(D) Bone remodeling* (day 28 onwards, lasting months to years): The "coupled remodeling" results from a balance of resorption by osteoclasts and new bone formation by osteoblasts. The process of bone remodeling usually lasts for many months to years, ultimately resulting in the regeneration of the normal bone structure with reconstituted marrow [2–6]. Mirra dated more precisely the callus tissues of each phase based on pathologic specimens in which a specific fracture event occurred days to weeks before evaluation [7]. He described the microscopic findings of the healing process timed on a week-to-week basis during the first 2 months. The process begins with a primitive explosive growth of mesenchymal cells which can be easily confused with a sarcoma and finishes with completely normal lamellar bone and reconstituted marrow. The timing of the biopsy is very important because the histologic features of callus are quite different depending on the event stages after fracture. Particularly during the early phase, the callus tissue exhibits granulation tissue with reactive myofibroblastic cells, extensive local hemorrhage, or variable necrosis and primitive osteoid often with chondroid, which may distinguish an incipient stress or fatigue fracture from an OSA difficulty. However, the callus tissue matures significantly during the next 3 weeks after injury and does not simulate a sarcoma anymore. The callus may present with mixed areas of older and younger histologic features, possibly from unperceived repeated minor injuries. The normal histologic phases of fracture healing are summarized in Table 2.1 and presented in Fig. 2.1 based on Mirra's description with addition of exact dates after fracture from my experience. *(1) Within first week*: Immediately after injury (*less than 3 days*), extensive local hemorrhage, fibrin exudate, and varying degrees of necrosis occur in association with neutrophils and lymphocytes at 24 hours, and macrophages at 48–72 hours to remove damaged, necrotic tissue. *From 3 to 5 days*, granulation tissue is formed with explosive proliferation of mesenchymal cells embedded in a loose myxomatous and fibrinoid matrix. The cells are stellate or spindle-shaped which migrate and anchor to fibrin strands. The overall shape resembles a "tissue culture-like" appearance. The individual cells are plump with pleomorphic nuclei in size and shape, which may simulate an undifferentiated sarcoma (Fig. 2.1a). By the end of the week *(6–7 days)*, the mesenchymal cells are more spindled and higher in number, which are tightly packed together forming a mass of poorly differentiated cells and infiltrate surrounding muscle fibers. In addition, other ominous cytologic features of high nuclear to cytoplasmic ratio, larger nucleoli, and high number of mitoses can more easily make a misdiagnosis of high-grade sarcoma (Fig. 2.1b, c). *(2) 1–2 weeks*: Sometime between 7 and 10 days, early fine wisps of primitive osteoid surrounded by ominous stromal cells often with chondroid can be seen. The cells can

Table 2.1 The phases of callus formation

< 3 days	Hemorrhage and edema, fibrin exudate, inflammatory cell infiltration, varying degrees of necrosis
3–6 days	Granulation tissue in tissue culture-like appearance, explosive growth of mesenchymal cells, quite ominous by the end of the week
7–10 days	Early fine wisps of primitive osteoid often with chondroid or cartilage, increasing cellularity of ominous cells
10–14 days	Primitive woven bone occasionally with masses of primitive chondroid to cartilage
2–3 weeks	Broad seams of woven with beginning of osteoblast rimming, beginning of trabeculae to connect together with less cellular marrow
3–4 weeks	"Roman aqueduct" sign, exquisite osteoblastic rimming with prominent intertrabecular injury vessels
5–7 weeks	Lamellar bone production, beginning of marrow fat formation
> 8 weeks	Well-developed lamellar bone with marrow fat, near normal marrow

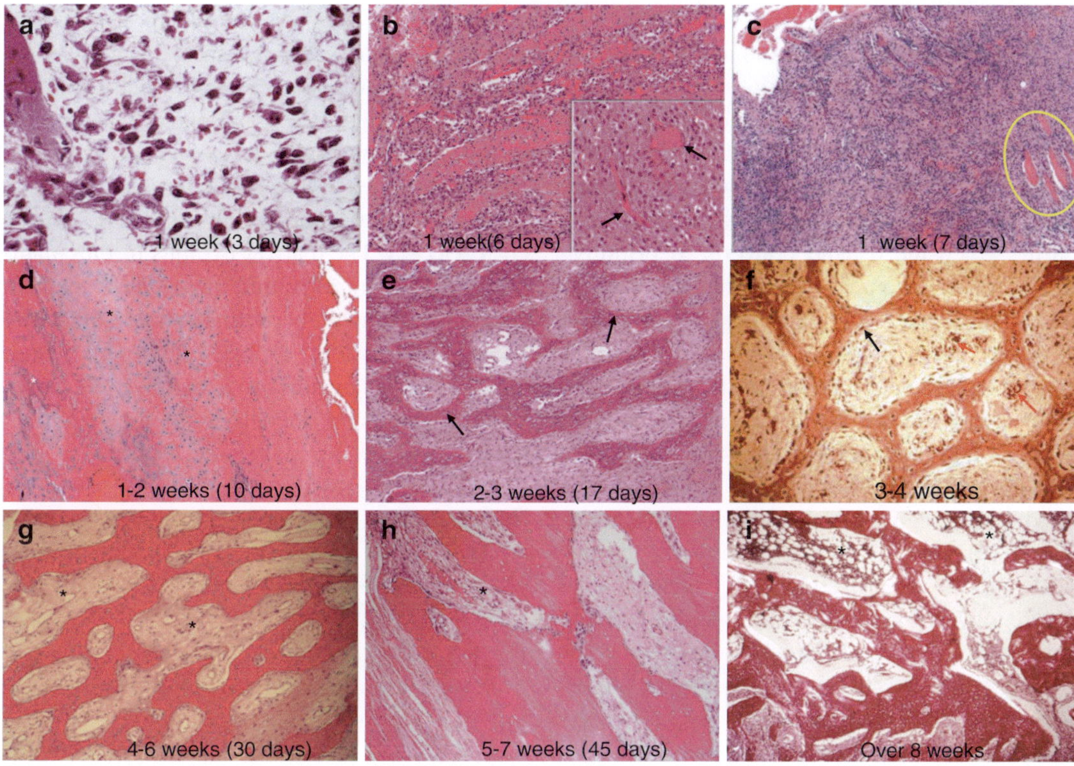

Fig. 2.1 Microscopic findings in exact age of the callus. (**a**) Granulation tissue with reactive myofibroblastic cells forms an overall shape of "tissue culture-like" appearance with cells embedded in a loose myxo-fibromatous matrix at 3 days after fracture. The cells are stellate or spindle-shaped, which migrate and anchor to fibrin strands. The individual cells are plump with pleomorphic nuclei in size and shape simulating an undifferentiated sarcoma. Edge of the lesion is diffusely infiltrative and even traps surrouding muscle fibers (yellow asterisk). (**b**) By the end of the first week, the mesenchyme cells grow explosively. The cellularity is strikingly increased, and most cells become spindle-shaped and tightly packed together forming a mass of poorly differentiated cells. There are a few wisps of primitive osteoid (inset). The individual cells appear ominous with high nuclear-to-cytoplasmic ratio, larger nucleoli, and high number of mitoses on higher-power magnification. (**c**) Several fine wisps of primitive osteoid surrounded by ominous stromal cells without osteoblastic rimming (circle) are seen as early as 7 days. With the mass of poorly differentiated cells and infiltration of surrounding muscle fibers, the fracture would be mistakenly diagnosed as OSA. However, the cells are monotonous from cell to cell, so-called *regularly ominous*, in contrast to "irregularly ominous" in OSA. (**d**) On 10 days' specimen, masses of primitive cartilage are emanated from a spindle cell stroma (black asterisks) mimicking a chondrosarcoma. The osteoid is beginning to convert to woven bone with calcium deposition (white asterisk). (**e**) On 17 days' specimen, woven bone trabeculae with osteoblast rimming and less cellular marrow are connecting together and begin to form variable-sized circles (arrows). The callus is no more mimicking sarcoma after this age. (**f**) During 3–4 weeks, most osteoid is converted trabeculae of mature woven bone with an exquisite *osteoblastic rimming* (black arrow). The bony trabeculae join each other forming variable-sized circles designated as the *Roman aqueduct* sign. Note prominent thin-walled, dilated capillaries, so-called injury vessels (red arrows), representing a maturate granulation tissue following the injury. (**g**) On 30 days' specimen, the intertrabecular tissues become less cellular with a few short spindle cells and prominent capillaries. The stroma exhibits a loose pre-marrow fat appearance. (**h**) On 45 days' specimen, the osteoblasts produce lamellar bone rather than woven bone producing a peripheral network of lamellar bone laid down over the primitive woven bone spicules, a pattern never seen in OSA. The stroma becomes bubbly to vacuolated and begins to produce primitive fat marrow (black sterisk). (**i**) After 8 weeks, the marrow exhibits further maturation with abundant fat cells and hematopoietic cells appearing completely normal (black asterisks)

be plump and chromatin rich, but nuclear and cytoplasmic features are monotonous from cell to cell, which seem to be, exhibitinh a "regularly ominous" appearance. Initially, the osteoid shows no osteoblastic no osteoblastic rimming, a pattern that observed in OSA. However, calcium deposition of the osteoid begins within 1–3 days, during which the osteoid converts to primitive woven bone. Some fields reveal masses of primitive chondroid to cartilage simulating chondrosarcoma (Fig. 2.1d). *(3) 2–3 weeks*: A single row of the plump osteoblasts begins to rim along the periphery of maturing woven bone spicules. Woven bone trabeculae with osteoblast rimming and less cellular marrow are connecting together and begin to form variable-sized circles (Fig. 2.1e). *(4) 3–4 weeks*: During this phase, most osteoid is converted into trabeculae of mature woven bone with a prominent osteoblastic rimming. The bony trabeculae join one another forming complete circles of variable size, referreed to as the "Roman aqueduct" sign. The sign may also be observed in osteoid osteoma, osteoblastoma, or injury-related lesions such as myositis ossificans. There are prominent thin-walled, dilated, capillaries, so-called *injury vessels* representing a maturate granulation tissue following the injury (Fig. 2.1f). After 2 weeks, the pathlogic findings are no more mimciking sracomas. *(5) 4–6 weeks*: The intertrabecular tissues become hypocellular with a few spindle cells, prominent capillaries, and loose pre-marrow fat appearance (Fig. 2.1g). *(6) 6–7 weeks*: The histologic features may overlap with those of 4–6 weeks after fracture. The osteoblasts produce lamellar bone rather than woven bone leading to a peripheral network of lamellar bone laid down over the primitive woven bone spicules, which pattern is an important sign of benign bone production and is never seen in OSA. The stroma becomes bubbly to vacuolated and begins to produce primitive fat marrow early in the sixth week (Fig. 2.1h). *(7) Over 8 weeks*: The marrow exhibits further maturation with fat cells and hematopoietic cells appearing completely normal. Over time, the bone is progressively replaced with pure mature lamellar bone spicules by a harmony of osteoblastic activity and osteoclastic remodeling.

References

1. Hoch B, Montag A. Reactive bone lesions mimicking neoplasms. Semin Diagn Pathol. 2011;28(1):102–12. https://doi.org/10.1053/j.semdp.2011.02.011.
2. Sheen JR, Garla VV. Fracture Healing Overview. In: StatPearls [Internet]. Treasure Island: StatPearls Publishing; 2023.
3. Frost H. The biology of fracture healing: an overview for clinicians. Part II. Clin Orthop Relat Res. 1989;248:294–309.
4. Ghiasi MS, Chen J, Vaziri A, Rodriguez EK, Nazarian A. Bone fracture healing in mechanobiological modeling: A review of principles and methods. Bone Rep. 2017;6:87–100.
5. Kostenuik P, Mirza FM. Fracture healing physiology and the quest for therapies for delayed healing and nonunion. J Orthop Res. 2017;35(2):213–23.
6. Marsell R, Einhorn TA. The biology of fracture healing. Injury. 2011;42(6):551–5.
7. Mirra JM. Callus and stress fracture. In: Mirra JM, editor. Bone tumors: Clinical, radiologic, and pathologic correlations. 2nd ed. Philadelphia: Lea & Febiger; 1989. p. 155–74.

3 Osteoma

(***osteo*** "bone" + ***ōma*** "forming")

3.1 Definition

Osteoma is a rare benign lesion mainly composed of dense and mature lamellar bone. It can arise either on the surface of the bone (parosteal or surface osteoma) or within the cancellous bone (medullary osteoma or enostosis). It is referred to as a "homoplastic osteoma" when occurs in bone, and it is referred to as a "heteroplastic osteoma" when arises in soft tissue. In 1951, Geschickter and Copeland [1] first described *parosteal osteoma* of bone as a new entity occurring in both benign and malignant forms in their collection of 16 patients with the lesion affecting long bones.

3.2 Incidence

Primary extracranial osteomas of long and flat bones are extremely unusual, occupying less than 0.03% of biopsied primary bone tumors [2].

3.3 Age

It occurs most frequently in adults, between the ages of 20 and 40 years [1].

3.4 Location

Parosteal osteoma most frequently affects bone formed by membranous ossification, such as calvaria, facial, and jaw bones. Rest of the parosteal osteoma can be found in the diaphysis or metaphysis of long bones [1, 3] or clavicle [4–6].

3.5 Clinical Features

Small lesions are usually slowly growing and asymptomatic and found incidentally, but larger lesions can lead to variable clinical presentations depending on their affected locations and subtypes, including: (1) calvarial and mandibular ivory exostoses, (2) osteomas of the paranasal sinuses, facial bones, and orbit (sino-orbital osteomas), (3) enostoses or bone islands, and (4) surface (juxtacortical) osteomas of long bones [7]. A mass or swelling and/or local pain for a long duration extending over months or years is the most common presentation. The other symptoms include limitation of joint motion, headache, paranasal sinuses (sinusitis, nasal discharge, mucocele), exophthalmos, double vision or loss of vision, or palpable hard mass. Bone islands are totally asymptomatic, although the size is giant

W.-J. Bahk, *Diagnosis and Management of Primary Bone Tumors*,
https://doi.org/10.1007/978-981-96-3484-2_3

enough. Osteoma is usually a solitary lesion, but multiple lesions may occur almost always in patients with Gardner syndrome with intestinal polyps, fibromatous and other lesions of connective tissue, and multiple sebaceous cysts.

3.6 Radiologic Findings

Plain radiograph Surface osteoma in the clavicle, pelvic, or long bones of the extremities is the rarest form which resembles ivory exostosis (surface osteoma) of the craniofacial bones [7] (Fig. 3.1a). Surface osteoma of long bone is usually seen as a well-circumscribed, mushroom-shaped, uniformly osteoblastic to dense ivory mass lesion attached to the underlying bone with broad base but no continuity between the mass and the host medullary cavity. In the early phase, the lesion is visible as a dense, irregular, or rounded mass which seems to be separated from the underlying skeletal structures (Fig. 3.1b). The underlying bone forms an irregular platform for further growth through the widening of the cortex with some periosteal reaction. In the late phase, the densely ossifying mass tends to circumscribe the underlying bone (Fig. 3.1c). Surprisingly, there is little destruction or reactive change in the adjacent bone in consideration of the density of the mass and its size [1]. **Bone scan** may reveal mildly increased or no uptake. **CT scan** shows

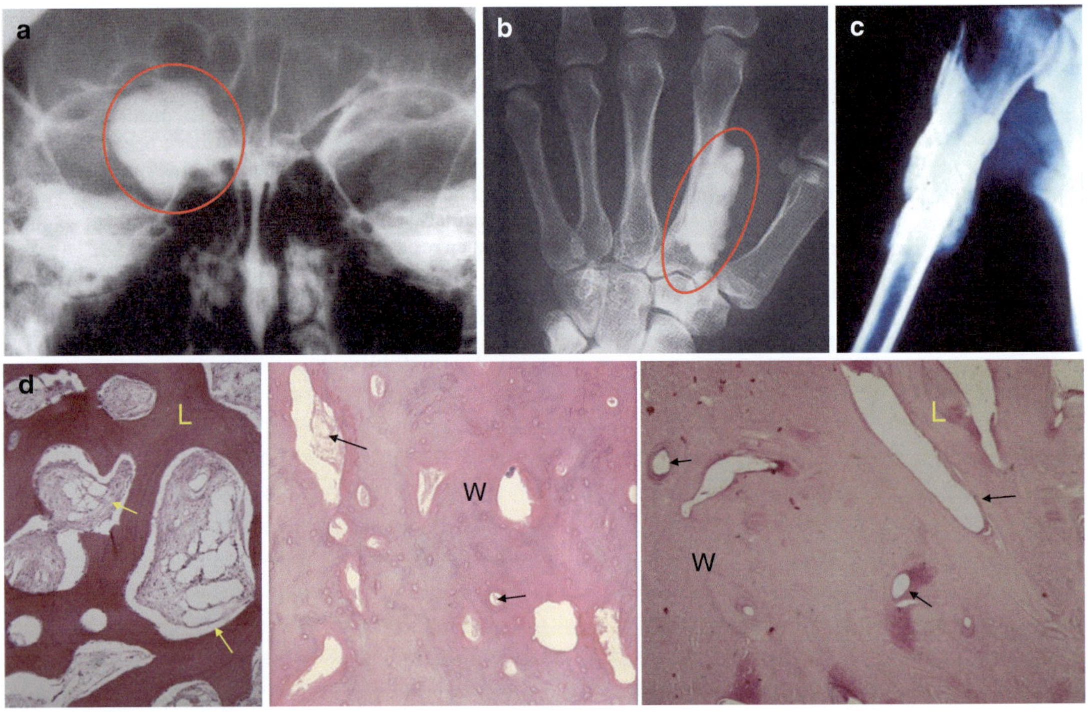

Fig. 3.1 (**a**) Radiograph of the skull shows a well-circumscribed, round to oval, uniformly dense lesion involving orbital floor (circle). (**b**) Radiograph reveals a well-defined heavily ossified mass that parallels the long axis of the fourth metacarpal bone and is broadly attached to the underlying cortex (circle). (**c**) Another radiograph notes an irregular, ivory-like, longitudinal mass paralleling the humerus axis attached to the underlying bone with a broad base. (**d**) Microscopic examination. (Left) The lesion predominantly consists of lamellar bones (L) with marrow spaces showing moderate cellularity, vessels, fibrous stroma, and fat cells (yellow arrows) indicating compact osteoma. (Middle) Another lesion reveals predominantly woven bones (W) with Harversian canal-like structure varying in size and shape (black arrows) indicating spongy osteoma. (Right) Note admixture of lamellar bones (L) and woven bones (W) with various haversian canal-like structures (arows), suggesting mixed subtype

a well-circumscribed, broad-based, homogeneously dense mass with cortical density on the surface of the bone. The cortical outgrowth is contiguous with intact and often thickened underlying bone. There is no visible separating membrane or cleavage plane. Infiltration into the surrounding soft tissue is not observed, and the adjacent bone marrow shows normal attenuation [3]. **MR finding** MR images duplicate the CT findings, with homogeneous appearance of the cortical outgrowth, normal surrounding soft tissue, and no abnormal signal intensity within the adjacent marrow [3]. The outer surface of the mass is covered by a thin fibrous tissue, but cartilage cap is not seen. The signal intensity is low on both T1- and T2-weighted images, and the lesion is not enhanced by contrast media.

3.7 Histologic Findings

Microscopically, osteoma is predominantly composed of mature lamellar or cortical bone with three histological subtypes, including: (1) very dense compact bone and paucicelullar fibrous stroma with or without Haversian system (compact osteoma), (2) ordinary trabecular bone with marrow component (spongy osteoma), or (3) mixed subtype with compact and spongy bones (Fig. 3.1d). The outer surface is surrounded by a thin layer of fibrous tissue without a cartilage cap. The bone itself is usually matured lamellar but can be woven to lamellar with recognizable haversian canals, which are typically not present in parosteal osteosarcoma. In addition, the fibroblastic stroma with spindle cells that is typical of parosteal osteosarcoma is not seen in osteoma [7]. However, Geschickter and Copeland [1] described that the tumor growth is more likely to show increased cellularity and, occasionally, the foci of fibro-spindle cell sarcoma at the periphery although mature bone and fibrous tissue predominate. Such foci may be readily chiseled away from the underlying bone by the surgeon and fail to show histologically malignant features on adequate examination.

3.8 Management

Asymptomatic lesion can be observed without any management. Excision is necessary for symptomatic lesion with mass effect (functional or cosmetic impairment). High incidence of recurrence was reported in half of the cases [1]. If there is histologic evidence of histologic evidence of spindle cell sarcoma at the periphery of the mass at the initial surgery or in the recurrent mass, more extensive revision surgery such as wide resection with or without reconstruction or amputation is necessary.

3.9 Clinical Course

Geschickter and Copeland [1] reported the lesions may have a malignant potential. The excised mass can recur and eventually tends to surround and invade the bone in frankly sarcomatous fashion. The lesion recurred in 7 of 13 (54%) patients who underwent a local excision. Four of these patients died of pulmonary metastases, with two occurring more than 5 years after the primary excision in their series. Thus, a close long-term follow-up examination or postoperative radiation to arrest residual growth is necessary after excision.

References

1. Geschickter CF, Copeland MM. Parosteal osteoma of bone: a new entity. Ann Surg. 1951;133(6):790.
2. Mirra JM. Osteoma. In: Mirra JM, editor. Bone tumors: clinical, radiologic, and pathologic correlation. 2nd ed. Philadelphia: Lea & Febiger; 1989. p. 174–82.
3. Lambiase R, Levine S, Terek R, Wyman J. Long bone surface osteomas: imaging features that may help avoid unnecessary biopsies. Am J Roentgenol. 1998;171(3):775–8.
4. Schajowicz F. Bone-forming tumors. In: Schajowicz F, editor. Tumors and tumorlike lesions of bone and joints. pathology, radiology, and treatment. 2nd ed. Berlin Heidelberg: Springer-Verlag; 1994. p. 29–140.
5. Yamamoto Y, Nishiyama Y. SPECT/CT imaging in bone scintigraphy of a case of clavicular osteoma. Asia Ocean J Nucl Med Biol. 2014;2(1):73–4.
6. Inokuchi T, Hitora T, Yamagami Y, Nishimura H, Yamamoto T. Parosteal osteoma of the clavicle. Case Rep Orthop. 2014;2014
7. Czerniak B. Sclerosing bone lesions. In: Dorfman HD, Czerniak B, editors. Dorfman and Czerniak's bone tumors (eBook). 2nd ed. Elsevier; 2016. p. 1317–45.

4 Enostosis (Bone Island) – Osteopoikilosis

(***En*** "in" + ***osteo*** "bone" + ***-sis*** "morbid process") – (***osteo*** "bone" + ***poikil(o)*** "spotted" + ***-sis*** "morbid process")

4.1 Definition

Enostosis is a commonly found focus of varible-sized, dense, mature compact (cortical) bone within the medullary cancellous bone (spongiosa), which is considered to be a misplaced hamartomatous cortical bone in the in the medulla. Osteoma is also composed of dense, compact cortical bone, but arises on the surface of bone instead of the mudullary cavity. *Osteopoikilosis* is a benign, autosomal dominant sclerosing dysplasia of bone typified by the presence of multiple bony lesions which are indistinguishable from a solitary enostosis.

4.2 Synonym

Bone island or meduallry osteoma for enostosis; spotted bone disease for osteopoikilosis.

4.3 Incidence

It is common but the exact incidence is not known because a vast majority of cases are asymptomatic and incidentally found. However, osteopoikilosis is only very rarely described in the literature.

4.4 Age

Enostosis is usually found in adults but occurs only rarely in children. However, osteopoikilosis may develop during childhood and persist throughout life, and therefore may be found in all age groups.

4.5 Location

It occurs anywhere in the skeleton, although there is predilection for the pelvis, long bones, spine, and ribs (Figs. 4.1, 4.2, and 4.3). The symmetric, peri-articular distribution and predominant meta-epiphyseal location of long tubular bones (hip, knee, and ankle) (Figs. 4.4 and 4.5) and carpal or tarsal bones are common locations for osteopoikilosis.

W.-J. Bahk, *Diagnosis and Management of Primary Bone Tumors*,
https://doi.org/10.1007/978-981-96-3484-2_4

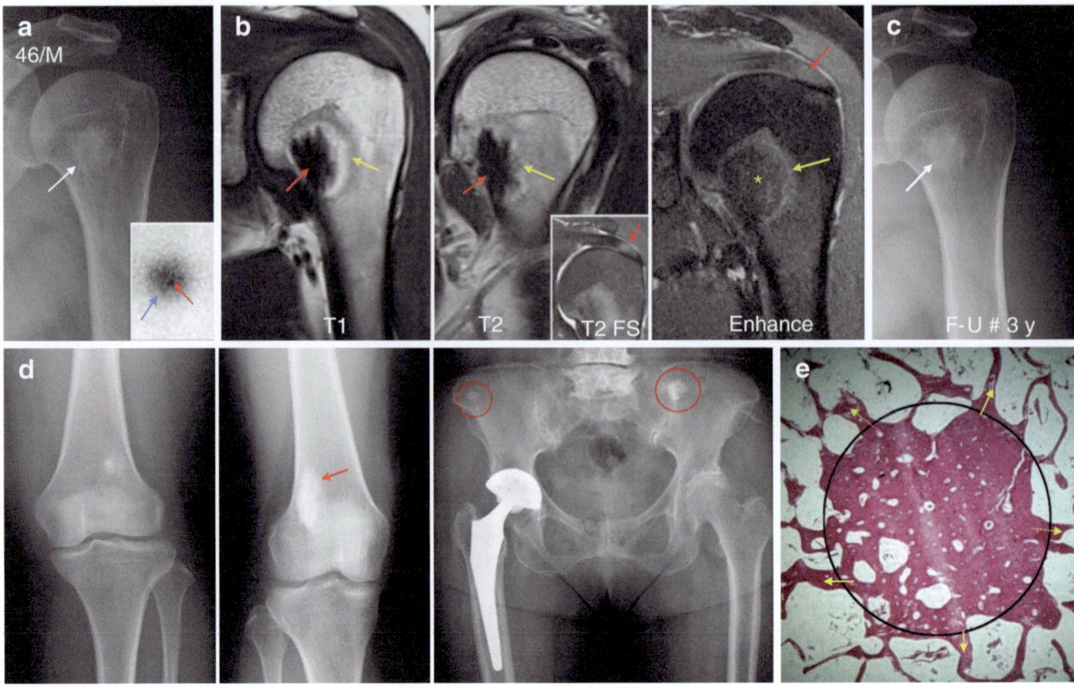

Fig. 4.1 (**a**) Radiograph taken for left shoulder pain in a 46-year-old woman man shows a round to oval densely radiopaque lesion merging into the host bone and exhibiting a spiculated margin, so-called *brush-like* or *thorn-like* border (white arrow). Pinhole bone scan (inset) reveals a focal central hot uptake (red arrow) with a peripheral weak uptake (blue arrow) suggesting a spiculated margin or reactive area (inset). (**b**) MR images demonstrate a medullary lesion having a *brush-like* or *thorn-like* margin with dark SI on both T1- and T2-weighted images (red arrows) and surrounding intermediate to high SI suggesting peri-tumoral reactive change (yellow arrows). The lesion itself presents focally dotted enhancement (asterisk) with a peripheral thin enhancement of the surrounding reactive lesion (arrow). There is an intermediate SI at supraspinatus tendon insertion on fat-saturated T2-weighted image (inset), which is focally enhanced (red arrow), indicating a partial tear or tendinopathy and likely accounting for the shoulder pain. (**c**) Follow-up radiograph at 3 years after biopsy notes no interval change of the lesion. (**d**) You can see incidentally found bone islands of variable size and locations. (**e**) Histologically, enostosis is composed of a main cortical bone spicule (black circle) with varibely sized and shaped Harversian canal-like structures within a normal host medullary cavity that is merged into the adjacent host cancellous bone (yellow arrows). These histologic findings correspond to a small dense leson within the meduallry cavity, showing characteristic (red arrow) on radiograph and MRI

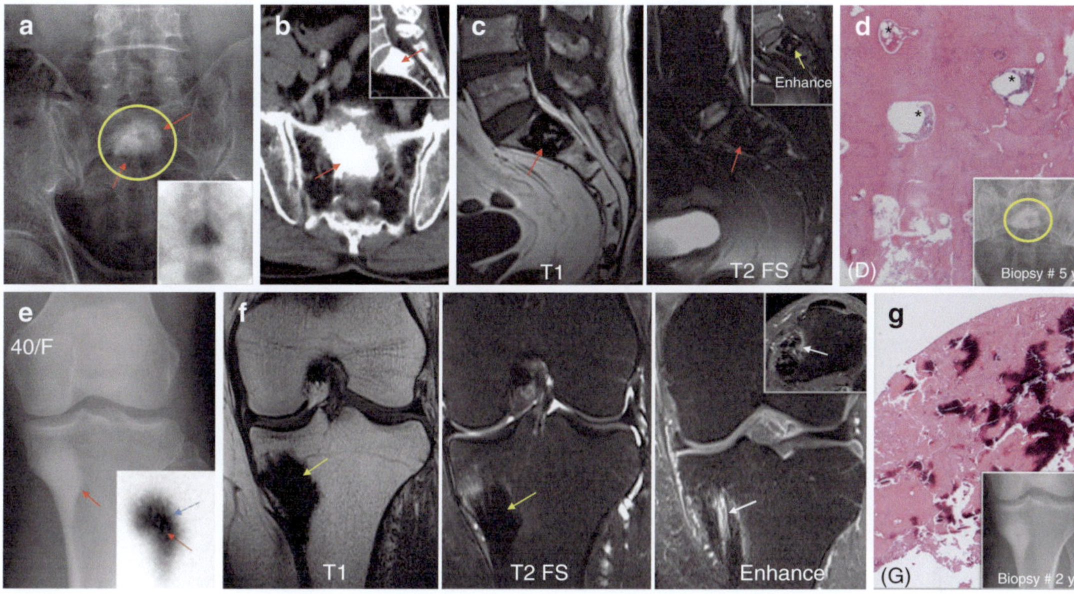

Fig. 4.2 Giant bone island. (**a**) Radiograph taken for low back pain of 1 month's duration in a 68-year-old man incidentally shows a large, homogeneously dense, round to oval lesion (yellow circle) with a spiculated margin merging into the host bone, so-called *brush-like* or *thorn-like* boder in the upper sacrum (red arrows). The densely calcified intraosseous lesion shows heterogeneously increased uptake localized in the upper sacrum on bone scan (inset). (**b**) CT scan reveals a uniformly dense lesion with irregularly spiculated border (arrows) within the medullary cavity of S1 segment of the sacrum. (**c**) MR images demonstrate a well-defined intramedullary lesion with mainly low SI and focal high signal on both T1- and T2-weighted images. The lesion is only focally enhanced (inset). (**d**) Microscopic examination notes predominantly thickened lamellar bone containing loose fibrous and fat tissues in the Harversian-like canals and intratrabecular spaces (black asterisks), indicating remodeling. Follow-up radiograph at 5 years after biopsy without surgical removal shows no interval change of the lesion (inset). (**e**) Radiograph taken for right knee pain by blunt trauma in a 40-year-old woman incidentally shows a homogeneously dense, oblong lesion having a spiculated margin (red arrows). The long axis is parallel to the direction of mechanical stresses on bone, representing adaptation to Wolff's law. There is no visible periosteal reaction. Pinhole scan reveals a localized central hot uptake (red arrow) with peripheral weak uptake (blue arrow) indicating a spiculated margin merging into the host bone in the medial proximal metaphysis of the left tibia (inset). (**f**) MR images demonstrate an irregularly shaped heavily calcified lesion with dark SI on T1- and T2-weighted fat saturation images (arrows). The cortex appears intact intact with no periosteal reaction. The lesion is heterogeneously well enhanced (white arrow). (**g**) Microscopic examination shows cortical-type bone containing Haversian-like canals with some woven bones and heavy calcification, heavy calcification, consistent with a final diagnosis of giant bone island. Follow-up radiograph at 2 years after biopsy without other treatment shows no interval change of the lesion, with a hazy biopsy hole (inset)

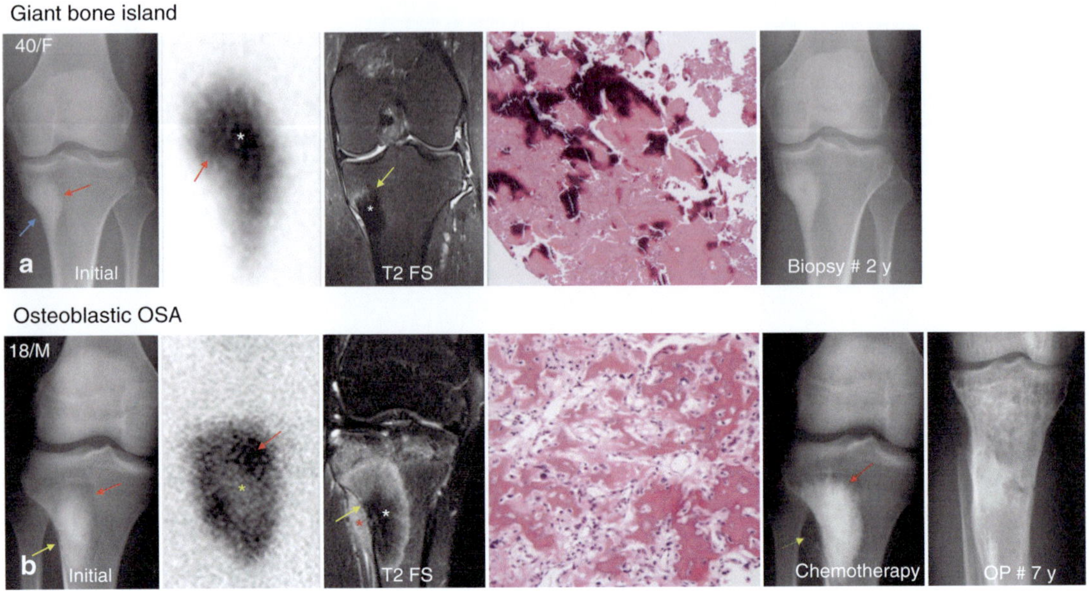

Fig. 4.3 Comparison of giant bone island and sclerotic OSA. (**a**) *Giant bone island* (same case in Fig. 4.2e): Radiograph taken for right knee pain by blunt trauma in a 40-year-old woman incidentally shows a homogeneously dense, oblong lesion having a spiculated margin (red arrow). The cortex is intact with no periosteal reaction (blue arrow). Pinhole bone scan reveals a localized central hot (white asterisk) with peripheral weak uptake (red arrow). MR image reveals a heavily calcified lesion with intact cortex and no periosteal reaction (yellow arrow), which is only partially enhanced by contrast medium (yellow arrow in inset of Fig. 4.2C). Microscopic examination reveals heavily calcified lamellar bone spicules containing varibly sized Haversian-like canals. Follow-up radiograph at 2 years after biopsy shows no interval change of the lesion. (**b**) *Sclerotic OSA*: Another radiograph taken for left knee pain in a 18-year-old adolescent shows a similar dense lesion with a spiculated margin as (**a**). However, there are surrounding radiolucent zone (red arrow) and cortical destruction with a subtle soft tissue mass, and a hazy periosteal reaction (yellow arrow). Pinhole bone scan reveals strongly increased uptake (red arrow) with internal photon defect, suggesting possible necrosis (yellow asterisk). Fat-saturated T2-weighted image demonstrates an intramedullary lesion with intermediate to high SI with a central dark signal of heavy calcification (white asterisk). Note cortical destruction (arrow) and soft tissue mass formation (red asteriks), idicating a locally aggressive to malignant tumor. Pathologic examination notes pleomorphic tumor cells being deeply embedded in abundant osteoid/woven bone, indicating sclerosing OSA. Follow-up radiograph after neoadjuvant chemotherapy demonstrates more prominently radiating bony streaks (red arrows) and more certain periosteal reaction with reactive bone formation (yellow arrow). Follow-up radiograph at 7 years after wide resection and reconstruction with allograft reveals the union of the grafted bone without a local recurrence

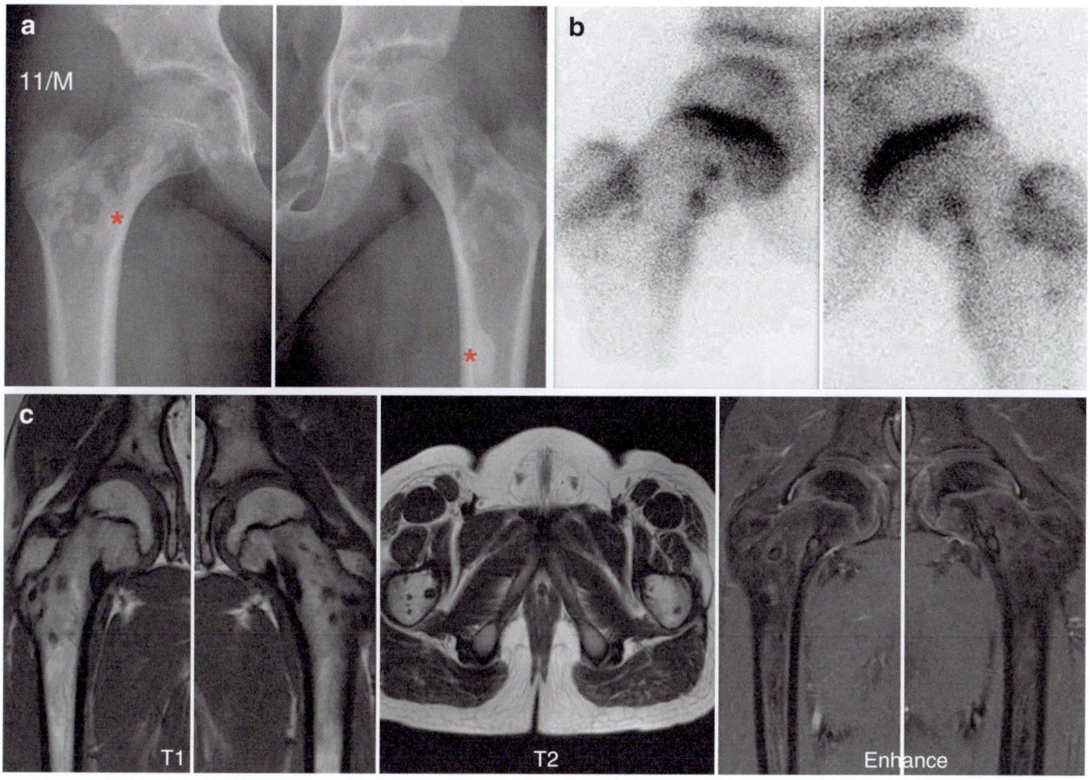

Fig. 4.4 Osteopoikilosis. (**a**) Radiograph taken for right hip pain after slip in an 11-year-old boy shows multiple round to oval dense, varying size of sclerotic nodules, which are symmetrically located in the neck and trochanteric area of the both femurs as well as acetabular areas. Note individual lesions are equivalent to those of enostosis. Some lesions are coalesced to become larger (asterisks). (**b**) On pinhole bone scan, some of the nodular lesions reveal increased uptake with discrete margins in both femoral bones, but not in acetabular lesions. (**c**) MR images demonstrate multiple small, well-defined, homogenous round to oval nodular foci with low to dark SI on both T1- and T2-weighted images clustered in both femurs, ilium, ischium, and symphysis pubis. Most lesions are not enhanced, but some are peripherally or internally enhanced

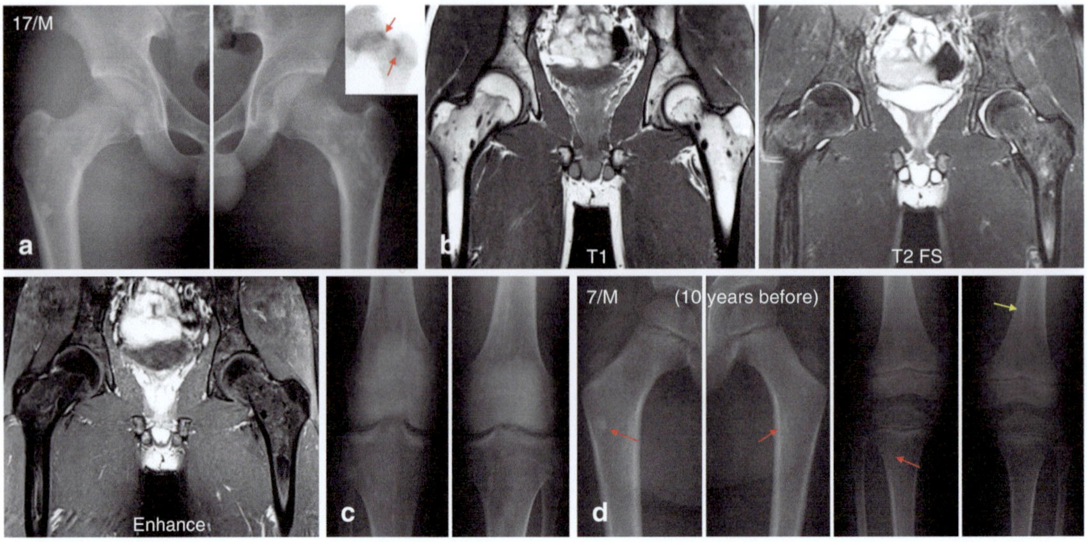

Fig. 4.5 Osteopoikilosis. (**a**) Radiograph taken for intermittent pain of the left hip in a 17-year-old adolescent incidentally shows multiple scattered small sclerotic foci of variable size in both proximal femurs and pelvic bones. Bone scan notes mild uptake in several foci (inset). (**b**) MR images reveal symmetrically distributed multiple small nodular foci with dark SI on both T1- and T2-weighted images in the proximal femurs and pelvic bones. Some lesions are peripherally or internally enhanced. (**c**) Additional radiograph of both knees for further evaluation of another involvement show similar numerous foci in both knee areas. (**d**) Previous radiographs taken for limping gait 10 years ago when he was 7 years old show a few similar small foci around the hips and knees (arrows), which were not recognized at that time by the initial pediatric orthopedist. After 10 years, the lesions have been significantly increased in number and size (**a**, **c**)

4.6 Clinical features

Most lesions are asymptomatic and are detected incidentally on radiographs taken for unrelated reasons. They are usually small, less than 1 cm, and the majority are between 2 mm and 2 cm in size. The lesion is called a *giant bone island* when the diameter is greater than 2 cm [1, 2], which may be painful and should be differentiated from sclerosing osteosarcoma (OSA).

4.7 Radiologic Findings

Plain radiograph reveals a homogeneously dense, round to oval sclerotic nodular or mass-like lesion of variable size with no bone destruction within the cancellous bone. Long axis of the oval lesion is usually parallel to the direction of mechanical stresses on bone, representing adaptation to Wolff's law. The lesion shows distinctive radiating bony streaks that merge with the surrounding host cancellous bone, creating *thorny radiation*, *speculated*, or *brush-like* border (Figs. 4.1a, 4.2a, and 4.3a). OSA can also produce similar peripheral radiating streaks which blend into the host bone. Thus, a large giant bone island should be differentiated from sclerosing OSA by incision biopsy (Fig. 4.3). *Osteopoikilosis* (spotted bone disease) is typified by the presence of multiple to numerous scattered small sclerotic nodules or foci of variable-size lesions which are indistinguishable from solitary enostosis (Figs. 4.4 and 4.5). **Bone scan** Enostosis is typically "cold" on skeletal scintigraphy, and thus, bone scan has been used for differentiating bone islands from the more aggressive entities. However, enostosis can be scintigraphically active, and thus it should be careful in the differential consideration of lesions otherwise characteristic of bone islands [3]. Giant bone island reveals a moderately to significantly increased uptake (Figs. 4.1, 4.2, and 4.3). **CT scan** shows a low-attenuation focus of small nodular or larger cortical-type bone showing characteristic sharp radiating bony streaks, so-called *pseudopodia* or *thorny radiation* within the medullary cavity. **MRI** The signal intensity (SI) is low on both T1- and T2-weighted images, equivalent to normal cortical bone with surrounding intermediate to high SI on both sequences suggesting peri-tumoral reactive changes in some cases (Figs. 4.1, 4.2, 4.3, 4.4 and 4.5). The lesion itself and surrounding reactive changes may be heterogeneously enhanced.

4.8 Histologic Findings

Enostosis and osteopoikilosis consist of predominantly compact (cortical-type) lamellar bone with a focal area of woven bone in some cases. Variably thickened trabeculae which radiate from the main lamellar bone mass blend with the adjacent host cancellous bone (Fig. 4.1e), representing *thorn-like* projection on radiograph and MRI. Enostosis may have prominent Haversian canals and loose fibro-vascular and fat tissues in the marrow cavity, indicating remodeling more commonly seen in larger lesions, so-called *giant bone island*. The increased turnover is usually presented as an increased uptake on bone scan (Figs. 4.1, 4.2, 4.3, 4.4 and 4.5).

4.9 Management

Asymptomatic lesion with classic radiographic finding can be observed without any management, and simple excision is necessary for symptomatic lesion. Biopsy is necessary for large lesions or those in adolescents, or growing lesions on follow-up evaluation to exclude more aggressive lesions such as osteoblastic OSA, and sclerotic metastases in adults. Simple excision is indicated for a large symptomatic lesion.

4.10 Clinical Course

Some lesions may slowly increase in size and number (Fig. 4.5). Prognosis is excellent with no recurrence when excised for pain.

References

1. Smith J. Giant bone islands. Radiology. 1973;107(1):35–6.
2. Gold RH, Mirra JM, Remotti F, Pignatti G. Case report 527: giant bone Island of tibia. Skeletal Radiol. 1989;18(2):129–32.
3. Greenspan A. Bone Island (enostosis): current concept—a review. Skeletal Radiol. 1995;24:111–5.

5 Melorheostosis

(***Melo*** "limb" + ***rheos*** "current" "to flow" + ***ostosis*** "osteogenesis")

5.1 Definition

Melorheostosis is a rare, non-hereditary, sclerosing bone dysplasia, sclerosing hyperostosis characterized by diffuse thickening of the cortical bone in a limited segment with a typical *dripping*, *flowing*, or *melting candle wax* appearance.

5.2 Synonym

Leri's disease/flowing periosteal hyperostosis.

5.3 Incidence

It is exceptionally rare.

5.4 Age

The condition usually begins in childhood and insidiously progresses for many years. Thus, it is often manifested later in adolescence or early adulthood before the age of 20 but can occur at any age.

5.5 Location

Melorheostosis can affect one bone (monostatic form) or multiple bones in one extremity (monomelic form), and rarely, multiple bones in more than one limb (polyostotic polymelic form). The lesion can be found almost anywhere with a predilection for short and long tubular bones of the limbs. Typically, it occurs on the surface of the affected bone but rarely encroaches on the medullary cavity.

5.6 Clinical Features

It often remains occult until young adulthood when significant hyperostosis results in clinical symptoms such as chronic pain, stiffness, swelling or mass effect, or joint motion limitation by soft tissue contracture. In the majority of monomelic forms, the anatomical distribution of the lesions was reported to be approximated to the sclerotomes [1, 2]. It is frequently accompanied by various lesions of the skin and underlying soft tissues (Fig. 5.4a). Morris et al. [3] reported cutaneous manifestations in 17% of 131 patients in a

W.-J. Bahk, *Diagnosis and Management of Primary Bone Tumors*,
https://doi.org/10.1007/978-981-96-3484-2_5

review of the literature. Skin lesions include circumscribed scleroderma, hyperpigmentation, edema, or fibrosis [4]. Uncommonly, it can present with a mineralized peri-articular mass.

5.7 Radiologic Findings

Plain radiograph A sclerotic cortical bone in various patterns with eccentric and segmental distribution is a typical radiographic finding (Figs. 5.1, 5.2, 5.3, and 5.4). The lesion usually involves the periosteal surface of either single or multiple adjacent bones often with endosteal thickening in many cases, but it may be purely intramedullary location-simulating medullary ostoma (enostosis or bone island) (Figs. 5.1e and 5.2a,d). The lesion usually shows a clear demarcation between the affected and unaffected bones. It is usually confined to sclerotomes but can follow across joints to the next bone. Five radiographic pattern, including classic, osteoma-like, myositis ossificans-like, osteopathia striata-like, and mixed patterns have been described [4]. The classic pattern is characterized by periosteal cortical thickening with thick undulating ridges of bone, reminiscent of molten wax, so-called *dripping or flowing candle wax* appearance (Fig. 5.1a). The classic pattern is reported to be seen only in 20–30% of cases [4, 5]. Features of melorheostosis, osteopathia striata, and osteopoikilosis often come together in the form of *mixed sclerosing bone dystrophy* [6]. Indeed, the precise boundary between melorheostosis and other sclerosing bone conditions including osteopoikilosis, osteopathia striata, hyperostosis, or osteosclerosis is overlapped, and it is difficult to exactly separate them [7–10]. However, they can be differentiated with careful history taking, clinical examination, and appropriate radiologic interpretation [5]. **Bone scan** usually reveals a mild to marked uptake [11–14], but no uptake in some cases (Figs. 5.2, 5.3, and 5.4). **CT scan** shows more details of the sclerotic alterations with high attenuation and encroachment of the medullary cavity. Soft tissue involvement may be observed with variable degrees of calcification. **MRI** The SI is usually dark on all sequences being equivalent to normal cortical bone sometimes with internal heterogeneous signals corresponding to variable other components such as vascularized fibrous tissue, collagen content, or mineralization. The lesion notes no or minimal enhancement by contrast medium (Figs. 5.1, 5.2, 5.3, and 5.4).

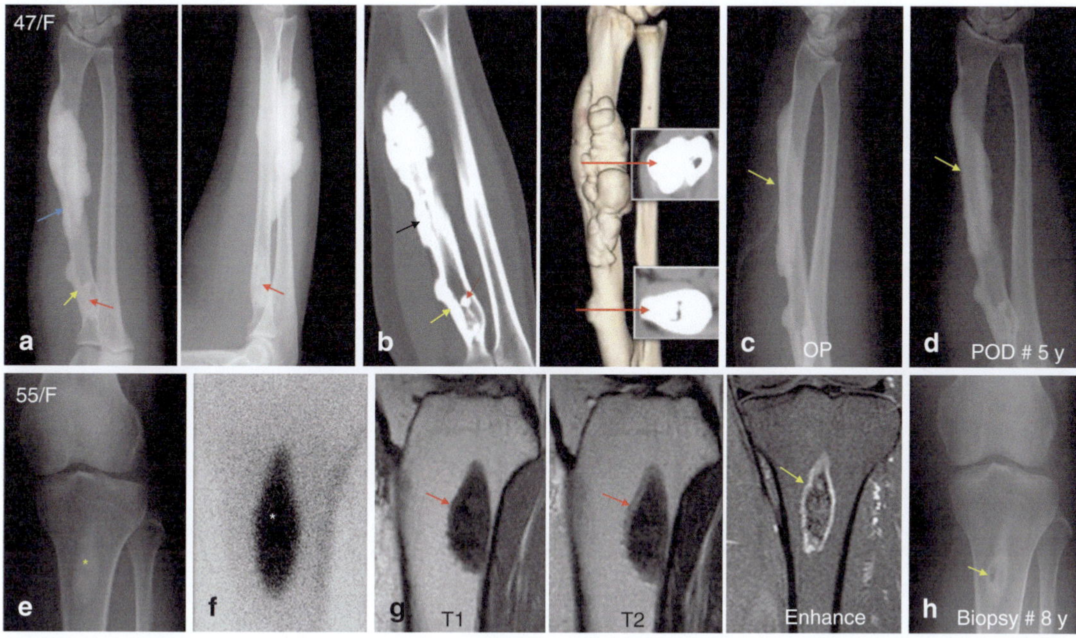

Fig. 5.1 *Classic pattern.* (**a**) Radiograph taken for a longstanding painless hard mass of the left forearm of 10 years duration with recently developed pain and tenderness over the mass in a 47-year-old woman shows a long, eccentric, densely ossifying, lobulated mass. The lesion exhibits a characteristic "melting" or "dripping" candle wax appearance, with irregular cortical thickening (blue arrow) involving dorso-radial side of radius shaft. There is also an intramedullary sclerotic lesion (red arrows) with a cortical thickening (yellow arrow) in the more proximal radius. (**b**) CT scan reveals an eccentric, irregularly extensive, lobulated, projecting mass-like high density in *melting down* appearance with an irregular cortical thickening (black arrow) affecting mid-shaft of radius. In addition, the cortical thickening (yellow arrow) with intramedullary high-density lesion (red arrow) is also seen in the proximal radius (Left). 3D CT scan notes a typical *dripping candle wax* appearance (Right). Axial images show a uniformly dense producing mass associated with cortical thickening and marked obliteration of the marrow cavity (insets). (**c**) The protruding part of the lesion was excised because of tenderness with pain over the mass. Microscopic examination demonstrates thick cortical bones composed of dense lamellar or lamellar to woven bone within the marrow spaces containing normal Haversian systems. (**d**) Follow-up radiograph at 5 years after excision reveals no evidence of recurrence or no further growth of the mass (yellow arrow). The patient is free of symptoms. *Giant bone island-like pattern:* (**e**) Radiograph taken for both knee pain of 2 years duration in a 55-year-old woman incidentally shows a well-defined large ovoid homogeneous sclerotic lesion in the medullary space simulating osteoma or giant bone island (asterisk). However, there is no *speculated* or *brush-like* border which typifies giant bone island. (**f**) Pinhole bone scan reveals a homogeneously strong uptake within the elongated medullary leson, simulating osteoma or giant bone islnad (asterisk), and weak uptake alsong the periphery of the lesion. (**g**) MR images demonstrate a relatively well-defined intramedullary lesion with heterogeneous dark SI with focal intermediate signals on both T1- and T2-weighted images. There is peripheral intermediate SI on T1-weighted image and intermediate to high SI on T2-weighted image surrounding the main lesion (red arrows). The main lesion exhibits heterogeneous enhancement and the periphery of the lesion is strongly enhanced by contrast medium (yellow arrow), suggesting a less immature melorheostosis lesion with fibrovascular reactive tissue and abundant collagen content around the dark signal of aberrant bone proliferation. (**h**) Follow-up radiograph at 8 years after incision biopsy shows a hazy biopsy hole (arrow) but no definite interval changes of the lesion

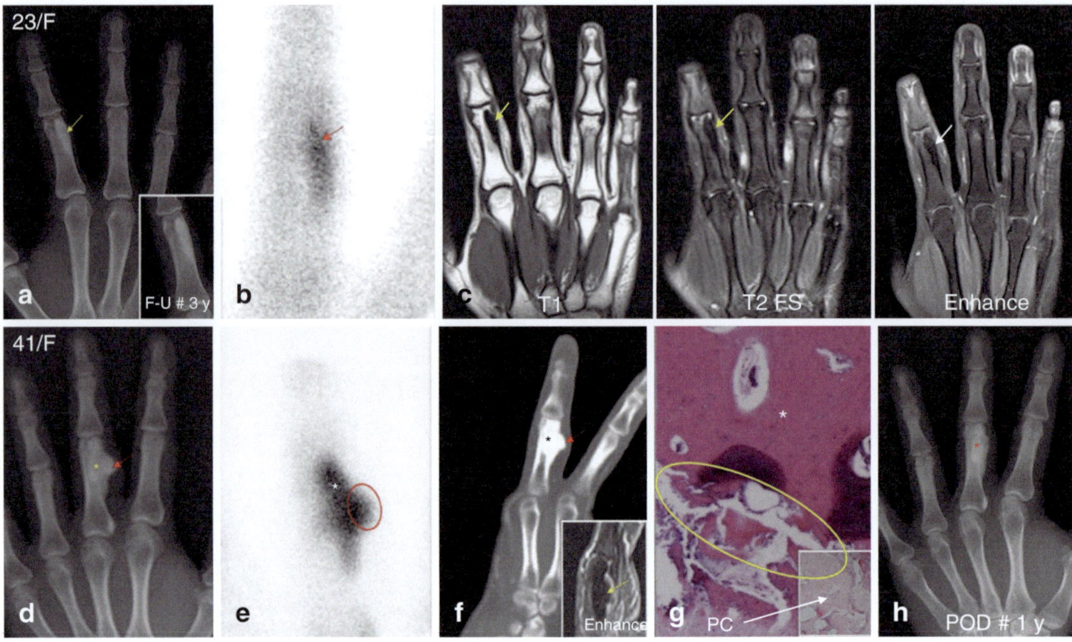

Fig. 5.2 *Medullary osteoma (enostosis)-like pattern.* (**a**) Radiographs taken for right wrist pain in a 23-year-old young woman show a well-defined, eccentric, purely intramedullary, oblong, sclerotic lesion in the radial side of the proximal phalanx of the index finger (arrow). Follow-up radiograph 3 years later notes no interval change of the lesion (inset). (**b**) Pinhole bone scan reveals a segmental, mild uptake in the lesion. (**c**) MR images demonstrate a well-defined, eccentric purely intramedullary, oblong lesion with dark SI (yellow arrows) on both T1- and T2-weighted images. The lesion is not enhanced at all (white arrow). *Osteoma-like pattern with periosteal chondroma:* (**d**) Radiograph taken for hard mass of the left middle finger of several months' duration in a 41-year-old woman shows a similar intramedullary sclerotic lesion (asterisk) in association with a small, round, dense mass protruding beyond the cortex (red arrow) of radial side of the third proximal phalanx. (**e**) Pinhole bone scan reveals an intense, segmental uptake (red asterisk), and an additional focal uptake (red circle), corresponding to the protruding lesion on radiograph (red arrow in (d). (**f**) CT scan demonstrates a significantly sclerotic lesion in the medulla (asterisk) with a tiny protruding sclerotic mass beyond the cortex (red arrow). MR image notes no surrounding soft tissue reaction and no enhancement of the lesion (inset). (**g**) Microscopic examination of the excised protruding mass shows hyaline cartilage nodules mostly with bland chondrocytes (inset), suggesting a concomitant periosteal chondroma (PC). Note several fragmented bone particles (yellow circle) made by curettage during surgical excision of the PC mass and underlying thickened cortex containing Haversian system, suggesting a part of melorheostosis (white asterisk). (**h**) Follow-up at 1 year after surgery reveals no evidence of the PC lesion, with no interval change in the melorheostosislesion (red asterisk)

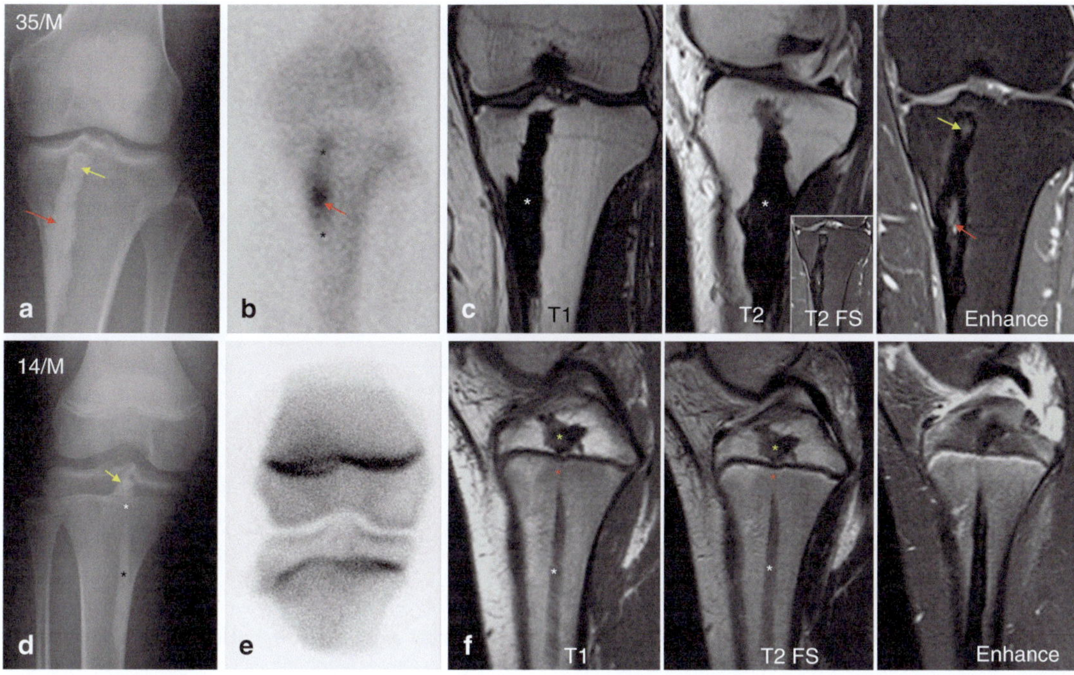

Fig. 5.3 *Osteopathia striata-like pattern.* (**a**) Radiograph taken for left knee pain of a 35-year-old man after a traffic accident incidentally shows a well-defined, dense, thick longitudinal striation (red arrow) which extends to the epiphysis (yellow arrow) crossing the medullary space of the left proximal tibia. The margin is quite clear and undulating between the affected and unaffected bones. (**b**) Bone scan reveals an elongated heterogeneous moderate uptake (asterisks) with a focal strong uptake (arrow). (**c**) MR images show a longitudinal thick lesion of irregularly marginated striation from the diaphysis of the proximal tibia through metaphysis to epiphysis with dark SI (white asterisks) on both T1- and T2-weighted images. There are focal areas of high SI in the center of the lesion on fat-saturated T2-weighted suggesting fat component (inset). There is a stronger enhancement in the center (red arrow) and a milder enhancement in the periphery (yellow arrow). (**d**) Another radiograph taken for both knee pain of 2 weeks duration in a 14-year-old boy incidentally shows a similar narrower lesion with clear margin in the diaphysis and metaphysis of the right proximal tibia (black asterisk). The lesion appears to terminate in the proximal metaphysis (white asterisk) without crossing the growth plate. A focal sclerotic lesion, similar in density, is confined to the epiphysis (arrow). (**e**) Pinhole bone scan reveals no uptake in both lesions of the meta-diaphysis and epiphysis. (**f**) MR images note a longitudinal, clear-margined, narrower striation with low SI (white asterisks) in the proximal diaphysis, which is discontinued in the metaphysis (red asterisks). Note a focal lesion confined to the epiphysis with the same SI (yellow asterisk). The lesion is not definitely enhanced

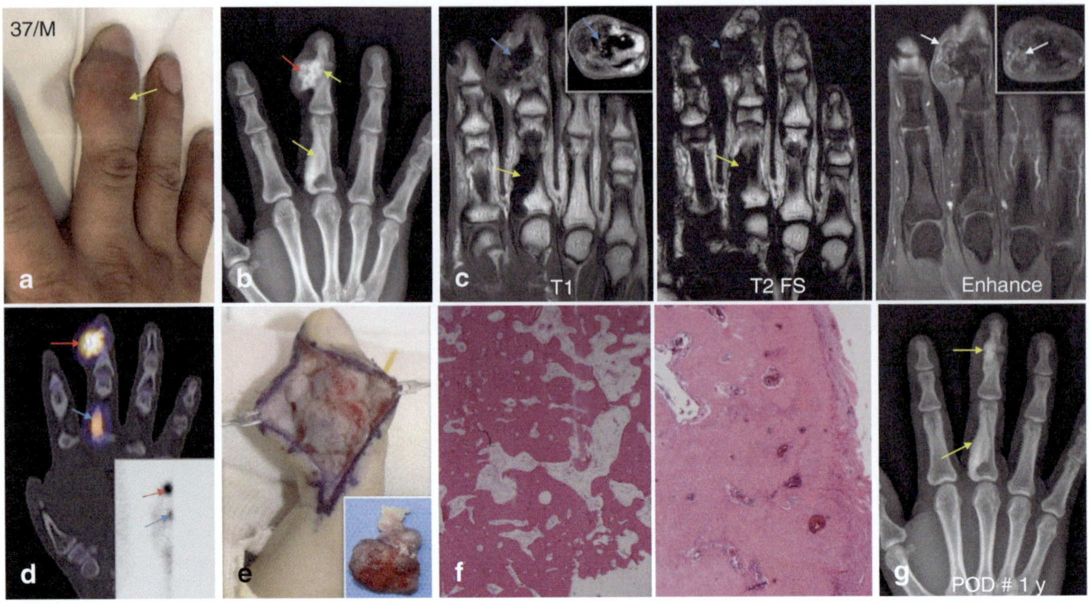

Fig. 5.4 *Osteoma-like and myositis ossificans-like mixed pattern.* (**a**) A 37-year-old man presents with a palpable mass and hyperpigmentation of the skin (arrow) as well as joint motion limitation of the right middle finger for 1.5 years. (**b**) Radiograph shows a densely mineralized exophytic dense mass (red arrow) at the lateral aspect of the distal interphalangeal joint and other eccentric sclerotic medullary lesions (yellow arrows), suggesting osteoma-like melorheostosis with concomitant periosteal osteoma or chondroma. (**c**) MR images demonstrate an irregularly mineralized, multilobulated, exophytic mass (blue arrows) and another sclerotic lesion at the medulla of the proximal phalanx (yellow arrows) with low SI on both T1- and T2-weighted images. There is also medullary sclerosis of dark signal (asterisk) with exophytic mass (blue arrow) at the middle phalanx on the T1-weighted axial image (blue arrow in inset). The exophytic, dense mass exhibits internal focal and peripheral enhancement (white arrows). However, the medullary sclerotic lesions are not enhanced. (**d**) Bone SPECT and bone scan show a strong uptake in the exophytic mass lesion (red arrows) and weaker uptake in the medullary lesion of the proximal phalanx (blue arrows). (**e**) The exophytic soft tissue mass was excised. (**f**) Microscopic examination: (Left) The center of the lesion shows thick cortical bone composed of dense lamellar or lamellar to woven bone with normal-looking marrow spaces. An osteoma or even normal cortex could not be differentiated without radiographic correlation. (Right) Another lesion toward the periphery reveals vascularized fibrous tissue with abundant collagen content, reflecting the focal and peripheral enhancement on MRI. (**g**) Follow-up radiograph at 1 year after surgery clearly shows no evidence of local recurrence with no interval change of the osteoma-like melorheostosis lesions (arrow)

5.8 Histologic Findings

The lesion consists of thick dense lamellar or lamellar to woven bone containing normal Haversian systems. However, the Harversian systems can be obliterated by significantly thickened trabeculae. Occasionally, osteoid and fibrous tissue may be interspersed in the marrow cavity. Cellular atypia or mitotic figures are absent. The lesion toward the periphery may exhibit fibrous tissues with abundant vessels and collagen content, corresponding to the focal and peripheral enhancement on MRI (Fig. 5.4f).

5.9 Management

Treatment options are conservative and symptomatic rather than curative, primarily aiming at relieving pain and restoring range of motion. Bisphosphonate may be useful for relieving pain and reducing swelling. A case of successful pain relief accompanied by long-term suppression of the bone resorption marker β cross-laps has been reported by prolonged treatment with the intravenous bisphosphonate zoledronic acid [15]. A continuous remission of disabling pain after treatment with denosumab has been reported in a patient whose symptom did not respond in the long term to zoledronic acid [16]. Surgical options includie resection of hyperostotic bone, excision of soft tissue masses, tendon lengthening, release of joint are indicated for severe contractures, limited joint motion, or pain. Even amputation can be carefully considered for significant deformity with disability or intractable pain.

References

1. Murray R, McCredie J. Melorheostosis and the sclerotomes: a radiological correlation. Skeletal Radiol. 1979;4(2):57–71.
2. Campbell C, Papademetriou T, Bonfiglio M. Melorheostosis: a report of the clinical, roentgenographic, and pathological findings in fourteen cases. J Bone Joint Surg. 1968;50(7):1281–304.
3. Morris JM, Samilson RL, Corley CL. Melorheostosis: review of the literature and report of an interesting case with a nineteen-year follow-up. J Bone Joint Surg. 1963;45(6):1191–206.
4. Freyschmidt J. Melorheostosis: a review of 23 cases. Eur Radiol. 2001;11(3):474–9.
5. Wordsworth P, Chan M. Melorheostosis and osteopoikilosis: a review of clinical features and pathogenesis. Calcif Tissue Int. 2019;104(5):530–43.
6. Walker GF. Mixed sclerosing bone dystrophies. J Bone Joint Surg Br. 1964;46(3):546–52.
7. Boulet C, Madani H, Lenchik L, Vanhoenacker F, Amalnath DS, De Mey J, et al. Sclerosing bone dysplasias: genetic, clinical and radiology update of hereditary and non-hereditary disorders. Br J Radiol. 2016;89(1062):20150349.
8. Abrahamson MN. Disseminated asymptomatic osteosclerosis with features resembling melorheostosis, osteopoikilosis, and osteopathia striata: case report. J Bone Joint Surg. 1968;50(5):991–6.
9. Green A Jr, Ellswood W, Collins J. Melorheostosis and osteopoikilosis, with a review of the literature. Am J Roentgenol Radium Therapy, Nucl Med. 1962;87:1096–111.
10. Pacifici R, Murphy WA, Teitelbaum SL, Whyte MP. Mixed-sclerosing-bone-dystrophy: 42-year follow-up of a case reported as osteopetrosis. Calcif Tissue Int. 1986;38(3):175–85.
11. Davis DC, Syklawer R, Cole RL. Melorheostosis on three-phase bone scintigraphy. Case report. Clin Nucl Med. 1992;17(7):561–4.
12. Drane WE. Detection of melorheostosis on bone scan. Clin Nucl Med. 1987;12(7):548–51.
13. Janousek J, Preston DF, Martin NL, Robinson RG. Bone scan in melorheostosis. J Nucl Med. 1976;17(12):1106–8.
14. Mahoney J, Achong DM. Demonstration of increased bone metabolism in melorheostosis by multiphase bone scanning. Clin Nucl Med. 1991;16(11):847–8.
15. Hollick RJ, Black A, Reid D. Melorheostosis and its treatment with intravenous zoledronic acid. BMJ Case Rep. 2010;2010:bcr0420091757.
16. Byberg S, Abrahamsen B, Kassem M, Ralston S, Schwarz P. Clinical improvement in a patient with monostotic melorheostosis after treatment with denosumab: a case report. J Med Case Rep. 2018;12(1):1–6.

6 Osteoid Osteoma

(***Osteo*** "bone" + ***oid, eidos*** "resemblance" ***oste(o)*** "bone" + ***ōma*** "forming")

6.1 Definition

Osteoid osteoma (OO) is a benign bone-producing tumor typified by painful, tiny to small, well-demarcated nidus consisting of osteoid and woven bone, which is surrounded by a thin layer of loose fibro-vascular connective tissue. Most nidi are less than 1–1.5 cm in diameter, with limited growth potential [1–3].

6.2 Subclassification

Based on the radiographic localization of the nidus, OO can be categorized into three types: the most common *cortical type* (Figs. 6.1, 6.2, 6.3, 6.4, 6.5, 6.6, 6.7, 6.8, and 6.9), the second most common *subcortical or medullary type* (Fig. 6.10), and the rarest *subperiosteal type* [4].

6.3 Incidence

OO is relatively common, accounting for about 2–3% of all excised primary bone tumors and 10–13% of benign bone tumors [2, 5, 6].

6.4 Age

The lesion can affect patients at any age but occurs most commonly in children, teenagers, and young adults between the ages of 10 and 25 years, occupying about 90% of patients. Patients are rarely younger than 5 years and older than 30 years [7, 8].

6.5 Location

OO may occur in any bone on the axial and appendicular skeleton, but over half of the cases affect long bones of the lower extremities (Figs. 6.1, 6.2, 6.3, 6.4, 6.5, 6.6, 6.7, 6.8, 6.9, 6.10, and 6.11). The femoral neck is the single most common site. The diaphysis of the mid-tibia is also frequently involved, but the lesion rarely occurs within the epiphysis. Intra-articular OO is most commonly seen in the hip joint. Most lesions are located in or near the cortex rather than being buried deep within the medullary space [2]. Cancellous and subperiosteal OO typically arise at the ends of the long bones adjacent to the joints [4], but may also occur in the diaphysis (Fig. 6.10). The lesion is

W.-J. Bahk, *Diagnosis and Management of Primary Bone Tumors*,
https://doi.org/10.1007/978-981-96-3484-2_6

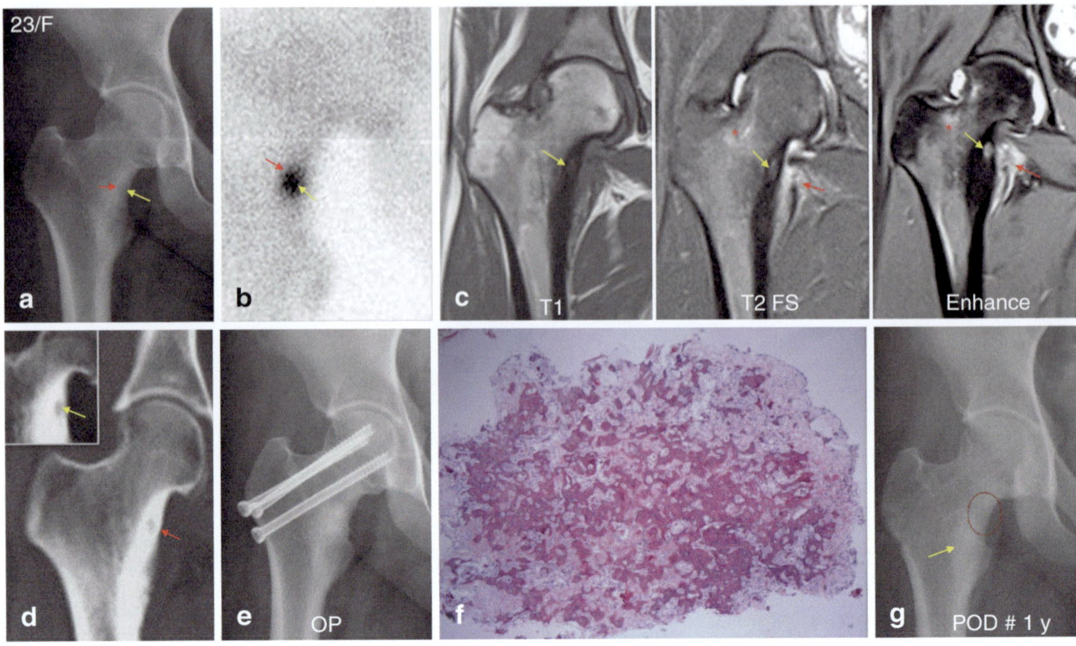

Fig. 6.1 (**a**) Radiograph taken for right hip pain which was severe at night and relieved by NSAID of 6 months duration in a 23-year-old young woman shows an intracortical, hazy, tiny sclerotic lesion (yellow arrow) surrounded by a very thin radiolucent line (red arrow), so-called *target-like* appearance, in the thickened medial cortex of the femroal neck. (**b**) Pinhole bone scan reveals a central small hot uptake (yellow arrow) with a peripheral blurred uptake (red arrow), so-called *rim sign*. (**c**) MR images demonstrate a tiny round to oval nidus confined to a thick sclerotic cortex (yellow arrows) with low to intermediate SI on T1-weighted image and heterogeneous high SI on fat-saturated T2-weighted image. Diffuse edema is seen in the adjacent bone marrow (red asterisk) and surrounding soft tissue (red arrow) on T2-weighted image. The nidus is more intensely enhanced along the periphery than in the center (yellow arrow). In addition, the edema of bone marrow (red asterisk) and soft tissue (red arrow) is diffusely enhanced. (**d**) CT scan shows an oval small radiolucent lesion with internal tiny sclerotic dots buried in the significantly thickened cortex (arrows). (**e**) Enucleation using *burr-down* technique was performed, followed by cannulated screw fixation to prevent perioperative fracture. (**f**) Low-power microscopic examination of the enucleated nidus shows a well-defined typical nidus consisting of haphazardly anastomosing trabeculae of pinkish primitive osteoid and purple woven bone with intertrabecular fibro-vascular tissues, which is surrounded by a thin FVZ, corresponding to the *rim sign* on pinhole bone scan. (**g**) Follow-up radiograph at 1 year after surgery reveals a barely discernible small lucent shadow (circle) with unchanged thickness of the sclerotic cortex (arrow). She is completely free of pain

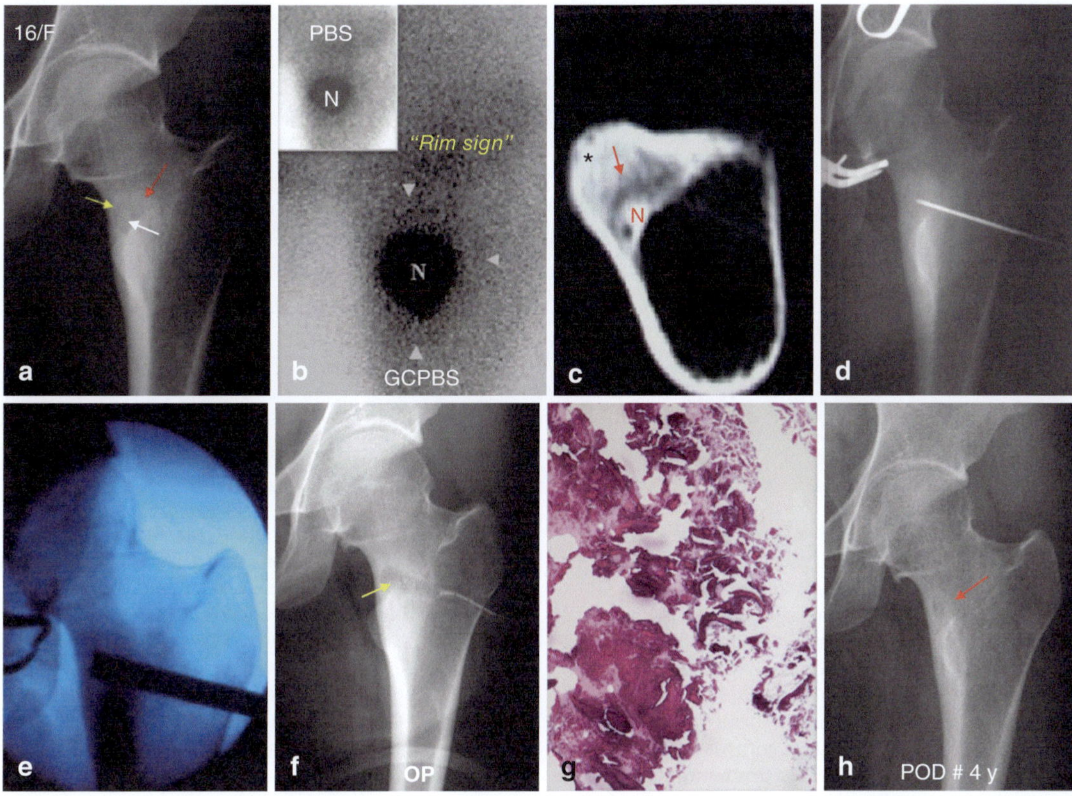

Fig. 6.2 (**a**) Radiograph taken for left hip pain of 3 years' duration that was relieved by ingestion of NSAID and recurred without medication in a 16-year-old female adolescent shows a dense, round to ovoid, small nidus (white arrow) surrounded by a thin radiolucent circle (yellow arrow), so-called *target-like* appearance. The outermost area presents a thick reactive sclerotic bone (red arrow). (**b**) PBS reveals a strong uptake in the nidus (N) with a surrounding blurred uptake (inset). GCPBS more clearly depicts a central strong uptake of the nidus (N) surrounded by a weak stippled uptake of the FVZ (arrow heads), so-called *rim sign*, which is indicative of OO. (**c**) CT scan also shows a dense nidus in the center (N) circumscribed by a thin radiolucent area (arrow). Note the outermost markedly thickened cortex (asterisk). (**d**) A guide K-wire for trephine insertion was targeted to the nidus under C-arm image intensifier. (**e**) A trephine was inserted from the lateral cortex along the guide K-wire to remove the nidus. (**f**) Immediate postoperative radiograph shows a complete removal of the nidus (arrow). (**g**) Microscopic examination of the obtained specimen demonstrates severely fragmented bony tissues by crush effect and necrotized by heat during trephining, which is comparable to the well-demarcated typical nidus obtained by enucleation using burr-down technique in Fig. 6.1f. (**h**) Follow-up radiograph at 4 years after surgery reveals no evidence of recurrence with a tiny hazy radiolucent defect and significant reduction of the thick surrounding sclerosis (arrow)

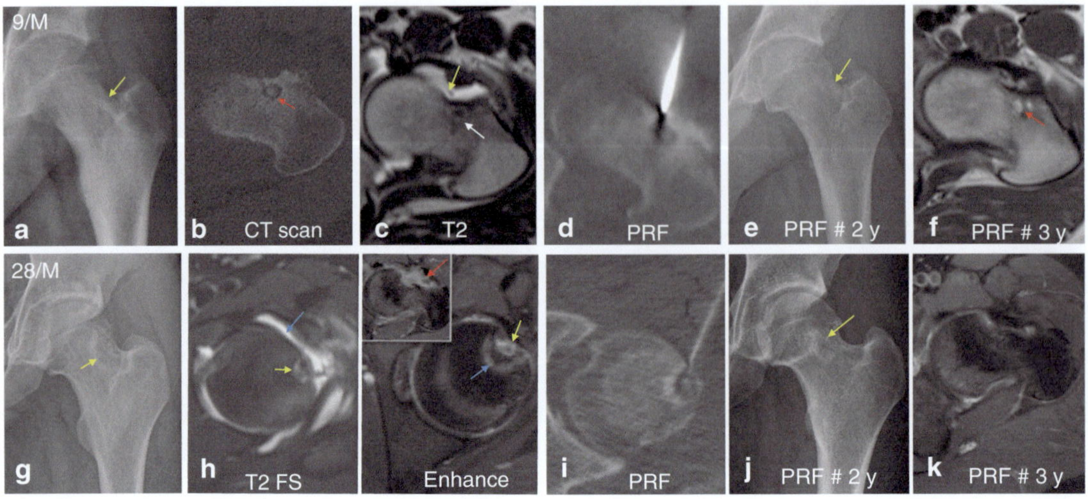

Fig. 6.3 *Percutaneous PRF ablation.* (**a**) Radiograph taken for left hip pain of 5 months without nocturnal aggravation in a 9-year-old boy shows a thickened cortex of the left femoral neck with a hazy tiny nidus (arrow). (**b**) However, CT scan clearly reveals a tiny dense nidus surrounded by a thin radiolucent area (red arrow). (**c**) T2-weighted MR image demonstrates a central tiny dark signal of small nidus with a peripheral intermediate SI (white arrow). There is a significant reactive effusion in the neighboring hip joint (yellow arrow). (**d**) CT-guided PRF ablation was performed under general anesthesia. (**e**) Radiograph at 2 years after the procedure shows a normalized cortex with clear margin (yellow arrow). (**f**) Follow-up MR image at 3 years after ablation shows healing of the lesion (arrow). *Recurrent lesion:* (**g**) Another radiograph taken for recurrent left hip pain at 1 year after curettage of histologically proven OO in a 28-year-old man shows a mixed osteolytic and osteoblastic lesion surrounded by a rim of sclerotic bone in the femoral neck (arrow). (**h**) MR images reveal a round intracortical lesion with heterogeneously intermediate and high SI and central dark signal on fat fat-saturated T2-weighted image (yellow arrow). A large amount of reactive joint effusion is also noted (blue arrow). The lesion is heterogeneously enhanced (yellow arrow), suggesting local recurrence of the nidus. Adjacent soft tissue (red arrow) as well as surrounding reactive rim (blue arrow) is well enhanced by contrast medium. (**i**) CT-guided PRF was performed under general anesthesia. (**j**) Radiograph at 2 years after the procedure notes that the lesion becomes consolidated with sclerotic change (arrow). (**k**) Follow-up MRI at 3 years after ablation shows no evidence of local recurrence and absence of joint effusion

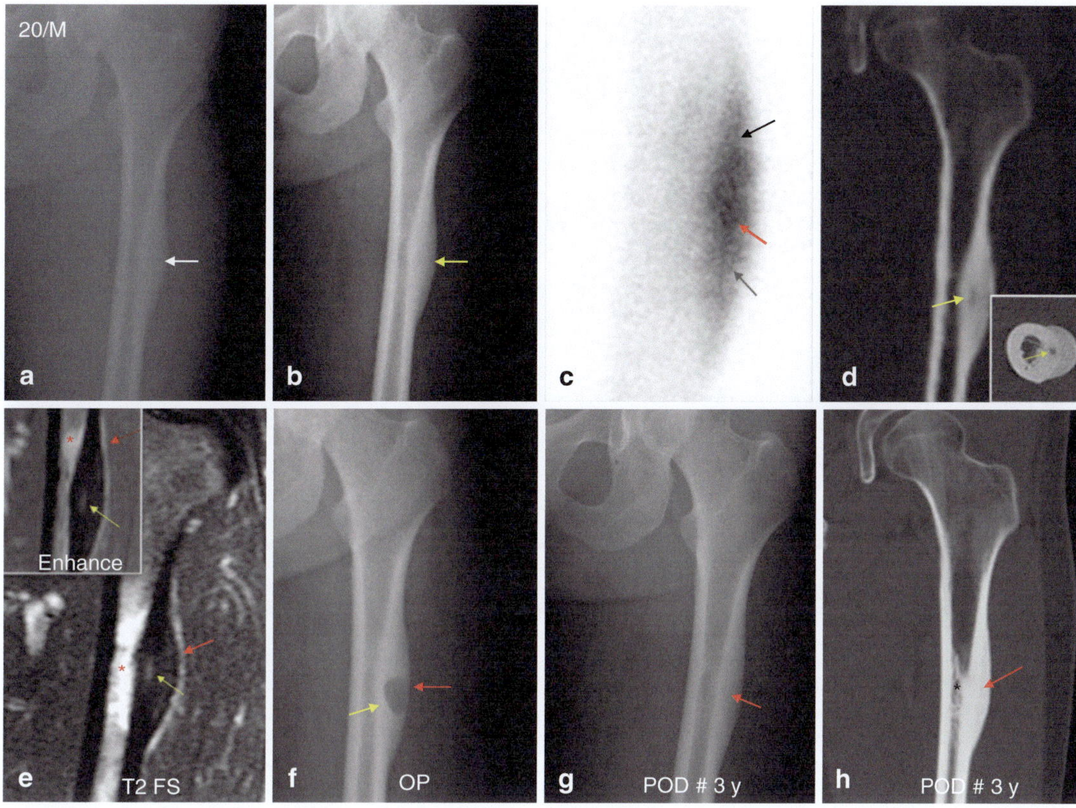

Fig. 6.4 *Greater penetration radiograph.* (**a**) Radiograph taken for the left thigh with nocturnal aggravation of 2 months' duration in a 20-year-old young man shows a fusiform-shaped extensive cortical thickening without a discernible internal radiolucency in the lateral aspect of the femoral mid-shaft (arrow). (**b**) However, another radiograph with greater penetration using higher kilovoltage reveals a hazy radiolucent nidus buried in the thickened dense cortex (arrow). (**c**) PBS reveals a diffusely increased activity along the thickened lateral cortex (black arrows) with a focal strong uptake (red arrow). (**d**) CT scan more clearly demonstrates a tiny, radiolucent nidus buried in the extensively thickened cortex (arrows). (**e**) MR image shows a tiny nidus of high signal (yellow arrow) with extensive bone marrow (red asterisk) and soft tissue edema (red arrow) on fat-saturated T2-weighted image. The nidus is only weakly enhanced (yellow arrow), but the edemas are strongly enhanced (inset). (**f**) The nidus was completely removed by *burr-down* technique (red arrow). Normal thickness of the cortex (yellow arrow) remained after surgery which would not allow a fracture. (**g**) Follow-up radiograph at 3 years after surgery reveals no evidence of recurrence with a mild decrease in cortical thickness (arrow). (**h**) Follow-up CT scan also shows no evidence of recurrence (arrow) with postoperative medullary change (asterisk)

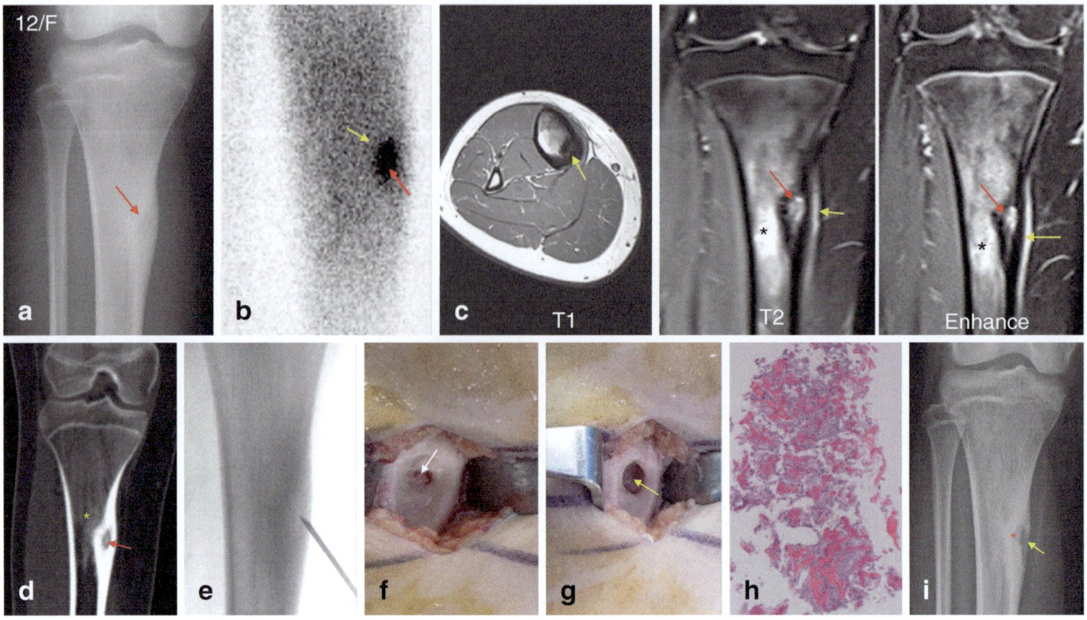

Fig. 6.5 *Burr-down technique.* (**a**) Radiograph taken for right proximal leg pain which became severe at night occasionally disturbing her sleep, and was relieved by NSAID, with a duration of 4 months in a 12-year-old girl shows a markedly thickened cortex with an internal hazy oval radiolucent lesion (red arrow). (**b**) PBS reveals a nodular hot uptake (red arrow) with a lesser increased uptake along the periphery (yellow arrow), the so-called rim sign. (**c**) MR images reveal an oval nidus buried in the thickened cortex with low SI on T1-weighted axial image (yellow arrow) and high SI with focal dark dots on T2-weighted image (red arrow). The nidus is strongly enhanced (red arrow). Edema is extensively presented in the adjacent bone marrow (asterisks) as well as soft tissue (yellow arrows), which is also well enhanced. (**d**) CT scan more clearly demonstrates a tiny low-attenuation nidus with a surrounding radiolucent area of FVZ (red arrow) buried in the markedly thickened cortex. Bone marrow edema is also seen (asterisk). (**e**) The nidus with reactive sclerotic bone is localized with C-arm image intensifier. (**f**) Using burr-down technique, the tiny reddish to yellowish nidus is beginning to appear in the crater made by a gradual peeling of the reactive thick sclerotic bone (arrow). (**g**) A clear defect with intact underlying host cortex is noted after complete removal of the nidus by curette (arrow), which allows avoidance of preventive fixation and bone graft. (**h**) Microscopic examination shows a well-defined typical nidus with overall intact contour. (**i**) Postoperative radiograph reveals a radiolucent defect (arrow) from enucleation of the nidus with an intact underlying cortex (asterisk). She is informed by a phone call to be completely free of pain at 2 years after surgery

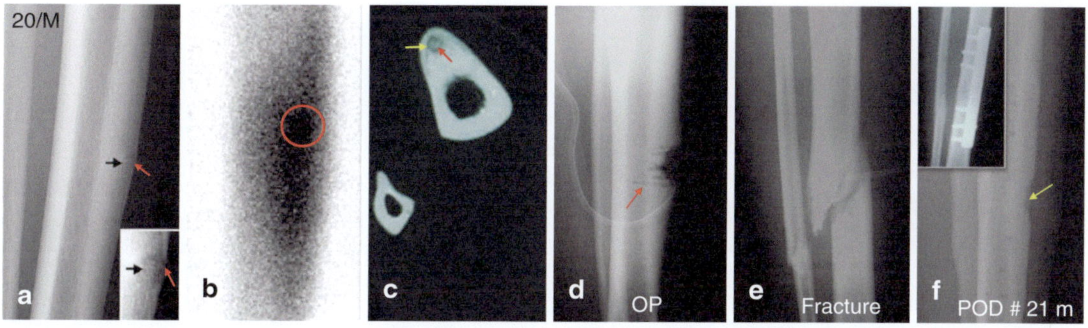

Fig. 6.6 *Postoperative fracture.* (**a**) Radiograph taken for left leg pain of 1 month's duration which is significantly aggravated after a military drill in a 20-year-old soldier shows tiny hazy round radiopaque nidus (black arrow) surrounded by a thin radiolucent circle (red arrow) that is more discernible on gamma correction radiograph (inset). (**b**) PBS reveals a diffuse strong uptake along the thickened cortex suggesting reactive sclerosis a focal hotter uptake indicating a small nidus (circle), so-called *hotter spot within hot area* sign. (**c**) CT scan typically notes a well-defined round dense nidus (red arrow) surrounded by a thin radiolucency (yellow arrow) within the thickened cortex. (**d**) Enucleation of the nidus was performed using a drill bit and osteotome by inexperienced surgeon. Note multiple deep drill holes through the reactive and normal cortex even with a penetrating hole in the cortex through the medullary cavity (arrow), all of which can weaken the mechanical strength of the tibia. (**e**) Radiograph taken for severe pain by simple torsional force during basketball playing shows pathologic fracture through the drill holes. (**f**) Open reduction with plate fixation was done (inset). Follow-up radiograph at 21 months after surgical excision shows no evidence of local recurrence and gradual remodeling of the cortex (arrow)

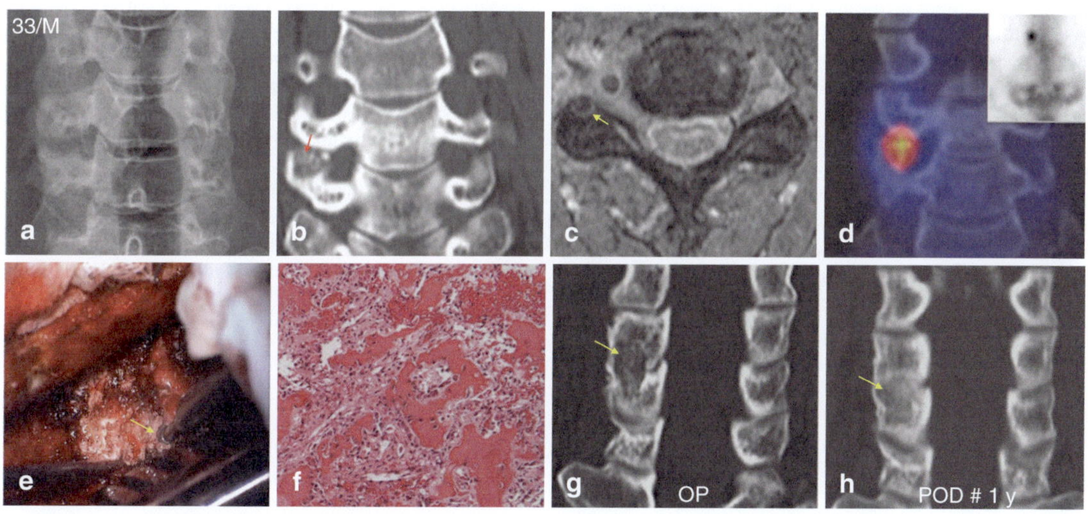

Fig. 6.7 (**a**) Radiograph taken for neck pain of 2 years' duration in a 33-year-old man shows no discernible abnormal finding suggesting a tumorous condition. (**b**) However, CT scan reveals a radiolucent lesion with small round to oval sclerotic nidus and several dots in the lateral mass of C6 vertebra (arrow). (**c**) MR image demonstrates a small round to oval mass with low SI surrounded by a thin high signal (yellow arrow). (**d**) Bone SPECT and bone scan (inset) show a focal hot uptake in the right side of the lower cervical vertebra. (**e**) Enucleation was performed using burr-down technique. (**f**) Microscopic examination shows irregularly serrated thick woven bone trabeculae with osteoblastic rimming arranged in a random manner as well as spindle cell proliferation with prominent hemorrhage and vascularity between the bone trabeculae. (**g**) After enucleation, autogenous bone graft was done between C5 and C6 vertebrae for fusion (arrow). (**h**) Follow-up radiograph at 1 year reveals solid fusion with no evidence of recurrence (arrow)

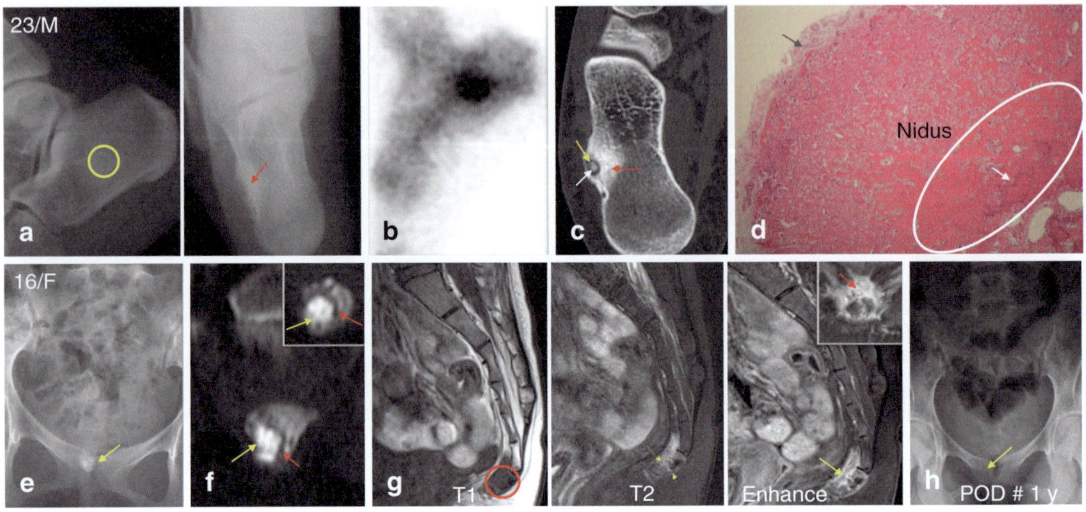

Fig. 6.8 *Rare locations: calcaneus.* (**a**) Radiographs taken for ankle pain that suddenly developed after military drill in a 23-year-old soldier show a small radiolucent lesion with a central sclerotic nidus and surrounding sclerosis in the calcaneus (circle) on anteroposterior (AP) view and associated thickened cortex on calcaneus axial view (red arrow). (**b**) Bone scan reveals a central focal strong uptake with lesser active uptake along the periphery. (**c**) CT scan clearly notes a typical finding of tiny, dense nidus in the center (white arrow) with radiolucent peripheral thin ring (yellow arrow), typical *target-like* appearance, surrounded by prominent reactive sclerotic bone (red arrow). (**d**) Microscopic examination of enucleated specimen reveals a well-defined nidus consisting of randomly interconnecting woven bone trabeculae surrounded by FVZ with poor vascularity (black arrow) that is reflected as a thin or thick radiolucent ring on radiograph and CT scan as well as mild peripheral uptake on bone scan. However, the intertrabecular spaces are filled with fibrous tissues and prominent vessels, presenting as a central focal hotter uptake on bone scan and heterogeneous strong enhancement on MRI. The woven bone tissue is more matured with cement lines (white arrow) in the center (circle). *Coccyx:* (**e**) Radiograph taken for coccygodynia of 2 years' duration of a 16-year-old girl shows a well-defined small highly dense mass in the coccyx (arrow). (**f**) CT scan clearly reveals a 1 cm-sized, round to oval, highly dense mass (yellow arrow) surrounded by a thin radiolucent zone (red arrow). (**g**) MR images demonstrate a tiny round to oval mass lesion (circle) with low SI on T1- and heterogeneous high SI on T2-weighted image. There is a significant perilesional soft tissue edema (arrows). The lesion itself is focally and peripherally enhanced (yellow arrow), and soft tissue edema is diffusely enhanced (red arrow) by contrast media. (**h**) Follow-up radiograph at 1 year after enucleation does not demonstrate previously seen mass lesion (yellow arrow). The patient is totally free of pain

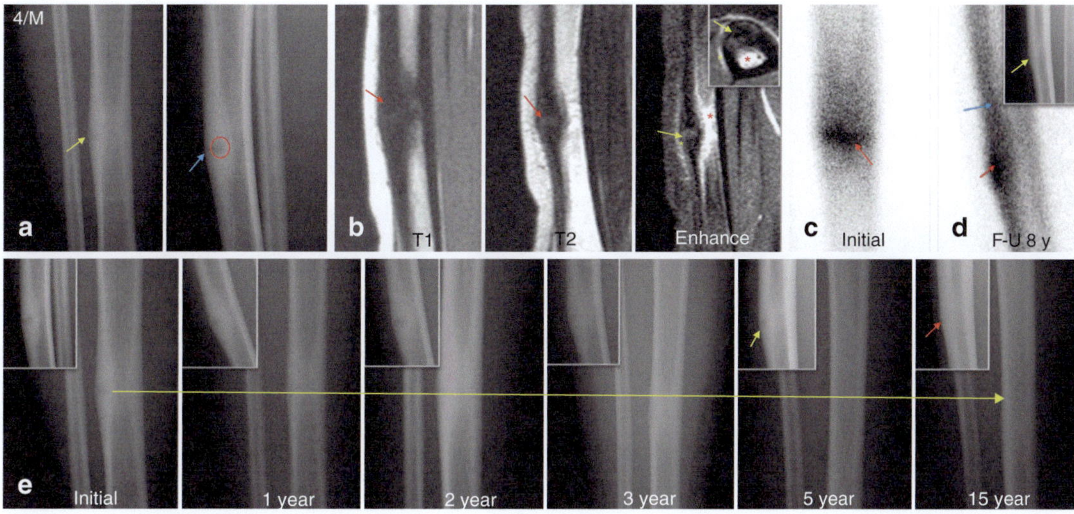

Fig. 6.9 *Spontaneous regression of cortical type.* (**a**) AP radiograph taken for right leg painful swelling with nocturnal aggravation in a 4-year-old boy shows a hazy tiny radiolucent lesion within the thickened cortex (yellow arrow). Lateral view reveals a tiny round radiolucent lesion with sclerotic dot (circle) and a short, transverse lucent line (blue arrow), suggesting OO with a linear fracture line. (**b**) MR images demonstrate an intracortical tiny nodular lesion with low SI on T1-weighted image and intermediate to high SI on T2-weighted image (red arrows). The nidus is heterogeneously and peripherally enhanced (yellow arrows). The diffuse perilesional bone marrow and periosteal edema (asterisks) are strongly enhanced. (**c**) Initial PBS notes an increased transverse bandlike uptake crossing the medullary space (red arrow), which would obscure the hot uptake in the nidus and surrounding weak uptake of OO, raising the possibility of insufficiency or stress fracture with preexisting OO. His parents wanted to manage the pain by intermittent use of analgesics without surgical removal. (**d**) Eight years later, follow-up pinhole scan shows a changed pattern initially from a linear transverse uptake to a long segmental uptake along the thickened anterior cortex (blue arrow) with a focal hot uptake suggesting a nidus (red arrow). The changed finding suggests a healing of the linear fracture with still active nidus reflecting the focal thickening of cortex with central hazy radiolucency on lateral radiograph (inset). (**e**) Long-term follow-up radiographs note a chronologic regression and disappearance of the nidus and reactive cortical sclerosis. Note the cortex appears to become normal with no discernible nidus on the AP view, but the cortex is still mildly thickened with a hazy nidus on the lateral view at 5 years follow-up (inset). Radiograph at 15 years follow-up shows a normalized cortex without visible nidus even on lateral view (inset)

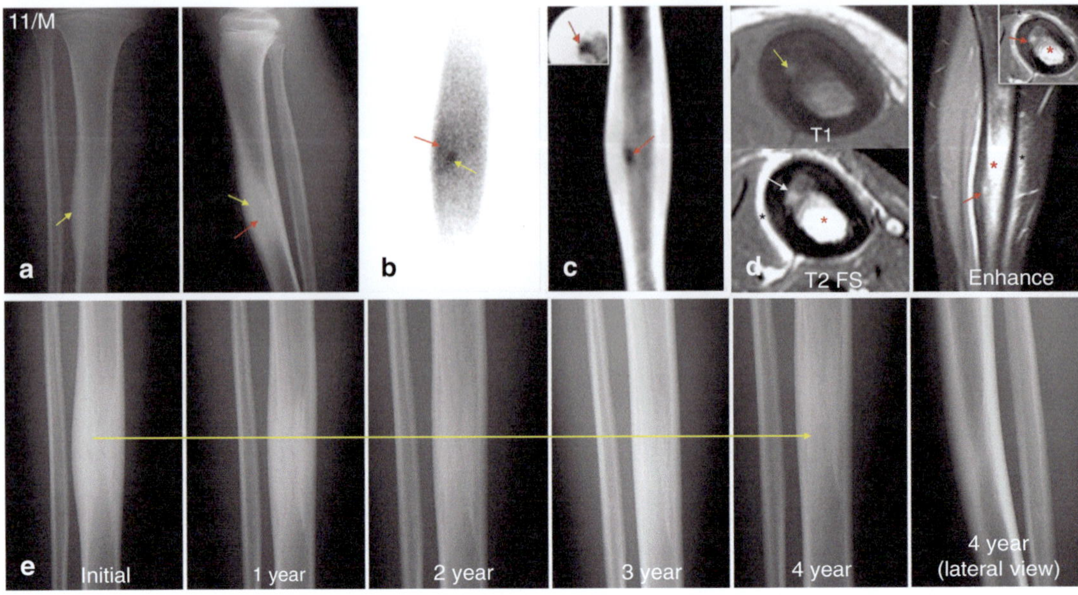

Fig. 6.10 *Spontaneous regression of medullary type.* (**a**) Radiograph taken for right leg pain that was severe enough to wake him from sleep in an 11-year-old boy shows only a markedly thickened cortex with no clearly discernible nidus (yellow arrows) in the mid-shaft of the right tibia. Note a hazy radiolucent lesion within the thickened cortex on the lateral view (red arrow). (**b**) PBS reveals a central tiny focal hot uptake (yellow arrow) with a peripheral lesser active uptake (red arrow), so-called *hotter spot within hot area* sign, in the subcortical medullary cavity. (**c**) CT scan excellently clarifies a tiny round to oval, radiolucent nidus (4 mm in diameter) located subcortically at the cortex-medulla junction, mainly medullary space (arrows), so-called *subcortical or medullary* type. (**d**) MR images reveal a subcortical tiny round nidus (arrows) with low to intermediate SI on T1-weighted image and heterogeneous high SI on fat-saturated T2-weighted image. The perilesional bone marrow and periosteal soft tissue edema are prominent (asterisks). Post-contrast image shows a well-enhanced tiny nidus itself (red arrows) and the edema is also clearly well-enhanced (asterisks). (**e**) His patients did not want surgical management despite the severe pain bothering sleep, and he was managed conservatively by taking NSAIDs only when the pain was severe. Mid-term follow-up radiographs show a chronological regression of the nidus and cortical sclerosis year by year. There is a near normal to mildly thickened cortex with no discernible radiolucent nidus at 4 years follow-up. He is free of symptoms

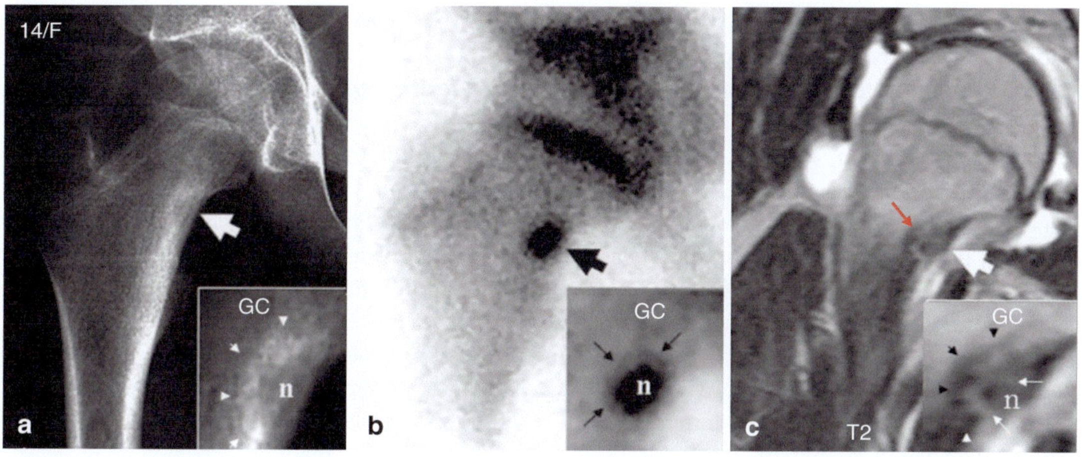

Fig. 6.11 *Gamma correction.* (GC) (**a**) Radiograph taken for right hip pain with limping gait of 9 months duration in a 14-year-old girl shows a hazy, elliptical, radiolucent lesion buried in thickened medial cortex of the right femoral neck (arrow). GC CR better defines a half-opaque nidus (n) and reactive peri-nidal sclerosis (arrows), but the FVZ: is not visible even on this radiograph (inset). (**b**) PBS depicts an oval lesion with a central hot uptake circumscribed by a blurred 2-mm thick ring-like zone of less intense uptake (arrow). GCPBS more clearly depicts a central strong uptake of the nidus (n) and peri-nidal ring-like milder uptake of FVZ, a typical *rim sign* (arrows in inset). (**c**) Coronal T2-weighted MR image shows an oval nidus with high SI with focal low signal surrounded by a blurred low signal suggesting FVZ (red arrow). There is associated periosteal soft tissue edema (white thick arrow). GC MRI (inset) more clearly portrays a slightly clearer nidus (n; white arrows) with central, low to dark signal of calcification, which is surrounded by a low signal of the FVZ (black arrows)

occasionally found in the small bones of hands and feet. Approximately 10–20% of the cases are located in the spine [9, 10], and they are mostly found in the posterior elements.

6.6 Clinical Features

Patients quite often present with a typical pain of continuously increasing severity over a period of months to years. The pain is initially mild to intermediate typically with a nocturnal aggravation, gradually worsens, and may eventually become severe enough to disturb sleep. The pain can be aggravated by physical activity such as exercise or military drill. Often, pain is dramatically relieved by aspirin or nonsteroidal anti-inflammatory drugs (NSAID), even in small doses, which is a virtual diagnostic symptom particularly if nocturnal aggravation is associated. The typical response of the pain to the drugs occurs in about 70–90% of patients, so the response is not universal [2, 11, 12]. Pain is not usually well-localized and may refer to an adjacent joint or radiate to a distal part of the extremity. Thus, pain can be present in the distal thigh when the lesion affects the femoral neck or trochanter area or even in the more distal extremity (sciatica) when involving the spine. Spinal lesions can lead to painful scoliosis with concavity on the side of the lesion due to unilateral spasm of paravertebral muscles. Other presentations may include joint pain and effusion simulating arthritis, painful swelling of the adjacent soft tissue, limping, or muscles atrophy. The lesion close to a growth plate in a growing child may cause length discrepancy by increased growth rate presumably related to hyperemia. However, several lesions without pain have been sporadically reported in various locations and summarized in a review of the literature [13], some of which is totally asymptomatic and incidentally discovered on radiographs for other reasons. The prevalence of painless OO was 1.6% in a review of 860 cases in the English literature and 5% in AFIP series [14, 15]. Several case reports on multifocal nidi have been published, most of which were within a single bone [16–24]. Sherman and McFarland [25] identified nerve fibers in the fibro-vascular zone (FVZ) around the nidus which were believed to be part of the autonomic nervous system. Years later, free nerve fibers were observed close to the blood vessels in the nidus by silver stain, which were thought to be a source of the typical pain [26, 27]. Makley and Dunn [28] observed increased prostaglandin (PG) synthesis, particularly of PGE2, in three patients having a pathologically proven OO with a typical history of bone pain, which was substantially relieved by aspirin or indomethacin. Vasodilation mediated by PGE2 and PG12 was thought to cause expansion of the OO and compression of the abundant nerve endings in the lesion. Since PGE can induce hyperalgesia, the 1000-fold increase of PGE2 synthesis probably cause the intense pain produced by the lesion. The hypothesis can be reinforced by the significant analgesic effects of NSAIDs in this condition. Greco et al. [29] also observed that PGE 2 and PG12 synthesis in fragments of the nidus were 33 and 26 times greater than in fragments of normal bone. However, the level of peripheral reactive sclerotic bone was nearly the same as that in normal bone. PG production was inhibited by using NSAIDs in the incubation medium, which suggested that PGs are locally synthesized by the tumor tissue. They verified the original report and strongly supported a theory of the pathophysiological role of PG as a mediator of pain. PGE 2 and PG12 are powerful vasodilators and determine the extent of inflammation and edema. More recently, Mungo et al. [30] found a strong immunohistochemical stain for cyclooxygenase-2 (COX-2) in the tumor osteoblasts, but it was scanty in the surrounding host osteoblasts of the reactive bone. Significant COX-1 staining was detected in both tumor itself and host osteoblasts. However, very limited amounts of COX-2 were detected in the tissues of fibrous dysplasia, osteoblastoma, and osteofibrous dysplasia. Therefore, the increased production of PG by OO would implicate that COX-2 is one of the mediators of the characteristic pain. The authors concluded that the newly developed selective COX-2 inhibitors can be used safely for pain control of OO.

6.7 Radiologic Findings

Plain radiograph shows a characteristic finding of a well-defined small round or oval to elliptical nodular lesion called *nidus*, which is usually less than 1–1.5 cm in diameter and surrounded by a thin, 1–2 mm, radiolucent fibrovascular (FVZ). The density of the nidus can be variable from radiolucent with or without central sclerotic dots (Figs. 6.4, 6.5, and 6.10) to homogeneously dense surrounded by a thin radiolucent circle, so-called *target-like* appearance (Figs. 6.1, 6.2, 6.3, 6.6, 6.8, and 6.9), depending on the amount of osteoid and more matured woven bone or degree of mineralization. Most lesions present surrounding reactive thick cortical sclerosis, some of which may be so extensive that the nidus cannot be seen. Often, the nidus, not visible on routine radiograph, can be demonstrated on radiographs with greater penetration using higher kilovoltage in some cases (Fig. 6.4a and b). In the shaft of long bones, the cortical thickening is usually fusiform-shaped, extensive, and markedly dense that may frequently result in the typical nidus hazy or indiscernible (Figs. 6.4a, 6.5a, and 6.9a). Such cortical OOs are usually associated with much more thick reactive sclerosis than medullary tumors. Intracapsular OO is difficult to identify because there is no periosteum and hence a periosteal reaction does not occur. Such cases may be confusing with a complicated synovial herniation pit which is one of skeletal "don't touch" lesions (Fig. 6.12). **Bone scan** is valuable for detecting OO revealing a focal hot uptake (Fig. 6.7d). More precisely, pinhole bone scan (PBS) presents a central focus of intense uptake (the nidus) within a surrounding mildly increased uptake, so-called *double density*, *rim*, or *hotter spot within hot area* sign (Figs. 6.1, 6.2, 6.4, 6.5, 6.6, 6.8, 6.9, 6.10, and 6.11), which is pathognomonic if presents [31]. The central "hotter" area represents the highly vascular nidus and the outer "less hot" area may suggest FVZ or less active reactive sclerosis [32, 33]. Conventional radiograph (CR) with a greater penetration using higher voltage in combination with PBS is economical and widely available. A *gamma correc-*

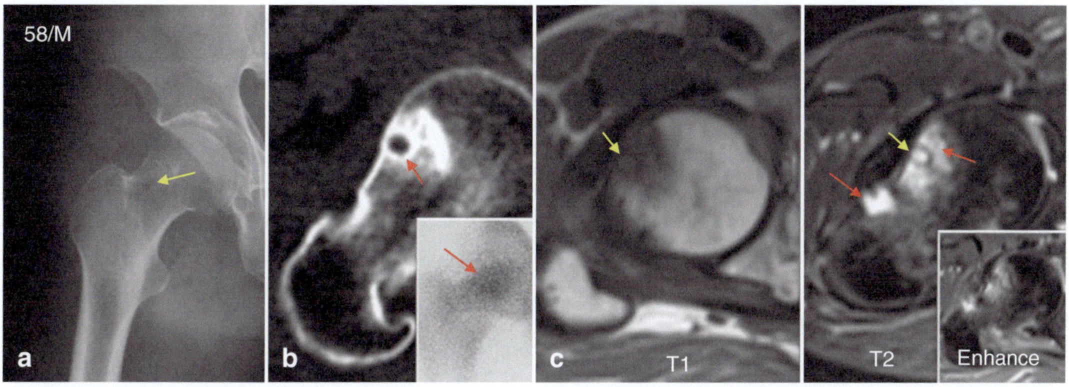

Fig. 6.12 *Symptomatic herniation pit.* (**a**) Radiograph taken for intermittent right hip pain of 4 months' duration in a 58-year-old man shows a tiny radiolucent round hole surrounded by a thin sclerotic rim in the femoral head (arrow). (**b**) CT scan reveals a well-defined tiny about 0.8 cm-sized hypodense cystic lesion surrounded by a thin sclerotic rim (arrow) with adjacent sclerotic change in the femoral head. Its subchondral location with pure cystic nature indicates a herniation pit rather than OO. PBS reveals diffuse mild reactive uptake (inset). (**c**) MR images demonstrate a subcortical tiny round lesion with low to intermediate SI on T1-weighted image and high SI on T2-weighted image with a surrounding dark signal of reactive sclerosis on both sequences (yellow arrows). There is a prominent perilesional edema of high signal (red arrows). The lesion itself is not enhanced, but the reactive lesion is well enhanced by contrast medium (inset), suggesting a reactive inflammation with edema, which is thought to be a possible cause of the hip pain

tion (GC) is useful to enhance the resolution of PBS, CR, and MRI in OO so that both the nidi and FVZ can be separately imaged (Fig. 6.11). The use of GC PBS and CR in combination is recommended for the specific diagnosis of oo, providing information about bone metabolism and anatomical characteristics. It can easily differentiate OO from sequestrum of osteomyelitis, abscess, osteogenic sarcoma, hemangioma, and even malignant metastasis [34]. The GCPBS is easy to perform and can substitute for CT scan producing a high-ionizing radiation, paticularly in the pediatricpopulation, as well as high-cost MRI. **CT scan** is the modality of choice to excellently detect and characterize OO lesions, particularly which are obscured or deeply buried in the markedly thickened cortex on routine radiographs (Fig. 6.4). Typically, it exhibits dense, oval to round nidus surrounded by a thin radiolucent area of FVZ, so-called *target-like* appearance (Figs. 6.2, 6.3, 6.5, 6.6, 6.7, and 6.8) or small radiolucent lesion with internal dots (Fig. 6.1d) as well as outermost thick sclerotic reactive bone in both occasions. The mineralization of nidus is clearly seen as punctate dots or ring-like, and it is usually regular. CT scan is particularly useful for the detection of spinal OO. However, CT scan has the disadvantage of exposure to high ionizing radiation, and it can be substituted by GCPBC as mentioned above at the end of radiologic findings section. **MR findings** can be nonspecific with variable signals depending on the amount of osteoid and more matured woven bone or degree of mineralization. Most frequently, the tumor exhibits low to intermediate SI on T1-weighted image and heterogeneous high SI on T2-weighted images (Figs. 6.1, 6.4, 6.5, 6.7, 6.8, 6.9, 6.10, and 6.11). The nidus is sometimes unable to be identified when it is too small or surrounding sclerosis and/or inflammatory changes are significant enough to obscure the nidus. Typically, the nidus may present a *target-like* appearance with intermediate to high central signal often with focal low to dark signal of calcification, which is surrounded by variable thickness of low signal suggesting FVZ on T2-weighted image (Fig. 6.11c). The nidus is heterogeneously enhanced with more intense enhancement at the periphery due to the surrounding FVZ, but the mineralization portion of the low signal is not enhanced (Fig. 6.1c). Occasionally, the lesion may be misinterpreted as aggressive lesion particularly if extensive bone marrow and surrounding soft tissue edema is associated without demonstration of the nidus. Therefore, MRI may not be recommended as a routine evaluation for the diagnosis of OO. However, MRI might be preferred to CT, especially in the pediatric population, to prevent exposure to high ionizing radiation.

6.8 Histologic Findings

The lesion is characteristically composed of a well-demarcated, round to oval nidus representing the neoplastic process and surrounding dense thick reactive bone which is not a part of the tumor. There is a distinct demarcation between nidus and reactive bone by a thin FVZ. The intertrabecular spaces are filled with fibrous tissues and prominent vessels, presenting as a central focal hotter uptake on bone scan and heterogeneous strong enhancement on MRI. In contrast, the thin FVZ has poor vascularity (Fig. 6.13a–c) and is reflected as a thin radiolucent zone surrounding a sclerotic nidus on image studies (Figs. 6.2, 6.6, 6.7, 6.8, and 6.11) or *rim sign* on pinhole bone scan (Figs. 6.1, 6.2, 6.5, 6.8, and 6.11). The nidus contains a variable amount of osteoid and woven bone seams in a random manner with osteoblastic rimming, and is surrounded by a thin FVZ. However, there is no true lamellar bone or cartilage. The osteoid tissue is usually more mature and denser with mineralization or ossification in the center because this part is older than the peripheral area, which appears as tiny radiopaque dot(s) within the nidus on radiograph or CT scan. If the nidus is less matured and contains prominent osteoid and scanty to no woven bone, the lesion can appear as a tiny hazy lucent defect on radiograph or CT scan. The osteoblasts are uniformly plump and have regular-shaped nuclei with abundant cytoplasm. Varying degrees of proliferation of spindle cells and osteoclasts with hemorrhage and prominent vascularity occur between irregularly serrated thick woven bone with osteoblastic rimming, which is identical to those in osteoblastoma except overall size of the lesion (Fig. 6.13d). Thus, radiologic correlation is mandatory to differentiate those entities by the location and size of the lesion. With time, the nidus becomes more

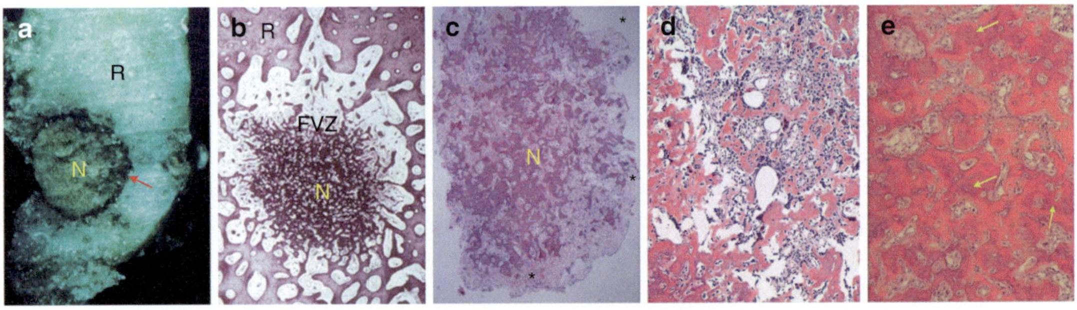

Fig. 6.13 *Microscopic features.* (**a**) Gross specimen from en-bloc resection shows a round to oval, yellowish-colored nidus (N) surrounded by a 1–2 mm thin, black, ring-like FVZ (red arrow). A dense reactive sclerotic bone (R) surrounding the nidus is significantly thickened. All of these findings are reflected more clearly in GC of PBS, CR, and MRI, which is pathognomonic for a diagnosis of OO without histologic confirmation. (**b**) Scanning view microscopic examination reveals a nidus (N) surrounded by reactive thick host cortical bone (R). There is a thin FVZ between the nidus and reactive bone. (**c**) Low-power magnification demonstrates a well-defined tiny nidus (N) consisting of randomly interconnecting trabeculae of osteoid and woven bones surrounded by a thin FVZ (asterisks). (**d**) Medium-power magnification presents a marked cellular proliferation between irregularly anastomosing woven bone trabeculae, prominently rimmed by osteoblasts. The intertrabecular stroma consists of loose connective tissues with prominent bland spindle cells, dilated vascular channels, and even scattered osteoclast-like giant cells. The histologic findings are identical to those in osteoblastoma. Thus, clinical, radiological, and histologic correlation is mandatory for differentiation of both entities. (**e**) Sclerotic nidus with a confluence of mineralized osteoid to lamellar bone trabecular is observed. Note prominent cement lines mimicking a pagetoid mosaic pattern, suggesting more maturation bones (yellow arrows)

sclerotic with confluence of mineralized osteoid even to lamellar bone trabeculae with prominent cement lines in pagetoid mosaic pattern, suggesting an older nidus (Fig. 6.13e).

6.9 Management

Although many authors reported spontaneous resolution of pain and healing of the lesions in a long period of several years [35–40], complete surgical removal of the nidus has been considered a standard option for patients with unremitting pain despite conservative treatment or those who could not tolerate long-term use of NSAID. Nonoperative management including periodic observation or pain control by NSAID medication can be considered as an option owing to the natural history of spontaneous healing (Figs. 6.9 and 6.10). However, it takes such a long period of 2–4 years that it is usually not tolerated to take the drugs, especially for children, and not suitable for possible adverse events such as gastrointestinal bleeding or renal dysfunction. Atar et al. [41] described two stages of the disease. The first stage is characterized by pain lasting 18–36 months, during which continuous use of analgesics is necessary. The second stage includes the healing of the nidus, which usually takes 3–7 years. The pain was relieved with NSAID after an average of 33 months ranging from 30 to 40 months of treatment [38]. Goto et al. [39] reported mean period of time until spontaneous diminution of pain in the 14 patients without NSAID was 75 months (range 24–180 months), but 8 out of the 12 patients with regular use of NSAID were free of pain even after discontinuing the drugs in the average of 18.3 months (range 2–36 months). They concluded ingestion of NSAID accelerates spontaneous healing, and it can be an important option alternative to surgical excision. Aspirin is contraindicated in children younger than 12 years old because of the possible development of Reye syndrome. Despite the lack of histological proof, recent development of high-quality CT scan and GCPBS in correlation of clinical history of a characteristic pain can make a correct diagnosis. Hazards of development of side-effects due to the prolonged course of medications can be expected, but the morbidity has been reported to be lower than that associated with operative treatment. More recently, newly developed selective COX-2 inhibitors are used to treat OO more safely [30]. The surgical procedure includes excision of the nidus (enucleation), curettage, or en-bloc resection. Despite the small size of lesion, the operative procedure can be extensive to find the small nidus buried in the thickened cortex, and sometimes residual nidus remains due to incomplete removal. Local recurrence rate is inversely related to the aggressiveness of the surgery. Intralesional curettage has the highest recurrent rate because of possibility of incomplete nidus excision, and en-bloc resection has the lowest recurrence rate. Enucleation or En-bloc surgical resection has a reported success rate between 88% and 100%, but with several disadvantages, such as difficulty to identify the precise location of the nidus and excision of a substantial volume of bone to ensure complete removal of the nidus, substentially leading to pathologic fracture (Fig. 6.6e). However, the nidus can be easily and completely removed by a simple *burr-down* technique with minimal removal of the host bone. An adequate localization and delineation of the nidus on high-quality C-arm image intensifier are crucial for correct exposure of the nidus deeply buried within markedly thick, reactive scelrotic bone (Fig. 6.5e). Using high-speed burr, the reactive thick sclerotic bone can be continuously and safely peeled off until the nidus begins to appear as a red-colored small round to oval spot (Fig. 6.5f). Then, the ridge of surrounding reactive bone needs to be removed with caution to preserve the nidus intact for a complete removal by curette (Fig. 6.5g). During the past decade, efforts were deployed to minimize bone removal, reduce the risk of pathologic fracture, and decrease the need forbone grafting. Recently, minimally invasive techniques such as CT-guided percutaneous radiofrequency (PRF) thermal ablation (Fig. 6.3d and i) or laser photocoagulation have become widely accepted methods of choice for the treatment of all localizations except those in contact with neural structures such as vertebral OO. PRF ablation under

CT guidance has been widely used with rapidly increasing frequency since the first successful result by Rosenthal et al. [42]. It provides rapid pain relief, early return to function with minimal morbidity, and shorter hospital stays when compared with traditional surgical removal. PRF ablation can be principally indicated in the deep-seated lesions of femoral neck or pelvis. It has a reported success rate close to 100% and lower recurrence rate of about 5% with almost negligible post-procedural complications [43–46]. Complications may include skin burns, skin and fat necrosis, soft-tissue infections, vasomotor instability, tendinitis, and hematoma, and another drawback is the inability to obtain biopsy specimens for microscopic examination.

6.10 Clinical Course

The nidus has a self-limited growing potential, which takes, however, a long period of several years to disappear. In some cases managed by analgesics, the pain was reported to be subsided with eventual regression of nidus after about 3 years of medication [3]. In my patients managed by an intermittent use of analgesic, it took about 4–5 years for healing of the lesion (Figs. 6.9e and 6.10e). The thick reactive zone of sclerosis gradually disappeared after removal of the nidus. Local recurrence will not occur if the nidus is completely removed by en-bloc resection and even marginal or intralesional procedure. Rarely, typical OO has been reported to progress into osteoblastoma [3, 47, 48]. Malignant transformation is not reported in the Mayo Clinic series [5]. However, one case of malignant transformation from OO to high-grade osteosarcoma has been reported in the cervical spine [49].

References

1. Czerniak B. Benign osteoblastic tumors. In: Dorfman HD, Czerniak B, editors. Dorfman and Czerniak's bone tumors. 2nd ed. eBook: Elsevier; 2016. p. 144–99.
2. Picci P, Mirra JM. Osteoid osteoma. In: Mirra JM, editor. Bone tumors: clinical, radiologic, and pathologic correlation. 2nd ed. Philadelphia, PA: Lea & Febiger; 1989. p. 248–438.
3. Campanacci M. Osteoid osteoma. In: Campanacci M, editor. Bone and soft tissue tumors. Wien, Austria: Springer-Verlag; 1999. p. 391–414.
4. Edeiken J, Depalma A, Hodes P. Osteoid osteoma (roentgenographic emphasis). Clin Orthop Relat Res. 1966;49:201–8.
5. Unni KK, Inwards Y. Osteoid osteoma. In: Dahlin's bone tumors: general aspects and data on 10,165 cases. Philadelphia: Lippincott Williams & Wilkins; 2010. p. 102–11.
6. Schajowicz F. Tumors and tumorlike lesions of bone and joints. Springer; 1994.
7. Habermann ET, STERN RE. Osteoid-osteoma of the tibia in an eight-month-old boy: a case report. J Bone Joint Surg. 1974;56(3):633–6.
8. Cohen MD, Harrington TM, Ginsburg WW. Osteoid osteoma: 95 cases and a review of the literature. Semin Arthritis Rheum. 1983;12(3):265–81.
9. Barlow E, Davies A, Cool W, Barlow D, Mangham D. Osteoid osteoma and osteoblastoma: novel histological and immunohistochemical observations as evidence for a single entity. J Clin Pathol. 2013;66(9):768–74.
10. Kan P, Schmidt MH. Osteoid osteoma and osteoblastoma of the spine. Neurosurg Clin N Am. 2008;19(1):65–70.
11. Healey JH, Ghelman B. Osteoid osteoma and osteoblastoma. Current concepts and recent advances. Clin Orthop Relat Res. 1986;204:76–85.
12. Pettine KA, Klassen R. Osteoid-osteoma and osteoblastoma of the spine. J Bone Joint Surg Am. 1986;68(3):354–61.
13. McDermott MB, Kyriakos M, McEnery K. Painless osteoid osteoma of the rib in an adult: a case report and a review of the literature. Cancer. 1996;77(8):1442–9.
14. Kransdorf M, Stull M, Gilkey F, Moser R Jr. Osteoid osteoma. Radiographics. 1991;11(4):671–96.
15. Jackson RP, Reckling FW, Mantz FA. Osteoid osteoma and osteoblastoma: similar histologic lesions with different natural histories. Clin Orthop Relat Res. 1977;128:303–13.
16. Glynn JJ, Lichtenstein L. Osteoid-osteoma with multicentric nidus: a report of two cases. J Bone Joint Surg. 1973;55(4):855–8.
17. Greenspan A. Multifocal osteoid osteoma. A case report and review of the literature. Am J Roentgenol. 1974;121(1):103–6. https://doi.org/10.2214/ajr.121.1.103.
18. Uehlinger E. Multizentrisches Osteoid-Osteom des Tibiaschaftes mit atypischem Röntgenbild. Archiv für orthopädische und Unfall-Chirurgie, mit besonderer Berücksichtigung der Frakturenlehre und der orthopädisch-chirurgischen Technik. 1977;89(1):101–7.
19. Keret D, Harcke HT, MacEwen GD, Bowen J. Multiple osteoid osteomas of the fifth lumbar vertebra. A case report. Clin Orthop Relat Res. 1989;248:163–8.

20. Allieu Y, Lussiez B, Benichou M, Cenac P. A double nidus osteoid osteoma in a finger. J Hand Surg Am. 1989;14(3):538–41.
21. Muren C, Höglund M, Engkvist O, Juhlin L. Osteoid osteomas of the hand: report of three cases and review of the literature. Acta Radiol. 1991;32(1):62–6.
22. Nelson M, Lack E, Freedman M. Multifocal osteoid osteoma in a 2.5 year-old child. Skeletal Radiol. 1994;23:465–7.
23. Schai P, Friederich N, Krüger A, Jundt G, Herbe E, Buess P. Discrete synchronous multifocal osteoid osteoma of the humerus. Skeletal Radiol. 1996;25(7):667–70.
24. Gonzalez G, Abril J, Mediero I, Epeldegui T. Osteoid osteoma with a multicentric nidus. Int Orthop. 1996;20(1):61–3.
25. Sherman M, McFarland G Jr. Mechanism of pain in osteoid osteomas. South Med J. 1965;58:163–6.
26. Schulman L, Dorfman HD. Nerve fibers in osteoid osteoma. J Bone Joint Surg. 1970;52(7):1351–6.
27. Byers PD. Solitary benign osteoblastic lesions of bone. Osteoid osteoma and benign osteoblastoma. Cancer. 1968;22(1):43–57.
28. Makley J, Dunn M. Prostaglandin synthesis by osteoid osteoma. Lancet. 1982;320(8288):42. https://doi.org/10.1016/s0140-6736(82)91174-6.
29. Greco F, Tamburrelli F, Ciabattoni G. Prostaglandins in osteoid osteoma. Int Orthop. 1991;15(1):35–7.
30. Mungo DV, Zhang X, O'Keefe RJ, Rosier RN, Puzas JE, Schwarz EM. COX-1 and COX-2 expression in osteoid osteomas. J Orthop Res. 2002;20(1):159–62.
31. Bahk YW. Benign bone tumors and tumorous conditions of bone. In: Bahk YW, editor. Combined scintigraphic and radiographic diagnosis of bone and joint diseases. 3rd ed. Berlin, Heidelberg: Springer; 2007. p. 401–55.
32. Helms C. Radionuclide skeletal survey for pediatric neoplasms. Radiology. 1984;151:779–85.
33. Kim JY, Chung SK, Park YH, Kim SH, Shinn KS, Bahk YW. Pinhole bone scintigraphic appearances of osteoid osteoma. Korean J Radiol. 1992;26(1):160–3.
34. Bahk YW, Kim SH, Chung YA, Bahk WJ, Park JM, Kang YM, et al. Depiction of nidi and fibrovascular zones of osteoid osteomas using gamma-correction Tc-99m HDP pinhole bone scan and conventional radiograph, and correlation with CT, MRI, and PVC phantom imaging. Nucl Med Mol Imaging. 2011;45(1):21–9.
35. Golding J. The natural history of osteoid osteoma; with a report of twenty cases. J Bone Joint Surg Br. 1954;36(2):218–29.
36. Moberg E. The natural course of osteoid osteoma. J Bone Joint Surg. 1951;33(1):166–70.
37. Vickers CW, Pugh DC, Ivins JC. Osteoid osteoma: a fifteen-year follow-up of an untreated patient. J Bone Joint Surg. 1959;41(2):357–8.
38. Kneisl J, Simon M. Medical management compared with operative treatment for osteoid-osteoma. J Bone Joint Surg Am. 1992;74(2):179–85.
39. Goto T, Shinoda Y, Okuma T, Ogura K, Tsuda Y, Yamakawa K, et al. Administration of nonsteroidal anti-inflammatory drugs accelerates spontaneous healing of osteoid osteoma. Arch Orthop Trauma Surg. 2011;131(5):619–25.
40. Simm R. The natural history of osteoid osteoma. ANZ J Surg. 1975;45(4):412–5.
41. Atar D, Lehman W, Grant A. Tips of the trade. Computerized tomography–guided excision of osteoid osteoma. Orthop Rev. 1992;21(12):1457–8.
42. Rosenthal DI, Alexander A, Rosenberg AE, Springfield D. Ablation of osteoid osteomas with a percutaneously placed electrode: a new procedure. Radiology. 1992;183(1):29–33.
43. Lanza E, Thouvenin Y, Viala P, Sconfienza LM, Poretti D, Cornalba G, et al. Osteoid osteoma treated by percutaneous thermal ablation: when do we fail? A systematic review and guidelines for future reporting. Cardiovasc Intervent Radiol. 2014;37(6):1530–9.
44. Çakar M, Esenyel CZ, Seyran M, Tekin AÇ, Adaş M, Bayraktar MK, et al. Osteoid osteoma treated with radiofrequency ablation. Adv Orthop. 2015;2015:807274. https://doi.org/10.1155/2015/807274.
45. Lassalle L, Campagna R, Corcos G, Babinet A, Larousserie F, Stephanazzi J, et al. Therapeutic outcome of CT-guided radiofrequency ablation in patients with osteoid osteoma. Skeletal Radiol. 2017;46(7):949–56.
46. Motamedi D, Learch TJ, Ishimitsu DN, Motamedi K, Katz MD, Brien EW, et al. Thermal ablation of osteoid osteoma: overview and step-by-step guide. Radiographics. 2009;29(7):2127–41.
47. Bruneau M, Polivka M, Cornelius JF, George B. Progression of an osteoid osteoma to an osteoblastoma: case report. J Neurosurg Spine. 2005;3(3):238–41.
48. Chotel F, Franck F, Solla F, Dijoud F, Kohler R, Berard J, et al. Osteoid osteoma transformation into osteoblastoma: fact or fiction? Orthop Traumatol Surg Res. 2012;98(6):S98–S104. https://doi.org/10.1016/j.otsr.2012.03.017.
49. Sugiyama T, Fushimi K, Nagano A, Tsugita M, Nozawa S, Iwai C, et al. The malignant transformation of osteoid osteoma in the cervical spine to high-grade osteosarcoma: a case report and review of literature. Br J Neurosurg. 2023;37(5):1023–7. https://doi.org/10.1080/02688697.2020.1842326.

Osteoblastoma

(***osteo*** "bone" + ***blastos*** "germ" + ***ōma*** "forming")

7

7.1 Definition

Osteoblastoma (OB) is a rare benign, locally aggressive bone tumor producing osteoid and woven bone, which is histologically identical to osteoid osteoma (OO), but OB exceeds 2 cm in diameter with a higher growth potential.

7.2 Synonym

Giant ostoid osteoma (non-preferred histological term).

7.3 Incidence

The incidence is rare, accounting for about 3% of all benign bone tumors and less than 1% of all bone tumors [1–5]. Its frequency is at least five times less than OO and 10 times less than osteosarcoma (OSA) [6].

7.4 Age

The lesion occurs most commonly in children, teenagers, and young adults between the ages of 10 and 30 years with a peak incidence in the second decade of life, being similar to that of OO and OSA. Up to 90% of patients are less than 30 years old [2, 3, 7].

7.5 Location

It may occur in any bones of the body but has an evident predilection for the axial skeleton, including the spine and sacrum , in more than 40% of cases [4–6] (Figs. 7.1 and 7.2). In the spine, posterior elements including lamina and pedicles are most frequently involved. The next common location is the jaw and other cranial bones. Other locations include long tubular bones (Fig. 7.3), pelvic bones, and short tubular bone of the foot (Fig. 7.4). In the long bones, OB involves the medulla rather than the cortex frequently in the meta-diaphysis of the proximal femur and humerus, where its overall distribution is similar to that of OO. However, OO is usually in or near the cortex rather than being buried deep within the medullary space (Fig. 7.5). In Mayo Clinic series, approximately 80% were metaphyseal and diaphyseal location, and the remaining 20% were located within the epiphysis [3] (Fig. 7.6a). OBs are mostly solitary, but they can only rarely be multicentric (involving more than one bone) or multifocal (having more than one nidus within a single bone) (Fig. 7.6).

W.-J. Bahk, *Diagnosis and Management of Primary Bone Tumors*,
https://doi.org/10.1007/978-981-96-3484-2_7

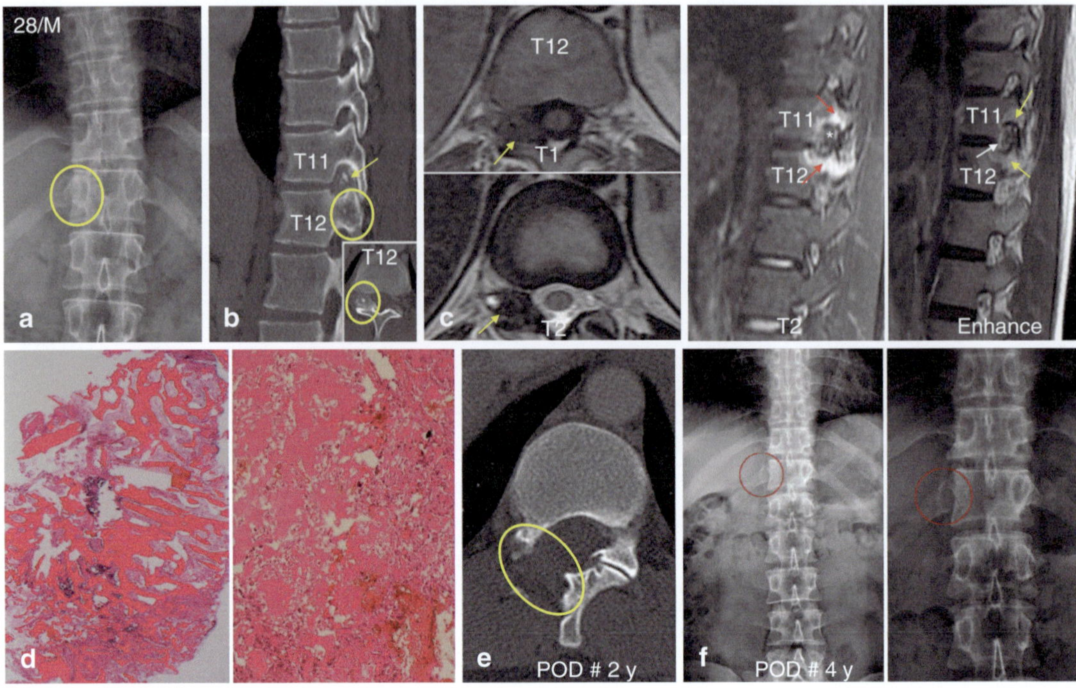

Fig. 7.1 *Spinal location.* (**a**) Radiographs taken for back pain of 6 months' duration in a 28-year-old man show a radiolucent lesion with internal fine, dense spots at the right costovertebral junction of T12 spine (circle) with mild listing curvature of the D-L spine. (**b**) CT scan more clearly reveals a relatively well-defined lytic lesion with tiny central calcification foci, which is partially surrounded by reactive sclerotic bone mainly affecting the right pedicle and focally facet joint of the D12 spine (circles). The lesion extends into the intervertebral foraminal space between T11 and T12 spines with internal calcific foci (arrow). (**c**) MR axial images demonstrate a relatively well-defined mass-like lesion with low to intermediate SI on T1-weighted and heterogeneous low SI with focal high signal on T2-weighted image (yellow arrows). Note an ill-defined, extensive, reactive inflammatory response including edema fluid of high signals (red arrows) surrounding the 2.3 × 2.5 cm sized soft tissue mass with heterogeneous signal (asterisk), so-called *flare phenomenon* on sagittal view, that obscures the actual bone tumor of T12 pedicle (lower red arrow). The phenomenon simulates a malignant process such as lymphoma or Ewing sarcoma. The tumor itself is peripherally and focally enhanced (white arrow), and the surrounding inflammatory areas in the pedicles of T11 and T12 spines are diffusely well enhanced (yellow arrows). (**d**) Microscopic examination: (Left) Low-power magnification notes a loose fibroblastic stroma with an interconnecting network of woven bone trabeculae. (Right) Higher-power magnification shows hypocellular bland stroma and extensive bone formation with prominent dilated capillary-type blood vessels and hemorrhage. A diagnosis of DB was rendered in consideration of the tumor size of more than 2 cm in diameter. (**e**) Follow-up CT scan at 2 years after en-bloc resection with laminectomy and facetectomy notes no evidence of local recurrence. (**f**) Follow-up radiographs at 4 years after surgery show no evidence of local recurrence (red circles) and resolution of the listing curvature

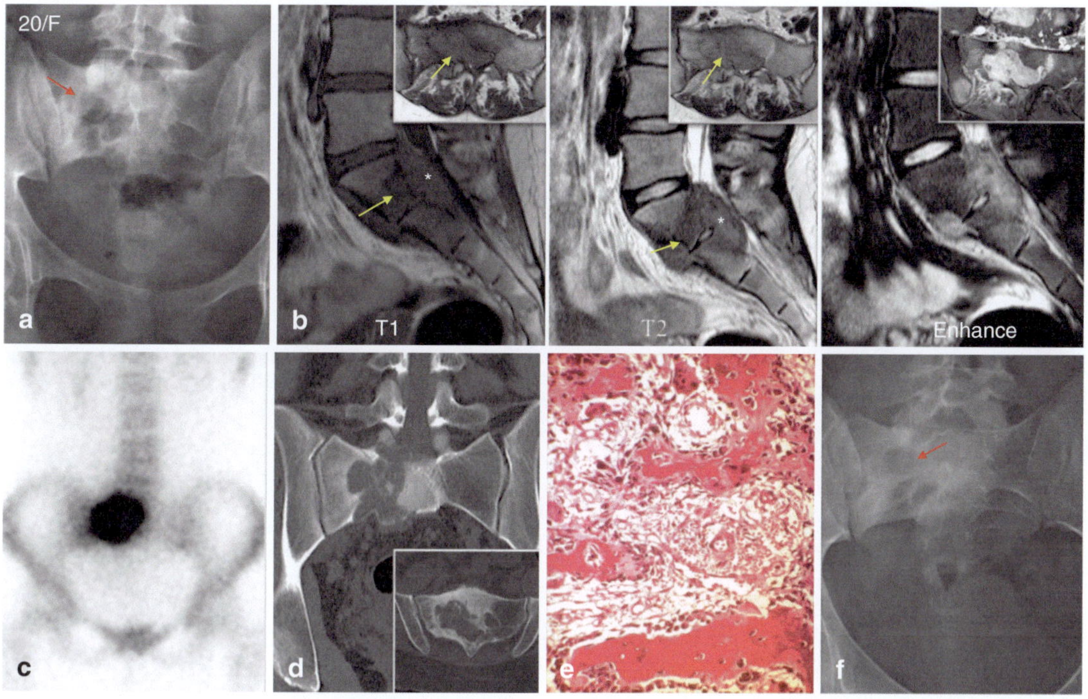

Fig. 7.2 *Sacral location.* (**a**) Radiographs taken for right buttock pain referred to proximal thigh of 1-year's duration in a 20-year-old young woman show a relatively well-defined osteolytic lesion with internal tiny, sclerotic foci, which is surrounded by a thin rim of sclerosis in the right upper sacrum (arrow). (**b**) MR images reveal a well-defined, approxiamtely 5 cm mass-like with low SI on T1- and heterogeneous intermediate SI on T2-weighted image in the first sacral body (yellow arrows). Note tumor extension into the spinal canal through cortical breakage compressing the cauda equina (asterisks). The bone and soft tissue lesion is well-enhanced by contrast medium. (**c**) Bone scan depicts a markedly intense uptake in the right side of the upper sacrum. (**d**) CT scan more clearly demonstrates a well-circumscribed large geographic destruction with internal tiny sclerotic foci. The surrounding bone demonstrates prominent sclerosis. (**e**) Microscopic examination notes interconnecting osteoid and woven bone trabeculae with a prominent osteoblastic rimming and loose, hypocellular intervening stroma with numerous capillaries. (**f**) Follow-up radiograph at 2 years after curettage shows no definite evidence of local recurrence with increased haziness (arrow)

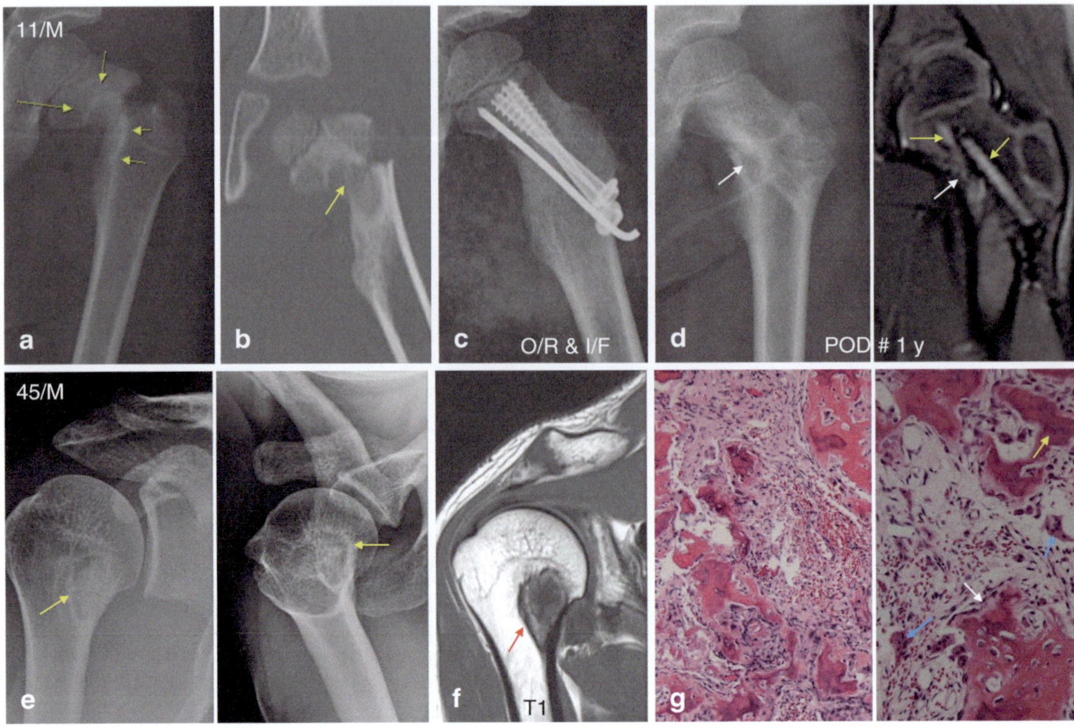

Fig. 7.3 *Long tubular bone. Femur:* (**a**) Radiographs taken for left hip pain after a slip in an 11-year-old boy show a pathologic fracture with severe angulation and gap. There is a concomittent finding of preexisting eccentric, well-defined, mixed lytic and blastic lesion which is surrounded by a thick rim of sclerosis in the intertrochanteric area of the femur (arrows). (**b**) CT scan more clearly reveals intralesional mineralization and the extent of the lesion with a thick surrounding sclerotic rim (arrow). (**c**) Thorough curettage followed by open reduction and multiple screw fixation was performed after histologic confirmation of OB by a frozen biopsy during surgery. (**d**) Follow-up radiograph at 1 year after surgery shows consolidation of the lesion (arrow). MR image reveals tracts of inserted screws (yellow arrows), but also show consolidation of the lesion without evidence of recurrence (white arrow). *Humerus:* (**e**) Radiographs taken for right shoulder pain of 1 year's duration in a 45-year-old boy show a well-defined, eccentric, mostly blastic, and partially lytic lesion surrounded by a thin sclerotic rim of reactive bone (arrows) in the humeral neck. (**f**) T1-weighted image reveals a well-defined eccentrically located medullary lesion with low and intermediate SI surrounded by a thin dark signal of sclerotic rim (arrow). (**g**) Microscopic examination. (Left) Low-power magnification notes an interconnecting network of osteoid and woven bone trabeculae with loose bland fibroblastic stroma and prominent hemorrhage and vasculature. (Right) Higher-power magnification shows bland stromal cells and fully matured woven bone spicules with multiple cement lines mimicking Paget bone (yellow arrow). Note the single layer of prominent osteoblastic rimming (white arrow), which is virtually never seen in high-grade OSA. A few multinucleated giant cells are also scattered (blue arrows)

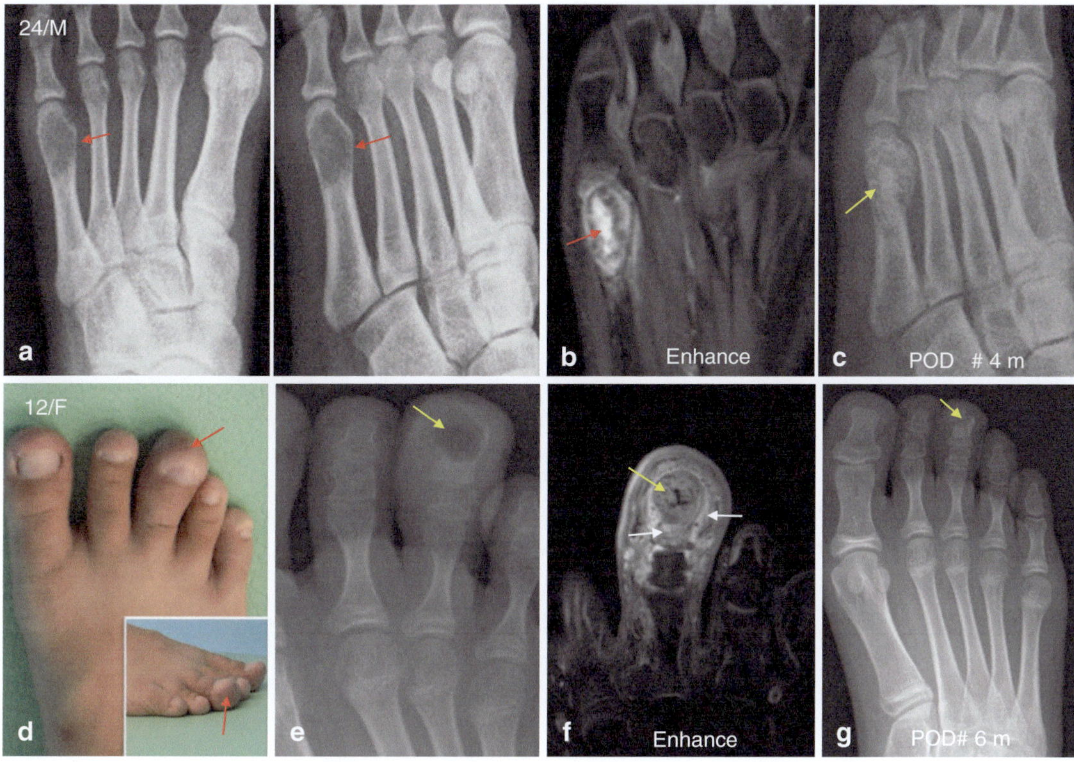

Fig. 7.4 *Short tubular bone. Metatarsal bone:* (**a**) Radiographs taken for left foot pain of 5 months' duration in a 24-year-old man show a concentric, well-defined, osteolytic lesion with multiple tiny sclerotic foci involving distal one-third of the fifth metatarsal bone. The underlying host bone is moderately expanding in fusiform shape with significant cortical thinning but no discernible destruction (arrows). (**b**) MR image reveals an expansile lesion but no cortical breakage with heterogeneous strong enhancement (red arrow) and weaker enhancement of adjacent marrow and soft tissue edema. (**c**) Follow-up radiograph at 4 months after curettage and autogenous bone graft 5 months' duration some consolidation of the lesion (arrow). *Distal phalanx*: (**d**) A 12-year-old girl presents with gradually enlarged right middle toe of 3 years duration (arrows). (**e**) Radiograph shows a well-defined expansile lytic lesion with possible cortical destruction and soft tissue extension in the distal phalanx (arrow). (**f**) However, the MR image reveals a well-defined, balloon-like expanding, mass-like lesion without discernible cortical destruction. The lesion is heterogeneously enhanced (yellow arrow), and adjacent marrow and soft tissue edema are well enhanced (white arrows). (**g**) Follow-up radiograph at 6 months after curettage and allografting demonstrates consilidation of the lesion (arrow)

Fig. 7.5 *A schema showing differences between OO and OB.* Most OOs are less than 2 cm in diameter with limited growth potential and are usually located in or near the cortex rather than being buried deep within the medullary space. In contrast, OBs mostly exceed 2–3 cm in diameter with higher growth potential, and typically affects the medullary space rather than the cortex

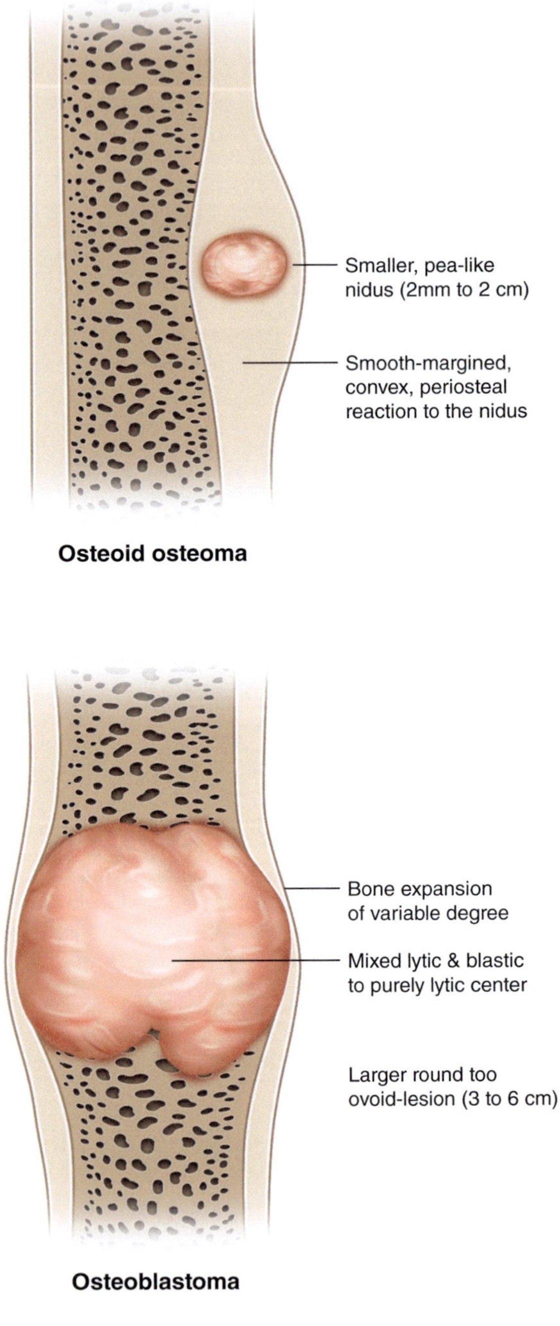

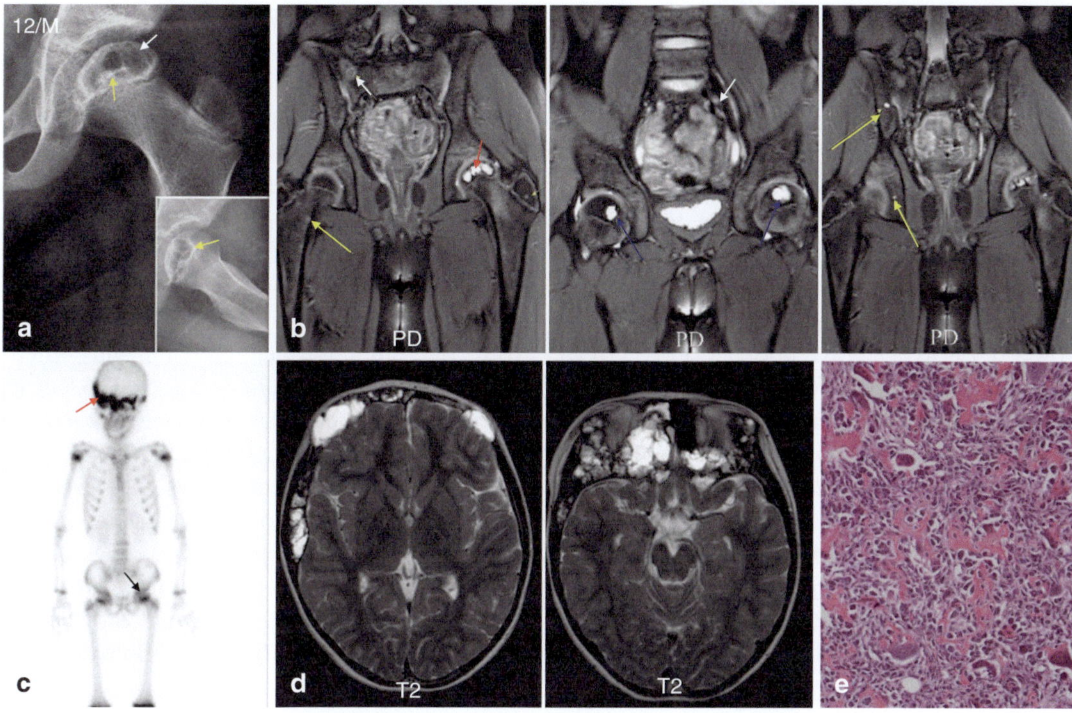

Fig. 7.6 *Multifocal OB.* (**a**) Radiographs taken for intermittent left hip pain of 5–6 months' duration in a 12-year-old man show a multilobulated osteolytic lesion (white arrow) and another well-defined, small, round to oval, more lucent lesion (yellow arrows), which is surrounded by a thin sclerotic rim. (**b**) MR images reveal multiple, round to oval lesions with bright SI in the epiphysis of the left femoral head (red arrow). There are also incidentally found small foci in the sacrum (white arrows) as well as multiple tiny to small lesions in the right femur and iliac bone (blue and yellow arrows), suggesting polyostotic bone tumor. (**c**) Bone scan depicts a focal tiny mild uptake at the left femoral head (black arrow) as well as a thick transverse band-like strong uptake in the temporal bone (red arrow). There is no uptake in other areas. (**d**) Skull MR images note multifocal lobulated mass-like lesions with high SI in the clivus, bifrontal skull base, bilateral sphenoid, and left temporal bones on T2-weighted image. (**e**) Microscopic examination of the biopsy specimen from the temporal bone shows interconnecting osteoid and woven bone trabeculae with prominent osteoblastic rimming and intervening bland spindle cells with numerous capillaries and a few multinucleated giant cells. Considering multiple variable-sized lesions with identical signal involving the femurs, ilium, sacrum, and skull bones, a diagnosis of multifocal OB was rendered. Surgical management was not performed due to the absence of pain or functional impairment in the temporal bone, and only intermittent mild pain in the hip

7.6 Clinical Features

Conventional OB differs from OO in that it has a higher growth potential to grow more than 2 cm in diameter. Moreover, the pain does not respond dramatically to aspirin or NSAIDs and is not most severe at night unlike OO [3, 7]. The incidence of night pain and sweats was reported to be only about 10% [2, 8]. A dull pain of insidious onset over 1–2 years often with progression in intensity is the most common symptom. However, an *aggressive* OB grows more rapidly and may produce severe symptoms such as intractable pain, joint stiffness or contracture, muscle wasting, or soft tissue swelling of short duration due to a severe peri-tumoral inflammatory reaction [6]. Unusually, conventional OB can also induce a pronounced inflammatory reaction in the surrounding soft tissue as in OO [5]. Localized swelling or tenderness is associated when the lesion is superficial. Spinal lesions can cause muscle spasms resulting in scoliosis or torticollis and compress the spinal cord or nerve roots producing neurologic deficits. Pathologic fracture is occasionally associated (Fig. 7.3a). Rarely, even systemic symptoms such as anorexia, fever, and weight loss can be presented due to immune response [8]. Multifocal OBs in a single bone or multicentric lesions in different bones have been mostly described as a single case report [9–13]. However, Lucas et al. [3] reported 43 cases (14%) in their large series of 306 cases of OB that were multifocal, including 4 cases that became multifocal after recurrence. OB can be exceptionally associated with oncogenic phosphaturic syndrome, which clearly regresses by surgical removal of the tumor [14, 15]. An extraordinary case of OB with severe systemic toxicity leading to impeding death secondary to cachexia, so-called *toxic OB* was also reported [16].

7.7 Radiologic Findings

Plain radiograph The lesion shows a wide range of radiographic patterns with varying ratios of osteolytic and osteoblastic densities. The tumor may be purely lytic, mixed lytic and sclerotic, or densely sclerotic (Figs. 7.1, 7.2, 7.3, 7.4, 7.6, 7.7, and 7.8), depending on the ratio of primitive osteoid to mature woven bone production as in OO. However, the nidus usually shows a relatively well-circumscribed, predominantly osteolytic lesion often containing variable extent of internal opaque density. A varying degree of reactive sclerosis may surround the nidus, but it may be minimal or absent unlike OO. The size of the nidus is greater than 2 cm in size often, but most OBs do not exceed 5–6 cm [4, 6]. Unfortunately, radiographic features are often nonspecific and suggest OB in only about 30–40% of cases [2, 3, 7]. When OB involves the

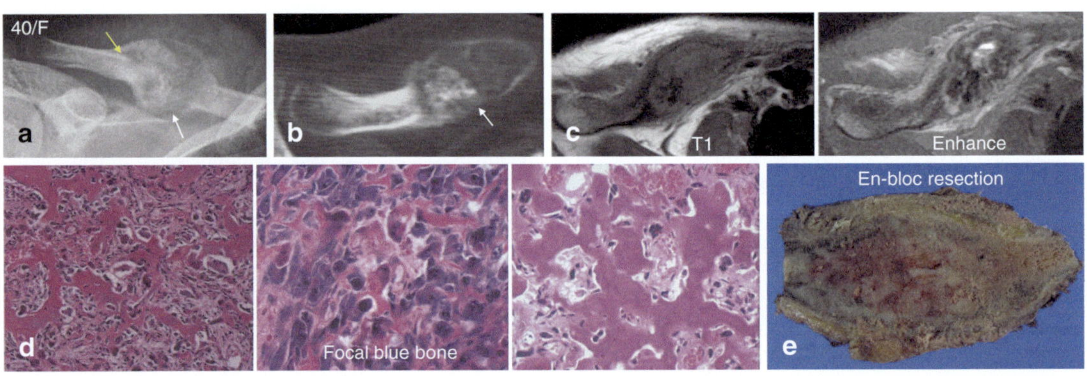

Fig. 7.7 *Aggressive OB*. (**a**) Radiographs taken for a slowly growing hard mass with pain in the right midclavicular area of 5 months' duration in a 40-year-old woman show a relatively well-defined, mixed lytic and sclerotic lesion with expansion in a fusiform shape. There is cortical destruction (white arrow), along with a Codman's triangle (yellow arrow) simulating a malignant bone tumor. (**b**) CT scan more clearly reveals a well-defined expansile lytic and sclerotic lesion with internal mineralization and partial cortical destruction (arrow). (**c**) MR images demonstrate a well-defined mass lesion with low and intermediate SI with focal dark signal of calcification, which is heterogeneously enhanced by contrast medium. (**d**) Microscopic examination. (Left) Medium-power magnification notes interconnecting osteoid to woven bone trabeculae rimmed by a prominent single layer of osteoblasts and an intervening bland loose hypocellular but highly vascular stroma. Many multinucleated giant cells are scattered throughout the lesion. (Middle) Higher-power magnification shows numerous large *epithelioid* osteoblasts at least twice the size of ordinary tumor osteoblasts with abundant eosinophilic cytoplasm and bizarre-shaped large vesicular nuclei with one or more prominent nucleoli. Note irregular osteoid to small trabeculae of immature woven bone that stain dark blue, so-called *blue speculated bone*. (Right) Some *epithelioid* osteoblasts are also seen within the trabeculae. (**e**) En-bloc resection was performed

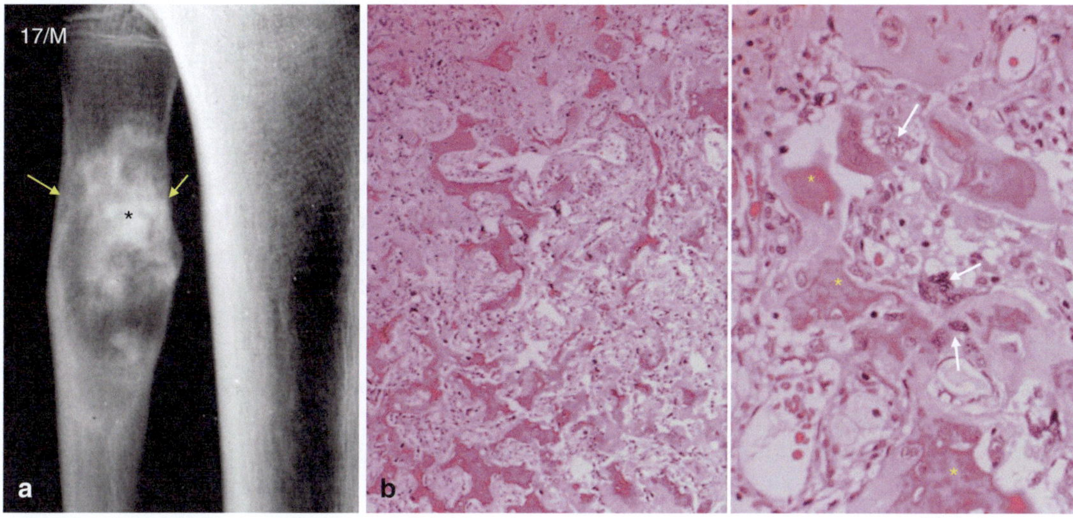

Fig. 7.8 *Pseudoanaplastic OB*. (**a**) Radiographs taken for acute knee pain during basketball playing in a 17-year-old boy incidentally show a fusiform, moderately expanded, osteolytic lesion mixed with intralesional sclerotic density (asterisk), indicating heavy mature woven bone production. There is a significant cortical thinning but no discernible breaches or destruction (yellow arrows), indicative of a benign bone-producing lesion, most consistent with OB. No significant change in the lesion was noted after 18 months without biopsy and any treatment due to the patient's initial refusal. (**b**) Microscopic examination. (Left) Moderate-power magnification shows an area conventional OB, which consists of irregularly interconnecting spicules of osteoid and woven bone with osteoblasts and numerous dilated capillary vessels. (Right) Higher-power magnification reveals osteoid to woven bone spicules and bizarre cells with extremely bizarre, huge nuclei (arrows), which were initially mistaken for OSA by the general pathologist. However, the surgeon decided to perform marginal excision without chemotherapy because the lesion had changed little during 18 months of follow-up without any treatment. And, the pathologic slides were sent to Professor Mirra for a second opinon. He made a final diagnosis of *pseudoanaplastic* OB based on total absence of true mitoses despite the presence of bizarre cells, following a thorough review of all sections and unchanged benign-looking radiographic pattern and clinical fact of incidentally found lesion. A diagnostic triangle of clinic, radiologic, and pathologic correlation is emphasized here for a correct diagnosis of this particular difficult case. The benign nature of the lesion was confirmed by patient's favorable outcome, without local recurrence or metastasis at 7 years after simple curettage

spine, it is usually localized within the posterior elements including lamina, pedicle, transverse, or spinous process. In contrast, OSA and giant cell tumor usually affect the spine body. The lesion is round to ovoid with focal cortical expansion and varying degree of fine, lacy network of intralesional densities, suggesting a bone-forming lesion. However, the abnormal bone density may not be seen when the quality of the radiograph is poor [4–6]. In the tubular bone, OB lesion is most often intramedullary, while OO is almost always intracortical, although either may occur in any portion of the bone. The lesion may be eccentric (Fig. 7.3) or centric particularly when affecting small bone (Fig. 7.4) and usually shows a relatively well-circumscribed, predominantly lytic lesion with variable extent of internal opacity. The lesion can exhibit a bubbly appearance with internal calcification, or patchy or cloud-like opacities, suggesting the bone-forming nature of the lesion. It also shows a varying degree of cortical expansion, usually eccentric, or often expands the host bone in a fusiform shape, and extends into soft tissues through the cortical breakage. However, the soft tissue components are usually contained by the intact periosteum. There can be a periosteal reaction with a tendency to produce a surrounding sclerotic shell which demarcates the tumor from the normal soft tissue [4, 6]. Occasionally, the lesion exhibits poorly demarcated destruction with Codman's triangle. Such locally aggressive-looking features simulating malignancy were found in about 25% of 123 patients in one series [2] and 12% of 306 patients in later series of the same institute [3]. The later series also reported that 72% of cases were thought to appear as benign, 10% malignant, and the remaining to be indeterminate in appendicular OB, based solely on their radiographic appearance. In contrast, 52% were thought to be benign, 33% indeterminate, and 15% malignant in vertebral OB. Rarely, multicentric (involving different bones) or multifocal (in a single bone) lesions can be presented (Fig. 7.6). Kyriakos et al. [17] reported two cases of histologically proven multifocal and multicentric OBs in the femur and tibia radiologically simulating a vascular tumor. An *aggressive* OB shares common radiographic features of conventional OB sometimes with a locally aggressive-looking appearance even including cortical breakage and adjacent soft tissue extension simulating a malignant tumor as well as larger size than conventional OB, usually exceeding 4 cm in diameter [18]. **Bone scan** usually reveals an intense focal uptake at the site of the lesion (Fig. 7.2c) and is very useful to detect rare case of multifocal or multicentric lesions (Fig. 7.6c). **CT scan** more clearly demonstrates a well-circumscribed expansile lytic and sclerotic lesion surrounded by varying degrees of reactive bone. It is useful to appreciate mineralization and to evaluate the extent of bone destruction (Figs. 7.1, 7.2, and 7.3). CT is reported to be superior to MRI in characterizing the morphology and matrix of tumor [19]. **MR findings** are nonspecific and MRI often overestimates the lesion. The lesion is usually well-defined with low to intermediate SI on T1-weighted image and heterogeneous intermediate SI with high signal of surrounding bone marrow and soft tissue edema on T2-weighted image. There are dark signals corresponding to the foci of calcification or rim of reactive sclerosis on both sequences. Rarely, extensive edema and inflammatory response in the adjacent bone marrow and soft tissues are so severe, which can be overestimated and often mistaken for a malignant tumor such as lymphoma or Ewing sarcoma. Crim et al. [20] described a severe inflammatory response involving several adjacent bones and soft tissue, occasionally producing a soft tissue mass, which is diffusely enhanced by contrast medium reflecting the inflammatory nature of the process and may cause overestimation of the size of the lesion. The soft tissue mass was histologically confirmed to be merely part of an inflammatory reaction but not tumor extension, and they called this *flare phenomenon*. Because of the extensive inflammatory response, the actual tumor site can be not appreciated on MR images (Fig. 7.1c), and this led to inadequate biopsy. Secondary aneurysmal bone cyst (ABC) is also associated in rare cases as in other benign bone tumors. The peri-tumoral bone and soft tissue lesion is diffusely enhanced by contrast medium reflecting the inflammatory nature of the process, which may cause an overestimation of aggressiveness and the size of the lesion (Fig. 7.1c). As a matter of course, the tumor itself is also avidly enhanced because OB is a highly vascular tumor (Figs. 7.1, 7.2, 7.3, 7.4, 7.6, and 7.7).

7.8 Histologic Findings

Microscopic features of OB are identical to those of OO. The tumor is characterized by a bland loose fibroblastic stroma with prominent vasculature and interconnecting network of osteoid and woven bone trabeculae, considerably rimmed by a single layer of osteoblasts, a feature virtually never seen in high-grade OSA. Degrees of maturation of the bone trabeculae vary from primitive osteoid to fully matured woven bone with multiple cement lines mimicking Pagetoid bone, but no true lamellar bone (Figs. 7.1, 7.2, 7.3, and 7.6). The osteoid or woven bone is usually deposited in coarse trabeculae or sparsely cellular sheets, but areas focally showing a lacelike appearance are occasionally identified in about 20% of cases [3]. The osteoblasts are usually uniform and bland. However, some lesions may consist of *epithelioid* osteoblasts occasionally proliferating in a multifocal pattern (more than one nidus within a single tumor), which can be mistaken for OSA particularly when combined with atypical bizarre cells, typical mitoses, and lace-like osteoid production. For diagnosis of OB, host lamellar bone destruction by *permeation* pattern, unequivocal anaplasia, and atypical mitosis which are characteristics of OSA should be absent. Focal areas containing chondroid matrix have been reported in about 6% of the patients [3, 21], but they have no clinical significance. Secondary ABC presenting multiple cystic spaces filled with blood may expand and enlarge the lesion. Multinucleated giant cells are often scattered, numerously or focally. Mitotic figures are mostly meager and typical. Those were nil to minimal in 89% of cases, moderate in 10%, and prominent in only 1% in a large series [3]. In 1973, Dorfman [22] first introduced the term *aggressive OB*, and two new cases were subsequently described by Revel and Scholtz [23]. Many histologic findings of aggressive and conventional OB may overlap. However, a hallmark of *aggressive OB* is the presence of *epithelioid* osteoblasts rimming the osteoid trabeculae as well as occasionally being within the trabeculae and forming loosely cohesive solid sheets that fill the intertrabecular spaces. In addition, one or more characteristic features such as bizarre-looking nuclei, more frequent mitotic activity as well as immature, small trabeculae staining dark blue, so-called *blue speculated bone* (Fig. 7.7d). The mere presence of *epithelioid* osteoblasts does not qualify the lesion as aggressive, and it is unable to identify any single histologic feature that could reliably predict aggressive behavior [3]. A large *epithelioid* osteoblast was defined as cells at least twice the size of ordinary tumor osteoblasts, with abundant eosinophilic cytoplasm and large vesicular nuclei with one or more prominent nucleoli by Dorfman and Weiss [18]. They also suggested that rare tumors can exist with histologic and radiographic features that straddle the border between OB and OSA and that most of these probably represent OB-like OSA. An *Aggressive OB* shows a more aggressive clinical course with a higher incidence of local recurrence than conventional OB, but no distant metastases. In 1976, Schajowicz and Lemos [24] described the clinical, radiographic, and pathologic features of eight cases of locally aggressive tumor under the name of *malignant OB*, which should be differentiated from OSA because of its peculiar histological pattern, diffrent radiographic findings, and clinical course with much better prognosis. The patients' ages varied widely from 6 to 67 years, with an average of 34 years. The lesion frequently recurs but does not metastasize with good prognosis. Radiologically, the lesion appeared extremely variable and was not diagnostic from expansion only with thinning of the cortex simulating giant cell tumor to destruction of the cortex with soft tissue extension mimicking sarcoma. The lesions present the typical histologic features of genuine OB and other aggressive features such as more abundant and larger osteoblasts with plump or bizarre hyperchromatic nuclei and frequent mitotic activity including rare atypical mitoses. There were foci alternating with fields rich in multinucleated giant cells. In addition, the authors described occasional zones of irregular, densely calcified immature osteoid (*spiculated blue bone*), which are lacking in conventional OB. However, it was observed in only 16% of 306 OBs in Mayo Clinic series [3]. In the same series, large epithelioid osteoblasts were identified in about one-fourth of cases, but they were the predominant cellular element only in 10% of cases. In addition, the authors observed a tendency for multifocal tumors to contain *epithelioid* osteoblasts, and two-thirds of the *epithelioid osteoblast-rich* tumors also had a multifocal pattern. Extraordinary, OB may histologically resembles a malignant tumor due to extremely bizarre histologic changes but is not aggressive form in biologic and clinical standpoints. Such cases have been called *pseudoanaplastic* OB because the lesion looks pleomorphic but is a naïve benign lesion which typically lacks abnormal mitoses and runs a benign clinical course [25, 26] (Fig. 7.8).

7.9 Management

Surgical management is the standard option because the lesion has potential for locally aggressive behavior and bone destruction. Surgical options depend on the stage and location of the tumor. Curettage is indicated for stage 1 (latent) and stage 2 (active) lesions, but resection is required for stage 3 (aggressive) lesion. Thorough curettage using high-speed burr or marginal resection is usually sufficient in most cases, but local adjuvant such as cryosurgery using liquid nitrogen or chemical cauterization with phenol may be considered after curettage to reduce the risk of local recurrence. The defect followed by surgical procedure need to be filled with bone graft or cement if it is large enough to threaten the mechanical stability of the bone with a possibility of perioperative fracture. En-bloc or wide resection with or without reconstruction may be indicated for locally aggressive large tumors or recurrent lesion following curettage. Preoperative embolization can be useful to reduce bleeding risk during the surgical procedure, particularly for large pelvic and vertebral lesions. More recently, percutaneous ablation procedures such as radiofrequency ablation [27, 28] or cryoablation [29, 30] have emerged for the treatment of OBs as in OOs, and have become more widely employed techniques with high clinical success rates and low complication rates.

7.10 Clinical Course

The lesion is benign but with a potential for progression (sometimes aggressive) and high local recurrence after incomplete curettage. Most patients can be cured by initial surgery with adequate treatment. Campanacci [6] suggested very low incidence of local recurrence by curettage with local adjuvant for Stage 1 and 2 lesions, or marginal resection for conventional OB and en-bloc resection or wide resection for Stage 3 lesion. However, Berry et al. [7] reported an overall local recurrence in 24% of the patients and most followed by curettage and packing. Lucas et al. [3] reported a single recurrence of 16% among Mayo Clinic patients and 21% in consultation patients. *Epithelioid* OB was initially reported with a more aggressive clinical course [18], but a more recent study suggested the histopathologic feature of *epithelioid* osteoblasts itself is not a reliable predictor of aggressiveness [3]. Campanacci [6] believed some OBs once thought to have trnasformed into OSA with metastases should be regarded as initially unrecognized OSA. In a large series of 306 OBs, only two cases (0.7%) underwent malignant transformation to high-grade OSA [3], which recurred multiple times in several years before becoming malignant. Other authors have sporadically documented this in case reports [31–33].

References

1. Greenspan A. Benign bone-forming lesions: osteoma, osteoid osteoma, and osteoblastoma. Skeletal Radiol. 1993;22(7):485–500.
2. McLeod RA, Dahlin D, Beabout J. The spectrum of osteoblastoma. Am J Roentgenol. 1976;126(2):321–5.
3. Lucas DR, Unni KK, McLeod RA, O'Connor MI, Sim FH. Osteoblastoma: clinicopathologic study of 306 cases. Hum Pathol. 1994;25(2):117–34.
4. Mirra JM, Picci P. Osteoblastoma. In: Mirra JM, editor. Bone tumors: clinical, radiologic, and pathologic correlations. Philadelphia: Lea & Febiger; 1989. p. 389–438.
5. Czerniak B. Benign osteoblastic tumors. In: Dorfman HD, Czerniak B, editors. Dorfman and Czerniak's bone tumors. 2nd ed. eBook: Elsevier; 2016. p. 144–99.
6. Campanacci M. Osteoblastoma. In: Campanacci M, editor. Bone and soft tissue tumors. Wien New York: Springer; 1999. p. 415–33.
7. Berry M, Mankin H, Gebhardt M, Rosenberg A, Hornicek F. Osteoblastoma: a 30-year study of 99 cases. J Surg Oncol. 2008;98(3):179–83.
8. Arkader A, Dormans JP. Osteoblastoma in the skeletally immature. J Pediatr Orthop. 2008;28(5):555–60.
9. Vensi E. Multiple benign osteoblastoma of the femur and frontal sinus. Ann Laringol Otol Rinol Faringol. 1965;64(6):768–77.
10. Michelacci M, Vasina P. A case of multifocal osteoblastoma at an unusual site. Arch Putti Chir Organi Mov. 1986;36:275–84.
11. Asada Y, Suzuki I, Suzuki M, Fukushima M. Atypical multiple benign osteoblastomas accompanied by simple bone cysts: a case report. J Craniomaxillofac Surg. 1991;19(4):166–71.
12. O'Connell JX, Rosenthal DI, Mankin HJ, Gudger GK, Dickersin GR, Schiller AL, et al. A unique multifocal osteoblastoma-like tumor of the bones of a single lower extremity. Report of a case. J Bone Joint Surg. 1993;75(4):597–602.
13. Adler C-P. Multifocal osteoblastoma of the hand. Skeletal Radiol. 2000;29(10):601–4.
14. Yoshikawa S, Nakamura T, Takagi M, Imamura T, Okano K, Sasaki S. Benign osteoblastoma as a cause

of osteomalacia. A report of two cases. J Bone Joint Surg Br. 1977;59(3):279–86.
15. Chun KA, Cho IH, Won KJ, Lee HW, Choi JH, Ahn JC, et al. Osteoblastoma as a cause of osteomalacia assessed by bone scan. Ann Nucl Med. 2003;17:411–4.
16. Mirra JM, Cove K, Theros E, Paladugu R, Smasson J. A case of osteoblastoma associated with severe systemic toxicity. Am J Surg Pathol. 1979;3(5):463–71.
17. Kyriakos M, El-Khoury GY, McDonald DJ, Buckwalter JA, Sundaram M, DeYoung B, et al. Osteoblastomatosis of bone. A benign, multifocal osteoblastic lesion, distinct from osteoid osteoma and osteoblastoma, radiologically simulating a vascular tumor. Skeletal Radiol. 2007;36:237–47.
18. Dorfman HD, Weiss SW. Borderline osteoblastic tumors: problems in the differential diagnosis of aggressive osteoblastoma and low-grade osteosarcoma. Ann Diagn Pathol. 1984;1(3):215–34.
19. Sundaram M, McGuire MH. Computed tomography or magnetic resonance for evaluating the solitary tumor or tumor-like lesion of bone? Skeletal Radiol. 1988;17:393–401.
20. Crim J, Mirra J, Eckardt J, Seeger L. Widespread inflammatory response to osteoblastoma: the flare phenomenon. Radiology. 1990;177(3):835–6.
21. Bertoni F, Unni KK, Lucas DR, McLeod RA. Osteoblastoma with cartilaginous matrix. An unusual morphologic presentation in 18 cases. Am J Surg Pathol. 1993;17(1):69–74.
22. Dorfman HD. Proceedings: malignant transformation of benign bone lesions. Proc Natl Cancer Conf. 1972;7:901–13.
23. Revell P, Scholtz C. Aggressive osteoblastoma. J Pathol. 1979;127(4):195–8.
24. Schajowicz F, Lemos C. Malignant osteoblastoma. J Bone Joint Surg Br. 1976;58(2):202–11.
25. Mirra JM, Kendrick RA, Kendrick RE. Pseudomalignant osteoblastoma versus arrested osteosarcoma. A case report. Cancer. 1976;37(4):2005–14.
26. Bahk WJ, Mirra JM. Pseudoanaplastic tumors of bone. Skeletal Radiol. 2004;33(11):641–8.
27. Weber M-A, Sprengel SD, Omlor GW, Lehner B, Wiedenhöfer B, Kauczor H-U, et al. Clinical long-term outcome, technical success, and cost analysis of radiofrequency ablation for the treatment of osteoblastomas and spinal osteoid osteomas in comparison to open surgical resection. Skeletal Radiol. 2015;44(7):981–93.
28. Arrigoni F, Barile A, Zugaro L, Fascetti E, Zappia M, Brunese L, et al. CT-guided radiofrequency ablation of spinal osteoblastoma: treatment and long-term follow-up. Int J Hyperth. 2018;34(3):321–7.
29. Kumasaka S, Miyazaki M, Tsushima Y. CT-guided percutaneous cryoablation of an aggressive osteoblastoma: a case report. J Vasc Interv Radiol. 2015;26(11):1746–8.
30. Cazzato RL, Auloge P, Dalili D, De Marini P, Di Marco A, Garnon J, et al. Percutaneous image-guided cryoablation of osteoblastoma. Am J Roentgenol. 2019;213(5):1157–62.
31. Dorfman H. Case records of the Massachusetts General Hospital: case 40. N Engl J Med. 1980;303:866.
32. Seki T, Fukuda H, Ishii Y, Hanaoka H, Yatabe S. Malignant transformation of benign osteoblastoma. A case report. J Bone Joint Surg. 1975;57(3):424–6.
33. Merryweather R, Middlemiss J, Sanerkin N. Malignant transformation of osteoblastoma. J Bone Joint Surg Br. 1980;62(3):381–4.

8 Low-Grade Central Osteosarcoma

(***Osteo(n)*** "Bone," ***sarco(s)*** "flesh," ***ōma*** "forming")

8.1 Definition

Low-grade central osteosarcoma (LGOSA) is a rare distinct form of low-grade malignant tumor arising from the medullary cavity of the bone, which consists of fibroblastic tumor cells with low-grade nuclear atypia and well-formed or relatively mature neoplastic bony trabeculae, typically showing an indolent clinical course. The World Health Organization endorses the use of a two-tier system designating an OSA as low grade (Grades 1 and 2 in Broder's four-grade system) and high grade (Grades 3 and 4) [1].

8.2 Synonym

Well-differentiated well-differentiated central osteosarcoma/low-grade intramedullary OSA.

8.3 Incidence

LGOSA is very rare, accounting for only 1–2% of all OSAs [2–6].

8.4 Age

The age distribution is between the second and fourth decades of life with a peak incidence in the third decade, during which nearly half of the cases occur [5, 6].

8.5 Locations

LGOSA most often affects the metaphysis of long bones of the lower extremities often extending into the epiphysis and/or diaphysis. The epi-metaphyseal area of the distal femur and the proximal tibia around the knee joint are the most frequent sites for involvement as in other variants of OSA, accounting for approximately 70% of the cases [5, 6]. Small tubular bones, jaw bones, and ribs are rarely involved.

8.6 Clinical Features

The most common symptom is pain of relatively milder intensity and longer duration than that of conventional high-grade OSA. The average dura-

W.-J. Bahk, *Diagnosis and Management of Primary Bone Tumors*,
https://doi.org/10.1007/978-981-96-3484-2_8

tion before diagnosis was reported to be 9 months [7] to 2 years [4]. Swelling with or without pain may also be present. Clinical importance of LGOSA is that it is often misdiagnosed as benign bone lesions. In the Mayo Clinic series, about one-third of the cases were diagnosed incorrectly at first, most commonly as fibrous dysplasia (FD) [5]. Thus, some patients have a history of local recurrences after previous curettage with a histologic diagnosis of benign bone tumor. Two cases closely simulating Pagetoid disease of bone were also reported [8]. Rarely, pathologic fracture is also associated.

8.7 Radiologic Findings

Plain radiograph Because LGOSA and FD are so similar histologically, a correlation with clinical and radiologic features is a mandatory rule for a correct diagnosis. However, radiographic features of LGOSA are variable, presenting a broad spectrum of varying degrees of lytic and blastic features. The lesion mainly in metaphysis often extends to the end of the bone. The lesion usually shows at least two of three radiographic findings of cortical destruction, soft-tissue extension, and cloud-like tumor matrix pattern that strongly suggest a bone-producing malignant tumor [7]. The density of the lesion can be presented as one of four patterns: (a) lytic with varying amounts of thick and coarse trabeculation (31%), (b) predominantly lytic with few thin, incomplete trabeculae (30%), (c) densely sclerotic (24%), or (d) mixed lytic and sclerotic (14%) [8]. By contrast, the mixed lytic and sclerotic pattern was reported in the majority of cases (80%) in other series [4]. Most lesions are poorly demarcated and expanded sometimes with a *trabeculated* or *soap-bubble* appearance. Periosteal new bone is distinctly uncommon. In the Mayo Clinic series, most cases (about 80%) seemed to be obviously malignant with poor margination, but the rest of the cases (about 20%) appeared benign [9]. Early lesions may mimic benign disease, whereas the older, larger lesions usually display evidence of malignancy. A careful analysis to detect evidence of their aggressiveness is required in the cases simulating benign bone tumors [5]. **CT scan** reveals cortical interruption and mineralization within the lesion, which is not definitely seen on radiograph. Chest CT is required to evaluate the presence of pulmonary metastases at initial presentation. **MR images** demonstrate intramedullary mass-like lesions with low to intimidated SI on T1-weighted image and heterogeneous low and high SI on T2-weighted image. It more clearly reveals cortical breaches or destruction and soft tissue mass of variable size from barely perceived to moderate, but typically small. Occasionally, cystic areas may be present in the tumor rarely with fluid levels. MRI is useful to evaluate soft tissue and neurovascular involvement as well as the extent of the tumor for planning a safe resection margin. It can also depict skip metastases. **Bone scan** usually reveals a heterogeneously increased uptake often with central void are of reduced or no uptake (Figs. 8.1, 8.2, and 8.3). It is also useful to evaluate the extent of local disease and the presence of a skip lesion as well.

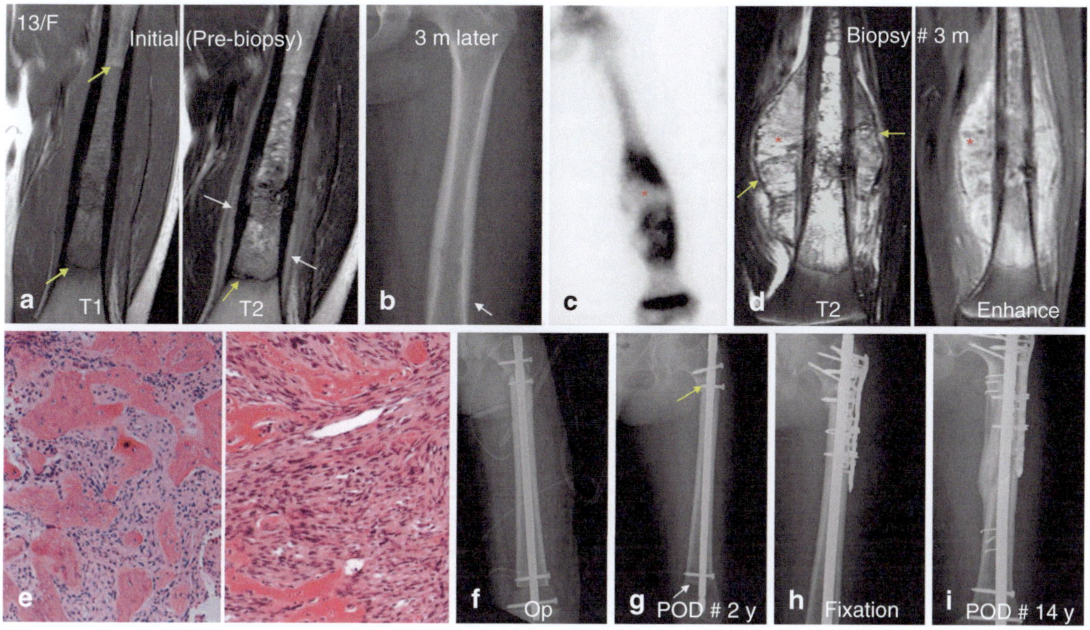

Fig. 8.1 *"FD-like" pattern with high-grade area.* (**a**) Initial MR images taken for intermittent thigh pain of 9 months' duration in a 13-year-old girl demonstrate a well-defined intramedullary lesion, extending over a long segment of the femoral shaft (yellow arrows). The lesion exhibits heterogeneous low SI on T1-weighted image and intermediate SI and multiple small nodular high and dark signal on T2-weighted image. There is a concentric, continuous lamellate periosteal reaction with edema (white arrows), but no discernible soft tissue mass. Incision biopsy was done in another hospital and she was managed by conservative with analgesics based on initial misdiagnosis of FD. (**b**) Radiograph taken for a gradual aggravation of the pain with significant increased thigh circumference for 3 months after incision biopsy shows an ill-defined moth-eaten destruction with a thin periosteal reaction (arrow) in the diaphysis of the distal femur, suggesting a locally aggressive or a malignan lesion. (**c**) Bone scan reveals a heterogeneously strong uptake with a central void area, suggesting possible central necrosis (sterisk). (**d**) Follow-up MR images note a marked progression of the lesion with cortical perforation and a huge mass (asterisks) surrounded by a thin rim of dark signal suggesting reactive bone (arrows). The intramedullary lesion as well as soft tissue mass is heterogeneously enhanced. (**e**) Microscopic examination: (Left) Medium-power magnification shows a mild to moderate number of fibroblastic spindle cells with mild atypia typically embedded in a dense collagenous stroma. Note irregular anastomosing bony trabeculae with variable thickness appearing curved and branching, so-called *alphabetic soup* appearance as seen in FD. (Right) Higher-power magnification of another area notes increased cellularity, moderate to severe nuclear atypia with frequent mitosis, and even occasional atypical mitoses, indicating high-grade pleomorphic area, occupying less than 50% of the tumor. (**f**) Wide resection followed by reconstruction using allograft fixed by intramedullary nail was performed. (**g**) Follow-up radiograph at 2 years after surgery reveals good union of the distal allo-host junction (white arrow), but nonunion of the proximal junction (yellow arrow). (**h**) The nail was changed to a larger size, followed by plate fixation with combined auto- and allograft. (**i**) Follow-up radiograph at 14 years after initial surgery shows no evidence of local recurrence with complete incorporation and consolidation of the graft

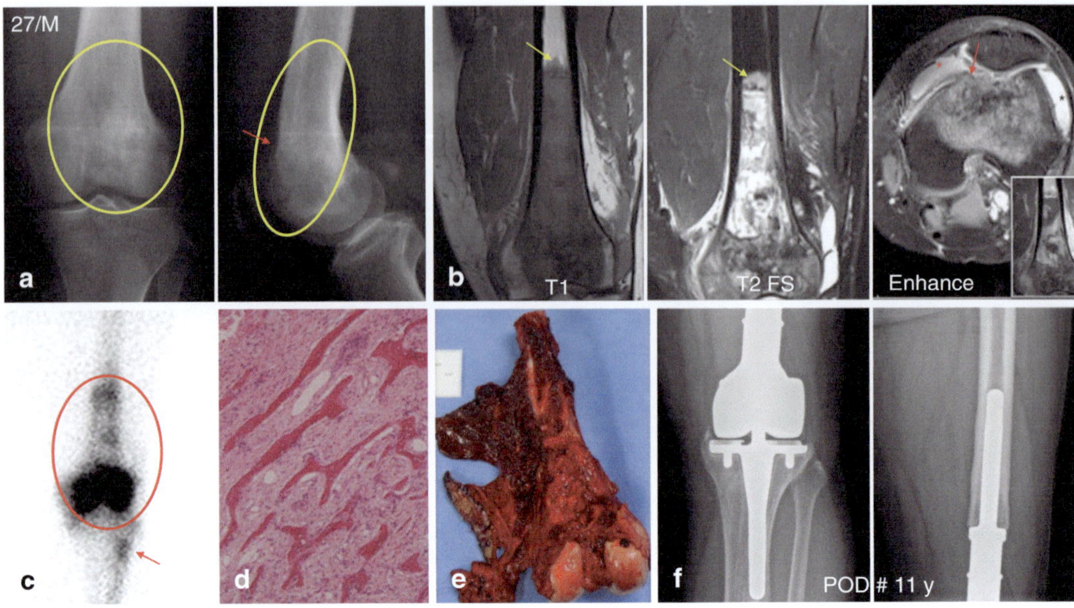

Fig. 8.2 *"Parosteal OSA-like" pattern.* (**a**) Radiograph taken for left knee swelling of 1 year's duration with recently developed pain in a 27-year-old man shows a poorly demarcated, intramedullary, concentric, mixed lytic, and sclerotic lesion (circles) with cortical disruption (arrow) in the epi-metaphysis of the distal femur. (**b**) MR images reveal a relatively well-defined, extensive, medulla occupying lesion in the epi-metaphysis of the distal femur, with extension to the diaphysis (yellow arrow), where the lesion is not seen on a plain radiograph. The SI is intermediate on T1-weighted image and heterogeneous high on fat-saturated T2-weighted image. Note focal articular destruction (red arrow) and tumor extension into the joint space (red asterisk) with heterogeneous enhancement by contrast medium. There is also extensive joint effusion (black asterisk). (**c**) Bone scan shows a strong uptake in the epi-metaphysis area and weaker focal uptakes in the diaphysis area (circle). There is another weak uptake in the proximal fibula (arrow), suggesting a reactive lesion because MRI shows no abnormal finding in this area. (**d**) Microscopic examination shows fibroblastic spindle cells of mild to moderate cellularity with mild atypia embedded in a dense collagenous stroma, which produces longitudinal seams of woven to lamellar-like bone in a parallel arrangement similiar to parosteal OSA. (**e**) A gross specimen obtained by wide resection including surrounding muscle and biopsy tract is shown. The margin was free of malignant tumor cells. (**f**) Follow-up radiograph at 11 years after surgery shows good maintenance of the tumor prosthesis with no evidence of local recurrence

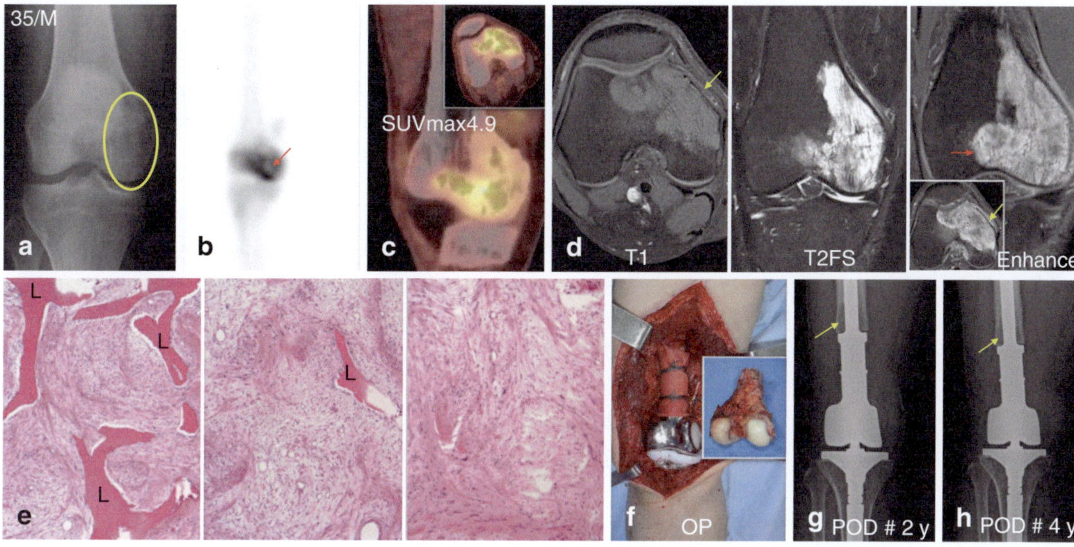

Fig. 8.3 *"Desmoid-like pattern."* (**a**) Radiograph taken for right knee pain of 10 months' duration in a 35-year-old man shows an ill-defined, eccentric, predominantly lytic lesion surrounded by a thin rim of sclerosis (arrow) in the medial condyle of the distal femur. There are a few thin incomplete trabeculae within the lesion. (**b**) Bone scan reveals a heterogeneously increased uptake with a small area of central void area, suggestive of necrosis (arrow), (C) PET/CT scan notes a heterogeneously increased FDG uptake (SUVmax 4.9) in the lesion. (**d**) MR images demonstrate a relatively well-defined but no sclerotic rim, intramedullary mass-like lesion in the epi-metaphyseal area of the distal fermur, with intermediate SI on T1-weighted and heterogeneous bright SI with internal several dark signals of trabeculation on fat-saturated T2-weighted image. Note clear cortical breaches and perforation producing a small soft tissue mass (yellow arrow), suggesting a locally aggressive tumor or a malignant lesion. The bony lesion and soft tissue mass are heterogeneously enhanced (arrows). (**e**) Microscopic examination: (Left) Low-power magnification shows fibroblastic stroma cells in a spindling fascicle pattern producing dense collagen and osseous material, which permeate and infiltrate the host lamellar bone (L). (Middle) Medium-power magnification reveals low to moderate cellularity producing minimal osteoid to primitive woven bone with encasement of a host lamellar bone spicule (L). (Right) Higher-power magnification notes spindle cell proliferation with mild to moderate cellularity and mild degree of atypia embedded within a dense collagenous stroma. The stroma cells are typically arranged in a spindling fascicle pattern which is reminiscent of a desmoid tumor. Given the minimal amount of osteoid, a diagnosis of LGOSA of *desmoid-like* pattern is made. (**f**) Wide resection followed by reconstruction using a tumor prosthesis was performed. (**g**) Radiograph at 2 years after surgery shows a radiolucency around the prosthesis-host junction (arrow), likely representing stress-shielding-related resorption, as the patient is free of any symptoms. (**h**) Follow-up radiograph at 4 years after surgery reveals no progression of the peri-prosthetic radiolucency, and the patient is still free of pain. The radiographic and clinical findings support the fact that the lesion would be a resorption by stress shielding rather than local recurrence. Chest CT scan shows no evidence of lung metastsis

8.8 Histologic Findings

LGOSA presents a well-differentiated fibroblastic stroma with mild atypia producing dense collagen and mature osseous material which are tremendously different from conventional high-grade OSA but similar to FD or parosteal OSA. Despite their similarities, tissue patterns of host lamellar bone permeation permeation or infiltrative growth pattern, with cytolgic findings of degree of atypia, mitotic activity, and pattern of bone production can provide clues to differentiate LGOSA from FD if presents. The stromal spindle cells produce abundant collagen in *interlacing* or *herring-bone* pattern and woven or woven to lamellar bone trabeculae in long parallel streamers with minimal to no osteoblastic rimming. To observe the tissue and cytologic patterns, an appropriate amount of adequate tissue sample is necessary, preferably via incision biopsy rather than needle or trocar biopsy. If a permeative growth pattern exists and/or the tumor destroys the cortex and invades soft tissue, it should be LGOSA. The spindle stromal cells arranged in a spindling fascicle pattern resembling those of low-grade fibrosarcoma are another clue for LGOSA. The mature fibroblastic spindle cells with mild to moderate cellularity are typically embedded in a dense collagenous stroma. The individual fibroblastic stromal cells are mildly plump with elongated nuclei containing prominent nucleoli in a uniform appearance. In general, atypia is mild and mitotic activity is low with rare to no abnormal mitosis. Neoplastic bone is usually woven or woven to lamellar bone arranged in one of the *FD-like* patterns (Fig. 8.1), *parosteal OSA-like* pattern (Fig. 8.2), and *desmoid-like* or *low-grade fibrosarcoma-like* pattern with minimal bone production (Fig. 8.3). True lamellar bone, if presents, implies residual host by tumor entrapment or permeation as in high-grade OSA. Typically, the bone component consists of irregular anastomosing long and thick bony trabeculae, often presenting as long longitudinal seams in parallel arrangement of lamellar-like bone as in parosteal OSA (Fig. 8.2d). Occasionally, the woven bone trabeculae arise directly from pure fibrous tissue and may appear curved and branching, producing the so-called *alphabetic soup* seen in FD (Fig. 8.1e). More rarely, amount of bone production is minimal and the fascicles of spindle-shaped cells resemble a desmoid tumor or low-grade fibrosarcoma (Fig. 8.3e). Extremely thickened irregular plates of bone with an irregular mosaic pattern of cement lines (Pagetoid bone) have also been presented posing a potential diagnostic pitfall as Paget's disease [8]. In some cases, high-grade pleomorphic areas can be seen within an LGOSA [5, 9, 10], so-called *dedifferentiated LGOSA*, which is more often observed in recurrent cases after incomplete removal of the tumor, but exceedingly rare in primary tumor. The low- and high-grade components are sharply demarcated, as in other low-grade tumors with dedifferentiation [6].

8.9 Management

Surgical excision with a wide margin is a generally accepted treatment of choice if technically feasible. A higher incidence of local recurrence sometimes with transformation to higher-grade OSA was reported after surgical excision with inadequate surgical margins [3]. Chemotherapy and radiotherapy are not routinely applied but can be reserved for dedifferentiated tumors to high-grade or recurrent tumors.

8.10 Clinical Course and Prognosis

Wide excision with adequate margin is almost never followed by local recurrence [9]. Practically, the local recurrence rate is, however, high due to high number of incorrect initial diagnoses and resultant inadequate surgical margin, mostly intralesional surgery such as curettage. Excision of tumor almost invariably led to local recurrences [4], and the recurrence can be delayed beyond 5–10 years after intralesional surgery [9, 11]. The recurrences are mostly related to inadequate intralesional surgery due to an incorrect diagnosis such as benign bone tumor. The transformation of LGOSA into a high-grade OSA was discovered in 15% of patients with recurrence in a large series, in whom the subsequent clinical course was similar to that of patients with conventional high-grade OSA [9]. In another series, four of the nine patients (44%) with a local recurrence had higher-grade tumors and three of these four patients developed metastases [4]. Although it is associated with a high incidence of local recurrence after inadequate surgery, the overall prognosis is excellent with an overall survival rate of 90% at 5 years and 80–85% at 10 years [4, 11]. The development of metastasis is strongly correlated with the transformation into high-grade OSA. In Rizzoli Institute clinic series, no patients with high-grade foci in less than 50% of the tumor showed metastatic lesions at the staging workup. They also have a very high probability of survival without adjuvant chemotherapy with evidence-free survival and overall survival of 88% and 95% at 5 years after surgery, respectively. However, the clinical behavior of the tumors with higher-grade foci in more than 50% overlaps with that reported for conventional high-grade OSA, with evidence-free survival and overall survival of 68% and 83% at 5 years after surgery and adjuvant chemotherapy, respectively [12].

References

1. Grimer RJ, Hogendoorn PCW, Vanel D. Tumours of bone: introduction. In: Fletcher CDM, Bridge JA, Hogendoorn PCW, Mertens F, editors. World Health Organization classification of tumours. Pathology and genetics of tumours of soft tissue and bone. 4th ed. Lyon: IARC Press; 2013. p. 244–7.
2. Bertoni F, Bacchini P, Fabbri N, Mercuri M, Picci P, Ruggieri P, et al. Osteosarcoma. Low-grade intraosseous-type osteosarcoma, histologically resembling parosteal osteosarcoma, fibrous dysplasia, and desmoplastic fibroma. Cancer. 1993;71(2):338–45.
3. Campanacci M. Cetral low-grade osteosarcoma. In: Campanacci M, editor. Bone and soft tissue tumors. Wien, Austria: Springer; 1999. p. 549–57.
4. Malhas A, Sumathi V, James S, Menna C, Carter S, Tillman R, et al. Low-grade central osteosarcoma: a difficult condition to diagnose. Sarcoma. 2012;2012:764796. https://doi.org/10.1155/2012/764796.
5. Unni KK, Dahlin DC, McLeod RA, Pritchard DJ. Intraosseous well-differentiated osteosarcoma. Cancer. 1977;40(3):1337–47.
6. Czerniak B. Osteosarcoma. In: Dorfman HD, Czerniak B, editors. Dorfman and Czerniak's bone tumors. 2nd ed. eBook: Elsevier; 2016. p. 200–355.
7. Ellis J, Siegel C, Martel W, Weatherbee L, Dorfman H. Radiologic features of well-differentiated osteosarcoma. Am J Roentgenol. 1988;151(4):739–42.
8. Franchi A, Bacchini P, Rocca CD, Bertoni F. Central low-grade osteosarcoma with pagetoid bone formation: a potential diagnostic pitfall. Mod Pathol. 2004;17(3):288–91.
9. Kurt AM, Unni KK, McLeod RA, Pritchard DJ. Low-grade intraosseous osteosarcoma. Cancer. 1990;65(6):1418–28.
10. Iemoto Y, Ushigome S, Fukunaga M, Nikaido T, Asanuma K. Case report 679. Central low-grade osteosarcoma with foci of dedifferentiation. Skeletal Radiol. 1991;20(5):379–82.
11. Choong P, Pritchard DJ, Rock MG, Sim FH, McLeod RA, Unni KK. Low grade central osteogenic sarcoma. A long-term followup of 20 patients. Clin Orthop Relat Res. 1996;322:198–206.
12. Righi A, Paioli A, Dei Tos AP, Gambarotti M, Palmerini E, Cesari M, et al. High-grade focal areas in low-grade central osteosarcoma: high-grade or still low-grade osteosarcoma? Clin Sarcoma Res. 2015;5(1):1–6.

High-Grade Central Conventional Osteosarcoma

9

(***Osteo(n)*** "Bone," ***sarco(s)*** "flesh," ***ōma*** "forming")

9.1 Definition

Osteosarcoma (OSA) is an intramedullary high-grade malignant bone tumor composed of malignant connective stroma that directly produces malignant osteoid and/or immature woven bone.

9.2 Classification

It is classified into primary, de novo, and secondary OSA resulting from malignant transformation of benign conditions such as Paget disease, extensive bone infarction, chronic osteomyelitis, various benign tumors, and irradiation, or from bone or soft tissue at the site of orthopedic metallic implants. In the early 1920s, a Broder's four-grade system was developed for grading oral squamous cell carcinoma [1]. The system includes Grade 1 (well-differentiated tumor) with 75–100% differentiated cells, Grade 2 (moderately differentiated tumor) with 50–75% differentiated cells, Grade 3 (poorly differentiated tumor) with 25–50% differentiated cells, and Grade 4 (anaplastic tumor) with less than 25% differentiated cells. The grading of malignant bone tumors has traditionally been based on Broder's grading system, which assesses cellularity and degree of anaplasia [2]. The seventh edition of the *AJCC Cancer Staging Manual* recommends a four-grade system, with Grades 1 and 2 as *low-grade* and Grades 3 and 4 as *high-grade*. The World Health Organization recommends a two-tier system designating as low grade (Grades 1 and 2 in Broder's four-grade system) and high grade (Grades 3 and 4) [3]. Primary OSA is divided into two main types depending on the location affected: intramedullary or central type and surface type. The intramedullary or central type includes low-grade or well-differentiated, conventional high-grade (osteoblastic, chondroblastic, and fibroblastic), telangiectatic, and small cell OSA. The surface type includes parosteal, periosteal, and high-grade surface OSA.

9.3 Incidence

OSA is the second most common primary malignant bone tumor ranking behind multiple myeloma, accounting for about 20% of primary bone sarcomas excluding multiple myeloma and other hematopoietic neoplasm and 15% of all primary bone tumors [4, 5]. Nonetheless, it is very rare, representing less than 1% of all cancers [6, 7]. Low-grade OSA is very rare, representing only 1% of all OSA [5].

W.-J. Bahk, *Diagnosis and Management of Primary Bone Tumors*,
https://doi.org/10.1007/978-981-96-3484-2_9

9.4 Age

The age distribution of the *primary form* shows typically bimodal peaks, the first major peak during adolescence younger than 20 years of age, and the second minor peak in older adulthood older than 50 years. *The secondary form* occurs in the elderly, with a incidence in adults older than 65 years. Low-grade OSA most commonly occurs during the third decade of life, occupying nearly half of the cases [5].

9.5 Locations

Primary OS typically occur at the metaphysis of long tubular bones, most frequently distal femur, proximal tibia, and proximal humerus in that order (Figs. 9.1, 9.2, 9.3, 9.4, 9.5, 9.6, 9.10, 9.11, 9.12, 9.14, 9.15, 9.16, 9.17 and 9.18), which represent nearly 70% of the cases [6]. The knee area is affected in about 50% of the patients [5]. Diaphysis is infrequently involved (Fig. 9.15), and the epiphysis is only rarely affected. Other sites less commonly affected include the fibula, pelvic bones especially ilium (Figs. 9.7, 9.8, 9.9, and 9.13), the axial skeleton including mandible, maxilla, and vertebrae. It is rare in bones of the forearm and small tubular bone of the hands and feet. The axial skeleton and flat bones are more commonly affected in older patients over 50 years of age [5]. Secondary OSA can occur in any bone, largely reflecting the combined incidence of their underlying conditions, with a higher incidence in the pelvic bone (a favorite site of Paget disease).

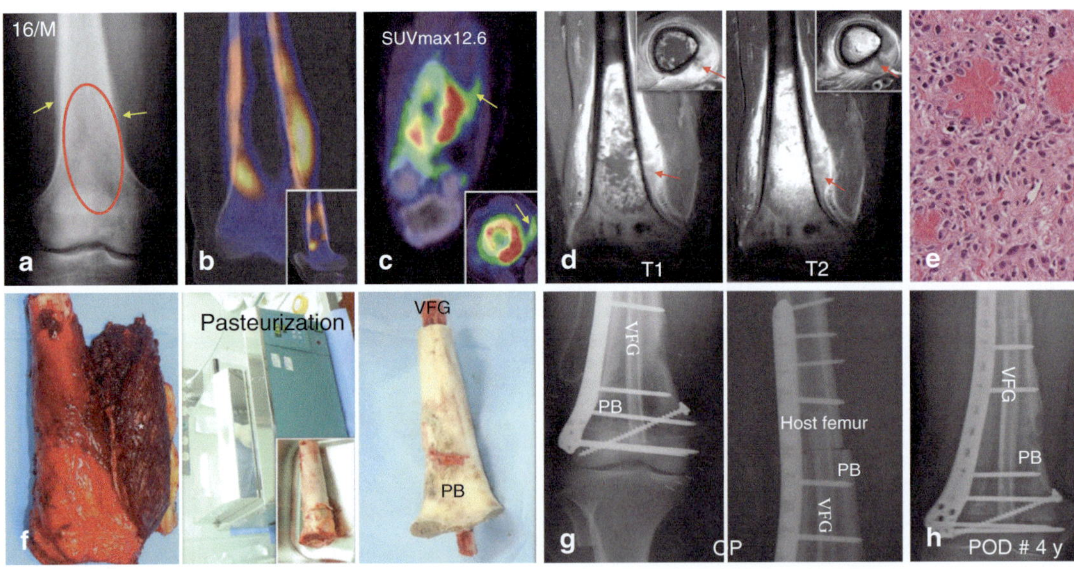

Fig. 9.1 Osteoblastic OSA. *Pasteurization.* (**a**) Radiograph taken for right knee pain of 1 mont's duration in a 16-year-old boy shows an ill-defined lytic and sclerotic lesion affecting the meta-diaphysis of the distal femur (circle). There is solid periosteal reaction on both the medial and lateral aspect of distal femur (arrows). (**b**) Bone SPECT reveals increased uptake in the distal femur corresponding to intramedullary lesion as well as periosteal reaction. (**c**) PET/CT scan demonstrates a heterogeneously intense FDG uptake (SUVmax 12.6) in the lesion with mild uptake in the medial aspect (yellow arrow) suggesting a biopsy tract. (**d**) MR images note an intramedullary mass-like lesion with heterogeneously low and intermediate SI with focal high signal on T1- and diffuse high SI on T2-weighted image. There are thick periosteal reactions on both medial and lateral sides and sub-periosteal soft tissue mass of similar SI on the posteromedial aspect (red arrows). (**e**) Microscopic examination shows pleomorphic stromal cells with severe nuclear atypism, and filigree osteoid and patch-like osteoid to immature woven bone indicating osteoblastic OSA. (**f**) Wide resection including surrounding muscle and soft tissue as well as biopsy tract was performed (Left). The resected femur was pasteurized after removal of surrounding soft tissue (Middle). And then, the pasteurized bone (PB) was augmented with vascularized fibula graft (VFG) obtained from the contralateral leg, which was used for reconstruction of the defect (Right). (**g**) Postoperative radiograph reveals the PB augmented with VFG securely fixed to the remaining normal femur by plate and screws. (**h**) Follow-up radiograph at 4 years after surgery notes no evidence of local recurrence with good maintenance of the PB with VFG

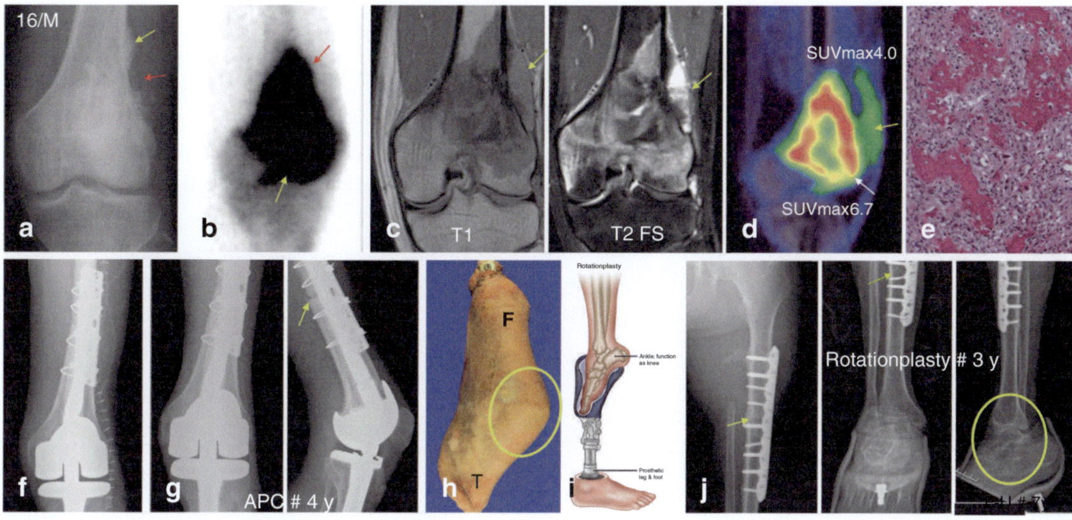

Fig. 9.2 **Osteoblastic OSA**. *APC and rotationplasty.* (**a**) Radiograph taken for left knee pain of 2 months duration in a 16-year-old boy shows an ill-defined mostly sclerotic and focally lytic medullary lesion with an interrupting Codman's triangle of aggressive periosteal reaction (yellow arrow) and a possible soft tissue mass (red arrow) mainly involving metaphysis of left distal femur. (**b**) Bone scan reveals a homogeneous strong uptake in the corresponding distal femur (yellow arrow) and soft tissue mass (red arrow). (**c**) MR images demonstrate an intramedullary lesion showing low SI on T1- and heterogeneously low and intermediate with focal high SI on T2-weighted image. Dark signals on both images suggest the mineralization of the tumor. Note cortical perforation with a soft tissue mass (yellow arrows) having intermediate SI on T1- and high SI on T2-weighted image. (**d**) PET/CT scan notes a heterogeneously intense FDG uptake (SUVmax 6.7) with less intense uptake in the surrounding soft tissue (SUVmax 4.0) suggesting a biopsy tract. (**e**) Microscopic examination shows pleomorphic stromal cells with severe nuclear atypism, and filigree to lace-like osteoid as well as sheets of coalescing trabeculae of more mature woven bone. (**f**) Wide resection and reconstruction with allograft-tumor prosthesis composite was performed. (**g**) Follow-up radiograph at 4 years after surgery shows no evidence of local recurrence but nonunion (red arrow). He suffered postoperative repeated, uncontrollable infection with resultant complete ankylosis of the knee joint and significant shortening of the extremity. (**h**) Resection of the infected distal femur (F) and proximal tibia (T) was performed for eradication of the repeated infection as strongly requested by the parents. Note completely fused knee (circle). (**i**) Rotationplasty was followed as one option for a mobile joint by an ankle functioning as the knee (circle) and recovery of limb length using prosthesis. (**j**) Follow-up radiographs at 3 years after rotationplasty reveal no evidence of local recurrence with radiologic union at attached sites of the femur and tibia (yellow arrows). The rotated foot and ankle fuction well as a knee joint (circle)

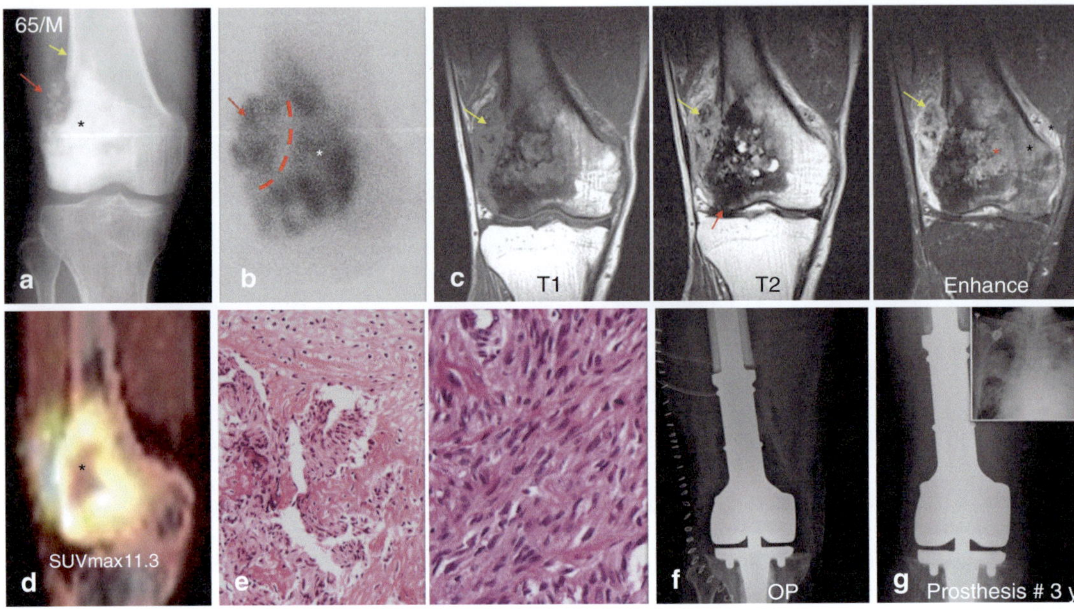

Fig. 9.3 Osteoblastic OSA. *Tumor prosthesis.* (**a**) Radiograph taken for right knee pain of 5 months duration in a 65-year-old man shows an ill-defined intramedullary sclerotic lesion (asterisk) with cortical destruction and soft tissue mass having internal calcification (red arrows) in the epi-metaphysis of the distal femur. There is a typical Codman's triangle with new bone deposition (yellow arrow). (**b**) Pinhole bone scan reveals inhomogeneous strong uptake in the medullary lesion (white asterisk) as well as in the soft tissue mass lesion (red arrow). (**c**) MR images demonstrate a relatively ill-defined intramedullary mass lesion (asterisk) with low to intermediate SI on T1- and heterogeneously intermediate and high SI on T2-weighted image. There are dark signals both in the medullary and soft tissue mass on both images, representing heavy mineralization. Note cortical destruction with a soft tissue mass with similar signal to medullary lesion (yellow arrows). Articular destruction is subtle (red arrow). The medullary lesion (red asterisk) and soft tissue mass (yellow arrow) are heterogeneously well enhanced. Adjacent marrow and soft tissue edema are diffusely well enhanced (black asterisk). (**d**) PET/CT scan demonstrates inhomogeneous high FDG uptake (SUVmax 11.3) in the distal femur and adjacent soft tissue with a central FDG-void area (black asterisk), suggestive of spontaneous possible spontaneous tumor necrosis. (**e**) Microscopic examination: (Left) Medium-power microscopic examination shows haphazardly arranged osteoid to immature woven bone spicules with a lace-like pattern, which are merged to form broader trabeculae with more pronounced mineralization. (Right) Higher-power examination reveals bizarre pleomorphic stromal cells with mitoses. (**f**) Wide resection and reconstruction with tumor prosthesis was performed with neoadjuvant and adjuvant chemotherapy. (**g**) Follow-up radiograph at 3 years after surgery notes good maintenance of the tumor prosthesis with no evidence of local recurrence. However, he died of disseminated pulmonary metastasis (inset)

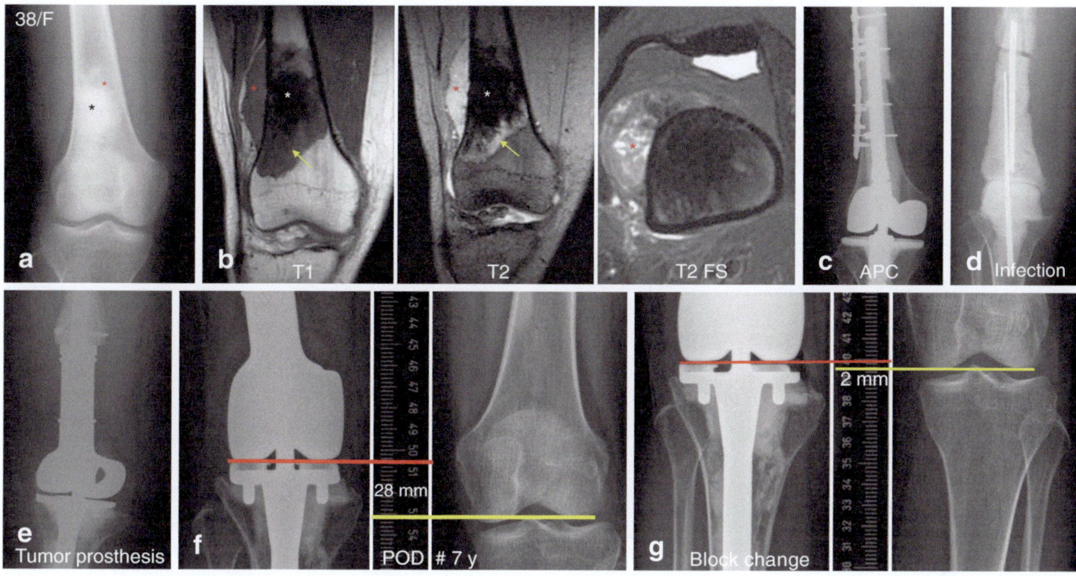

Fig. 9.4 **Osteoblastic OSA**. *Wear of prosthesis.* (**a**) Radiograph taken for right knee pain of 9 months duration in a 38-year-old woman shows an ill-defined fluffy intramedullary lesion (black asterisk) associated with surrounding focal radiolucent areas (red asterisk) in meta-diaphysis of the distal femur. (**b**) MR images reveal relatively well-defined intramedullary mass-like lesion with a large dense sclerotic area of dark signal of severe mineralization in the center of the lesion on both sequences (white asterisks) and small peripheral areas of low to intermittent signal (yellow arrow) on T1-weighted image and intermediate to high SI (white arrow) on T2-weighted image. There is extra-osseous mass formation (red asterisks) though the cortical breaches, which shows intermediate SI on T1-weighted image and intermediate to high SI on T2-weighted image being identical to that of peripheral signal of the bone lesion. The mass is more prominent (red asterisk) on the fat-saturated T2 axial view. Microscopic examination notes predominantly osteoblastic component mixed with focal chondroblastic areas indicating osteoblastic (not shown). (**c**) Wide resection and reconstruction with allograft-prosthesis composite (APC) was performed. (**d**) Removal of APC with debridement was done followed by insertion of temporary cement spacer due to postoperative infection at 1 year after initial surgery. (**e**) After control of infection, the temporary cement insertion was removed and the defect was reconstructed with tumor prosthesis. (**f**) The patient complains of knee pain and limping gait with gradual shortening of right thigh. Follow-up lower extremity scanogram at 7 years after initial surgery demonstrates shortening of right femur by 28 mm compared to contralateral side. (**g**) The discrepancy was reduced to 2 mm by femoral component block change. She is doing well with shoe correction of the residual shortening

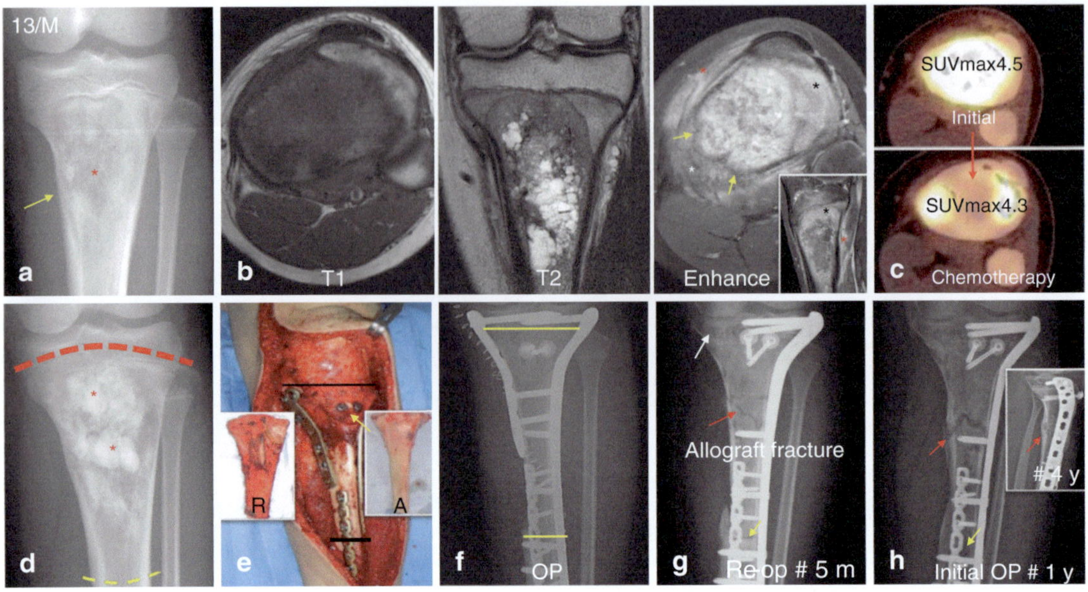

Fig. 9.5 Osteoblastic OSA. *Allograft*. (**a**) Radiograph taken for left knee pain of 3 week's duration in a 13-year-old boy shows an ill-defined radiolucent lesion (asterisk) with osteoblastic nodules involving the proximal tibia. There is a cortical thinning with a possible disruption, but no defiite periosteal reaction (arrow). (**b**) MR images reveal a concentric intramedullary lesion with intermediate SI with focal low signal on T1- and heterogeneously intermediate and high SI on T2-weighted image, affecting the meta-diaphysis of the proximal tibia. The lesion is heterogeneously enhanced, and perilesional bone marrow edema (black asterisks) and surrounding soft tissue edema (red asterisk) are also enhanced. Note cortical destruction (yellow arrows) with soft tissue mass, which is weakly enhanced (white asterisk). (**c**) Initial PET/CT scan demonstrates heterogeneously intense FDG uptake (SUVmax 4.5), which is not changed in intensity but significantly decreases in size after chemotherapy. (**d**) Follow-up radiograph after chemotherapy notes significant bone formation in the lesion (red asterisk). Wide segmental resection including a part of the epiphysis (dotted curved line), preserving the tibia tuberosity, was performed. (**e**) Allogeneic tibia (A) adequately matched to resected segment (R) was prepared, and placed in the defect (between proximal and distal black lines). It was securely fixed with plates, and the preserved tibial tuberosity was fixed using screws (yellow arrow). (**f**) Immediate postoperative radiograph shows a well-fixed allograft (from proximal to distal yellow lines) to the remaining epiphysis and diaphysis of host tibia using plates and screws. Removal of medial plate and autogenous bone graft was performed for nonunion at the host bone and allograft junction at 17 months after initial surgery. (**g**) Follow-up radiograph at 5 months after reoperation reveals union of proximal junction (white arrow) but nonunion of distal junction (yellow arrow) with newly developed fracture line emanating from the site of a previous screw hole in the middle of allograft (red arrow). Autogenous bone graft was performed again 1 year after development of fracture due to nonunion of the graft fracture. (**h**) Follow-up radiograph at 1 year after bone graft notes a visible fracture gap with some bone formation at fracture site of the graft on AP view (red arrow) and complete union of distal junction (yellow arrow). There is radiologic union with a bridging callus of the graft fracture on lateral view (red arrow in inset) with no evidence of local recurrence at 4 years after initial surgery

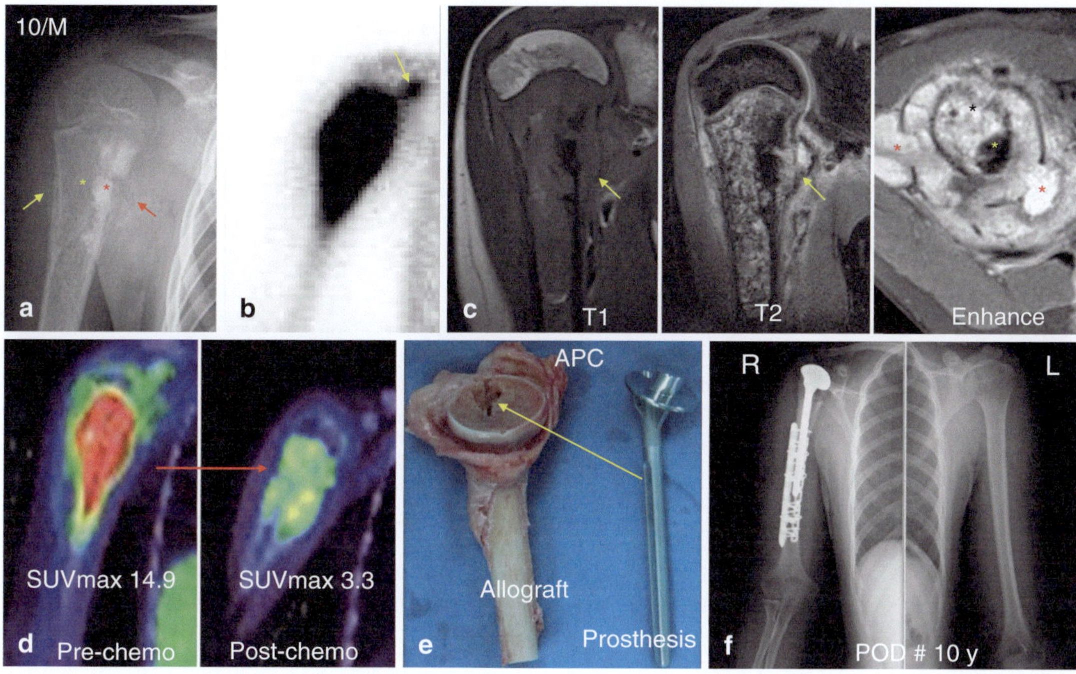

Fig. 9.6 **Osteoblastic OSA**. *APC*. (**a**) Radiograph taken for right shoulder pain for 2 months' duration in a 10-year-old boy shows a sclerotic lesion (red asterisk) with ill-defined moth-eaten to permeative radiolucent lesion (yellow asterisk) affecting meta-diaphysis of the proximal humerus. Note cortical destruction with a soft tissue mass (red arrow) and solid periosteal reaction (yellow arrow). (**b**) Bone scan reveals a homogeneous strong uptake in the meta-diaphysis as well as a focal uptake in the epiphysis suggesting a possible reactive uptake because there is no abnormal signal in the epiphysis on MRI. (**c**) MR images demonstrate an ill-defined medullary lesion with low SI on T1- and heterogeneously high SI with numerous dark signals on T2-weighted. There is cortical destruction with soft tissue mass (yellow arrows). The bony lesion is heterogeneously enhanced (black asterisk) but the dark signal focus is not enhanced indicating calcification (yellow asterisk). The soft tissue mass lesions are also strongly enhanced (red asterisks). (**d**) PET/CT scan notes an intense FDG uptake (SUVmax 14.9) in the corresponding area, which is markedly reduced (SUVmax 3.3) by chemotherapy. (**e**) Allograft-prosthesis composite (APC); An allograft is prepared for insertion of the tumor prosthesis augmented with bone cement to reconstruct the defect followed by wide resection. (**f**) Follow-up radiograph at 10 years after surgery shows good maintenance of APC with no evidence of local recurrence, but significant shortening of the arm length compared to contralateral left arm. However, the patient has no physical or mental discomfort regarding the arm length discrepancy

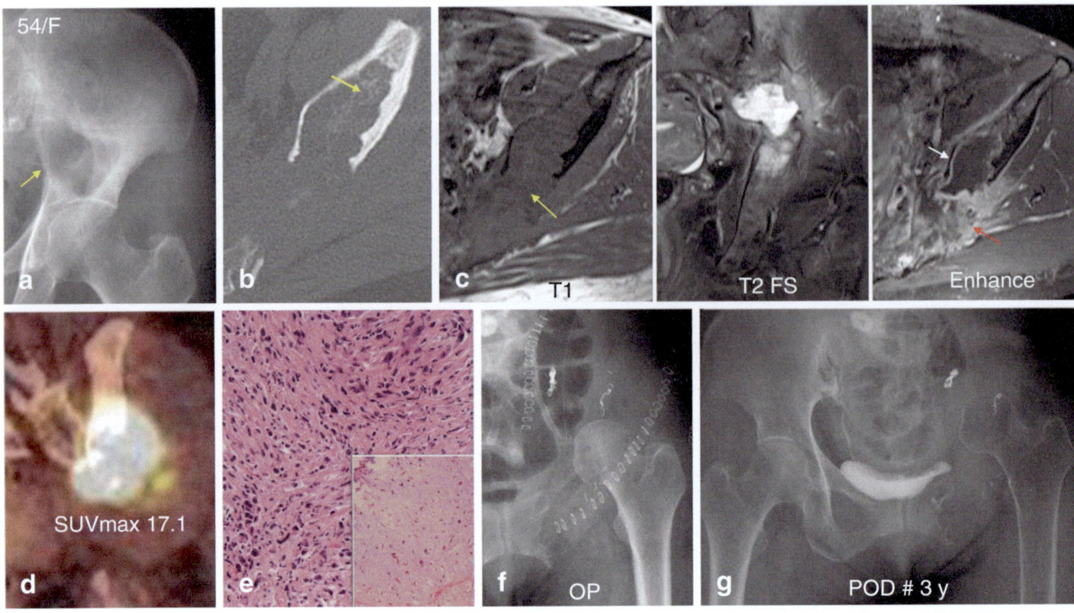

Fig. 9.7 Osteoblastic OSA. *Internal hemi-pelvectomy.* (**a**) Radiograph taken for left hip pain for 1 year's duration in a 54-year-old woman shows an ill-defined, geographic destruction with sclerotic density and possible cortical disruption (yellow arrow) in the acetabulum and iliac bone. (**b**) CT scan reveals an aggressive osteolytic lesion containing internal chondroid or osteoid matrix (yellow arrow) with marked cortical destruction and soft tissue mass formation. (**c**) MR images demonstrate an intramedullary mass lesion with low to intermediate SI on T1-weighted image and heterogeneously high SI on fat-saturated T2-weighted image. There is significant cortical destruction as well as huge soft tissue mass formation (yellow arrow). The medullary lesion is peripherally enhanced (white arrow) and the soft tissue mass (red arrow) is heterogeneously well enhanced. (**d**) PET/CT scan notes an intense FDG uptake (SUVmax 17.1) in the corresponding area including soft tissue mass, which is markedly reduced (SUVmax 3.6) by chemotherapy. (**e**) Microscopic examination shows pleomorphic stromal cells with severe nuclear atypism, and mostly filigree to lace-like osteoid production as well as focal areas of malignant cartilage formation (inset). (**f**) Internal hemi-pelvectomy was performed without reconstruction. (**g**) Radiograph at 3 years after surgery as well as MRI and CT scan shows no evidence of local recurrence with mild upward migration. However, the patient is tolerable to walk with a mild limp

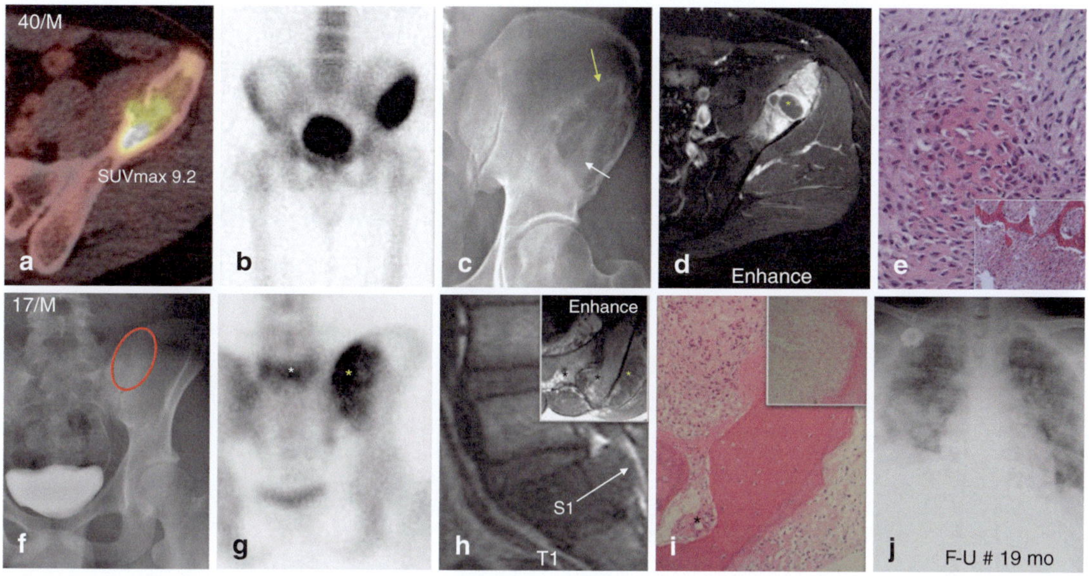

Fig. 9.8 **Osteoblastic OSA**. *Incidentally found OSA*. (**a**) PET/CT scan taken for routine medical examination in a 40-year-old man shows a foal heterogeneous FDG uptake (SUVmax 9.2) in the left iliac bone. (**b**) Bone scan reveals a homogeneously strong uptake. (**c**) Radiograph notes a large well-defined, multilobulated, oval, radiolucent lesion with internal dense areas (white area), surrounded by a rim of sclerosis (yellow arrow), affecting the left iliac wing. (**d**) Enhanced MR image demonstrates a well-enhanced expansile intramedullary mass lesion with internal nonenhancing cystic or necrotic area (asterisk). (**e**) CT-guided biopsy shows spindle cell proliferation with osteoid production. *Untreated patient with OSA* (**f**) Radiograph taken for lower back pain and left buttock painful swelling of 3 months' duration in a 17-year-old adolescent shows a suspicious hazy radiopaque lesion with obliteration of upper part of left sacroiliac (SI) joint (red circle). (**g**) Bone scan reveals strong uptake in the medial part of left iliac bone around the S-I joint (yellow asterisk) and less strong uptake in the upper part of sacrum (white asterisk). (**h**) T1-weighted MR image notes a posteriorly outgrowing mass lesion from the sacrum compressing cauda equina (white asterisk). Enhanced axial view shows heterogeneously enhanced medullary lesion (black asterisks) and soft tissue mass (yellow asterisk). (**i**) Microscopic examination demonstrates pleomorphic spindle cells producing abundant osteoid, which permeates host lamellar bone (black asterisk). Note malignant cartilage formation in the focal area (inset). (**j**) Despite the under age, he strongly refused wide resection because of the anticipated risk of bladder and bowel dysfunction. He and his parents decided to receive chemotherapy only. After 3 cycles of chemotherapy at 19 months after initial visit, he died of disseminated spread of the disease including pulmonary metastasis

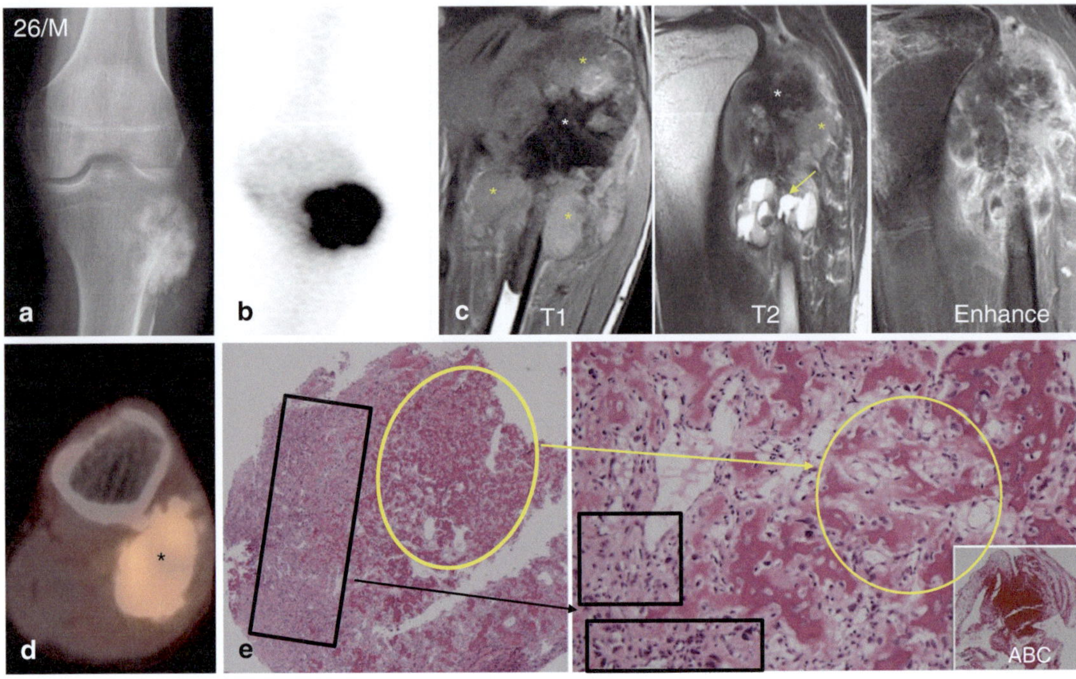

Fig. 9.9 **Sclerosing OSA**. (**a**) Radiograph taken for left knee pain and limitation of motion of several months' duration in a 26-year-old man shows an ill-defined, densely sclerotic, outgrowing mass in the proximal fibula. (**b**) Bone scan reveals a homogeneous strong uptake in the corresponding lesion of proximal fibula and soft tissue mass. (**c**) MR images demonstrate meduallary lesion (white asterisk) with low to dark SI on both T1- and T2-weighted images, as well as large extra-osseous masees (yellow asterisks) showing intermedaite to high SI on T1- and T2-weighted images. Note fluid-fluid levels suggesting possible secondary aneurysmal bone cyst (yellow arrows). The meduallry and soft tissue lesions are heterogeneously enhanced. (**d**) PET/CT scan notes an intense FDG uptake in the proximal fibula and surrounding soft tissue (asterisk). (**e**) Microscopic examination: (Left) Low-power magnification shows a mesh-work-like pattern of heavily mineralized tumor bone (circle) and less dense peripheral area with higher cellularity (rectangle). (Right) High-power magnification reveals the tumor cells deeply embedded within the more mature central tumor bones are scanty, smaller, and less malignant looking, a phenomenon reffered to as "normalization" (yellow circle). However, those in the peripherally located tumor osteoid have a high number of cells with bizarre and anaplastic nuclei (black rectangles). The heavily mineralized tumor bone is excessive to the proportion of tumor cells, indicating sclerosing OSA. A-K amputation was performed and he died of lung and multiple spine metastases 1 year after surgery

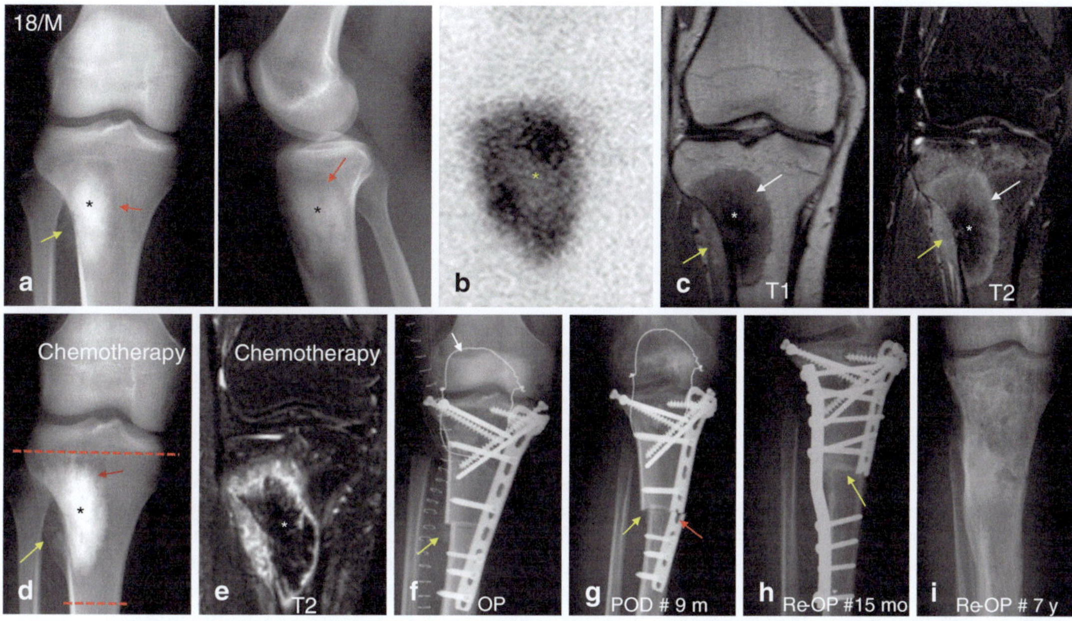

Fig. 9.10 **Sclerosing OSA**. (**a**) Radiograph taken for right knee pain for 5 months in an 18-year-old adolescent shows an eccentric, significantly sclerotic lesion (asterisk) exhibiting an "ivory-like" density, (asterisk) with a *brush-like* radiation and a radiolucent transitional zone (red arrow). Note thinning of the medial cortex with a subtle, hazy soft tissue mass in the medial aspect of the proximal tibia (yellow arrow). (**b**) Bone scan shows strongly increased uptake with central decreased uptake (red arrow). (**c**) MR images demonstrate a well-defined eccentric intramedullary lesion with low SI on T1- and intermediate to high SI on T2-weighted image with central dark signal of heavily mineralized tumor bone on both sequences (white asterisks). There are cortical breaches with a soft tissue mass (yellow arrows). (**d**) Follow-up radiograph after neoadjuvant chemotherapy notes increased size of the dense lesion (black asterisk) with more prominent radiating bony streaks (red arrow) and more clear visible soft tissue mass having periosteal reaction and reactive bone formation (yellow arrow). (**e**) Follow-up MR image after neoadjuvant chemotherapy shows markedly increased size of the central dark signal (asterisk) suggesting internal maturation of the most tumor bones. (**f**) Wide resection of proximal tibia and fibular head was performed with reconstruction using allograft fixed by plate and tension band wiring (white arrow). Autogenous chip bone graft was additionally applied to the at allograft and tibia junction (yellow arrow) to promote union. (**g**) Radiograph at 9 months after surgery shows nonunion (yellow arrow) with metallic failure (red arrow). A distal part of the broken plate was removed and stronger fixation was performed using an additional lateral plate with autogenous bone graft. (**h**) Radiograph at 15 months after re-operation reveals consolidation between allograft and tibia junction (yellow arrow). (**i**) The plate and screws were removed at 3 years after re-operation due to chronic infection. Follow-up radiograph 7 years after re-operation notes no evidence of local recurrence with complete union of the allograft to the host bone

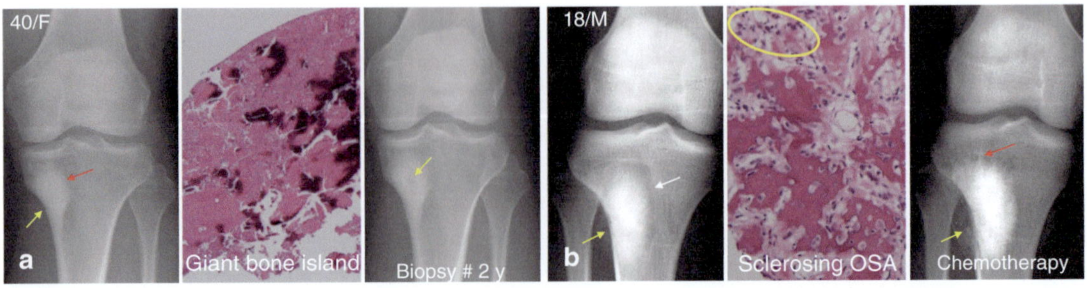

Fig. 9.11 *Sclerosing OSA* vs. *giant bone island.* (**a**) Radiograph taken for right knee pain by blunt trauma in a 40-year-old woman shows a homogeneously dense, oblong lesion having a spiculated margin with peripheral radiating streaks, "brush-like" pattern of radiation (red arrow). The long axis is parallel to the direction of mechanical stresses on bone, representing adaptation to Wolff's law. There is no periosteal reaction (yellow arrow). Trocar biopsy reveals a cortical-type bone containing Haversian-like canals in association with woven bones indicative of enostosis/bone islands. Radiograph at 2 years later notes no interval change with a hazy radiolucent hole made by biopsy trocar. (**b**) Another radiograph taken for left knee pain in an 18-year-old male patient reveals a similar dense lesion with *brush-like* radiation and radiolucent transitional zone (white arrow). Note a subtle, hazy periosteal reaction which is not observed in giant bone island (yellow arrow). Microscopic examination reveals pleomorphic stromal cells with osteoid (circle) and profusely mineralized tumor bone, indicating sclerosing OSA. Follow-up radiograph after neoadjuvant chemotherapy demonstrates more prominently radiating bony streaks (red arrow) and soft tissue mass with more clearly seen periosteal reaction and reactive bone formation (yellow arrow)

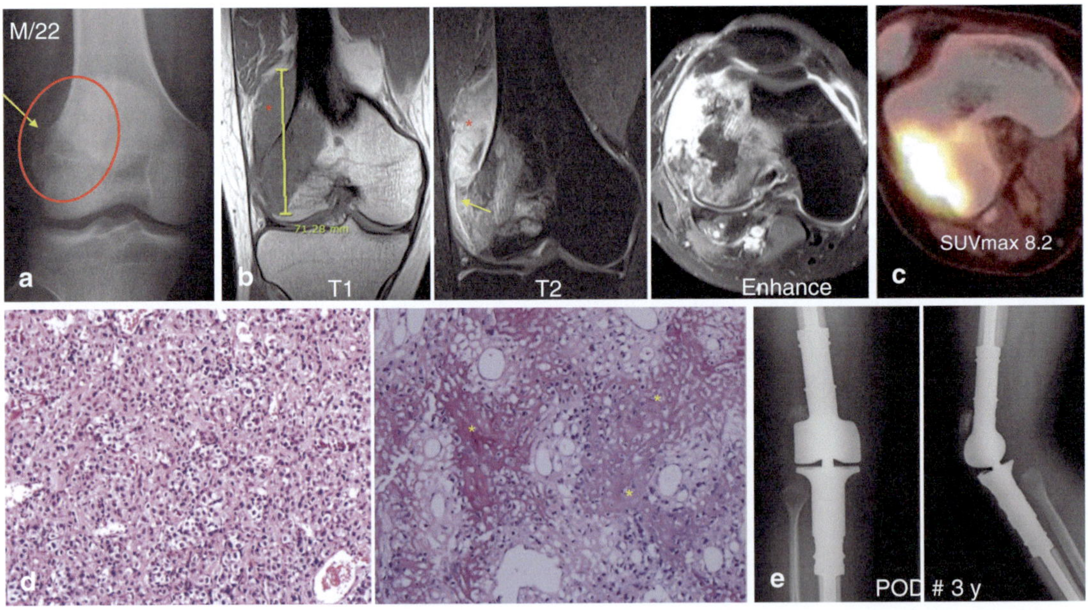

Fig. 9.12 **Chondroblastic OSA**. (**a**) Radiograph taken for right pain of 1 month's duration in a 22-year-old young man shows a a subtle, mottled, eccntric radiolucent lesion (red circle) with hazy soft tissue mass (yellow arrow) in the lateral condyle of the femur. (**b**) MR images reveal an ill-defined eccentric intramedullary lesion with low SI on T1- and heterogeneously high SI on T2-weighted image affecting the epi-metaphysis of the lateral femoral condyle. There is cortical destruction with extra-osseous soft tissue extension (red arrows). The medullary lesion and soft tissue mass are heterogeneously enhanced. (**c**) PET/CT scan demonstrates a heterogeneously intense FDG uptake in the medullary lesion as well as in the soft tissue mass (SUVmax 8.2). (**d**) Microscopic examination notes extensive and predominant malignant cartilage matrix throughout the lesion with severely atypical chondrocytes, which is intimately admixed with neoplastic bone (asterisks on right). (**e**) Follow-up radiograph at 3 years after wide resection and reconstruction shows good maintenance of the prosthesis with no evidence of local recurrence

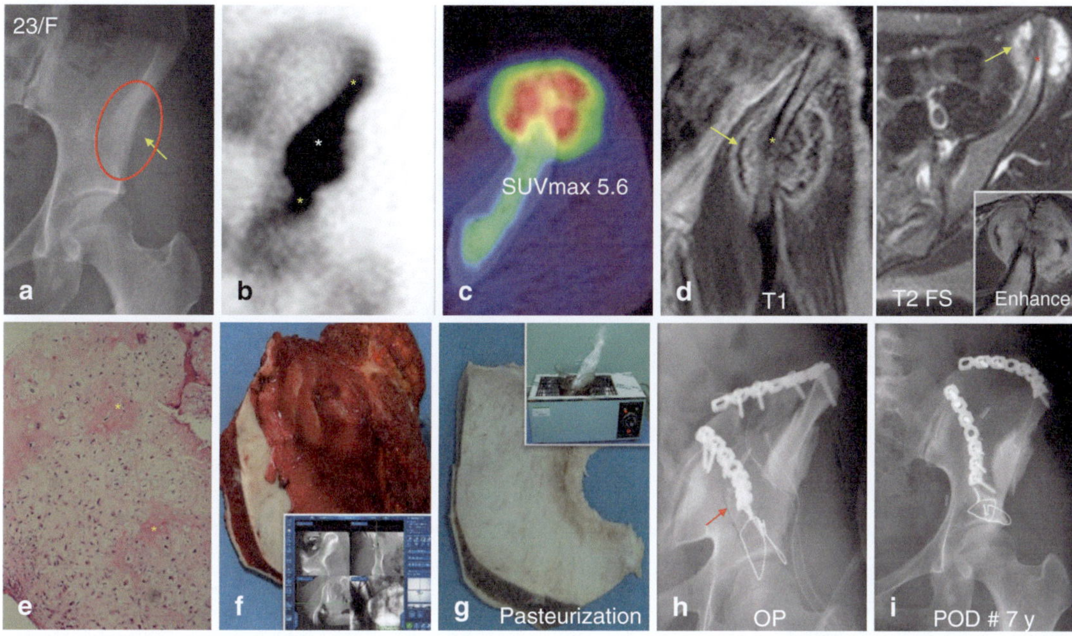

Fig. 9.13 **Chondroblastic OSA**. (**a**) Radiograph taken for left pelvis pain of 1 month's duration in a 23-year-old young woman shows an ill-defined sclerotic lesion (circle) with focal radiolucent holes as well as a hazy soft tissue mass (arrow) involving left iliac bone. (**b**) Bone scan reveals a homogeneously strong uptake in the corresponding bone and soft tissue lesions (white asterisk) as well as along the lateral margin of the iliac wing (yellow asterisks). (**c**) PET/CT scan notes a heterogeneously intense localized FDG uptake in the bony lesion and soft tissue mass (SUVmax 5.6). (**d**) MR images demonstrate an ill-defined intramedullary lesion (yellow asterisks) and larger soft tissue masses (yellow arrows) with heterogeneously low and high SI on T1- and high SI on fat-saturated T2-weighted image. The lesions are heterogeneously enhanced (inset). (**e**) Microscopic examination shows extensive production of cartilage matrix throughout the lesion with pleomorphic chondrocytes, which are intimately admixed with tumor osteoid (asterisks). (**f**) Wide resection using computer assisted navigation system was performed with negative margin. (**g**) The soft tissue and muscle were clearly removed from the resected iliac bone for pasteurization. (**h**) Subsequently, the recycled bone was repositioned and fixed with plate and wiring. (**i**) Follow-up radiograph at 7 years after surgery reveals good maintenance of the recycled bone without evidence of local recurrence.

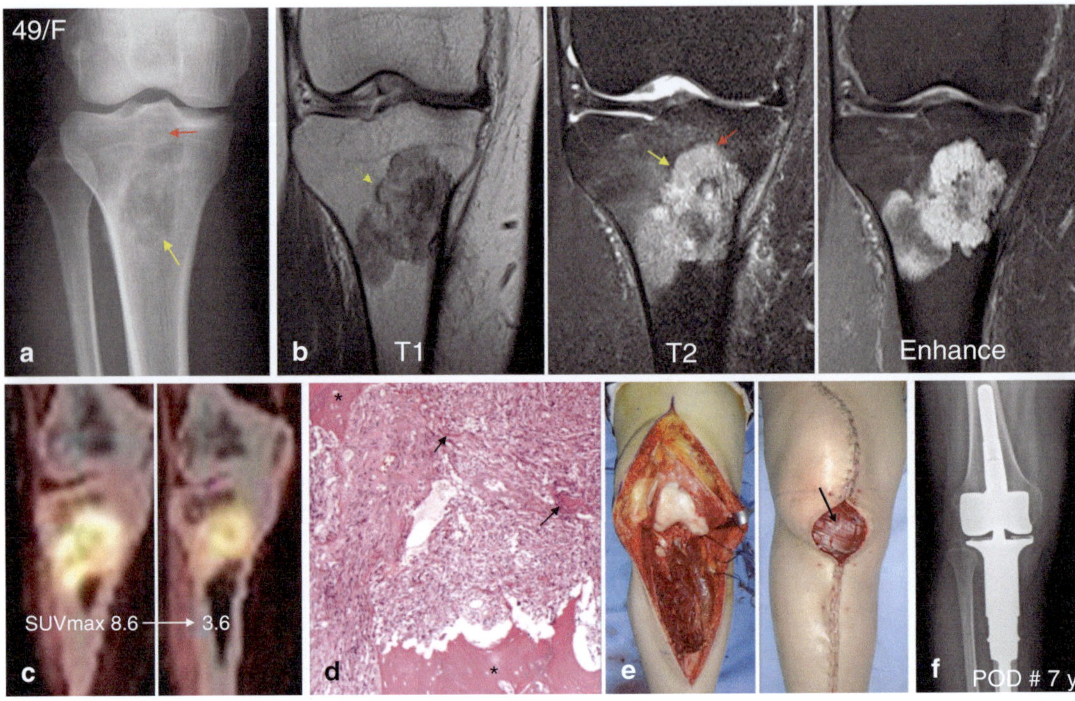

Fig. 9.14 Fibroblastic OSA. (**a**) Radiograph taken for right knee pain of 10 months' duration in a 49-year-old woman shows a relatively well-defined lytic lesion with internal hazy densification, surrounded by thin, incomplete rim of sclerosis (yellow arrow), mainly affecting the metaphysis of the proximal tibia and possibly extending to part of the epiphysis (red arrow). (**b**) MR images reveal a relatively well-defined intramedullary mass lesion mainly involving the metaphysis and focally extending to the epiphysis (red arrow) of the proximal tibia with low to intermediate SI on T1- and intermediate to high SI on T2-weighted image, showing focal areas of dark signal. There is a thin dark signal surrounding the lesion (yellow arrow). The lesion is heterogeneously well enahnced. (**c**) PET/CT scan demonstrates a heterogeneously intense FDG uptake (SUVmax 8.6) in the proximal tibia. The SUVmax is dropped to 3.6 by neoadjuvant chemotherapy. (**d**) Low-power microscopic examination notes tumor mass permeating the host lamellar bone (black asterisks), which consists of pleomorphic stromal cells producing abundant fibrous tissues or collagen matrix with only a minimal bone formation (arrow). (**e**) Wide resection with reconstruction using tumor prosthesis was performed. The soft tissue defect was covered by a medial gastrocnemius muscle flap (arrow). (**f**) Follow-up radiograph at 7 years after surgery reveals good maintenance of the tumor prosthesis with no evidence of local recurrence

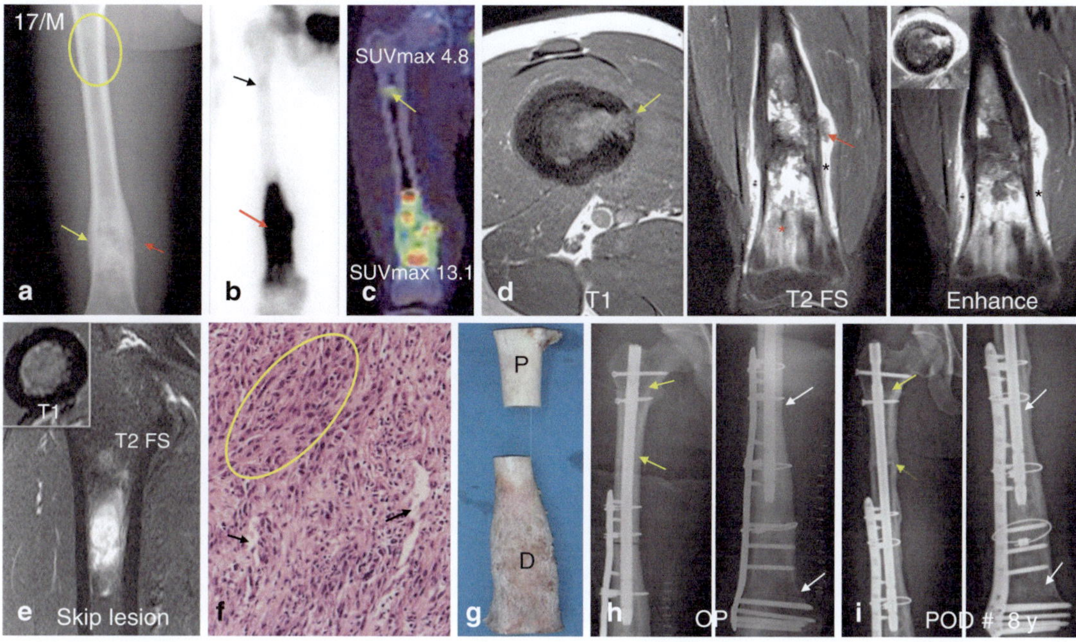

Fig. 9.15 **Fibroblastic OSA**. (**a**) Radiograph taken for right thigh pain of 4 months' duration in a 17-year-old boy shows an ill-defined expanding radiolucent lesion with some sclerotic areas in the meta-diaphysis of the distal femur. There is a thick periosteal reaction (yellow arrow) as well as hazy soft tissue mass (red arrow). However, plain radiograph shows no definite skip lesion in the proximal femur (yellow circle). (**b**) Bone scan reveals segmental area of intensely hot uptake in the distal femur (red arrow) and area of subtle mild uptake in the proximal femur (black arrow). (**c**) PET/CT scan notes a heterogeneously intense FDG uptake in the distal femur (SUVmax 13.1) and less active uptake (yellow arrow; SUVmax 4.8) in the proximal femur, suggesting a possible skip lesion. (**d**) MR images of the distal femur demonstrate an ill-defined extensive, expansile, intramedullary lesion with heterogeneously low to intermediate SI on T1- and mixed low, intermediate, and high SI on T2-weighted image with extensive adjacent bone marrow edema (red asterisk). Cortical perforation is more clearly visible on an axial image (yellow arrow), and a soft tissue mass is more clearly noted on coronal images (red arrow). Prominent periosteal reaction with reactive edema is also well visible (black asterisks). The lesion itself and adjacent bone marrow edema are heterogeneously enhanced, and periosteal edema is strongly enahnced (black asterisks). (**e**) MR images of the proximal femur show another nodular lesion with SI similar to the distal lesion, indicating a skip lesion. There is no definite cortical perforation. (**f**) Microscopic examination reveals predominant pleomorphic spindle stromal cells producing fibrous tissues or collagen matrix as well as osteoid production in a filigree pattern (circle), corresponding to sclerotic areas on radiograph. There are pericytoid vascular spaces (arrows) mimicking hemangiopericytoma. (**g**) Wide resection of the proximal and distal femur was performed after neoadjuvant chemotherapy, and the surrounding muscle and soft tissue were removed from the proximal (P) and distal (D) femur for pasteurization. (**h**) The recycled segments were put back to the original sites and fixed with an intramedullary nail and plate. The junction sites are clearly visible in the proximal segment (yellow arrows) and distal segment (white arrows). (**i**) Follow-up radiograph at 8 years after surgery shows no evidence of local recurrence with radiologic healing at the (yellow arrows) and distal (white arrows) segments and the host bone

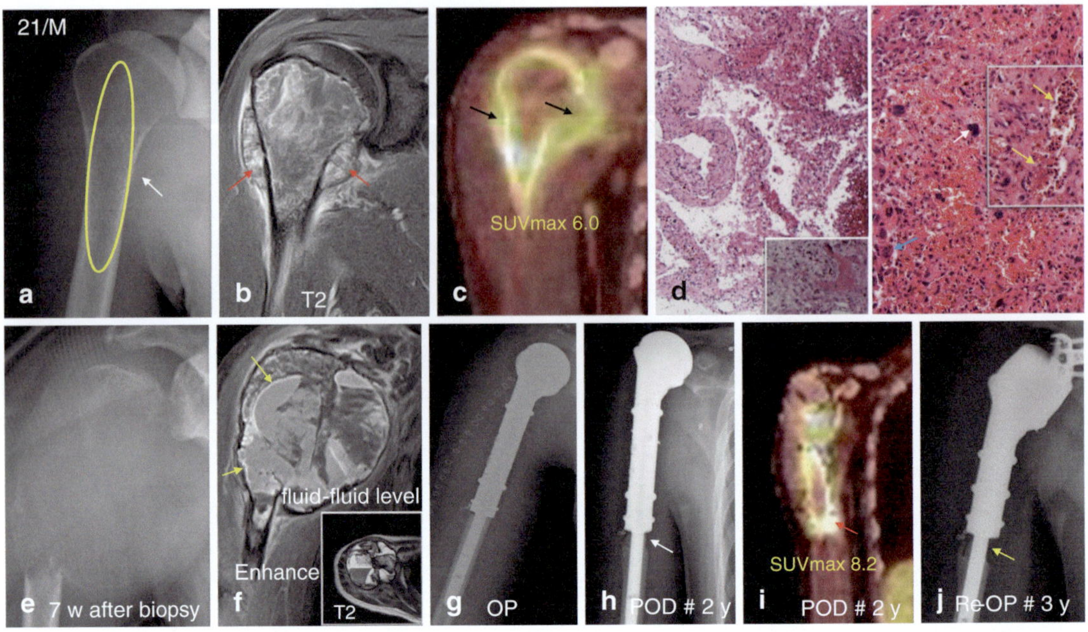

Fig. 9.16 Telangiectatic OSA. (**a**) Radiograph taken for right shoulder pain of 10 days' duration in a 21-year-old man shows an ill-defined moth-eaten to permeative destruction in the meta-diaphysis of proximal humerus (circle). A hazy soft tissue extension is suspected (arrow). (**b**) T2-weighted MR images reveal a multichambered mass-like lesion extending to adjacent soft tissues (red arrows) through medial and lateral cortical breaches. (**c**) PET/CT scan reveals a heterogeneously intense FDG uptake (SUVmax 6.0) in the proximal humerus and soft tissue mass (arrows). (**d**) Microscopic examination: (Left) Low-power magnification demonstrates blood-filled and empty vascular spaces surrounded by septa with variable thickness, which are histologically indistinguishable from ABC. Osteoid production is focal and osteoclast-type multinucleated giant cells are frequently found. (Right) Higher-power magnification of a septum reveals bizarre pleomorphic spindle cells with severely atypical nuclei, producing osteoid, and frequent atypical mitotic figures. Malignant-looking multinucleated giant cells with bizarre nuclei (white arrow) are scattered together with distinctly bland-looking giant cells (blue arrow). Some malignant cells are seen free-floating within the extensive hemorrhagic areas. Note atypical stromal cells free-floating in the vascular space (yellow arrows in inset). (**e**) Radiograph taken for severely aggravated pain with swelling of right shoulder, accompanied by fever and headache at 7 weeks after biopsy during the third cycle of neoadjuvant chemotherapy shows significant progression of the tumor with extensive cortical destruction and huge soft tissue mass formation. (**f**) Enhanced MR image reveals that the tumor extends to the epiphysis with significantly increased overall size. The intramedullary tumor as well as soft tissue mass is composed of peripherally enhancing lobules and septa. T2-weighted axial image demonstrates several fluid-fluid levels (inset). (**g**) Wide resection with reconstruction using tumor prosthesis was performed. (**h**) Follow-up radiograph at 2 years after surgery shows bone resorption at the distal humerus and tumor prosthesis junction (white arrow). Incision biopsy shows chronic inflammation with abundant granulation tissue but no malignant cells. (**i**) PET/CT scan notes a diffuse intense FDG uptake (SUVmax 8.2) around the tumor prosthesis, particularly at the junction between the distal humerus and the prosthesis (red arrow), suggesting a possible local recurrence or extensive granulation tissue formation around the tumor prosthesis. The patient suffered recurrent dislocation of the shoulder prosthesis and revision surgery was done at this time. (**j**) Follow-up radiograph at 3 years after revision surgery reveals bone resorption at the distal humerus and tumor prosthesis junction (yellow arrow) probably due to stress shielding but no evidence of local recurrence

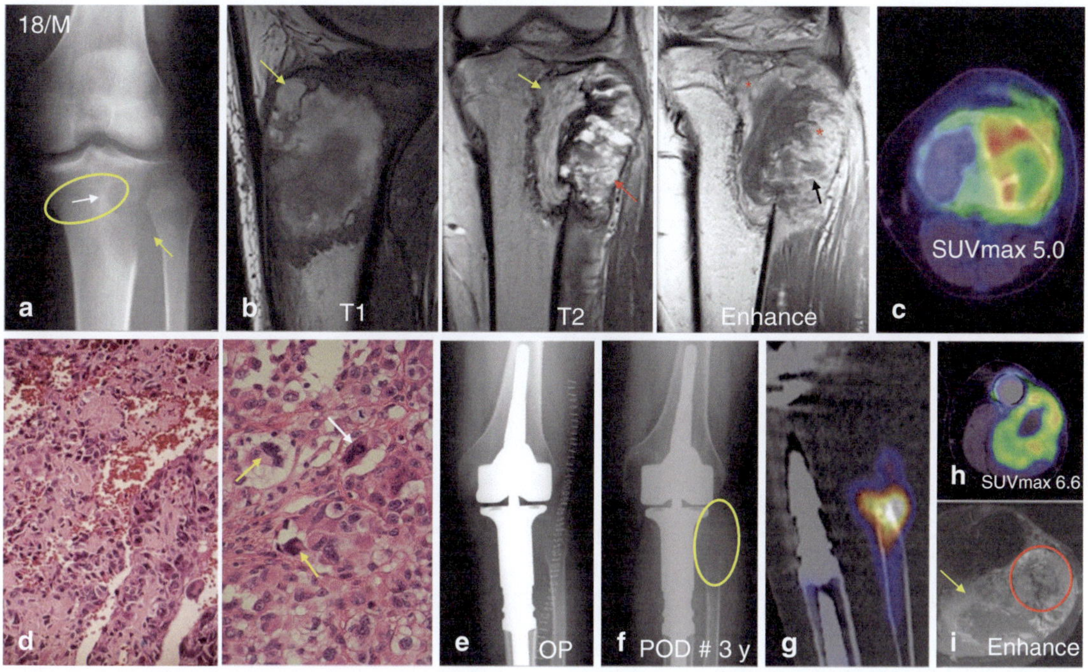

Fig. 9.17 **Telangiectatic OSA**. (**a**) Radiograph taken for right knee pain of 4 months' duration in an 18-year-old boy shows an ill-defined eccentric purely lytic lesion with an incomplete rim of sclerosis (white arrow) in the epimetaphysis of proximal tibia. There is significant cortical destruction, possibly accompanied by soft tissue mass formation (yellow arrow). (**b**) MR images reveal an eccentric intramedullary mass lesion mainly affecting the metaphysis and extending to the epiphysis (yellow arrows) with heterogeneous intermediate and slightly high SI on T1- and heterogeneously high SI with central dark signal on T2-weighted image. Note cortical breakage and large soft tissue mass with internal hemorrhage and multichambered cystic lesions with fluid-fluid levels (red arrow). The medullary and soft tissue mass lesion is heterogeneously enhanced (asterisks) with thin nodular septal enhancement (yellow arrow). (**c**) PET/CT scan notes a heterogeneously increased FDG uptake in the proximal tibia (SUVmax 5.0). (**d**) Microscopic examination: (Left) Medium-power magnification demonstrates blood-filled and empty vascular spaces surrounded by septa composed of pleomorphic spindle cells. (Right) High-power examination shows highly bizarre pleomorphic cells (yellow arrow) that exceed the cytologic range typically seen in ABC, producing osteoid. Atypical mitosis is also observed (white arrow). (**e**) Wide resection followed by reconstruction with tumor prosthesis was performed. (**f**) Follow-up radiograph at 3 years after surgery reveals destruction of the proximal fibula with soft tissue extension (red arrow). (**g**) Bone SPECT notes an intensely hot uptake in the left proximal fibula. (**h**) Follow-up PET/CT scan demonstrates a heterogeneously increased FDG uptake (SUVmax 6.6) in the peri-prosthetic area as well as proximal fibula and soft tissue of calf, suggesting a local recurrence of the tumor invading the adjacent fibula. (**i**) Enhanced MR image shows an intramedullary mass lesion totally destructing proximal fibula and forming a large soft tissue mass with peripheral thick wall (arrow) and nodular enhancement (circle). The patient died of lung metastasis 3 years after surgery

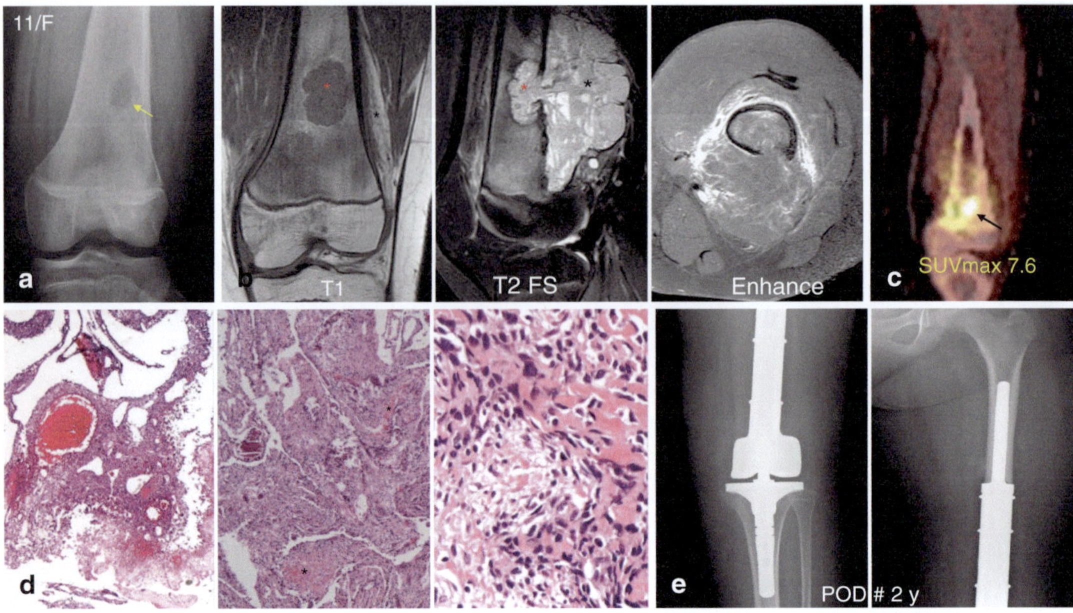

Fig. 9.18 Telangiectatic OSA. (**a**) Radiograph taken for right distal thigh pain of several months' duration, which is aggravated 10 days prior to medical attention in an 11-year-old girl shows a well-defined oval purely lytic lesion with a hazy thin surrounding sclerosis (arrow) and periosteal reaction in the diaphysis rather than the metastasis of the distal femur. (**b**) MR images reveal a well-defined small intramedullary lesion (red asterisks) with a huge soft tissue mass formation (black asterisk) through cortical breakage. The SI is low to intermediate on T1- and heterogeneously intermediate and high SI with multiple fluid-fluid levels in the soft tissue mass on fat-saturated T2-weighted image. The intramedullary lesion and soft tissue mass lesion are heterogeneously enhanced. (**c**) PET/CT scan demonstrates a heterogeneously increased FDG uptake with internal focal intense uptake (arrow), appearing disproportionately small relative to the actual tumor volume, referred to as the "iceberg" pattern, in the left distal femur (SUVmax 7.6). (**d**) Microscopic examination: (Left) Low-power magnification notes blood-filled and empty vascular spaces surrounded by variably thickened wall-like septa with scattered multinucleated giant cells simulating ABC. (Middle) Medium-power magnification shows atypical spindle cells producing focal osteoid deposition (black asterisks) within thickened septa. (Right) Higher-power magnification reveals bizarre pleomorphic stromal cells with frequent atypical mitotic figures, which directly produce primitive osteoid. (**e**) Follow-up radiograph at 2 years after wide resection and reconstruction with a tumor prosthesis notes good maintenance of the tumor prosthesis without evidence of local recurrence

9.6 Clinical Features

The most frequent presentation is bone pain associated with progressively enlarging soft-tissue mass or swelling of short duration, usually a few weeks to months. At first, the pain is usually mild and intermittent, which gradually increases in severity probably due to progression of bone weakness with minimal to larger stress fracture. Swelling is the next common presentation, which develpos as the lesion progresses and destructs the cortex to form a soft tissue mass. Limitation of adjacent joint or joint contracture can be associated in more advanced cases. Joint effusion may herald epiphyseal extension or involvement. The overlying skin may be warm, erythematous, edematous, and prominent engorged superficial veins. At times, pathologic fracture is accompanied most frequently in the femur and humerus. Extremely rare patients have no symptoms and are incidentally found on images for various reasons including routine medical check-up (Fig. 9.17). Constitutional signs such as weight loss, general weakness, pallor or anorexia-related tumor spread, or metastasis can occur, usually in later stages and rarely even in the initial evaluation of patients.

9.7 Serologic Findings

Serum alkaline phosphatase is the only laboratory determination with significant alteration in OSA and is often elevated depending on the amount of new-bone formation and osteoid deposition, which is particularly high in patients with a heavy tumor burden or in those with prominent osteoblastic differentiation. The serum value tends to return to normal after surgical ablation or after extensive tumor necrosis induced by preoperative chemotherapy. It will increase again with tumor recurrence. McKanna et al. [8] reported about 80% of patients, who had phosphatase determinations recorded, showed an elevation at the time of local recurrence or metastasis.

9.8 Secondary OSA (Figs. 9.22, 9.23, 9.24, and 9.25)

Paget's disease of bone (PDB) is common in Western countries and those immigrating from these countries, but it is rare in Scandinavia or the Far East. OSA is estimated in approximately 1% of patients with PDB, which is several thousand-fold times more frequent than in the general population. The associated OSA is usually high-grade, and most frequently occurs in the pelvis, femur, and humerus, followed by the tibia and skull, where are favorite locations for PDB. These OSA occur most frequently in patients in their seventh decade with longstanding or polyostotic disease, at a time when primary conventional OSA is extremely rare in the general population [9]. A sudden onset or worsening of may herald development of secondary OSA. The prognosis is significantly poorer when compared to that of primary conventional OSA. ***Radioation-induced OSA*** Earlier, the development of bone sarcoma by ionizing radiation was

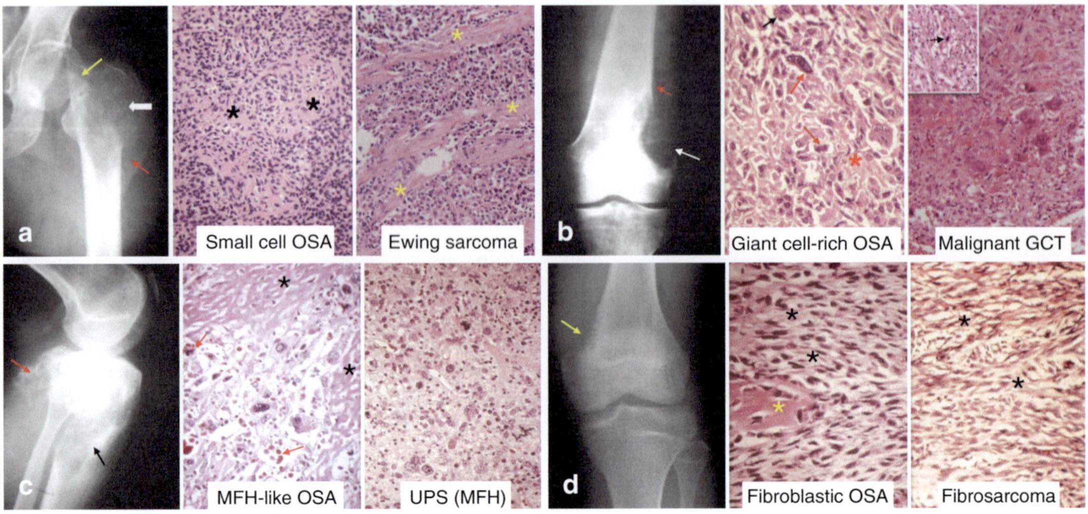

Fig. 9.19 *OSA often producing minimal osteoid which requires extensive samples.* (**a**) *Small cell OSA:* Radiograph shows an ill-defined radiolucent geographic lesion with moth-eaten to permeative destruction and internal multiple dotted densification (white arrow) involving the trochanteric area of the proximal femur. Pathologic fracture (yellow arrow) is associated with a large soft tissue mass (red arrow). Microscopic examination reveals uniform small-sized round to oval cells with scanty cytoplasm. Osteoid matrix deposition (black asterisks) is often scanty and inconspicuous, but it is indispensible for differentiating small cell OSA from other small round cell malignancies such as lymphoma and Ewing's sarcoma. In Ewing's sarcoma, tumor cells typically grow in sheet-like or irregular islands delineated by dense fibrous tissue (yellow asterisks) with no osteoid production. (**b**) *Giant cell-rich OSA:* Radiograph shows an ill-defined radiolucent geographic lesion with cortical destruction and a soft tissue mass (white arrow) affecting mainly the metaphseal of the distal femur. Radiologic findings of mainly metaphyseal location, Codman's triangle (red arrow), and intralesional density of fluffs are clues to a giant cell-rich OSA rather than conventional GCT. Microscopic examination reveals bizarre pleomorphic stromal cells (red arrows) with multinucleated giant cells, some of which can be anaplastic, derived from anaplastic stromal cells (black arrow). However, the stromal cells and multinucleated giant cells may be deceptively benign-looking which easily lead to an erroneous diagnosis of conventional GCT, particularly when radiographic features are not correlated. The amount of osteoid deposition is variable but usually scanty (red asterisk). In malignant GCT, microscopic examination demonstrates proliferation of atypical round to oval mononuclear stromal cells with typical and atypical multinucleated giant cells as well as abnormal mitosis (black arrow in inset). However, there is no definite tumor osteoid or woven bone formation. (**c**) *UPS (MFH)-like OSA:* Radiograph shows an ill-defined radiolucent lesion with internal densities (black arrow) and a soft tissue mass (red arrow). Microscopic examination reveals bizarre phagocytic or histiocytic stromal cells resembling undifferentiated pleomorphic sarcoma (UPS) (former malignant fibrous histiocytoma; MFH) often with minimal tumor osteoid (black asterisks). This variant is often associated with considerable hemorrhage and erythro-phagocytosis, which may produce pink droplet or globules (red arrows) by deposition of lipoprotein breakdown products of erythrocytes in the cells, referred to as *sarcoma bodies* [4]. (**d**) *Fibroblastic OSA:* Radiograph also reveals an ill-defined, geographic destruction and discernible cortical destruction ill-defined geographic bone destruction and discernible cortical disruption with a soft tissue mass formation (arrow). Microscopic examination demonstrates atypical tumor cells arranged in a "herringbone" pattern, as in FSA, producing abundant fibrous tissue and collagen matrix (black asterisks), with focal minimal deposition of primitive bone (yellow asterisk). FSA also exhibits fibrous tissue and collagen bundles with atypical tumor cells arranged in a "herringbone" pattern (black asterisks), but no osteoid or primitive bone is observed throughout the entire field. The above-mentioned variants of OSA, often producing minimal or scanty osteoid, request an extensive sample by incision biopsy rather than needle or trocar biopsy

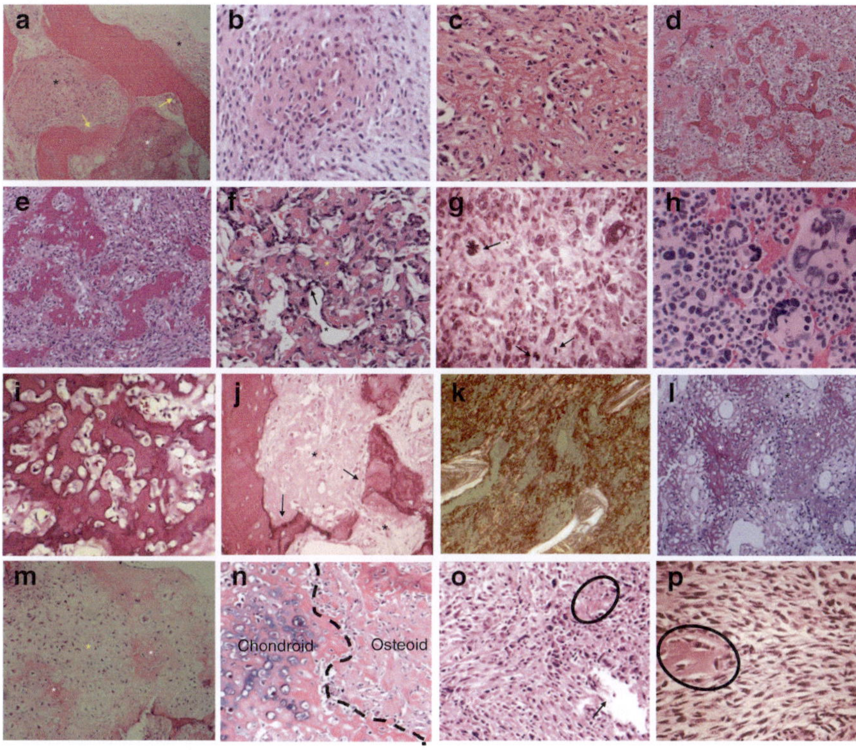

Fig. 9.20 *Microscopic examination of conventional OSA: Osteoblastic OSA* (**a**) Low-power view shows atypical spindle cells producing osteoid, which occupies bone marrow space (black asterisk) and permeate the host lamellar bone (yellow arrows), referred to as *permeative or encasement* pattern. (**b**) High-power view reveals pleomorphic spindle cells in size and shape with irregular hyperchromatic nuclei, which directly produce a fibrillar pinkish collagenous matrix and osteoid. (**c**) A more advanced case shows clear-cut anaplastic spindle cells with nuclear pleomorphism, abnormal chromatin clumping, high nuclear to cytoplasmic ratio, and prominent nucleoli with atypical mitoses, producing a deliate lace-like osteoid matrix. (**d**) In another case, the anaplastic stromal spindle cells are producing abundant haphazardly distributed primitive osteoid (black asterisk) toward mature Pagetoid bone with deposited cement lines in a random manner, referred to as a *mosaic pattern* (white asterisks) making an anastomosing network. (**e**) A further advnaced case reveals definitely anaplastic spindle cells collaborating clearly recognizable trabeculae of woven bone with more advanced mineralized (white asterisks). (**f**) Hemangiopericytoma-like pattern of tumor growth can be recognized as in another high-grade sarcoma such as mesenchymal chondrosarcoma, fibrosarcoma, or undifferentiated pleomorphic sarcoma. Note a prominent characteristic *staghorn* pattern or pericytoid vascular spaces (black asterisks) surrounded by pleomorphic spindle cells (black arrows) producing an osteoid matrix (yellow asterisks). (**g**) Higher-power view demonstrates tumor cells with frequent atypical mitoses (black arrows). (**h**) Extraordinarily bizarre cells can be observed. *Sclerosing OSA:* (**i**) The heavily mineralized tumor bone is excessive in proportion to the tumor cells. The tumor cells deeply embedded in the bone matrix are scarce and small resembling normal osteocytes. The cytology features of malignancy are subtle to absent, the so-called *normalizing* effect by Jaffe, which can make a diagnosis of OSA difficult if there is no permeation pattern on examining histologic slide as well as no radiologic correlation. (**j**) Deceptively bland-looking "normalized" tumor cells embedded in osteoid (black asterisk) permeate the preexisting host bone spicules and trap it in its wake (black arrows), absolutely indicating malignant tumor despite the bland-looking stromal cells. (**k**) Polarized microscope shows typical lamellar bones that are permeated by tumor cells. *Chondroblastic OSA* (**l**) Low-power view shows light pink chondroid areas containing tumor cells in lacunar spaces (white asterisks) are intimately intermingled with purple sheet-like osteoid areas (white asterisks). (**m**) Medium-power view reveals bizarre pleomorphic tumor cells in lacunar spaces producing chondroid and osteoid. There are islands of osteoid (white asterisks) within the chondroid matrix (yellow asterisk). (**n**) Higher-power view notes a gradual transition zone between chondroid and osteoid (black dotted line) where it is difficult to differentiate the matrices (osteochondroid). *Fibroblastic OSA:* (**o**) Bizarre highly pleomorphic spindle cells with striking nuclear atypia and frequent mitoses produce mostly fibrous tissue or collagen matrix and scant focal osteoid (circle). Note highly vascular stroma with variable-sized pericytoid vascular spaces which resembles hemangiopericytoma (arrow). (**p**) The tumor cells can be arranged in a *herringbone* or *storiform* pattern containing conspicuous deposition of homogenous eosinophilic material in the majority of the field, which closely resembles pure fibrosarcoma. However, a minimal focal deposition of osteoid directly by tumor cells (black circle) is seen. Such small foci of osteoid production can be only observed on careful examination, and may be absent in limited specimens obtained by inadequate biopsy, which finding is easily mistaken for fibrosarcoma

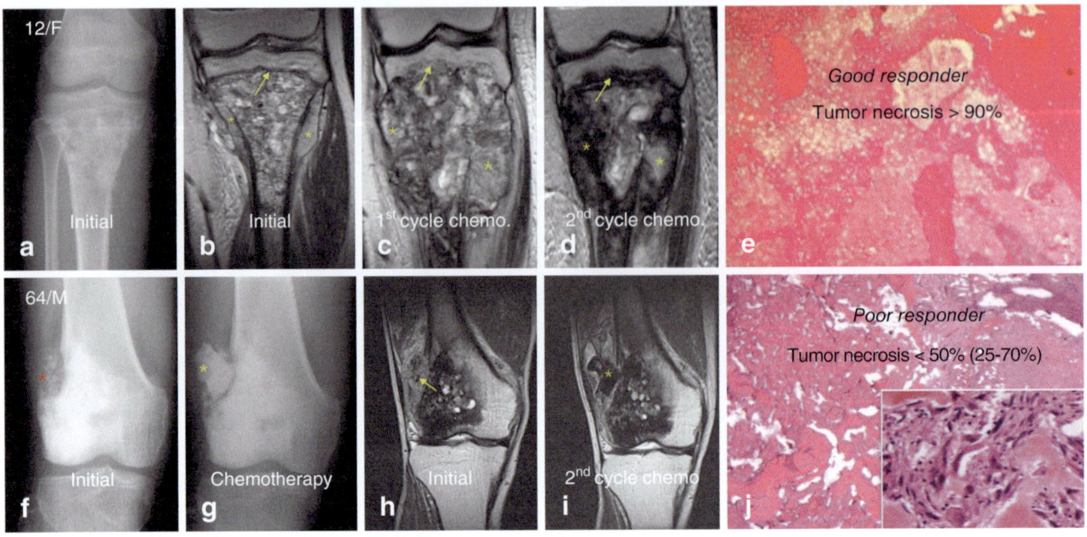

Fig. 9.21 Pathologic assessment of neoadjuvant chemotherapy. *Good responder* (**a**) Radiograph taken for right knee pain of 3 months' duration in a 12-year-old girl shows an ill-defined mixed osteoblastic and osteolytic mass lesion with hazy periosteal reaction mainly in the metaphyseal area of the proximal tibia. (**b**) Initial T2-weighted MR image reveals an intramedullary mass lesion mainly in the metaphysis with heterogeneously high SI which extends to the diaphysis. However, the epiphysis seems to be not involved (yellow arrow). There is soft tissue mass formation both at lateral and medial aspects (asterisks). (**c**) MR image after first neoadjuvant chemotherapy notes further progression, particularly with markedly increased size of the soft tissue masses (yellow asterisks) as well as focal epiphyseal extension (yellow arrow). (**d**) However, follow-up MR image after another cycle of chemotherapy demonstrates an interval decrease in size and extent of the lesion especially with shrinkage of the soft tissue masses (yellow asterisks) and progression of tumor necrosis with calcification. The epiphyseal lesion reveals a dark signal of mineralization (yellow arrow). (**e**) Microscopic examination of the resected specimen shows nearly complete tumor necrosis with scattered foci of viable tumor cells less than 10%, classified as a good responder. *Poor responder* (**f**) Radiograph taken for right knee pain of 4 months' duration in a 64-year-old man shows an ill-defined intramedullary sclerotic lesion with cortical destruction resulting in soft tissue mass formation with scattered internal calcifications (red asterisk) in the epi-metaphysis of the distal femur. (**g**) Radiograph after neoadjuvant chemotherapy reveals no definite interval change of the bone lesion. There is a cement plug inserted for bleeding control during incision biopsy (yellow asterisk). (**h**) Initial T2-weighted MR image reveals an intramedullary mass lesion with heterogeneously intermediate and high SI. There is lateral cortical bone destruction with a nacked soft tissue mass (yellow arrow). (**i**) Follow-up MR image after the second cycle of neoadjuvant chemotherapy notes an increse in tumor size, particularly of the soft tissue mass, especially soft tissue mass, containing a non-enhancing area indicating tumor necrosis. A dark signal (yellow asterisk) is visible within the soft tissue mass indicating a cement plug inserted for bleeding control during incision biopsy. (**j**) Microscopic examination of the resected specimen shows a varying degree of tumor necrosis depending on the location (25–70% with average less than 50%), classified as poor responder

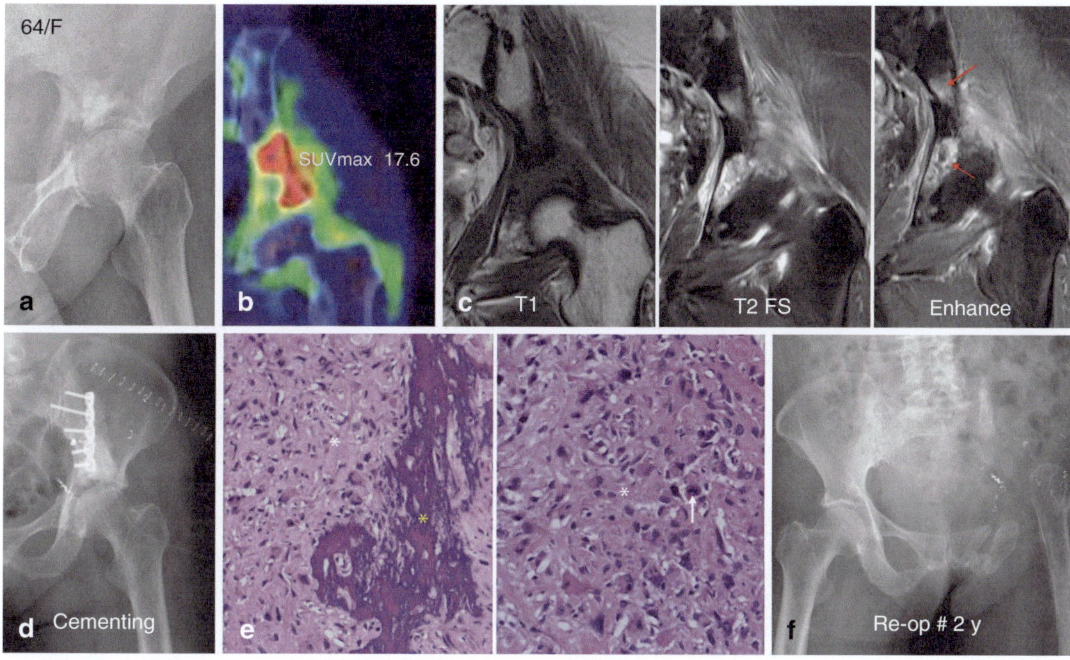

Fig. 9.22 **Secondary OSA**. *Radiation-induced OSA*. (**a**) Radiographs taken for left hip pain of 2 months' duration with no history of trauma in a 64-year-old woman show ill-defined radiolucent destruction with osteoblastic densities and pathologic fracture in left acetabulum and part of ilium. The patient had a history of irradiation for cervical cancer 23 years ago. (**b**) PET/CT scan demonstrates a heterogeneously intense FDG uptake in the acetabulum and ilium (SUVmax 17.6) along with less intense uptake in the adjacent soft tissue and around the hip joint. A focal intense uptake wasobserved in both lungs, suggesting possible multiple pulmonary metastases (not shown). (**c**) MR images reveal an ill-defined intramedullary mass lesion with cortical breakthrough and soft tissue extension. The SI is low on T1- and heterogeneously intermediate and high on fat-saturated T2-weighted image. The medullary lesion is heterogeneously well-enhanced (red arrows). (**d**) Curettage and cementing followed by open reduction and internal fixation with a plate was performed under the impression of metastatic cancer possibly from the known cervical cancer. (**e**) However, microscopic examination notes atypical spindle cells producing osteoid (white asterisk) and calcified woven bone (yellow asterisk) indicating OSA rather than than carcinoma. (Right) Higher-power view shows pleomorphic spindle cells with bizarre nuclei and atypical mitoses (white arrow) directly producing abundant osteoid (white asterisk). The final diagnosis was secondary OSA, by definition induced by prior irradiation for cervical cancer. Internal hemipelvectomy was performed. (**f**) She died of disease spread 2 years after internal hemipelvectomy

first described following irradiation for tuberculous arthritis [10]. Subsequently, a causative link between irradiation and sarcoma has been strengthened, and diagnostic criteria for radiation-induced sarcoma have been proposed [11]: (1) Radiologic and/or microscopic evidence of nonmalignant nature of initial bone condition before irradiation should exist. (2) Irradiation is given to the lesion and the subsequently developed sarcoma should arise in the irradiated area. (3) A long asymptomatic latent period between irradiation and the development of the secondary sarcoma should have elapsed. The latent period has been reported to range from 3 to 33 years with a mean of 8 to 12 years [12–16]. (4) All sarcomas should be histologically proven (Figs. 9.22 and 9.23). Radiation-induced bone sarcoma has been allegedly reported much more aggressive than its conventional counterpart, and its prognosis was also markedly worse with shorter survival in the past [17, 18]. However, more recently, the prognosis has become reasonable using modern adjuvant chemotherapy and surgery with an adequate wide margin, and in the absence of metastases [19]. ***Fibrous dysplasia (FD)*** very rarely can undergo malignant change, especially in patients with polyostotic FD in the setting of McCune-Albright syndrome, Mazabraud syndrome (4–5%), or in those with prior irradiation for treatment. ***Liposclerosing myxofibrous tumor (LSMFT)*** may also undergo malignant change more commonly than FD, up to 10–16%. ***Bone infarct*** rarely can be associated with various types of sarcomas including OSA (Fig. 9.24). Histologically, we observed a definite transition zone to exist in the space between the ancient infarct and the trnasformed sarcoma, supporting the assumption that sarcoma may rise from the reparative tissues at the periphery of old infarcts [20]. The transition zone consisted of granulation tissues including interlacing fascicle of spindle cells, capillary proliferation with foamy macrophage and chronic inflammatory cells as well as atypical cells of varying degree. Furthermore, in the sarcoma side of transition zone, atypical spindle cells imperceptibly merged into high-grade sarcoma including OSA (Fig. 9.24d). Bahk et al. [21] reported an extremely rare case of OSA associated with osteochondritis dissecans and described similar transition zone between the sarcoma and the preexisting benign lesion, which contained bland, atypical repair tissue imperceptibly emerged into frank OSA. Malignant transformation has been also well documented in ***Involutional lipoma of bone*** [22]. *LSMFT and involutional intraosseous lipoma* contain similar cellular constituents of fat cell necrosis with focal calcification and reactive ischemic bone formation ("pseudopagetoid" or "mosaic" bone) as *bone infarct* does. The mechanism of malignant transformation within preexisting LSMFT is also unclear, but it has also been observed that malignant change may begin from the reparative tissue adjacent to the bone infarct area (Fig. 27.51 in Chap. 27). ***Bone marrow transplantation*** (BMT) has been widely performed for treatment in patients with malignant and nonmalignant hematologic disease (Fig. 9.25). An increasing number of recipient patients can expect long-term survival, but they may have a risk of developing secondary malignancies. Various patient- and/or treatment-related factors can predispose BMT patients to have the development of secondary malignancies, among which alkylating chemotherapeutic agents, genetic predisposition, and total body radiotherapy are thought to be the most important factors. In addition, immunosuppressive therapy, immunodeficiency, viral infection, or GvHD may also contribute to tumorigenesis following BMT [23]. Most reported cases of secondary malignancies after BMT are hematopoietic malignancies such as non-Hodgkin lymphoma. Solid tumor are rare after BMT, and OSA has been extraordinarily reported in the literature [24, 25].

9.9 Diagnosis and Staging

Plain radiographs and MRI are the first-line imaging tools to describe and define the extent of OSA. High-resolution CT scan, bone scan, and PET/CT scan are also mandatory tools for detecting metastases or skip lesions for staging.

9.10 Radiologic Findings

Plain radiograph provides various presentations with protean findings but plays an important role in diagnosis. Typically, it shows an ill-defined intramedullary moth-eaten to permeative destruction usually with cortical destruction mainly affecting metaphysis and frequently extending to epiphysis or diaphysis. A pure diaphyseal location is rare and may suggest Ewing's sarcoma or lymphoma. A naked soft tissue mass formation through a broken cortex is usual. The margin is ill-defined without a slerotic rim, with a wide zone of transition. The lesion usually shows a mixture of lytic and sclerotic appearance but is entirely lytic or sclerotic in some cases. A rare form of purely lytic appearance is characteristic of telangiectatic OSA, and can also be seen in fibroblastic, chondroblastic, small cell, or giant cell-rich variants which often produce only minimal focal osteoid. The intralesional opacities can be variably presented as "fluffy" or "cumulus cloud-like" to irregularly sclerotic masses or one large, uniformed area of ivory density depending on the amount, shape, and degree of tumor bone production, calcified matrix, and osteoid. Such a single, large, intramedullary, eccentric opacity with an ivory density can also be seen in a rare case of giant bone islands. Differentiation of sclerotic OSA from giant bone island can be impossible only by conventional radiograph, if OSA does not present aggressive periosteal reaction such Codman's triangle or cortical destruction with a soft tissue mass formation because both entities may show peripheral thorny, or brush-like radiation (Fig. 9.11). Aggressive periosteal reaction by deposition of reactive woven bone between cortex and periosteum displaced by the tumor as it transgresses, and this most commonly appears as one or more of multiple lamella (onion skinning), radiating (sun bursting), or centrally interrupting Codman's triangle. **MRI** is essential to determine accurate *local staging* and to evaluate for limb sparing surgery by assessing intraosseous tumor extension to growth plate, epiphysis, and diaphysis or skip lesions. In addition, it clearly shows a relationship between the soft tissue involvement and the neurovascular structures as well as the effects of neoadjuvant chemotherapy. MRI shows a medullary mass lesion with heterogeneous low SI of mineralized/ossified components and intermediate SI of nonosteoid components on T1-weighted image, and low SI of mineralized/ossified components and high SI of nonmineralized/osteoid soft tissue components on T2-weighted image. Peritumoral edema and hemorrhage show low to intermediate SI on T1- and high on T2-weighted images. In most cases, the cortex is significantly destroyed with soft tissue extension having similar signals of medullary tumor, and new bone formation by periosteal reaction with low signal. The solid viable component of the tumor is heterogeneously enhanced to varying degrees depending on vascularity, and the chondroblastic component can be enhanced with a septal and nodal pattern as in chondrosarcoma. Chest CT, bone scan, and PET/CT scan have an important role in staging by detecting skip lesions or distant metastases. **CT scan** clearly demonstrates cortical destruction and soft tissue mass formation but adds no or little to plain radiography and MRI for an assessment of the tumor itself. In addition, it may be useful in identifying a small amount of ossification in poorly mineralized lytic lesions, which are not seen on radiographs or MRI, and those in complex anatomical locations including pelvis and spine as well as for detecting lung metastases. **Bone scan** shows a homogeneous or heterogeneous strong uptake in the primary tumor, reflecting active osteoblastic activity and tumor-induced bone formation (Figs. 9.2, 9.3, 9.6, 9.7, 9.8, 9.9, 9.10, 9.11, 9.12, and 9.13) and metastatic or skip lesion (Fig. 9.15b). **PET/CT scan** shows a heterogeneously intense FDG uptake at the primary bone lesion due to high metabolic activity, suggesting a malignant lesion. In addition, it can provide not only skip lesions (Fig. 9.15c) and distant metastases but also histological response to neoadjuvant chemotherapy. PET/CT scan is very useful for primary staging, tumor grading, neoadjuvant chemotherapy monitoring, and follow-up evaluation to detect local recurrence (Fig. 9.17h).

9.11 Histologic Findings

Histologic findings of OSA are tremendously variable in histologic patterns and in the degree of cytologic atypia from minimal (low-grade) to markedly ominous (high-grade). High-grade OSA is composed of two main constant elements of (1) *malignant stromal cells* with clear-cut anaplasia and (2) *extracellular osteoid and bone matrix* produced directly by the tumor cells, which are admixed with varying proportions (Fig. 9.20). The tumor cells aggressively grow with moth-eaten to permeative pattern gradually replacing the marrow space and invading the preexisting trabeculae of medullary bone. Then, the tumor cells permeate and encase the host bone, finally trapping it in its wake, the so-called *permeative* or *encasement* pattern (Fig. 9.20a and j). Finally, the cortical bones are totally destructed and the tumor cells extend into the adjacent soft tissue to form naked masses. Reactive multinucleated giant cells are often observed particularly in hypervascular and hemorrhage areas. Spontaneous tumor necrosis is a common event. In a series of 20 patients who received only surgical resection without chemotherapy, 30% of the patients showed greater than 20% necrosis (range 25–67%; mean 43%) and 70% had less than 20% necrosis (range 0–19%; mean 4%) [26]. In another study, about 45% of the 76 tumors from patients who had not received preoperative chemotherapy had no evidence of spontaneous necrosis, 41% had less than 24% necrosis, and only one patient had more than 50% necrosis [27]. It can be assumed that over 60% of necrosis can be spontaneous and may not necessarily reflect a chemotherapy effect. However, near complete or complete necrosis equivalent to good responder in chemotherapy cannot occur spontaneously in OSA and is attributed to neoadjuvant chemotherapy [5]. (1) *The malignant stromal cells* are the main clue for diagnosis of OSA, which show clear-cut anaplasia such as nuclear atypism or pleomorphism in size and shape, abnormal chromatin clumping, high nuclear to cytoplasmic ratio, prominent nucleoli with numerous mitoses frequently including atypical mitoses (Fig. 9.20g). The stromal cells have densely eosinophilic cytoplasm resembling osteoblasts but are usually much larger than normal, even activated osteoblasts. The cell morphology can vary and include epithelioid, plasmacytoid, spindled, small round cells, clear cells, and giant cells. (2) *Neoplastic bone matrix* directly produced by malignant stromal cells, which should be separated from reactive bone, fracture callus or periosteal reaction, is another essential feature for the diagnosis of OSA. The neoplastic bone matrix begins with the elaboration of fibrillar collagenous matrix, which is shown as a dense, fibrillar pinkish material between the malignant stromal cells (Fig. 9.20b). As the lesion progresses, it appears as immature, primitive, unorganized trabeculae a forming filigree to lace-like disorganized pattern with early mineralization (Fig. 9.20c), and wide sheets of coalescing trabeculae of more matured woven bone with calcification in later stage, intimately associated with neoplastic cells. The color is pinkish (eosinophilic) if unmineralized, but it is purple (basophilic) if mineralized. It can appear as Pagetoid bone with deposited cement lines in a random manner, so-called *mosaic pattern* (Fig. 9.20d). A characteristic "staghorn" or *antler-like* pattern or pericytoid vascular spaces mimicking *hemangiopericytoma*, which is surrounded by pleomorphic spindle cells producing osteoid matrix, can be recognized (Fig. 9.20f) as in other high-grade sarcomas such as mesenchymal chondrosarcoma. Other matrix such as malignant cartilage or fibrous tissue can be also produced with varying proportions from focal to extensive. By definition, the lesion is OSA no matter what the extent of other matrices and how meager the bone matrix is if presents. If cartilage or fibrous tissue is extensive, it is classified as cartilaginous or fibroblastic OSA, respectively. A broad spectrum of different histologic subtypes may present depending on the prominent ce types and produced matrices, such as osteoblastic, chondroblastic, fibroblastic, telangiectatic, small

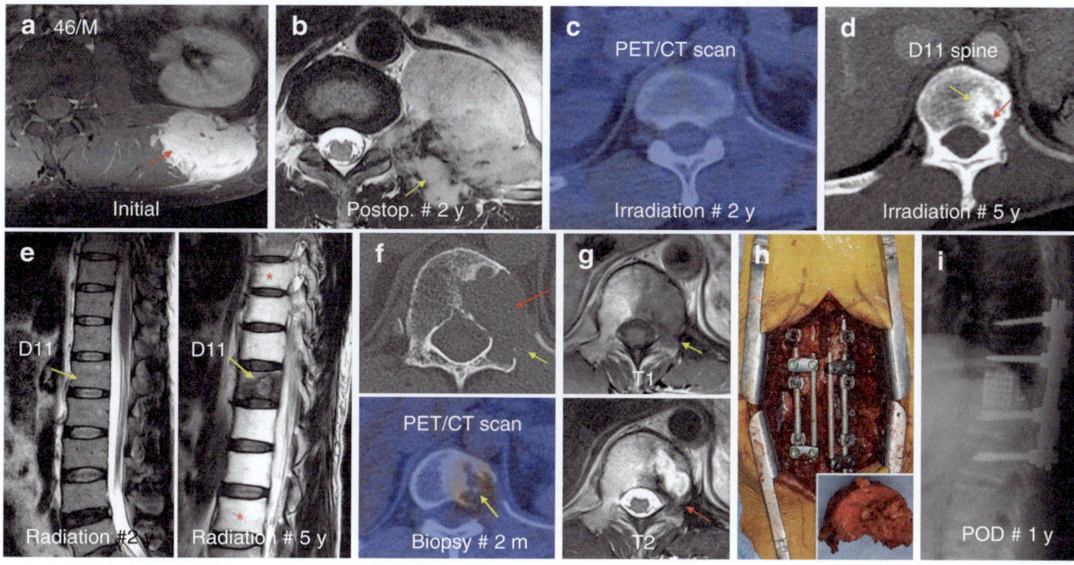

Fig. 9.23 **Secondary OSA**. *Radiation-induced OSA*. (**a**) MR image taken for a left paravertebral mass in a 46-year-old man shows an infiltrative soft tissue mass (arrow). En-bloc resection was performed based on a diagnosis of fibromatosis made by incision biopsy at another university hospital. (**b**) MR image taken for recurrent mass at 2 years after surgical resection reveals an ill-defined mass at previously resected area (arrow). After re-excision of the mass with subsequent 10th through 12th rib resection, external beam irradiation with 72.6Gy/33Fx was performed on the left paravertebral region. (**c**) Follow-up PET/CT scan at 2 years after re-excision notes no evidence of local recurrence. (**d**) However, CT scan taken for left paravertebral pain at 5 years after irradiation demonstrates a focal destructive lesion (red arrow) with a thick surrounding sclerotic area lesion (yellow arrow) involving vertebral body. (**e**) (Left) Sagittal MR image at 2 years after irradiation demonstrates no evidence of abnormal signals in the spine including D11 spine (yellow arrow). (Right) However, MR image at 5 years after irradiation notes a focal medullary lesion in the D11 spine body (red arrows) as well as diffuse post-irradiation bone marrow change in the D-L spines (between red asterisks). (**f**) (Top) Follow-up CT scan 2 months later shows marked progression of destruction (red arrow) with destruction of pedicle and extension to soft tissue (yellow arrow). (Bottom) PET scan reveals increased FDG uptake in the corresponding lesion without any distant metastasis. Microscopic examination of pedicle biopsy reveals pleomorphic epithelioid and spindle cells with abundant osteoid to woven bone consistent with osteoblastic OSA (not shown). (**g**) MR images reveal medullary lesion in the posterior aspect of the body with low SI on T1- and heterogeneously intermediate and high SI on T2-weighted image, which destroys the pedicle and extends into soft tissue (arrows). (**h**) Total en-bloc spondylectomy followed by posterior interbody fusion using mesh-cage with allo-fibula bone and instrumentation was performed. (**i**) Follow-up radiograph at 1 year after surgery notes good maintenance of the mesh-cage and instrumentation

cell, and others. In addition, other histomorphologic variants such as giant-cell rich, osteoblastoma-like, undifferentiated pleomorphic sarcoma (UPS)-like, and epithelioid variants are also rarely presented. On the basis of the predominant matrix produced by the tumor cells, conventional OSA is divided into osteoblastic (80%), chondroblastic (10%), and fibroblastic (10%) types [28, 29]. Each subtype may have varying proportions of the matrix, not only from case to case but also from area to area within the same case. The majority of cases (70–75%) are *mixed from OSA* consisting of two or more components, and the remaining cases (20–25%) may produce one predominant component which is usually more difficult to diagnose due to closely simulating other bone tumors [4]. Those variants producing only focal minimal osteoid such as chondroblastic, fibroblastic, telangiectatic, small cell, and giant cell-rich OSA require adequate incision biopsy rather than needle or trocar biopsy to obtain extensive and adequate samples (Fig. 9.19). A clinical, radiologic, and pathologic correlation, so-called *diagnostic triangle*, is necessary for a correct diagnosis for such tumors. *Osteoblastic OSA* (Figs. 9.1, 9.2, 9.3, 9.4, 9.5, 9.6, 9.7, and 9.8) predominantly produces a filigree to lace-like osteoid and/or disorganized woven bone or wide sheets of coalescing trabeculae of more matured woven bone. When the matrix is heavily mineralized tumor bone which is excessive to the proportion of tumor cells, it can be designated as *sclerosing OSA* (Figs. 9.9 and 9.10), which accounts for approximately 10% of primary high-grade OSA [4]. After becoming incarcerated in the trabeculae of tumor osteoid and woven bone, the originally plump tumor cells tend to become smaller resembling normal osteoblasts and less malignant looking than those being outside the osteoid, a phenomenon described as *normalizing* influence by Jaffe [30]. These deceptively bland looking tumor cells with banal appearance of the neoplastic bone matrix may make the diagnosis of OSA more difficult without pathologic finding of "permeation" or "trapping" of host lamellar bone and radiologic feature of cortical destruction with soft tissue masses. *Normalization* can can also be used in a wider sense to describe highly ossified areas in a more mature OSA [5]. *Chondroblastic OSA* (Figs. 9.12 and 9.13) predominantly produces malignant cartilage matrix, which is intimately merged with the noncartilage component of neoplastic bone. The cartilaginous component may be quite extensive and dominant throughout the tumor being more than 90% in some cases. Less than 5% of OSA produce this degree of chondrosarcomatous tissue [4]. The cartilage matrix is usually hyaline, but myxoid and other forms of cartilage are rare, except in the jaws and pelvis. Only a highly malignant cartilage can be observed without neoplastic bone if the biopsy specimen is inadequately small by core or trocar biopsy. If such finding of malignant cartilage without neoplastic bone component is found especially in adolescent or young adult patients who are inadequate age for chondrosarcoma, chondroblastic OSA should be suspected and excluded by a scrutinized examination to find at least meager neoplastic osteoid or woven bone. Even re-biopsy should be considered to obtain enough specimens to find even meager neoplastic bone. *Fibroblastic OSA* (Figs. 9.14 and 9.15) abundantly produces fibrous tissues or collagen matrices that can be extensive. Osteoid/woven bone production is usually minimal and observed focally. The stromal cells are mostly spindled, and less commonly forms areas of epithelioid cells, which are usually significantly pleomorphic and atypical, indicating high-grade, but may show moderate atypica, indicating intermediate-grade malignancy. On occasion, it resembles pure fibrosarcoma containing inconspicuous foci of homogeneous eosinophilic material, which are often arranged in a *herringbone* or *storiform* pattern. Fibroblastic OSA tends to produce a neoplastic bone in a filigree pattern [4]. This variant is often highly vascular with *staghorn* or pericytoid vascular spaces resembling hemangiopericytoma. *Telangiectatic OSA* (Figs. 9.16, 9.17, and 9.18), accounting for variable ranging of 2.5–12% of all OSAs [4, 5, 29, 31–34], consists of multiple blood-filled or empty vascular spaces surrounded by septa with variable thickness simulating aneurysmal bone cyst (ABC). However, the septa consist of bizarre pleomorphic spindle cells with severely atypical

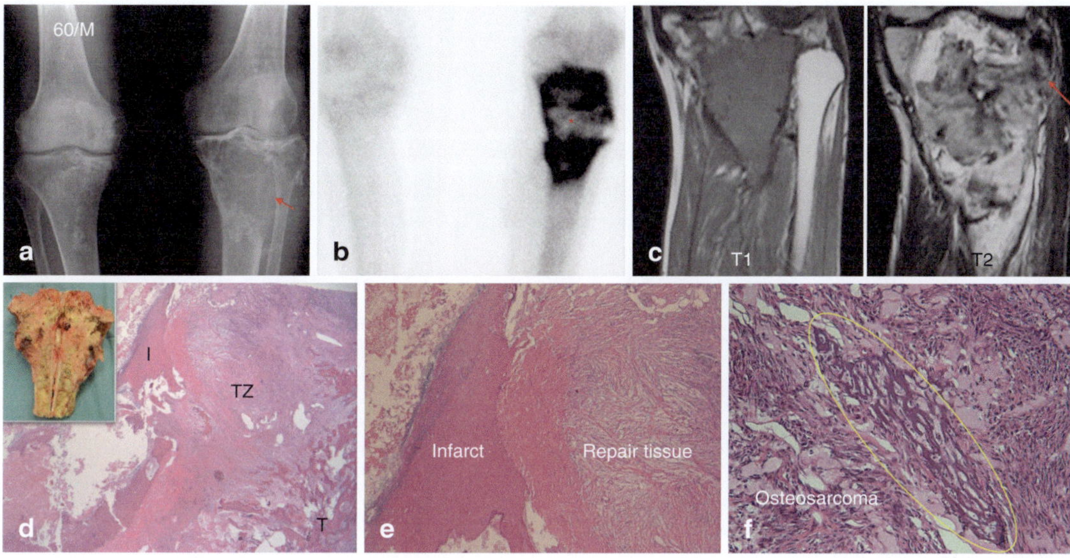

Fig. 9.24 **Secondary OSA**. *Infarct associated OSA*. (**a**) Radiograph taken for left knee pain of 5 months' durtion and acute swelling of 10 days' duration in a 60-year-old man shows an ill-defined expansile multilobulated geographic destruction with cortical destruction and soft tissue extension (red arrow) involving the left proximal tibia. Note multiple serpiginous lesions involving both distal femurs and proximal tibia, suggestive of preexisting multiple bone infractions. (**b**) Bone scan reveals a heterogeneously strong uptake with a central photon defect (asterisk), suggestive of cnetral tumor necrosis or poor vascularity, in the aggressive lesion affecting the left proximal tibia. However, there is no uptake in other areas of bone infarcts. (**c**) MR images demonstrate an ill-defined intramedullary expansive space-occupying mass lesion with cortical destruction and soft tissue extension (red arrow) having low to intermediate SI on T1- and heterogeneous intermediate, high SI with focal dark signals on T2-weighted image. (**d**) Low-power microscopic examination notes bone infarction (I) and bone-forming spindle cell tumor (T). There is a clear *transition zone* (TZ) of fibrous tissue between areas of infarct (I) and tumor (T). (**e**) Medium-power examination shows a host lamellar bone spicule with empty lacunae, indicative of bone infarct and adjacent zone of repair tissue. (**f**) Higher-power examination of tumor area reveals bizarre anaplastic stromal cells, producing lace-like osteoid interspersed among those cells indicating osteoblastic OSA arising from a preexisting bone infarct. A below-knee amputation was performed and adjuvant chemotherapy was not instituted because of poor performance of the patient. The patient died of metastases 11 months after the initial diagnosis

nuclei and frequent atypical mitotic figures. If septa are broken down, individual malignant stromal cells may be identified as free-floating in the hemorrhagic area. The lesion is frequently associated with massive hemorrhage and necrotic debris. Osteoid production is usually scanty, focal, and confluent, and may be absent in inadequate specimen, especially when needle or trocar biopsy was done. In addition to malignant-looking multinucleated giant cells, definitely benign-looking multinucleated giant cells are frequently found in the septa simulating ABC. *Small cell OSA* (Fig. 9.19a) is one of the rarest subtypes, only occupying about 1.3–1.9% of all OSAs [35–37]. It is typified by a proliferation of undifferentiated uniform small to intermediate-sized cells with scant cytoplasm. The tumor cells exhibit high nuclear/cytoplasmic ratio, focal pleomorphism, round to oval nuclei and cytoplasmic vacuoles. The amount of osteoid or bone matrix is quite variable, but usually scanty and inconspicuous. In a Mayo series [36], it was scanty in about half of the cases (51.4%), but prominent in about 11%. The pattern of osteoid production was usually lace-like, but a broad sheet pattern was not seen. Thus, it can often be difficult to differentiate small cell OSA from other small round cell malignancies such as lymphoma and Ewing's sarcoma, particularly with limited samples by inadequate biopsy usually

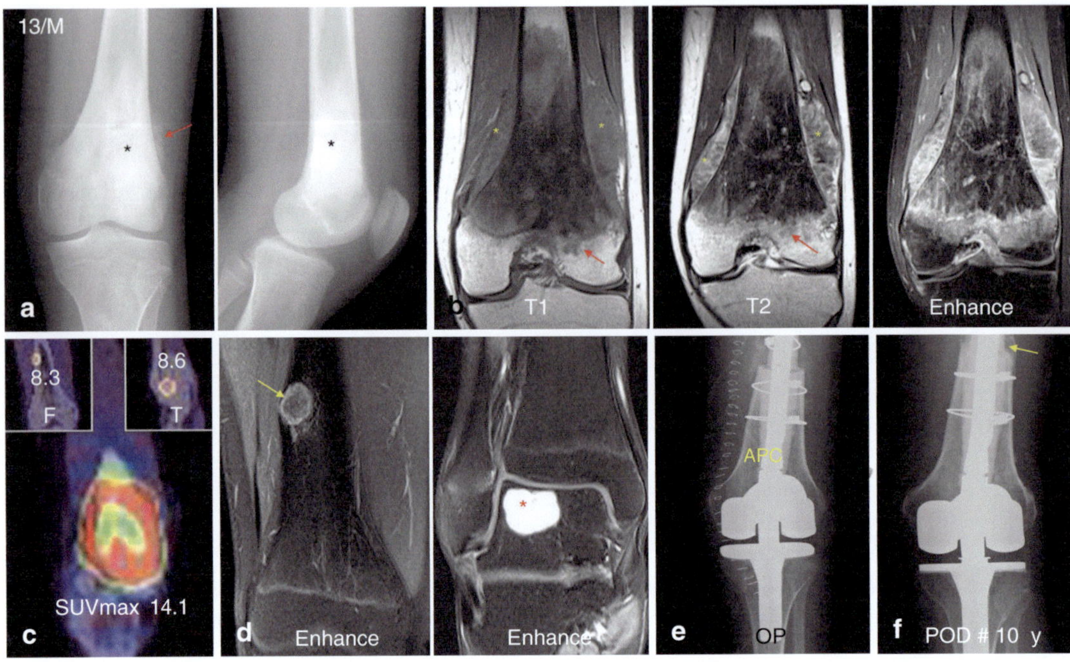

Fig. 9.25 **Secondary OSA**. *Bone marrow transplantation-related OSA*. (**a**) Radiograph taken for knee pain of 3 monts' duration in a 13-year-old boy shows an ill-defined large fluffy intramedullary lesion (black asterisks) with a hazy soft tissue mass (red arrow) affecting the meta-diaphysis of the distal femur. He has a history of acute lymphoblastic leukemia cured by chemotherapy, total body irradiation (Total 1200 cGy) followed by bone marrow transplantation (BMT) from the sibling donor 9 years ago when he was a 4-year-old. (**b**) MR images reveal an ill-defined medulla-occupying lesion mainly involving the meta-diaphysis with heterogeneously low and intermediate SI and internal dark signal on both T1- and T2-weighted images. Note focal epiphyseal extension through a breached epiphyseal plate (arrows) and extraosseous extension forming soft tissue masses (yellow asterisks). The medullary lesion and soft tissue mass lesions are heterogeneously well enhanced. Incision biopsy confirmed a diagnosis of osteoblastic OSA. (**c**) PET/CT scan demonstrates a heterogeneous intense localized FDG accumulation (SUVmax 14.1) in the left distal femur. There are other areas with intense FDG uptake at the right distal femur (F; SUVmax 8.3) and right talus (T; SUVmax 8.6) as well. (**d**) However, enhanced MR images note well-demarcated lesions with peripheral rim and central dotted enhancement (yellow arrow) in the distal femur and homogeneous enhancement (asterisk) in the talus suggesting benign lesion. (**e**) Wide resection and reconstruction with allo-prosthesis composite was performed. (**f**) Follow-up radiograph at 10 years after surgery with chemotherapy shows good union at allograft-host junction with no evidence of local recurrence. Follow-up radiographs of the right distal femur and ankle reveal little change in the benign lesions

using needle or trocar. A characteristic *staghorn* pattern mimicking hemangiopericytoma surrounded by pleomorphic spindle cells producing an osteoid matrix was observed in about one-third of cases [36]. Radiographic features are not distinctive, but the tumor location mainly in metaphysis extending to part of the diaphysis is suggestive of OSA rather than Ewing's sarcoma or lymphoma which mainly affects the diapysis. *Giant cell-rich OSA* (Fig. 9.19b) is also a very rare subtype, accounting for about 3% of all OSAs [38–40]. Osteoclast-like giant cells can be seen in hemorrhagic and perivascular areas in up to 25% of OSAs [41]. However, giant cell-rich or osteoclast-rich OSA exhibits numerous osteoclast-like giant cells uniformly scattered throughout the solid area of fibro-vascular stroma mimicking a giant cell tumor (GCT), which more or less masks the sarcoma cells. In addition, the mononuclear stromal cells show pleomorphism with variable nuclear atypia, which produce variable amounts of tumor osteoid or bone but are usually scanty. It can be easily mistaken for conventional or malignant GCT when tissue samples do not include osteoid deposition. The favorite sites of the lesion are diaphyseal and metaphyseal not crossing the physis, a pattern that helps distinguish it them from a conventional GCT [38].

9.12 Management

Standard treatment includes neoadjuvant (preoperative) chemotherapy, surgical resection, and adjuvant (postoperative) chemotherapy. Chemotherapy preceding surgery can shrink and downstage the tumor making a limb-sparing procedure more feasible as well as preventing the spread of cancer. Drugs used in the treatment of OSA include high-dose methotrexate (HDMTX), cisplatin (CDP), adriamycin (ADM), and ifosfamide (IF), generally used in combination with promising results. It is not clear if a four-drug combination (HDMTX, CDP, ADM, IF) offers advantages over a three-drug combination (HDTX, CDP, DM) treatment [42], but a two-drug chemotherapy regimen was reported as a poor prognostic factor [43]. However, a high incidence of nonhematologic toxicities was reported with ototoxicity, renal impairment, and cardiac failure [44]. Thus carboplatin [45] and pirarubicin [46] were introduced instead of cisplatin and doxorubicin, respectively, with less toxicity. A limb-sparing surgery involves tumor resection with an adequate wide margin including parts of normal bone and soft tissue, as well as the previous biopsy tract followed by reconstruction of the defect using various methods. Reconstruction options are biologic, nonbiologic, combined, or other methods. (1) Biologic methods are divided into *autograft* (bone from another part of a patient's own body or recycled patient's diseased bone) and *allograft* (bone taken from a donor). If a bone bank is not available, autograft including vascularized fibular graft, recycled bone using autoclave, pasteurization, and irradiation can be used in selective cases. (2) Nonbiologic reconstruction includes ready-made or custom-made tumor prosthesis. (3) In some cases, tumor prosthesis can be used in an allograft-prosthesis composite (APC) form. (4) Reconstruction can be achieved by distraction osteogenesis or expandable tumor prosthesis for growing children with an expected significant limb-length discrepancy. Rotationplasty, an unusual type limb-sparing procedure at present, was considered the best option for children younger than 12 years old with tumors around the knee who were expected to have significant leg length discrepancy due to so much growing potential left. Amputation can be the best option if the tumor is very large or if it extends into the neurovascular structures, it might not be possible to save the limb. Amputation is also indicated in cases with severely contaminated margins or local recurrence, which does not allow for adquate wide resection and reconstruction, or uncontrollable infection. In a long-term follow-up study on patients with endoprosthetic replacement for malignant bone tumors, the incidence of secondary amputation was 16% at 30 years [47].

9.13 Clinical Course and Prognosis

The prognosis depends on response to chemotherapy, tumor size, anatomic site, and surgical margin. As mentioned earlier, spontaneous necrosis usually occurs less than 20% of the tumor, but rarely up to 60% that is not necessarily considered to be chemotherapy effect. However, complete or subtotal necrosis over 90% almost never occurs spontaneously and is considered a good responder to chemotherapy. Pathologic grading system for evaluating the effect of current neoadjuvant chemotherapeutic regimen modified from the original criteria has been widely accepted, where the grades are defined as [32, 48]: *Grade I*, little or no effect of chemotherapy noted; *Grade II*, a partial response with more than *50%* tumor necrosis attributable to preoperative chemotherapy; however, some histologic sections demonstrated areas of viable tumor *Grade III*, greater than 90% tumor necrosis with foci of viable tumor in some histologic sections; and *Grade IV*, no viable-appearing tumor cells noted in any of the histologic sections. *Grades I and II* are considered as *poor responder* and *Grades III and IV* as *good responder* (Fig. 9.21). When treated properly, high-grade OSA of the extremities that is resectable without distant metastasis at presentation has a survival rate of about 60–70%, while that involving the axial skeleton has only about 30% of survival rate [42]. Metastases at presentation, localized tumor, anatomic site (extremity or axial), pathologic grade to preoperative chemotherapy, and serum levels of alkaline phosphatase are considered the most possible prognostic factors of survival. The survival rate is higher for patients with low-grade OSA, good response with over 90% tumor necrosis and adequate wide margin, but lower for patients high-grade with spread disease, poor response with less than 90% tumor necrosis, and inadequate margin. The 5-year relative survival rate of patients with OSA from the Surveillance, Epidemiology, and End Results (SEER) [49] program between 2010 and 2016 was 77% for localized, 65% for regional, 26% for distant disease with 60% for all SEER stages combined. *Small cell OSA* should be treated on a conventional OSA protocol including neoadjuvant chemotherapy, wide surgical resection with reconstruction, and adjuvant chemotherapy. The overall 5-year survival rate for the series of small cell OSA was 28.5%, whereas the cumulative 5-year survival rate was increased to about 69% with addition of chemotherapy since 1975 [36]. *Telangiectatic OSA* was considered to be the most lethal type [4]. Earlier, Mayo Clinic data reported that more than 80% of the patients died of the disease within 2 years after diagnosis if treated only with surgery [31]. But, later studies demonstrated telangiectatic OSA was responsive to combined chemotherapy and potentially curable [48, 50, 51]. More recent studies demonstrated that this subtype seemed to be even more sensitive to modern multimodality chemotherapy with better survival than conventional OSA. Bacci et al. [29] reported a significantly better histologic response to chemotherapy than conventional OSA (96% vs. 68% of good histologic response) and disease-free survival (83% vs. 55%) in the telangiectatic OSA group. Weiss et al. [52] also reported a comparable to better result of 5-year event-free and overall survival rates for telangiectatic OSA (58% and 67%, respectively) and for conventional OSA (44.3% and 58.3%, respectively). Over the recent decades, most altering or intensifying chemotherapy regimens for newly diagnosed OSA has failed to improve the former 60–70% long-term survival. The only success in improving patient outcomes was the addition of Mifamurtide (liposomal product) to the three- or four-drug regimen with an activation of their cytotoxic function against tumor cells by increasing circulating level of TNF alpha and interleukin-6 [53, 54]. Mifamurtide to multidrug chemotherapy increased long-term survival from 70 to 78% at 8 years [45] and improved the outcome of patients who presented with metastases at diagnosis [40]. For increased long-term survival, a more comprehensive understanding is necessary of the molecular and genetic heterogeneity and morphological adaptability of OSA, and the future treatment paradigm needs to shift from targeted anti-oncogenic therapy to immunological approach.

References

1. Broders AC. Squamous-cell epithelioma of the lip: a study of five hundred and thirty-seven cases. JAMA J Am Med Assoc. 1920;74(10):656–64.
2. Unni KK. Osteosarcoma of bone. In: Unni KK, editor. Bone tumors. New York, NY: Churchill Livingstone; 1988. p. 107–33.
3. Grimer RJ, Hogendoorn PCW, Vanel D. Tumours of bone: introduction. In: Fletcher CDM, Bridge JA, Hogendoorn PCW, Mertens F, editors. World Health Organization classification of tumours. Pathology and genetics of tumours of soft tissue and bone. 4th ed. Lyon: IARC Press; 2013. p. 244–7.
4. Mirra JM. Osteosarcoma. In: Mirra JM, editor. Bone tumors: clinical, radiologic, and pathologic correlations. 2nd ed. Philadelphia, PA: Lea & Febiger; 1989. p. 248–389.
5. Dorfman HD, Czerniak B. Osteosarcoma. In: Dorfman HD, Czerniak B, editors. Bone tumors. St. Louis: Mosby; 1998. p. 128–252.
6. Campanacci M. High grade osteosarcoma. In: Campanacci M, editor. Bone and soft tissue tumors. Wien New York: Springer; 1999. p. 463–515.
7. Mirabello L, Troisi RJ, Savage SA. Osteosarcoma incidence and survival rates from 1973 to 2004: data from the surveillance, epidemiology, and end results program. Cancer. 2009;115(7):1531–43.
8. McKenna R, Schwinn C, Soong K, Higinbotham N. Sarcomata of the osteogenic series (osteosarcoma, fibrosarcoma, chondrosarcoma, parosteal osteo-

genic sarcoma, and sarcomata arising in abnormal bone): an analysis of 552 cases. J Bone Joint Surg. 1966;48(1):1–26.
9. Hansen MF, Seton M, Merchant A. Osteosarcoma in Paget's disease of bone. J Bone Miner Res. 2006;21(S2):P58–63.
10. Beck A. Zur Frage des Roentogensarkoms, zugleich ein Beitrag zur Pathogenes des Sarkoms. MMW. 1922;69:623.
11. Cahan WG, Woodard HQ, Higinbotham NL, Stewart FW, Coley BL. Sarcoma arising in irradiated bone: report of eleven cases. Cancer. 1998;82(1):8–34.
12. Arlen M, Higinbotham NL, Huvos AG, Marcove RC, Miller T, Shah I. Radiation-induced sarcoma of bone. Cancer. 1971;28(5):1087–99.
13. Mark RJ, Poen J, Tran LM, Fu YS, Selch MT, Parker RG. Postirradiation sarcomas. A single-institution study and review of the literature. Cancer. 1994;73(10):2653–62.
14. Bechler J, Robertson W Jr, Meadows A, Womer R. Osteosarcoma as a second malignant neoplasm in children. J Bone Joint Surg Am. 1992;74(7):1079–83.
15. Meadows AT, Strong LC, Li FP, D'Angio GJ, Schweisguth O, Freeman AI, et al. Bone sarcoma as a second malignant neoplasm in children: influence of radiation and genetic predisposition. Cancer. 1980;46(12):2603–6.
16. Huvos AG, Woodard HQ, Cahan WG, Higinbotham NL, Stewart FW, Butler A, et al. Postradiation osteogenic sarcoma of bone and soft tissues. A clinicopathologic study of 66 patients. Cancer. 1985;55(6):1244–55.
17. Young J, Liebscher L. Postirradiation osteogenic sarcoma with unilateral metastatic spread within the field of irradiation. Skeletal Radiol. 1982;8(4):279–83.
18. Sim F, Cupps R, Dahlin D, Ivins J. Postradiation sarcoma of bone. J Bone Joint Surg. 1972;54(7):1479–89.
19. Kalra S, Grimer R, Spooner D, Carter S, Tillman R, Abudu A. Radiation-induced sarcomas of bone: factors that affect outcome. J Bone Joint Surg Br. 2007;89(6):808–13.
20. Bahk WJ, Lee AH, Kang YK, Park JM, Chung YG, Shin DS, et al. Infarct associated sarcoma: a possible pathogenesis based on histological observation of repair tissue origin in two cases. Acta Oncol. 2010;49(6):868–72.
21. Bahk WJ, Brien EW, Mirra JM. Osteosarcoma associated with osteochondritis dissecans. A case report and review of the literature. J Bone Joint Surg. 1997;79(12):1849–53.
22. Milgram JW. Malignant transformation in bone lipomas. Skeletal Radiol. 1990;19(5):347–52.
23. Deeg HJ, Socié GR. Malignancies after hematopoietic stem cell transplantation: many questions, some answers. Blood. 1998;91(6):1833–44.
24. Curtis RE, Rowlings PA, Deeg HJ, Shriner DA, Socié G, Travis LB, et al. Solid cancers after bone marrow transplantation. N Engl J Med. 1997;336(13):897–904.
25. Bielack S, Rerin J, Dickerhoff R, Dilloo D, Kremens B, von Stackelberg A, et al. Osteosarcoma after allogeneic bone marrow transplantation. A report of four cases from the Cooperative Osteosarcoma Study Group (COSS). Bone Marrow Transplant. 2003;31(5):353–9.
26. Björnsson J, Inwards CY, Wold LE, Sim FH, Taylor WF. Prognostic significance of spontaneous tumour necrosis in osteosarcoma. Virchows Arch. 1993;423(3):195–9.
27. Springfield D, Schakel M Jr, Spanier S. Spontaneous necrosis in osteosarcoma. Clin Orthop Relat Res. 1991;263:233–7.
28. Hauben E, Weeden S, Pringle J, Van Marck E, Hogendoorn P. Does the histological subtype of high-grade central osteosarcoma influence the response to treatment with chemotherapy and does it affect overall survival? A study on 570 patients of two consecutive trials of the European Osteosarcoma Intergroup. Eur J Cancer. 2002;38(9):1218–25.
29. Bacci G, Ferrari S, Ruggieri P, Biagini R, Fabbri N, Campanacci L, et al. Telangiectatic osteosarcoma of the extremity: neoadjuvant chemotherapy in 24 cases. Acta Orthop Scand. 2001;72(2):167–72.
30. Jaffe HL, editor. Tumors and tumorous conditions of the bones and joints. Phildelphia, PA: Lea & Febiger; 1958.
31. Matsuno T, Unni KK, McLeod RA, Dahlin DC. Telangiectatic osteogenic sarcoma. Cancer. 1976;38(6):2538–47.
32. Rosen G, Huvos AG, Marcove R, Nirenberg A. Telangiectatic osteogenic sarcoma. Improved survival with combination chemotherapy. Clin Orthop Relat Res. 1986;207:164–73.
33. Huvos AG, Rosen G, Bretsky SS, Butler A. Telangiectatic osteogenic sarcoma: a clinicopathologic study of 124 patients. Cancer. 1982;49(8):1679–89.
34. Larsson S-E, Lorentzon R, Boquist L. Telangiectatic osteosarcoma. Acta Orthop Scand. 1978;49(6):589–94.
35. Edeiken J, Raymond AK, Ayala A, Benjamin R, Murray J, Carrasco H. Small-cell osteosarcoma. Skeletal Radiol. 1987;16(8):621–8.
36. Nakajima H, Sim FH, Bond JR, Unni KK. Small cell osteosarcoma of bone: review of 72 cases. Cancer. 1997;79(11):2095–106.
37. Dahlin DC, Unni KK. Osteosarcoma of bone and its important recognizable varieties. Am J Surg Pathol. 1977;1(1):61–72.
38. Bathurst N, Sanerkin N, Watt L. Osteoclast-rich osteosarcoma. Br J Radiol. 1986;59(703):667–73.
39. Wang C, Yin Q, Liao J, Lou J, Ding X, Zhu Y. Giant cell-rich osteosarcoma in long bones: clinical, radiological and pathological features. Radiol Med. 2013;118(8):1324–34.
40. Chow LTC. Giant cell rich osteosarcoma revisited—diagnostic criteria and histopathologic patterns, Ki67, CDK4, and MDM2 expression, changes in response to bisphosphonate and denosumab treatment. Virchows Arch. 2016;468(6):741–55.
41. Troup J, Dahlin D, Coventry M, editors. The significance of giant cells in osteogenic sarcoma. Do they

indicate a relationship between osteogenic sarcoma and giant cell tumor of bone? Mayo Clin Proc; 1960.
42. Picci P. Osteosarcoma (osteogenic sarcoma). Orphanet J Rare Dis. 2007;2(1):1–4.
43. Bacci G, Longhi A, Versari M, Mercuri M, Briccoli A, Picci P. Prognostic factors for osteosarcoma of the extremity treated with neoadjuvant chemotherapy: 15-year experience in 789 patients treated at a single institution. Cancer. 2006;106(5):1154–61.
44. Ferrari S, Smeland S, Mercuri M, Bertoni F, Longhi A, Ruggieri P, et al. Neoadjuvant chemotherapy with high-dose Ifosfamide, high-dose methotrexate, cisplatin, and doxorubicin for patients with localized osteosarcoma of the extremity: a joint study by the Italian and Scandinavian Sarcoma Groups. J Clin Oncol. 2005;23(34):8845–52.
45. Meyers PA, Schwartz CL, Krailo MD, Healey JH, Bernstein ML, Betcher D, et al. Osteosarcoma: the addition of muramyl tripeptide to chemotherapy improves overall survival-a report from the Children's Oncology Group. J Clin Oncol. 2008;26(4):633–8.
46. Shinozaki T, Watanabe H, Yanagawa T, Shirakura K, Takagishi K. Pirarubicin-based versus doxorubicin-based osteosarcoma chemotherapy. Ann Pharmacother. 2002;36(6):996–9.
47. Grimer R, Aydin B, Wafa H, Carter S, Jeys L, Abudu A, et al. Very long-term outcomes after endoprosthetic replacement for malignant tumours of bone. Bone Joint J. 2016;98(6):857–64.
48. Huvos AG. Pathologic assessment of preoperative (neoadjuvant) chemotherapy. In: Huvos AG, editor. Bone tumors: diagnosis, treatment and prognosis. 2nd ed. Philadelphia, PA: WB Saunders; 1991. p. 122–8.
49. SEER (Surveillance, Epidemiology, and End Results (SEER) Program) Research Data, 18 Registries (2000–2018), released April 2021, Surveillance Research Program, National Cancer Institute, DCCPS, Bethesda, 2021. https://seer.cancer.gov/explorer/. Accessed 27 Sept 2021.
50. Rosen G, Caparros B, Huvos AG, Kosloff C, Nirenberg A, Cacavio A, et al. Preoperative chemotherapy for osteogenic sarcoma: selection of postoperative adjuvant chemotherapy based on the response of the primary tumor to preoperative chemotherapy. Cancer. 1982;49(6):1221–30.
51. Buzdar AU, Krakoff IH, Kakalec CA, Chawla SP, Benjamin RS. Effectiveness of chemotherapy in the management of metastatic telangiectatic osteosarcoma. Am J Clin Oncol. 1988;11(2):177–80.
52. Weiss A, Khoury JD, Hoffer FA, Wu J, Billups CA, Heck RK, et al. Telangiectatic osteosarcoma: the St. Jude children's research hospital's experience. Cancer. 2007;109(8):1627–37.
53. Kleinerman ES, Erickson KL, Schroit AJ, Fogler WE, Fidler IJ. Activation of tumoricidal properties in human blood monocytes by liposomes containing lipophilic muramyl tripeptide. Cancer Res. 1983;43(5):2010–4.
54. Kleinerman ES, Jia S-F, Griffin J, Seibel NL, Benjamin RS, Jaffe N. Phase II study of liposomal muramyl tripeptide in osteosarcoma: the cytokine cascade and monocyte activation following administration. J Clin Oncol. 1992;10(8):1310–6.

Parosteal Osteosarcoma

10

(***Par(a)*** "to, at, from the side of," ***Osteo(n)*** "Bone," ***sarco(s)*** "flesh," ***ōma*** "noun forming suffix")

10.1 Definition

Parosteal osteosarcoma (OSA) is a slow-growing, low-grade malignant bone-forming tumor (Grade 1–2) arising from the outer layer of the periosteum. Dedifferentiated parosteal osteosarcoma (DPOS) is a histologically higher-grade sarcoma (Grade 3–4) that coexists with a conventional low-grade parosteal OSA.

10.2 Synonyms

Juxtacortical OSA.

10.3 Incidence

Parosteal OSA rarely occurs and accounts for less than 1% of biopsy-proven primary bone tumors [1], about 3–7% of all OSAs [2–5], and 65% of the surface OSAs [5].

10.4 Age

The age at presentation usually is typically in early adulthood after skeletal maturation and middle-aged adults with a peak incidence in the third and fourth decades [3, 4]. About 80% of patients are between 20 and 50 years of age [1]. In consideration of a slowly growing tumor, age of onset should be, however, several years earlier.

10.5 Locations

Parosteal OSA has a unique propensity to occur in purely metaphyseal or meta-diaphyseal area of the distal femur in its posterior aspect (Figs. 10.1, 10.2, 10.3, and 10.4), accounting for about 70–80% of cases [1, 3]. The next frequent locations include proximal humerus, proximal tibia, and proximal femur [1, 2] (Fig. 10.3a, d). Diaphyseal location is

W.-J. Bahk, *Diagnosis and Management of Primary Bone Tumors*,
https://doi.org/10.1007/978-981-96-3484 2_10

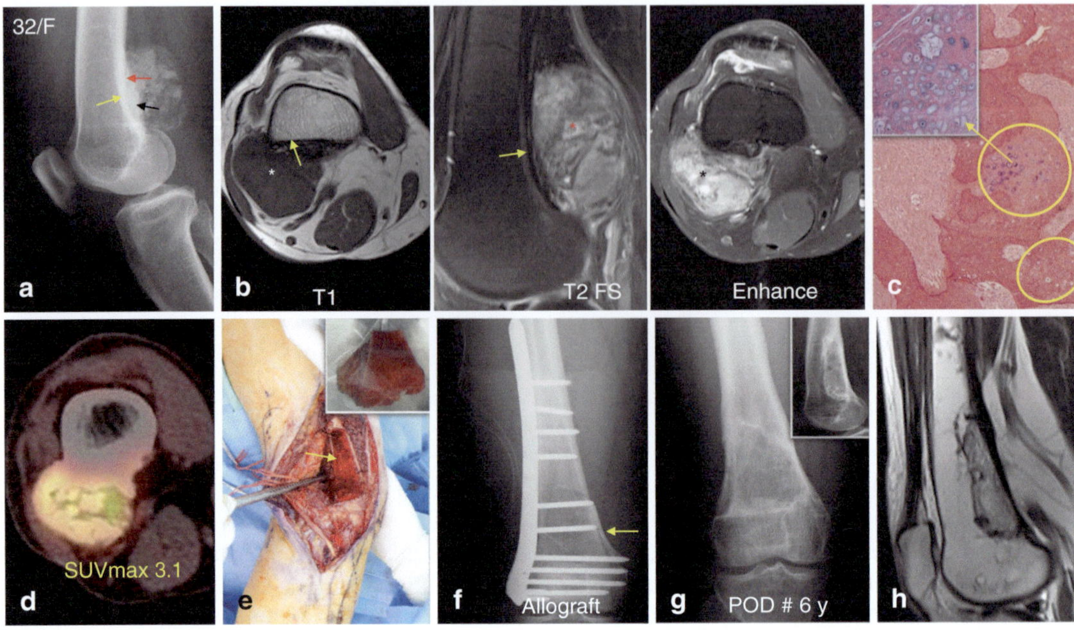

Fig. 10.1 ***Unique propensity in the distal femur.*** (**a**) Radiographs taken for a slowly growing, hard mass in right popliteal of 2 years' duration in a 32-year-old lady shows a well-demarcated, heavily mineralized, outgrowing *cauliflower-like* mass attached to the intact cortex in the posterolateral aspect of the distal femur. The mass is broadly fused to the intact and densely thickened underlying cortex (yellow arrow), so-called *paste-on* appearance. The deepest part of the mass near base adjacent to the cortex is maximal in density (black arrow), and less toward the mass surface, suggesting a fibrous, immature osteoid, or cartilage component. A thin radiolucent cleavage line is seen between the base of the tumor and the host cortex (red arrow), so-called *string sign*. However, periosteal reaction by its elevation is not observed. (**b**) MR images reveal a well-defined outgrowing mass on the intact cortical surface with low SI on T1-weighted image (white asterisk) and heterogeneous intermediate and high on fat-saturated T2-weighted image (red asterisk). The underlying cortex is preserved intact and there is no discernible abnormal signal in the medullary cavity (arrows). The lesion is heterogeneously well enhanced by contrast medium (black asterisk). (**c**) Although radiograph and MR images definitely indicate parosteal OSA, incision biopsy was perfomred because the patient strongly wanted a histologic confirmation before surgical resection. Microscopic examination demonstrates dense collagenous stroma with mildly atypical spindle cells producing well-formed osseous trabeculae with mosaic cement lines. There are also focal areas of cartilaginous differentiation with atypical chondrocytes in the form of nodules (circles). Higher-power view notes atypical chondrocytes of a grade similiar to the spindle cell component (inset). A histologic diagnosis of conventional parosteal OSA was confirmed. (**d**) PET/CT scan presents heterogeneously increased FDG uptake (SUVmax 3.1) in the mass but not in the medullary cavity. (**e**) Hemicondylar wide resection of the lateral condyle was performed (yellow arrow). The defect after resection (arrow), was reconstructed using a well-matched allograft from the bone bank (inset). (**f**) Postoperative radiograph shows a well-matched allograft securely fixed by plate and screws (arrow). (**g**) Follow-up radiograph at 6 years after initial surgery reveals a good incorporation of the allograft and well-preserved native knee joint without collapse of the allograft (arrow). (**h**) Follow-up MR image notes no evidence of local recurrence with a good incorporation of the allograft

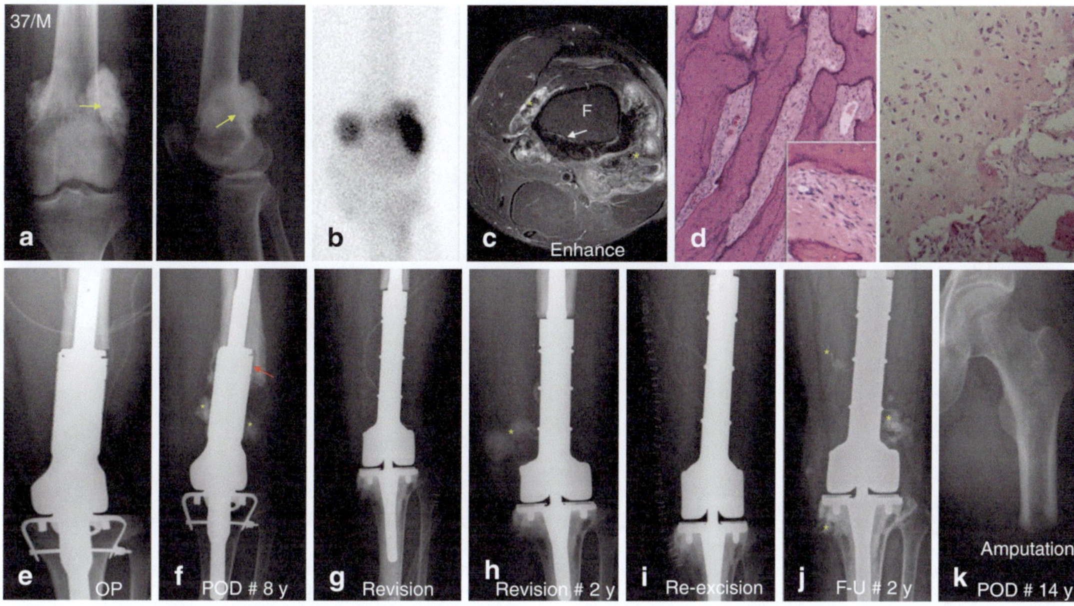

Fig. 10.2 ***Unique propensity of location in the distal femur***. (**a**) Radiographs taken for slowly growing, hard mass around the knee of 1 year's duration in a 37-year-old man shows irregularly lobulated, densely ossifying, exophytic masses, and intact underlying cortex, which wrap mainly around the metaphyseal area of the distal feur. There is a thin radiolucent cleavage line between the base of the tumor and the host cortex (arrows), a *string sign* for typical *paste-on* appearance of parosteal OSA. Periosteal reaction is not visible. (**b**) Bone scan reveals intense and more extensive uptake in the lateral portion, as well as relatively weaker and smaller uptake in the medial portion of the mass. (**c**) Axial MR image demonstrates a heterogeneously well-enhancing , outgrwoing, mutilobulated mass (asterisks), wrapping around the underlying femur (F). There is focal cortical obliteration and compression by the dark signal of the calcifying mass, suggesting a possible tumor invasion to the medullary cavity (arrow). (**d**) Microscopic examination: (Left) Medium-power magnification demonstrates an anastomosing pattern of well-formed woven bone trabeculae with cement lines, typically appearing as long streamer in parallel fashion. Note intervening stroma between the bone trabeculae consisting of mildly atypical spindle cells (inset). (Right) A focal area of cartilaginous differentiation with atypical chondrocytes is found in another field. (**e**) Wide resection and reconstruction with a tumor prosthesis were performed. (**f**) Follow-up radiograph at 8 years after surgery shows periprosthetic loosening and upward migration of the prosthesis into the femur (red arrow) associated with densely calcified soft tissue, suggesting a local recurrence (asterisks). (**g**) Wide excision of the soft tissue masses followed by revision of the tumor prosthesis was performed. (**h**) Follow-up radiograph at 2 years after revision surgery reveals another local recurrence in the soft tissue (asterisk). (**i**) Re-excision of the recurrent soft tissue mass was done. (**j**) Follow-up radiograph at 2 years after re-excision shows multiple recurrent soft tissue masses (asterisks). (**k**) Above-knee amputation was performed at 12 years after initial surgery. However, there was no evidence of dedifferentiation to higher grade on the last microscopic slides. The patient is doing well with no evidence of local recurrence and metastasis at 14 years after initial presentation despite the multiple local recurrence

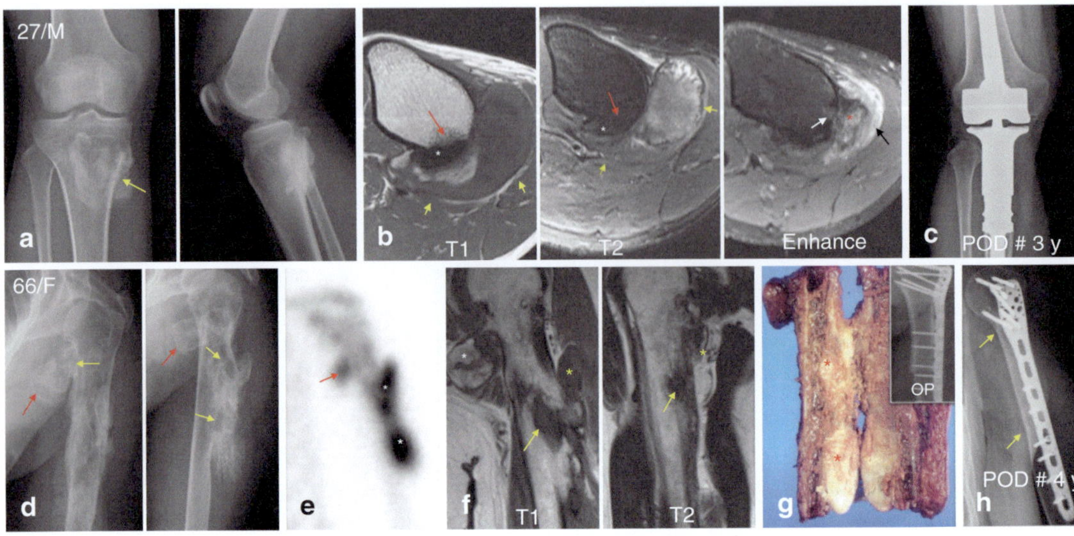

Fig. 10.3 ***The next common locations; proximal tibia***. (**a**) Radiograph taken for right knee pain with palpable hard mass of 6 months' duration in a 27-year-old man shows a well-defined, irregular, dense, exophytic, cauliflower-like mass attached to the surface of posterior aspect of proximal tibia. The underlying cortex appears to be focally breached (arrow). There is not clearly visible "string sign" and periosteal reaction. (**b**) MR images present a well-defined exophytic mass on the posterior cortex of proximal tibia (yellow arrows), showing predominantly low to intermediate SI on T1-weighted image and intermediate SI with a focal high signal suggesting cartilage component on T2-weighted image. There is a focal area low-to-dark signal of ossification on both sequences (white asterisks). Note a cortical breach in the posteromedial aspect of the distal femur with focal medullary extension (red arrows). The mass lesion is peripherally (black arrow) and centrally enhanced (asterisk). The meduallry coponent is weakly enhanced (white arrow). (**c**) Follow-up radiograph at 3 years after wide resection and reconstruction with a tumor prosthesis notes good maintenance with no evidence of local recurrence. ***Proximal humerus***: (**d**) Radiograph taken for left upper arm pain with palpable hard mass of 1 year's duration in a 66-year-old man shows an irregular, densely mineralized, longitudinal main mass outgrowing from the lateral cortex with disrupted underlying cortex (yellow arrows). There is another small mass from the medial cortex of the humerus (red arrows). (**e**) Bone scan reveals a hot uptake in the lateral main mass lesion (black asterisks) and focal mild uptake in the medial mass lesion (red arrow). (**f**) MR images reveal an irregularly shaped, exophytic, main mass (yellow asterisks) with low SI on T1 and heterogeneous low and high SI on T2-weighted image, which markedly invades into the medullary cavity (yellow arrows). There is another smaller medial mass with heterogeneous SI on T1-weighted image (white asterisk). (**g**) Wide resection followed by reconstruction with intercalary allograft was performed (inset). The resected specimen demonstrates a significant medullary invasion through the cortical destruction (asterisks). (**h**) Follow-up radiograph at 4 years after surgery notes radiologic union between the allogrft and the host humerus (arrows) with no evidence of local recurrence

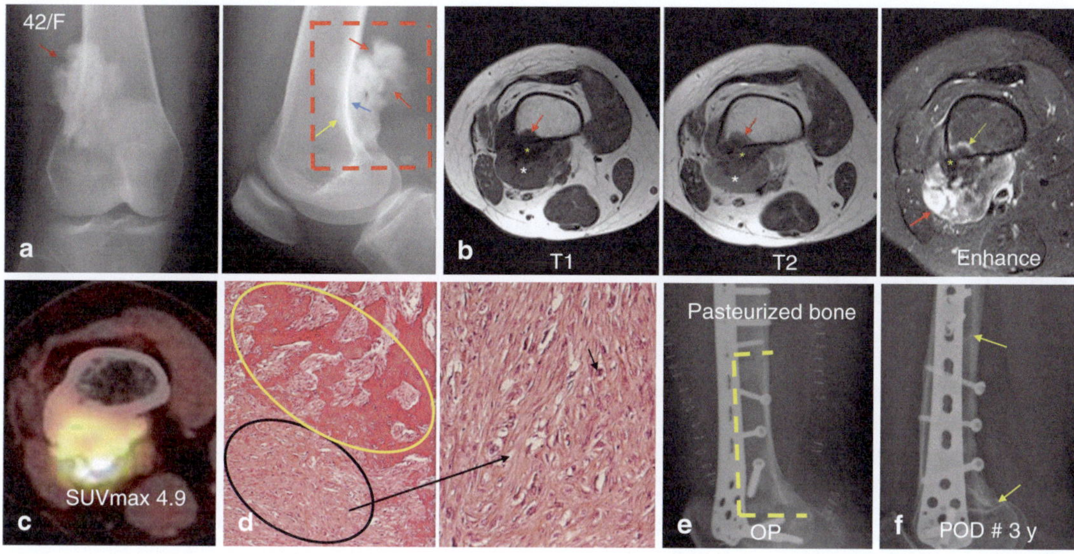

Fig. 10.4 ***DPOS at initial presentation (synchronous type).*** (**a**) Radiographs taken for slowly growing, hard mass of right knee of 1 year's duration with newly developed pain of 2 months' duration in a 42-year-old woman shows an exophytic cauliflower-like mass attached to the intact underlying cortex, with evenly dense central ossification in the posterolateral aspect of the distal femur. There is a thin radiolucent cleavage line (blue arrow) between the base of tumor and the host cortex, so-called *string sign*. Note minimal medullary extension (yellow arrow) and poorly defined additional radiolucent areas (red arrows) suggesting a possible dedifferentiation. However, there is no periosteal reaction. (**b**) MR images reveal a well-defined exophytic lobulated mass with low SI on T1-weighted image and intermediate SI on T2-weighted image (white asterisks) as well as a focal dark signal of heavy ossification in the base adjacent to the cortex on both sequences (yellow asterisks). There is small cortical destruction with focal medullary invasion (red arrows). The main mass lesion is strongly enhanced (red arrow) with a nonenhancing area of heavy ossification (asterisk). The focal medullary extending lesion is peripherally enhanced (yellow arrow). (**c**) PET/CT scan shows heterogeneously increased FDG uptake (SUVmax: 4.9) in the exophytic mass, but no definite uptake in the medullary lesion. (**d**) Microscopic examination: (Left) Medium-power magnification notes an area consisting of dense collagenous stroma with minimally atypical spindle cells producing woven bone spicules in anastomosing pattern (yellow circle), indicating a preexisting parosteal OSA and another area of more pleomorphic and atypical stromal cells producing primitive osteoid formation (black circle). Note abrupt transition area between the two components. (Right) Higher-power magnification notes more pleomorphic stromal cells with abnormal mitosis (black arrow) embedded in primitive ostoid, indicating dedifferentiation to higher-grade conventional OSA. (**e**) Hemicondylar wide resection of lateral condyle including main tumor mass and medullary extension was performed with chemotherapy (dotted rectangle in (**a**)). The defect was reconstructed with a pasteurized autogenic bone (dotted lines) and securely fixed with plate and screws. (**f**) Follow-up radiograph at 3 years after surgery reveals a complete union of the recycled autograft to the remaining host bone (arrows) with no evidence of local recurrence

very rare, in contrst to periosteal OSA, which is exclusively located in the diaphysis of tibia and femur. Exceedingly rarely, other bones including mandible, clavicle, and tarsal bones have been reported to be affected [5].

10.6 Clinical Features

Patients typcailly present with a firm and fixed mass usually without pain, which has been slowly growing for a long duration, often over 1–2 years or even 4–5 years (Figs. 10.1, 10.2, 10.3, and 10.4). On occasion, the mass causes dull or aching pain and may limit the motion of adjacent joint. Knee flexion can be restricted by a large tumor affecting posterior distal femur. Very rarely, it can be also incidentally found (Fig. 10.3).

10.7 Radiologic Findings

Plain radiograph typically shows a well-defined, outgrowing, irregularly lobulated, round to oval mass with dense mineralization attached to the intact cortex with a broad base but no periosteal reaction by its elevation (Figs. 10.1, 10.2, 10.3, and 10.4). Thus, there is no periosteal new bone deposition in parosteal OSA, while periosteal elevation by expansion of periosteal OSA stimulates prominent new bone deposition in the pattern of radiating striations ("*sun bursting*") or Codman's triangle. The size at presentation is usually large because of slow growth and lack of symptom, which prevent early medical seeking. The mass is uniformly dense or unevenly mineralized appearing as *cauliflower-like* or *mushroom-like* shape with denser ossification in the center and focal radiolucent areas in the periphery. The deepest part of the mass near the base, adjacent to the cortex, is meximal in density and less dense toward tumor surface, suggesting an immature bone or cartilage component (Fig. 10.1a). Characteristically, the tumor mass is broadly fused to the surface of the cortex without continuity to the medulla of the host bone, so-called *paste-on* appearance (Fig. 10.1a), while the host bone flares into the mass with loss of the underlying cortex which blends into the host medullary bone in osteochondroma (OC) (Fig. 13.1a in Chap. 13). The *paste-on* appearance is a typical finding that can easily distinguish a parosteal OSA from an OC to make preoperative biopsy unnecessary. A radiolucent cleavage line between the base of the tumor and the host cortex, so-called *string sign* representing the intact periosteum, is often observed (Figs. 10.1a, 10.2a, and 10.4a). It can be not clearly seen if the tumor stalk gradually grows within the tumor and obliterates the radiolucent cleavage plane in late stage (Fig. 10.3). Similar radiolucent cleavage line can also be seen in some cases of dysplasia epiphysealis hemimelica (Trevor's disea), which always affects, however, the epiphyses or epiphyseal equivalents of bone. The underlying host cortex is usually intact and thickened, but can be focally breached and the tumor may the medullary cavity. The cortex has been reported to be normal in about half of the cases, thickened in one-fourth, and destructed in the rest of the cases [5]. Medullary involvement is generally so minimal that it is usually difficult to recognize on plain radiographs. However, it is occasionally detected on plain radiographs in advanced cases (Fig. 10.3a), and is best appreciated by CT scan or MRI. The tumor mass tends to grow circumferentially along the cortical surface, and become huge enough to evntually wrap around the shaft of the involved bone (Fig. 10.2a). Poorly defined radiolucent areas may be observed within the heavily mineralized tumor mass with irregular cloudy opacities, suggesting possible dedifferentiation (Fig. 10.4a). In general, there is no periosteal reaction nor recognizable periosteal new bone formation. **MRI** reveals a well-circumscribed exophytic mass attached to the cortex with predominantly low SI and focal dark signals on both T1-weighted and T2-weighted images dut to a well-mineralized component (Figs. 10.1, 10.2, 10.3, and 10.4). Foci of high signal on T2-weighted image may be suggestive of higher-grade tumor or differentiation with fibroblastic or cartilaginous component. However, the T2 signal can vary depending on the presence of hemorrhage or necrosis. In the late stage, the exophytic multilobulated mass can grow large enough to wrap around the shaft of the underlying bone (Fig. 10.2c). In some cases, MR images can render a cartilaginous cap partially covering the tumor clearly visible. The extent of the medullary involvement is best appreciated on axial images (Figs. 10.3b, f and 10.4b). In the Mayo Clinic series, medullary involvement was observed in 22% of patients. It was estimated to be slight (less than 10% of the cross-sectional area) in 14% and moderate (10–25% of the cross-sectional area) in 8% of patients [5]. The mass lesion, as well as the medullaty extention, is heterogeneously enhanced. **CT scan** notes a well-defined mineralized mass with high signal intensity and low-attenuation signal, suggesting an unmineralized peripheral component in some cases. It is useful to evaluate involvement of the cortex, tumor intrusion into the medullary cavity, and extension into the soft tissues. However, detecting medullary and soft tissue intrusion is not as sensitive as MR images. CT scan also may visualize a cartilaginous cap partially covering the tumor mass if presents. **Bone scan** usually shows a hot uptake in the lesion (Figs. 10.2b and 10.3e). **PET/CT scan** generally shows a heterogeneously intense FDG uptake in the exophytic mass (Figs. 10.1d and 10.4c).

10.8 Histologic Findings

Parosteal OSA consists of a dense collagenous stroma with minimally atypical spindle cells simulating those of a low-grade fibrosarcoma (FSA), and also producing well-formed osseous trabeculae. Coalescence of bony trabeculae can form solid bony areas (Fig. 10.5a). The bone trabeculae formed directly from the pure fibrous stroma tissue can be arranged with irregularly anastomosing, well-formed, various shapes of curved bone (*alphabetic soap*) pattern without prominent osteoblastic rimming, referred to as *fibro-osseous metaplasia* as in fibrous dysplasia (FD) (Fig. 10.5b). Or, they are often regularly arranged as long steamers in a parallel pattern with normal-looking woven or finely lamellar bone with mosaic cement lines, so-called pagetoid bone (Fig. 10.5c). There is a lack of periosteal new

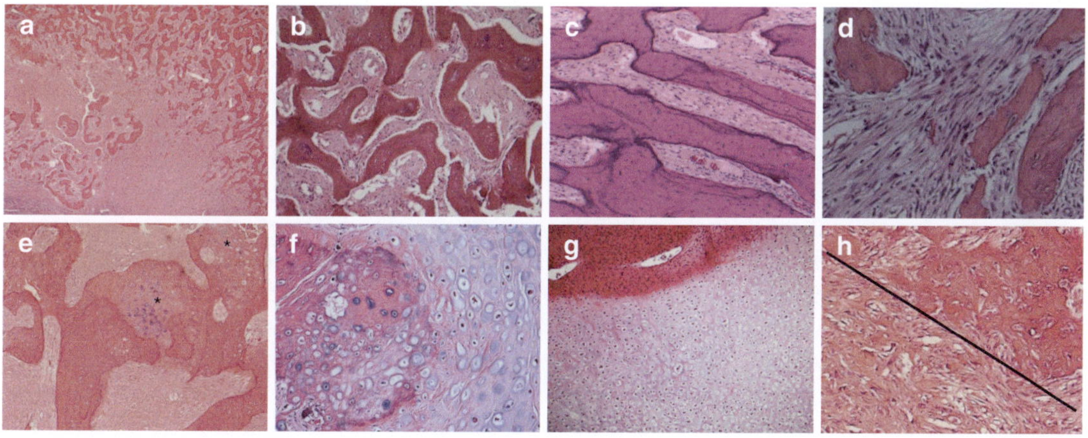

Fig. 10.5 Microscopic examination. (**a**) Low-power magnification shows a dense collagenous stroma with numerous irregular anastomosing and curved osseous trabeculae. (**b**) Medium-power magnification reveals irregularly anastomosing, well-formed, curved bone trabeculae without prominent osteoblastic rimming, referred to as *fibro-osseous metaplasia* as in FD, embedded in mild to moderate cellular fascicles of spindle cells. It is also called the *alphabetic soap* pattern. (**c**) Characteristically, long woven bone trabeculae with mosaic cement lines, so-called *Pagetoid bone*, are arranged in a parallel pattern with intervening fascicles of spindle cells. (**d**) Higher-power magnification demonstrates mild to moderate atypical stromal cells with increased mitotic activity, which are arranged in *herringbone* pattern between bone trbeculae, as in FSA. (**e**) Foci of cartilage differentiation are observed in the form of nodules (asterisks). (**f**) Higher-power magnification demonstrates mildly to moderately atypical chondrocytes in the hyaline matrix. (**g**) In some cases, cartilage differentiation is seen in the form of cartilaginous cap, mimicking OC. (**h**) The lower-grade tumor (upper right) is abruptly changed to higher-grade spindle cell sarcoma (lower left) with a sharp transition zone between the two components, indicating *dedifferentiation*

bone formation because parosteal OSA grows in exophytic fashion without periosteal elevation, while periosteal OSA elevates the periosteum by expansion of the tumor stimulating prominent new bone deposition. Higher-power magnification presents mild to moderate atypical stromal cells with increased mitotic activity (Grade 1 or 2), which are arranged in long sweeps of a parallel arrangement of the nuclei or *herringbone* pattern between bone trabeculae (Fig. 10.5d). Cartilage differentiation with mildly to moderately atypical chondrocytes, reflecting a similar grade to the spindle cell component is usually minimal in the form of scattered nodules if presents (Figs. 10.1c and 10.5e, f). When the cartilage component is more than 40–50%, periosteal OSA is more likely in which the cartilage component is characteristically profuse [1]. The lesion may produce a cartilage cap in the periphery which partially covers the tumor mass mimicking OC (Fig. 10.5g), which can be clearly visible on MR images in some cases. Medullary involvement was identified on macroscopic sections with a varying rate from 22% [5] to 36% (26.7% of low-grade tumors and 52% of intermediate-grade) [4], and up to 65% in DPOS [6]. The effect of medullary involvement on survival and local recurrence has been debated for many years. The rate of medullary involvement was reported to correlate with tumor grade of the tumor; 18% in the patients with Grade 1, 25% in Grade 2, and 43% in those with DPOS [5]. However, another studies [4] found that intramedullary involvement did not correlate with the grade of tumor, which accords with the findings of others who have found no correlation between intramedullary involvement and survival [2, 5, 7–10], local recurrence [5, 11, 12], or metastasis [5, 11]. Therefore, the authors considered medullary involvement would not be a feature of a more aggressive tumor. A progression to higher-grade sarcoma, so-called *dedifferentiation*, can occur either at initial presentation (synchronous type) or much more often at the time of recurrence (metachronous type), and most of these tumors were reported to occur after more than one local recurrence [13]. However, another series reported that most DPOS lesions are synchronous and most metachronous DPOS are detected in the first local recurrence. Thus, the authors addressed that the potential for dedifferentiation in parosteal OSA should be reconsidered [6]. Twenty-nine of 120 (24%) patients with POS in the Rizzoli Institute files [6] and 21 of 75 patients (28%) in the Mayo Clinic series [10] underwent dedifferentiation. The low-grade tumor is abruptly changed to higher-grade spindle cell sarcoma in some area with a sharp transition zone between the two different components as in dedifferentiated CSA (Figs. 10.4d and 10.5h). The phenomenon can be reflected as ill-defined radiolucent areas within the heavily mineralized tumor mass on radiograph (Fig. 10.5a).

10.9 Management

Wide resection with an adequate margin followed by reconstruction is a standard option for treatment. For typical low-grade tumor that does not wrap around the host bone or even DPOS with focal medullary invasion, geometric osteotomy (hemicylindric resection) of involved bone and reconstruction with allograft or recycled autograft bone can be considered (Figs. 10.1f and 10.4e). The hemicylindric resection saves a considerable part of meta-diaphysis as well as epiphysis and preserves the native joint. However, larger tumors with extensive medullary extension, encircling the host bone, locally recurrent tumor, or DPOS, require a complete resection of the affected bone and reconstruction with tumor prosthesis including joint replacement (Figs. 10.2e and 10.3c) or allograft (Fig. 10.3g). Amputation may be necessary for extensive tumor, disseminated or multiple local recurrences (Fig. 10.2k), or complications of prior surgery such as uncontrolled infection. Chemotherapy is not necessary for typical low-grade tumors is indicated for parosteal OSA progressing to high-grade DPOS. Early identification and surgical removal of metastasis as well as eradication of the disseminated tumor cells by adequate chemotherapy would improve the clinical outcomes in patients with dedifferentiation.

10.10 Clinical Course and Prognosis

The prognosis is excellent with a 5-year survival rate of up to 100% in Grade 1 and 80% in Grade 2 parosteal OSA (overall 85–90%) if surgical margin is adequate. In large series, the overall 5-year and 10-year survival rate were about 90% and over 80%, respectively [4, 5]. However, incomplete resection or inadequate margin result in a local recurrence and even dedifferentiation to higher-grade sarcoma. Local recurrence was reported to occur in 60% of patients with intralesional resection and about 20% of those with marginal resection, but only 3% of patients with wide resection [4] (Fig. 10.2). Dedifferentiation was reported in about 15–24% of patients [4–6, 13], and 80% of the local recurrences were histologically dedifferentiated high-grade [4]. Metastasis almost never occurs in Grade 1 tumors but the frequency of metastasis is increased in Grade 2 and dedifferentiated tumors. Dedifferentiation is significantly associated with an increased risk of metastasis (47% at 5 years compared to nil for patients without dedifferentiation) [5]. Distant metastasis is the major cause of treatment failure. DPOS behaves more malignantly than parosteal OSA but less malignantly than high-grade surface OSA. The prognosis of DPOS is better than that of dedifferentiated central and peripheral CSA [6].

References

1. Mirra JM. Parosteal osteosarcoma. In: Mirra JM, editor. Bone tumors: clinical, radiologic, and pathologic correlations. 2nd ed. Philadelphia: Lea & Febiger; 1989. p. 1688–721.
2. Campanacci M. Parosteal osteosarcoma. In: Campanacci M, editor. Bone and soft tissue tumors. Wien New York: Springer-Verlag; 1999. p. 525–48.
3. Czerniak B. Osteosarcoma. In: Dorfman HD, Czerniak B, editors. Dorfman and Czerniak's bone tumors. 2nd ed. (eBook): Elsevier; 2016. p. 200–355.
4. Unni KK, Osteosarcoma IY. Dahlin's bone tumors: general aspects and data on 10,165 cases. Philadelphia: Lippincott Williams & Wilkins; 2010. p. 122–57.
5. Okada K, Frassica FJ, Sim FH, Beabout JW, Bond JR, Unni KK, Parosteal osteosarcoma. A clinicopathological study. J Bone Joint Surg Am. 1994;76(3):366–78.
6. Bertoni F, Bacchini P, Staals EL, Davidovitz P. Dedifferentiated parosteal osteosarcoma: the experience of the Rizzoli Institute. Cancer. 2005;103(11):2373–82.
7. Ahuja SC, Villacin A, Smith J, Bullough P, Huvos A, Marcove R. Juxtacortical (parosteal) osteogenic sarcoma: histological grading and prognosis. J Bone Joint Surg Am. 1977;59(5):632–47.
8. Johnson K, Davies A, Mangham D, Grimer R. Parosteal osteosarcoma of a metatarsal with intramedullary invasion. Skeletal Radiol. 1999;28:111–5.
9. Picci P, Campanacci M, Bacci G, Capanna R, Ayala A. Medullary involvement in parosteal osteosarcoma. A case report. J Bone Joint Surg. 1987;69(1):131–6.
10. Unni KK, Dahlin DC, Beabout JW, Ivins JC. Parosteal osteogenic sarcoma. Cancer. 1976;37(5):2466–75.
11. Funovics PT, Bucher F, Toma CD, Kotz RI, Dominkus M. Treatment and outcome of parosteal osteosarcoma: biological versus endoprosthetic reconstruction. J Surg Oncol. 2011;103(8):782–9.
12. Han I, Oh JH, Na YG, Moon KC, Kim HS. Clinical outcome of parosteal osteosarcoma. J Surg Oncol. 2008;97(2):146–9.
13. Wold LE, Unni KK, Beabout JW, Sim FH, Dahlin DC. Dedifferentiated parosteal osteosarcoma. J Bone Joint Surg Am. 1984;66(1):53–9.

Periosteal Osteosarcoma

11

(***Peri*** "around," ***Osteo(n)*** "Bone," ***sarco(s)*** "flesh," ***ōma*** "noun forming suffix")

11.1 Definition

Periosteal osteosarcoma (OSA) is an intermediate-grade malignant bone forming tumor with predominant chondroblastic differentiation arising on the surface of bone, typically underneath the deep layer of the periosteum.

11.2 Synonym

Juxtacortical chondroblastic OSA, but not recommended.

11.3 Incidence

Periosteal OSA is the second most common type of surface OSA after the parosteal OSA, accounting for less than 2% of all OSAs [1–3] and about one-fourth of surface OSAs [4–6].

11.4 Age

The age at presentation is usually in adolescence and early adulthood with a peak incidence in the second decade which is similar to that for conventional OSA [1, 4].

11.5 Locations

Periosteal OSA exclusively occurs in the diaphysis of the tibia and the femur in contrast to parosteal OSA which has a unique propensity to occur in purely metaphysis or meta-diaphysis of the distal femur in its posterior aspect. More rarely, it is encountered in the humerus or ulna. Involvement of flat bones or short bones is exceedingly rare.

11.6 Clinical Features

Patients usually present with a palpable mass or selling, with or wihout pain of a relatively shorter duration than that of parosteal OSA (several weeks to months).

11.7 Radiologic Findings

Plain radiograph shows a predominantly radiolucent, fusiform, broader-based mass attached to the cortical surface with a strong propensity to occur in the diaphysis of long bone (Figs. 11.1 and 11.2). There are areas of nonmineralized matrix interspersed with the mineralized portions in the tumor mass, and the outer margin is the

W.-J. Bahk, *Diagnosis and Management of Primary Bone Tumors*,
https://doi.org/10.1007/978-981-96-3484-2_11

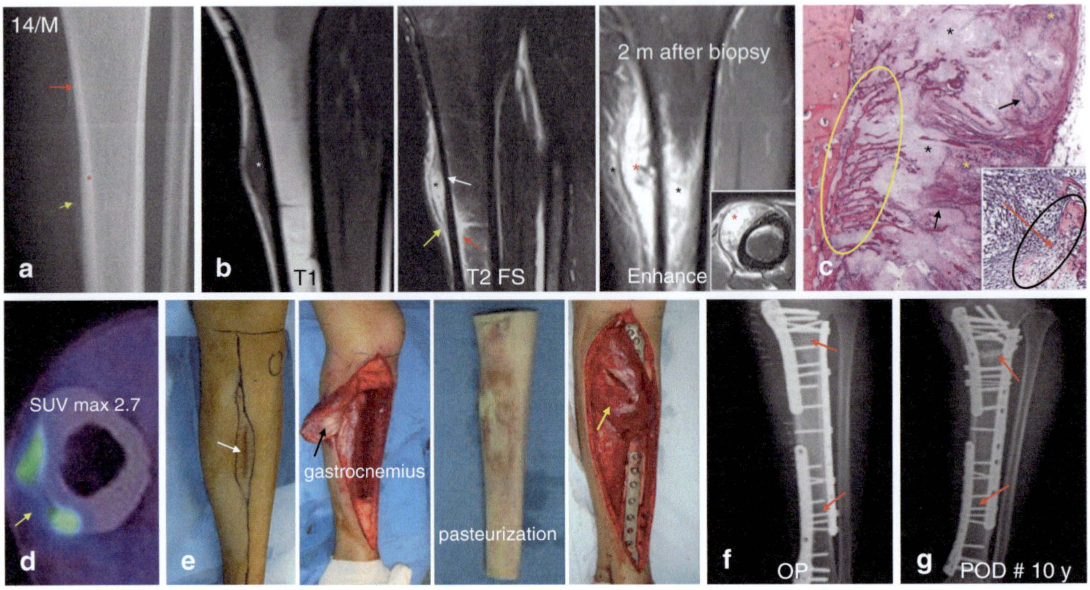

Fig. 11.1 (**a**) Radiograph taken for left leg pain of 4 months' duration in a 14-year-old boy shows a hazy radiolucent, fusiform, broad-based mass attached to the surface of the tibia diaphysis. The underlying host cortex is intact and mildly thickened without medullary involvement (red asterisk). Note the elevation of the periosteum with internal stippled hazy densification (yellow arrow) as well as Codman's triangle (red arrow). (**b**) MR images demonstrate a well-demarcated subperiosteal mass (asterisks) with low SI on T1- and high SI with partial intermediate signal on fat-saturated T2-weighted image, representing high water content of extensive chondroblastic component. A focal high signal is also noted at the medullary cavity, suggesting a mild peritumoral edema (red arrow). The underlying cortex is, however, intact without a tumor extension into the bone marrow (white arrow). Thin low SI of sclerotic rim surrounding the lesion has a continuity with underlying host cortex, creatin a *beak-like* appearance (yellow arrow). Follow-up enhanced MR image at 2 months after incision biopsy reveals progression of the tumor with marked enlargement that is strongly enhanced (red asterisk). In addition, peritumoral inflammation with edema in surrounding muscle, soft tissue, and medullary cavity becomes more significant and is well enhanced (black asterisks). Despite the progression of the lesion, the axial view shows that the tumor encircles less than half of the affected bone (inset). (**c**) Low-power microscopic examination shows a predominant cartilage component in the form of variable-sized multiple nodules (black asterisks) separated by bands consisting of malignant spindle cells at the periphery of the nodules (black arrows). The atypical spindle cells are more abundant at the outer part of the tumor mass (yellow asterisks). There are numerous tiny striations represented by reactive new bone which are perpendicular to the cortex (yellow circle), which can be seen as a *sunburst* appearance on radiograph. Higher-power magnification of the outer surface of the tumor demonstrates a high number of chondrocytes with atypical nuclei equivalent to Grade 2 to 3 CSA, which gradually blend into the undifferentiated spindle cell area with osteoid to woven bone formation (inset). (**d**) PET/CT scan reveals a mildly increased FDG uptake (SUVmax 2.7) in the periosteal mass with a post-biopsy change (yellow arrow), but not in medullary space. (**e**) A longitudinal incision was made including a previous biopsy scar (white arrow) for wide resection with adequate margin. Then, gastrocnemius flap was prepared for adequate coverage of the pasteurized bone (black arrow). Tumor, periosteum, surrounding muscles, and bone marrow were completely removed from the resected bone for pasteurization. The defect was reconstructed by pasteurized bone securely fixed with plates and screws, and properly covered by a prepared gastrocnemius muscle flap (yellow arrow). (**f**) Immediate postoperative radiograph shows well-matched pasteurized bone in the original site with visible osteotomy lines (arrows). (**g**) Follow-up radiograph taken at 10 years after surgery reveals no evidence of local recurrence and good maintenance of the recycled bone with complete union of osteotomy sites (arrows). He is disease-free at 10 years after surgery without chemotherapy

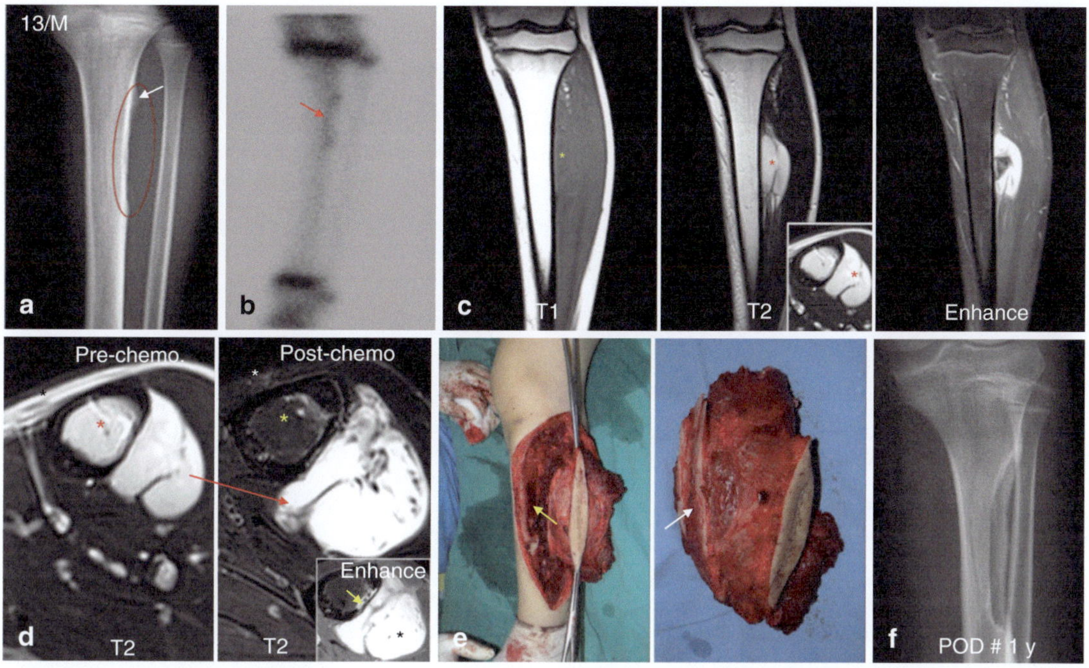

Fig. 11.2 (**a**) Radiograph taken for left leg pain of 3 months' duration in a 13-year-old boy shows a hazy fusiform radiolucent mass on the surface of the tibial diaphysis. The underlying cortex seems to be intact with irregular and superficial erosion by an external mass in a *saucer* shape without invasion of the medullary cavity (red circle). A Codman's triangle is also seen at the periphery of the lesion (red arrow). (**b**) Bone scan reveals mildly increased uptake along the *saucer*-shaped extrinsic erosion of the underlying cortex beneath the tumor mass (arrow). (**c**) MR images demonstrate a well-defined fusiform mass (asterisks) attached to the intact underlying cortex without any medullary signal change. The SI is iso to surrounding muscle on T1- and high SI with low to intermediate signal in the septa on T2-weighted image. Axial image notes that the tumor encircles less than half of the affected bone (inset). The mass is heterogeneously well enhanced. (**d**) Follow-up MR image after neoadjuvant chemotherapy demonstrates a moderately increased size of the tumor mass when compared to that of prechemotherapy. However, soft tissue and bone marrow edema (asterisks) disappeared after chemotherapy. After contrast injection (inset), the mass lesion is well enhanced (black asterisk) and a focal cortical invasion is still identified with heterogeneous enhancement (yellow arrow). (**e**) Wide hemi-cylindrical resection of tibia, including the tumor mass, surrounding healty muscle and soft tissuuse as well as previous biopsy scar, was performed. Note the surface of the remaining tibia (yellow arrow) and the resected segment of the tibia (white arrow). (**f**) Follow-up radiograph at 1 year after surgery shows no evidence of local recurrence in the absence of chomotherapy

least mineralized, giving the impression that the tumor blends into the surrounding soft tissue [5]. The mass is typically longer than it is wide. The underlying cortex can be intact, thickened, or extrinsically eroded by the pressure of the tumor mass in a *saucer* shape, but the medullary cavity is usually not invaded. The periosteum appears elevated due to the expansion of the tumor mass between the cortex and the deep layer of the periosteum. The periosteal new bones are formed in the form of fine striations perpendicular to the cortex, referred to as *sunburst* or *hair-on-end* appearance, and Codman's triangle at the periphery of the mass. In contrast, parosteal OSA cannot elevate the periosteum and does not produce new bone because it arises from the outer surface of the perioseum (Fig. 11.3). The sunburst appearance occurs when Sharpey's fibers stretch out perpendicularly to the bone instead of laying down a new layer because the lesion grows too fast. In addition to the linear or stippled densification, focal patchy calcification suggestive of calcification of the cartilage component can be seen. On the contrary to parosteal OSA, periosteal OSA has no tendency to encircle or wrap the involved bone, and it does not involve the medul-

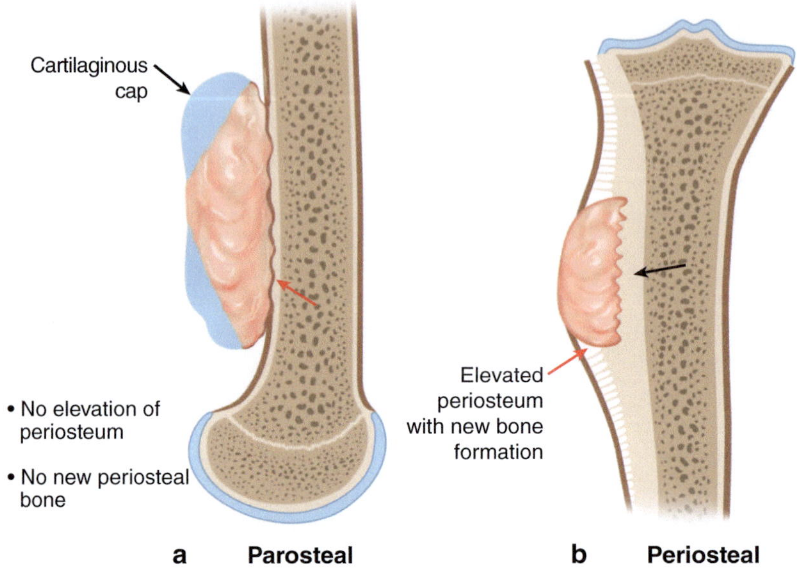

Fig. 11.3 ***Schema of differentiation between parosteal and periosteal OSA***. (**a**) ***Parosteal OSA*** arises from the outer layer of the periosteum. In some cases, a cartilaginous cap partially covers the tumor (black arrow), which can be clearly visible on MRI. The underlying cortex is usually intact, but occasionally thickened or focally destructed (red arrow). There is no periosteal reaction and periosteal new bone formation. (**b**) ***Periosteal OSA*** also originates from the surface of bone but typically underneath the deep layer of the periosteum. The underlying cortex can be intact, irregularly thickened, or extrinsically eroded by the pressure of the tumor mass in a *saucer* shape (black arrow). The periosteum is elevated by the tumor mass and new bones are frequently deposited in the form of numerous fine striations perpendicular to the cortex (red arrow), referred to as *sunburst or hair-on-end* appearance

lary cavity at least for a long time (Figs. 11.1 and 11.2). These findings are essential for the differential diagnosis of both entities and are best seen on CT scan and MRI. **Bone scan** usually shows mild to moderate uptake along the *saucer*-shaped extrinsic erosion of the underlying cortex beneath the tumor mass (Fig. 11.2b). **PET/CT scan** also shows a heterogeneously increased FDG uptake in the lesion (Fig. 11.1d). **CT scan** is useful for detecting cortical changes, associated medullary aberrations, calcification, and periosteal reaction extending into the soft-tissue mass. Additionally, a lower attenuation than that of muscle, reflecting the high water content of the extensive cartilage component, which is a histologic characteristic of periosteal OSA, can be seen. **MR images** typically reveal a subperiosteal soft tissue mass attached to the cortex underneath the stretched periosteum with low to intermediate (iso to surrounding muscle) SI on T1- and heterogeneous intermediate and high SI on T2-weighted image (Figs. 11.1b and 11.2c). Murphy and colleagues [7] reported high SI on T2-weighted image in 83% of 40 cases in AFIP series, representing high water content of chondroblastic component. The finding corresponded to the result of the pathologic review in which all periosteal OSA had a cartilage component, and it was the predominant tissue in 85% of the cases. Focal or extensive areas of surrounding soft tissue and adjacent marrow edema are often observed with intact cortex, representing reactive changes (Fig. 11.1b). Based on the original definition by Unni et al. who established this condition, periosteal OSA is limited to the periphery of the cortex. On radiograph, the endosteal surface is normal and the meduallry cavity is not involved. Periosteal OSA cannot be differentiated from the conventional OSA if these criteria are not met [5]. However, involvement of the medullary canal by periosteal OSA may be controversial subject if it does not occur or it can be present although extremely rare. In AFIP series, focal areas of adjacent marrow replacement were common on MR images but represented reactive changes if the signals were not directly continuous with the overlying soft-tissue mass that occurred in only one patient and confirmed as bone marrow invasion by histologic evaluation [7]. Thus, marrow invasion itself should not preclude the diagnosis if there are other distinctive features [7–9]. Axial image show that the tumor encircles less than half of the affected bone at most (Figs. 11.1b and 11.2d), in contrast to parosteal OSA, which tends to grow circumferentially and to become huge enough eventually to wrap around the involved in advanced cases. The lesion often presents septal and peripheral enhancement, suggesting a cartilage component as well as the nodular features with a prominent degree of enhancement related to the more vascularized malignant tissue and the intermixed fibrous and osteoid components [7]. It can also be diffusely and strongly enhanced (Figs. 11.1b and 11.2c).

11.8 Histologic Findings

Periosteal OSA is predominantly composed of a cartilage component in the form of irregular poorly marginated lobules separated by bands consisting of malignant spindle cells. Areas, even small and focal, of osteoid or primitive woven bone production directly from undifferentiated spindle cells at the outer surface of the tumor mass and periphery of the lobules should be identified for a diagnosis of OSA. However, the amount of bone component is often so minimal that may not be seen, particularly if the specimen is not adequately obtained by closed biopsy, such as needle or trocar biopsy. There can be numerous tiny striations representing spicules of reactive new bone formation which are perpendicular to the cortex (Fig. 11.1c). The tumor cartilage can undergo endochondral ossification often presenting a radiating speculation on radiograph, so-called *sunburst* appearance. The cartilage component usually has moderate to severe nuclear atypism equivalent to Grade 2 or 3 chondrosarcoma (CSA). When there is no osteoid/woven bone production, the tumor is classified as a CSA. The tumor osteoid or woven bone is usually lace-like rather than trabecular pattern. The outer margin of the tumor mass is rather well demarcated by a pseudocapsule occasionally with satellite nodules. Only reactive woven bone can be seen if biopsy material is obtained in the deeper part of the tumor mass near the cortex and Codman's triangle.

11.9 Management

Wide resection with an adequate margin, followed by reconstruction using various methods, is the cornerstone of treatment. For a small, localized tumor, hemicylindrical resection of the affected bone can be allowed with or without reconstruction (Fig. 11.2e). The role of chemotherapy and its timing remains still debatable.

11.10 Clinical Course and Prognosis

Local recurrence is almost always followed by marginal or incomplete excision but is rare when adequate wide margin is achieved. The prognosis is intermediate between parosteal OSA and conventional OSA. The overall survival rate at 5 years was 77–89% and 66–84% at 10 years [10–12]. Current guidelines and recommendations do not appear to have common consensus regarding the role of chemotherapy due to the rarity of the tumor, and multicenter studies are needed to provide calrification. The major series have not proven the efficacy of chemotherapy in improving survival outcomes [10, 11]. Another single-institutional study also failed to find the efficacy of chemotherapy in improving survival outcomes [12]. In a review article on the actual impact of chemotherapy, available data are in favor of administering chemotherapy only to patients with high-risk characteristics, such as high-grade tumor with medullary involvement. The authors concluded that chemotherapy plays a major role in high-risk patients to reduce the tumor size before excision, except for those with low-grade, chemoresistant tumors [13].

References

1. Czerniak B. Osteosarcoma. In: Dorfman HD, Czerniak B, editors. Dorfman and Czerniak's bone tumors. 2nd ed. eBook: Elsevier; 2016. p. 200–355.
2. Campanacci M. Periosteal osteosarcoma. In: Campanacci M, editor. Bone and soft tissue tumors. Wien New York: Springer-Verlag; 1999. p. 517–24.
3. Unni KK, Inwards Y. Periosteal osteosarcoma. In: Unni KK, Inwards CY, editors. Dahlin's bone tumors: general aspects and data on 10,165 cases. 6th ed. Philadelphia: Lippincott William & Wilkins; 2010. p. 145–7.
4. Murphey MD, Robbin MR, McRae GA, Flemming DJ, Temple HT, Kransdorf MJ. The many faces of osteosarcoma. Radiographics. 1997;17(5):1205–31.
5. Unni KK, Dahlin DC, Beabout JW. Periosteal osteogenic sarcoma. Cancer. 1976;37(5):2476–85.
6. Huvos AG. Juxtacortical osteogenic sarcoma. In: Huvos AG, editor. Bone tumors: diagnosis, treatment and prognosis. 2nd ed. Philadelphia: WB Saunders; 1991. p. 157–77.
7. Murphey MD, Jelinek JS, Temple HT, Flemming DJ, Gannon FH. Imaging of periosteal osteosarcoma: radiologic-pathologic comparison. Radiology. 2004;233(1):129–38.
8. Hall R, Robinson L, Malawar M. DuniWK. Periosteal osteosarcoma. Cancer. 1985;155:165–71.
9. Sonobe H, Iwata J, Furihata M, Ohtsuki Y, Mizobuchi H, Yamamoto H. Periosteal osteosarcoma of the femur with bone marrow involvement: a case report. Pathol Int. 1994;44(5):407–11.
10. Grimer RJ, Bielack S, Flege S, Cannon SR, Foleras G, Andreeff I, et al. Periosteal osteosarcoma–a European review of outcome. Eur J Cancer. 2005;41(18):2806–11.
11. Cesari M, Alberghini M, Vanel D, Palmerini E, Staals EL, et al. Periosteal osteosarcoma: a single-institution experience. Cancer. 2011;117(8):1731–5.
12. Chan CM, Lindsay AD, Spiguel AR, Gibbs CP Jr, Scarborough MT. Periosteal osteosarcoma: a single-institutional study of factors related to oncologic outcomes. Sarcoma. 2018;2018(1):8631237.
13. Assi T, Kattan J, Nassereddine H, Rassy E, Briand S, Court C, et al. Chemotherapy in the management of periosteal osteosarcoma: a narrative review. J Bone Oncol. 2021;30:100389.

High-Grade Surface Osteosarcoma 12

12.1 Definition

High-grade surface osteosarcoma (OSA) is exclusively high-grade malignant bone-forming tumor emerging from the surface of the long bone as parosteal or periosteal OSA without or with minimal medullary involvement at best.

12.2 Incidence

It is extremely rare, accounting for less than 1% of all OSAs [1–3] and about 9% of surface OSAs [4].

12.3 Age

The lesions usually occur in adolescents and young adults [5]. About 70% of patients were reported to occur in the second and third decades of life [4, 6].

12.4 Locations

The most frequent involvement sites include the diaphysis or meta-diaphysis of the femur, tibia, and humerus [4, 5]. The favorite ages (adolescents and young adults) and locations (the distal femur and proximal humerus being involved most frequently) are similar to those of high-grade medullary OSA.

12.5 Clinical Features

Patients most commonly present with a palpable mass or swelling and pain of varying duration from months to years [5, 6]. However, a relatively short duration of symptom (less than 1–3 months in about half of 27 patients with available information about duration) was usual in other series [4] (Fig. 12.1). Rarely, limited motion of joint adjacent to the tumor can occur.

W.-J. Bahk, *Diagnosis and Management of Primary Bone Tumors*,
https://doi.org/10.1007/978-981-96-3484-2_12

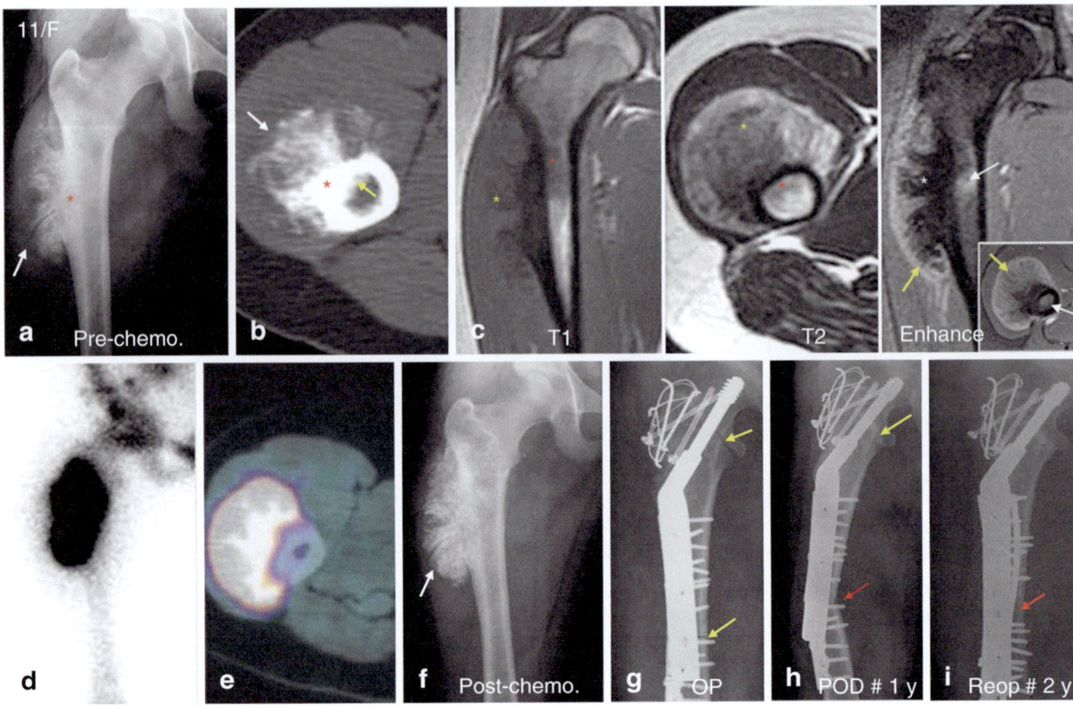

Fig. 12.1 (**a**) Radiograph taken for right proximal thigh mass with pain of 1 month's duration in a 11-year-old girl shows a large, fusiform, outgrowing mass with dense irregular opacities in a fluffy immature pattern and peripheral radiolucent area attached to the surface of the proximal femur, mainly the diaphysis. The outer margin of the mass is indistinct (arrow). Base of the mass is broad and the underlying cortex is thickened (asterisk). There is no "string sign" of discernible thin lucent zone between the tumor and the underlying cortex that is characteristic of parosteal OSA. (**b**) CT scan more clearly reveals an ill-defined exophytic soft tissue mass with multiple opacifications attached to the superficially eroded and irregularly thickened cortex (asterisk). The outer margin is irregular and indistinct (white arrow), and minimal medullary invasion is seen (yellow arrow). (**c**) MR images demonstrate an ill-defined, fusiform-shaped, exophytic mass (yellow asterisks) attached to the irregularly thickened cortex with superficial erosion by the mass, which minimally extends into the medullary cavity (red asterisks), corresponding to minimal medullary invasion on CT scan. The mass extensively circumscribes more than half of the underlying bone diameter (yellow asterisk) on T2-weighted axial image. The SI is intermediate (iso to surrounding muscles) on T1-weighted image and heterogeneous high SI on T2-weighted image with internal dark signals of dense bone on both sequences. The mass lesion is well enhanced (yellow arrows) except for the dark bone-forming areas (white asterisk). The focal medullary lesion is also enhanced (white arrows). (**d**) Bone scan notes a homogeneously strong uptake. (**e**) PET/CT scan shows heterogeneously increased FDG uptake in the exophytic mass lesion. (**f**) Follow-up radiograph after neoadjuvant chemotherapy reveals more prominent ossification of the mass including the previous lucent peripheral area (arrow). (**g**) Radiograph after wide resection with reconstruction using a pateurized femur notes good position with visible gaps between host bone and pasteurized bone (arrows). (**h**) Follow-up radiograph at 1 year after surgery and adjuvant chemotherapy shows a fracture with angulation at the distal host-graft junction "red arrow". The proximal junction is united well (yellow arrow). (**i**) Follow-up radiograph at 2 years after reduction and plate fixation reveals no evidence of local recurrence with complete healing of the fracture (arrow)

12.6 Radiologic Findings

High-grade surface OSA typically shows a poorly defined, dense to moderately mineralized, fusiform-shaped mass with a broad base, which is attached to the surface of the underlying bone without medullary involvement. The pattern of mineralization tends to simulate that of high-grade central OSA with fluffy, immature appearance to irregular cloud-cumulus opacities predominantly at the base of the lesion. The outer margin of the mass is irregular and indistinct

(Fig. 12.1a). However, a thin lucent zone between the tumor and the underlying cortex, so-called *string sign*, a characteristic of parosteal OSA, is quite rare. Radiating spicules of new bone perpendicular to the long axis of the bone, referred to as "*sun burst*" appearance, which is characteristic of periosteal OSA, are also rare [4]. The underlying cortex can be intact but is frequently altered by the extrinsic tumor mass (thickened, superficially eroded, or destructed). Periosteal reaction can be rarely associated, but Codman's triangle or spiculated periosteal reaction is usually not seen. **CT scan** more clearly exhibits an exophytic mass arising from the surface of the cortex with irregularly dense mineralization and indistinct outer margin. Additionally, it presents erosion or thickening of the underlying cortex as well as medullary extension if presents (Fig. 12.1b). **MR findings** MRI can accurately depict an exophytic main mass with or without medullary involvement, as well as peritumoral and medullary edema. MR images reveal a poorly defined fusiform mass adhered to the cortex underneath the periosteum with low (osteoid to woven bone) and intermediate SI (nonossified soft tissue components) on T1-weighted and low (osteoid to woven bone) and high SI (nonossified cartilage or soft tissue components) on T2-weighted images. The cartilage component scattered throughout the mass is clearly identified as focal or extensive high signal depending on the degree of cartilage production. Circumferential involvement of the host bone was reported in 28% of the cases on CT or MRI, half of which extensively encircled more than 50% of the underlying bone. Medullary involvement was observed in about 30% [4] (Fig. 12.1c). Circumferential involvement was also reported in another series with an average of 53% (range, 20–100%) [6]. The authors also detected medullary canal involvement in half of the patients who had cross-sectional studies. In another series, minimal medullary involvement was seen in one-third to half of the patients [7]. The lesion is strongly enhanced except for dark bone-forming areas. **Bone scan** shows homogenous strong uptake (Fig. 12.1d). **PET/CT scan** reveals a significantly intense FDG uptake in the lesiosn, suggesting a malignant lesion (Fig. 12.1e). In addition, it provides informations on distant metastases to other organs and the hitological response to neoadjuvant chemotherapy.

12.7 Histologic Findings

The microscopic features are identical to those of high-grade medullary OSA. Thus, the exophytic mass located on the bone surface is critical for a correct diagnosis. Individual stromal cells are highly pleomorphic, hyperchromatic, with large nuclei surrounded by a small amount of cytoplasm, and frequent mitoses including abnormal type (Grade 3 or 4 according to Broder's grading system). The stroma cells directly produce osteoid and immature bone in ribbon, nest, or filigree pattern, often with a prominent lace-like architecture. Varying degrees of cartilage differentiation are associated with bone production, and a cartilage component can be extensively deposited in up to 50% of the lesion by the malignant cells. There are no areas of low-grade spindle cells embedded between the stream of woven bone trabeculae seen in parosteal OSA, which finding can eliminate a dedifferentiated parosteal OSA [6].

12.8 Management

High-grade surface OSA is treated by the same protocol as for high-grade conventional central OSA. Wide resection and reconstruction combined with systemic chemotherapy is a standard option for treatment (Fig. 12.1f–i).

12.9 Clinical Course and Prognosis

Local recurrence is almost always followed by marginal or incomplete excision. The prognosis is the same as conventional high-grade central OSA. In the Mayo Clinic series, the overall survival was 58% at 3 years and 46% at 5 years [4]. However, the 5-year overall survival was 82% and disease-free survival was 70% in the Rizzoli

Institute study [6]. Surprisingly, the overall 5-year survival rate was higher than the overall survival reported for both conventional central OSA (67.5%) [8] and dedifferentiated parosteal OSA (72%) [9] in the same Institution's series. It was thought to be more likely because of the small number of the patient group rather than a different behavior of surface tumors and central lesions.

References

1. Wold LE, Unni KK, Beabout JW, Pritchard DJ. High-grade surface osteosarcomas. Am J Surg Pathol. 1984;8(3):181–6.
2. Klein MJ, Bonar SFM, O'Donnell PG. High grade surface osteosarcoma. In: Editorial board, editor. The WHO classification of tumours. 5th ed. Lyon: International agency for research on cancer; 2020. p. 417–8.
3. Unni KK, Inwards Y. Osteosarcoma. In: Dahlin's bone tumors: general aspects and data on 10,165 cases. Philadelphia: Lippincott Williams & Wilkins; 2010. p. 122–57.
4. Okada K, Unni KK, Swee RG, Sim FH. High grade surface osteosarcoma: a clinicopathologic study of 46 cases. Cancer. 1999;85(5):1044–54.
5. Czerniak B. Osteosarcoma. In: Dorfman HD, Czerniak B, editors. Dorfman and Czerniak's bone tumors. 2nd ed. (eBook): Elsevier; 2016. p. 200–355.
6. Staals EL, Bacchini P, Bertoni F. High-grade surface osteosarcoma: a review of 25 cases from the Rizzoli Institute. Cancer. 2008;112(7):1592–9.
7. Unni K, Inwards C, Bridge J, Kindblom L, Wold L. Maliganat bone-forming lesions. AFIP atlas of tumor pathology series 4. Tumors of the bones and joints. Washington: AFIP-ARP; 2005.
8. Bacci G, Longhi A, Versari M, Mercuri M, Briccoli A, Picci P. Prognostic factors for osteosarcoma of the extremity treated with neoadjuvant chemotherapy: 15-year experience in 789 patients treated at a single institution. Cancer. 2006;106(5):1154–61.
9. Bertoni F, Bacchini P, Staals EL, Davidovitz P. Dedifferentiated parosteal osteosarcoma: the experience of the Rizzoli Institute. Cancer. 2005;103(11):2373–82.

Part III

Cartilage-Forming (Chondrogenic) Tumors and Lesions

Osteochondroma

13

(***osteo*** "bone" **+** ***chondros*** "cartilage" **+** ***ōma*** "forming")

13.1 Definition

Osteochondroma (OC) is a developmental anomaly consisting of a bony protuberance covered with a cartilage cap of variable thicknesses, which emanates outwardly from the surface of bone and is continuous with the medullary cavity of the underlying bone. Actually, OC has been considered as a hamartomatous or developmental anomaly in the distinct clinical settings of either solitary form or multiple hereditary forms (osteochondromatosis). However, germline mutations in EXT1 and EXT2 genes have been found in the development of solitary and multiple forms of the disease [1–3], and thus, OC should be considered a unique form of a benign bone tumor rather than a hamartoma. Most patients (86%) are reported to have a solitary lesion [4]. Exostosis is a benign protuberance with a cartilage cap extending outward from an underlying bone, including two forms of OC and degenerative marginal osteophyte [5].

13.2 Synonym

(Osteocartilaginous) Exostosis.

13.3 Incidence

OC is one of the most common bone tumors, but the reported incidence is considerably variable from one series to another depending on the high subject to selection bias, patients' medical attention, and surgeon's surgical indication. The reported incidence ranges varies from 15% to 35% of benign bone tumors and about 10–15% of all bone tumors in the major series [4, 6–9]. The incidence should be much higher because many patients are asymptomatic and do not seek medical attention. Solitary OC can be incidentally detected in about 1–2% of individuals who had an extensive radiographic evaluation for other reasons [5].

13.4 Age

OC develops during the period of rapid skeletal growth and remains for the rest of the life. Thus, it can be found at any age, but most patients are diagnosed in their first two decades of life.

W.-J. Bahk, *Diagnosis and Management of Primary Bone Tumors*,
https://doi.org/10.1007/978-981-96-3484-2_13

13.5 Locations

The lesion can occur in the metaphysis of any long bones formed by endochondral ossification. The distal femur and proximal tibia around the knee joint are most commonly involved (in about half of the cases), followed by the proximal femur, humerus, or distal tibia, and flat bones such as ilium and scapula (Figs. 13.1, 13.2, 13.3, 13.4, and 13.5). Rarely, it affects small bones of hands and feet (Figs. 13.6 and 13.7), and even ribs, vertebrae, calcaneus, or talus (Fig. 13.8). Extremely rarely, it is even found within soft tissue without osseous/intra-articular involvement, so-called *extra-skeletal OC* [10, 11] (Fig. 13.9). Marginal osteophyes form as a consequence of degenerative process of the joints, typically also occurring at any bone but is mostly found in the hip and knee region, calcaneus or spines (Fig. 13.13c).

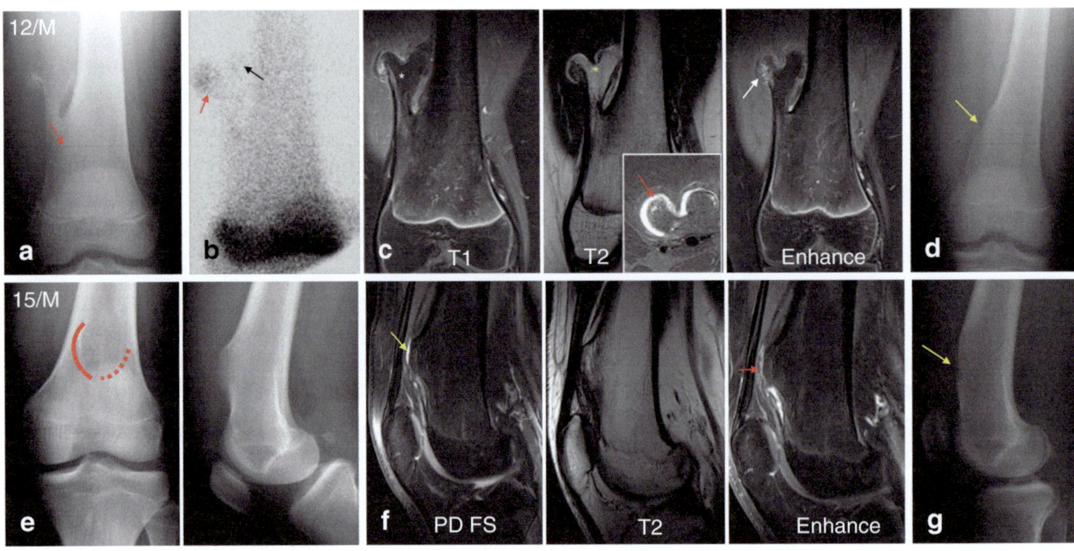

Fig. 13.1 ***Pedunculated types***. (**a**) Radiograph taken for left knee hard mass of 5 years' duration in a 12-year-old boy shows a bony projection on a narrow-based, pedunculated stalk with a bifurcated bulbous tip typically pointing away from the joint toward the diaphysis. The cortex of the host bone flares into the mass, and the spongy bone of the mass blends into the medulla of the host bone (arrow). This *flaring with medullary continuity* is pathognomonic for OC and allows diagnosis wihtout biopsy. A cartilage cap does not appear on the plain radiograph. (**b**) Pinhole bone scan reveals a focal mild uptake in one bulbous tip (red arrow) and no uptake in another tip (black arrow) of the bifurcated mass. (**c**) MR images show a bony projection with a bifurcated bulbous tip (asterisks), which flares into the cortex and medulla of the host bone. The SI of the mass is low on T1-weighted images and intermediate to high on T2-weighted images. A thin cartilage cap with a bright signal is clearly visible and measues 3.7 mm in thickness (inset). The cap presents focal and peripheral enhancement (white arrow). (**d**) The OC mass including cartilage cap is completely excised. ***Sessile type:*** (**e**) Anteroposterior radiograph taken for left knee protruding mass of 3 months' duration in a 15-year-old boy shows an incomplete "U"-shaped line (red line) which suggests that the mass is imaged en face. Lateral view shows a bony outgrowth on a broad sessile base without pedunculated stalk. (**f**) MR images demonstrate a bony outgrowth with a medullary continuation. A thin cartilage cap is clearly visualized, measuring less than 7 mm in thickness on fat-suppressed proton density image (yellow arrow) and is peripherally thin enhanced (red arrow). (**g**) The OC mass including cartilage cap is also completely excised

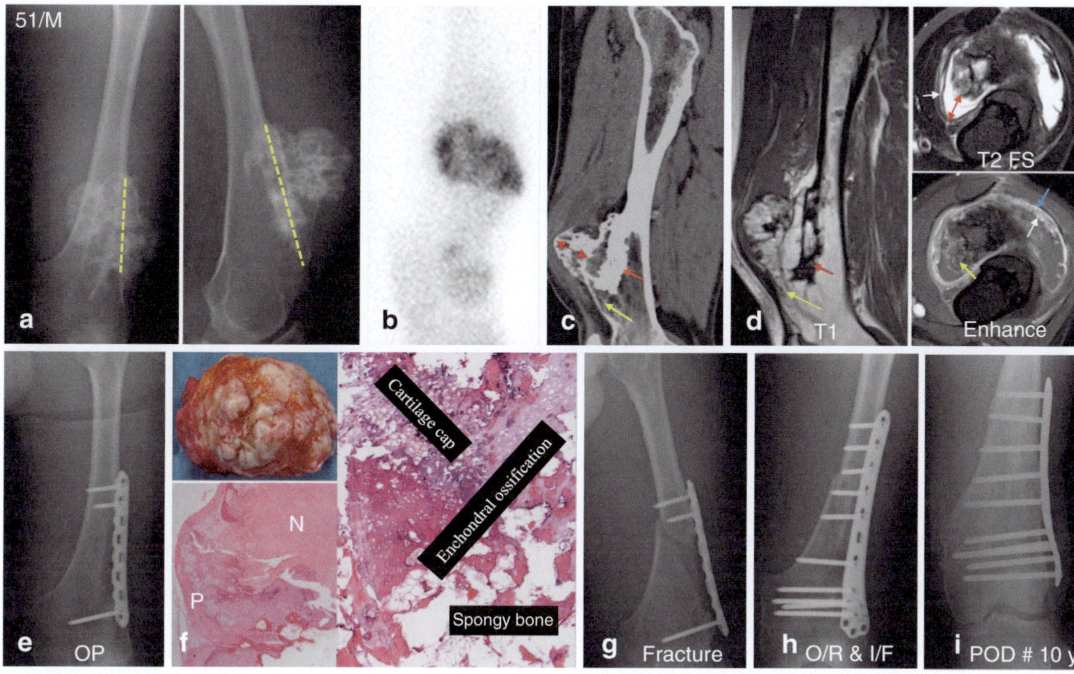

Fig. 13.2 ***Heavily calcifying OC.*** (**a**) Radiographs taken for left distal thigh hard mass of 40 years' duration and newly developed pain over the mass for 2 weeks in a 51-year-old man show a large protruding mass with lobulated margin and heavy calcification. The typical finding of *flaring with cortical and medullary continuity* for OC is obscured because of a significant calcification. (**b**) Pinhole bone scan reveals heterogeneously increased uptake in the protruding bony mass. (**c**) The heavily calcified portion simulates a thickened intact cortex and obscures the continuity to medullary cavity even on CT scan (red arrow). However, a small area of medullary continuation with host bone marrow is focally seen (yellow arrow). The thickness of the mineralized cartilage cap with calcification can be also accurately measured (double-headed arrow). (**d**) T1-weighted MR image shows dark signal of heavy calcification that obscures the typical continuity between the mass and host bone (red arrow). However, a focal area of the continuity is also clearly seen as CT scan (yellow arrow). A thick bright signal presenting cartilage cap is measured about 2.5 cm in maximum thickness (double-headed arrow) on fat-saturated T2-weighted image, suggesting a high possibility of malignant change in consideration of newly developed pain over a long-standing OC. There is a thin low signal outside the high signal surrounding the cartilage cap (white arrow), representing a fibro-vascular perichondrium covering the cap. Enhanced view presents septal (yellow arrow) and peripheral enhancement (white arrow) as well as a thin outermost enhancement outlining the cartilage cap, indicating the perichondrium (blue arrow). (**e**) En-bloc resection with prophylactic plate fixation was performed because of a probability of malignant transformation despite the histologic diagnosis of OC by incision biopsy. (**f**) (Left, top) Gross specimen of the excised mass exhibits an irregularly thickened, multilobulated, glistening, yellow-white cartilage surface covered by a thin fibrous tissue. The maximum thickness of the cartilage cap measures 3 cm on the cut surface. (Left, bottom) There are a focal area of cartilage necrosis (N) and a thin perichondrium covering the cartilage cap (P). (Right) Medium-power magnification presents a heavily calcifying cartilage cap with disorganized bland chondrocytes and spongy bones formed by endochondral ossification of the cartilage. (**g**) A radiograph taken for pain after slip 1 month after surgery shows a spiral fracture. (**h**) Open reduction followed by internal fixation with a stronger condylar locking plate was performed. (**i**) Follow-up radiograph at 10 years after surgery reveals no evidence of local recurrence

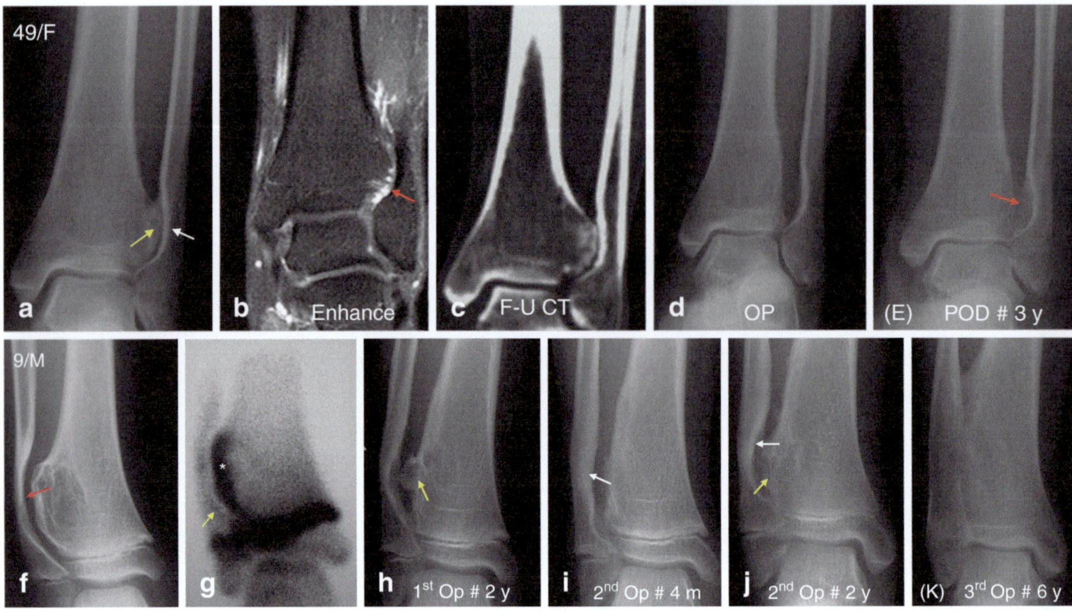

Fig. 13.3 ***Longstanding mass with an erosion of adjacent bone***. (**a**) Radiograph taken for intermittent ankle pain of 4 years' duration in a 49-year-old woman shows a protruding sclerotic mass in the lateral malleolus (yellow arrow), which produces a pressure erosion with thickened underlying cortex of the adjacent fibula (white arrow), suggesting a longstanding mass. (**b**) MR image reveals a pressure erosion of the distal fibula by a broad-based bony protrusion with a thin cartilage cap in the lateral malleolus. The cartilage cap presents multiple tiny nodular enhancements (arrow). (**c**) Two years later, CT scan taken for a more frequent and aggravated pain demonstrates the same findings with no interval change. (**d**) The mass was excised because of the aggravated pain nature. (**e**) Follow-up radiograph at 3 years after surgery reveals hazy bone formation in the erosion site of the fibula (red arrow). And she is free of pain. (**f**) Radiograph taken for palpable mass with intermittent pain of 2 years' duration in a 9-year-old boy shows a large, sessile, protruding mass having continuity with the host bone. Note pressure erosion with sclerotic margin and bending deformity in the controlateral distal fibula attributed to the longstanding extrinsic pressure by the mass (red arrow). (**g**) Pinhole bone scan reveals a strong uptake along the margin of the protruding mass (asterisk) and mild uptake along the erosion site in the controlateral fibula (arrow). (**h**) Radiograph taken for recurrent mass with pain at 2 years after initial surgical resection shows small recurrent mass (yellow arrow), which was re-excised. (**i**) Follow-up radiograph at 4 months after re-excision reveals correction of the bending deformity and remodeling of the erosion with new bone formation (white arrow). (**j**) However, a radiograph taken for recurrent ankle pain 2 years after re-excision shows a second recurrent mass (yellow arrow) with recurrent marked erosion (white arrow) in the controlateral fibula. (**k**) Last follow-up radiograph at 6 years after the third excision demonstrates bony ankylosis of the distal tibia-fibula joint (red arrows). He is doing well with no pain

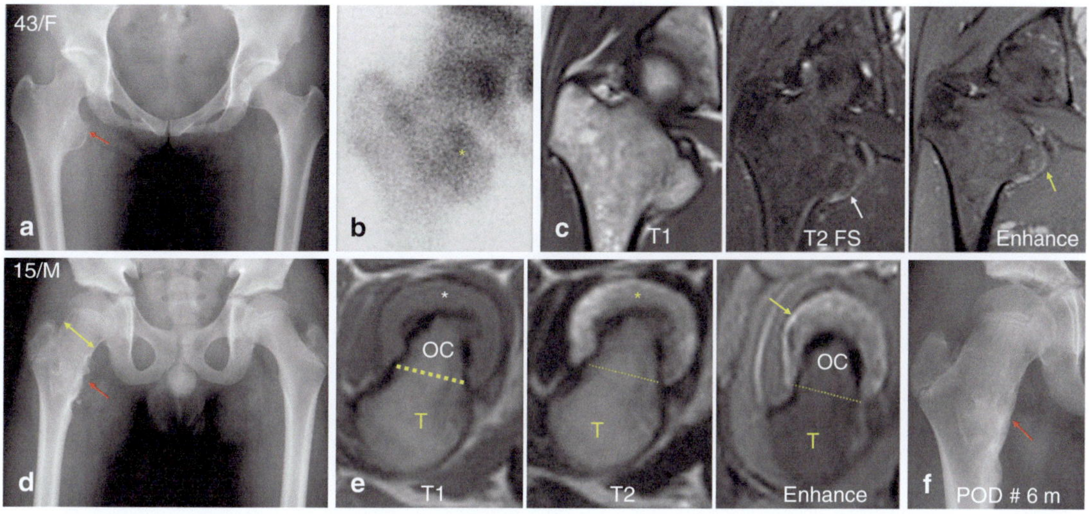

Fig. 13.4 ***Less common locations (lesser trochanter).*** (**a**) Radiograph taken for right snapping hip with intermittent pain of 1 month's duration in a 43-year-old woman shows asymmetricity of proximal femurs at a glance. The right femoral neck is much wider and the lesser trochanter seems to be much larger with an indistinct overlapping bony mass (red arrow), compared with the controlaterl left side. (**b**) Pinhole bone scan reveals heterogeneous mild and moderate uptake in the lesser trochanteric area (asterisk). (**c**) MR images reveal a bony protrusion with SI identical to that of the host medullary bone on both sequences, which has a continuity with the host bone at the lesser trochanter area. Fat-saturated T2-weighted image demonstrates a thin cartilage with high signal of less than 3 mm in thickness (white arrow). The mass presents a thin peripheral enhancement (yellow arrow). The mass was not excised because it did not severely bother the patient. (**d**) Radiograph taken for right hip discomfort in a 15-year-old boy shows an ill-defined, focally mineralized, outgrowing lesion with an undulated underlying cortex in the lesser trochanteric area (arrow). The femoral neck is markedly wider (double-headed arrow) when compared to that of the contralateral left side. (**e**) MR images demonstrate a bony projection (OC) blending into the medullary cavity of lesser trochanter (T) with identical signal to that of the host medullary bone on both sequences. The mass is covered by a cartilage cap of 12 mm in thickness (asterisks) with intermediate SI on T1-weighted image and heterogeneous high SI on T2-weighted image. The cap presents a peripheral thin enhancement with focal internal enhancement (arrow). (**f**) Follow-up radiograph at 6 months after excision reveals some remodeling of the underlying cortex with new bone formation (arrow)

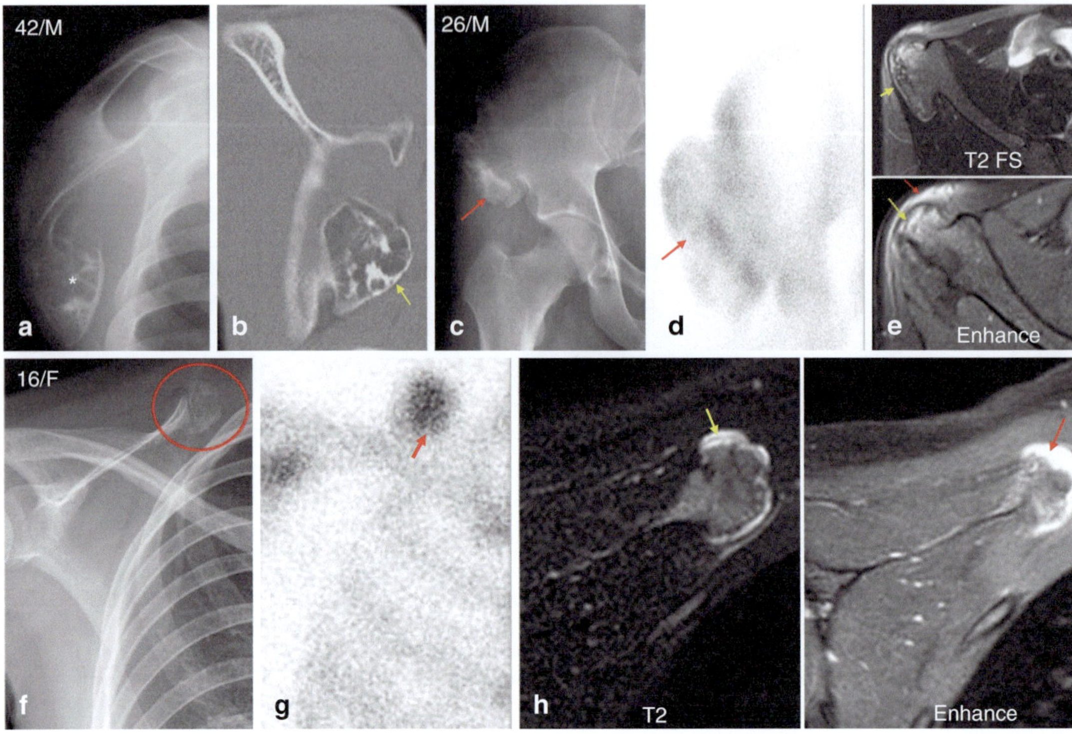

Fig. 13.5 ***Less common locations (flat bones).*** (**a**) Radiograph taken for right upper back pain on inspiration in a 42-year-old man shows a bubbly bony protuberance with internal septa and focal sclerotic areas in the inferior-medial aspect of the right scapula (asterisk). (**b**) CT scan reveals a trabeculated, focally calcified, extruding bony mass with a thin cartilage cap (yellow arrow). The inspiratory pain disappeared following surgical excision, with no evidence of local recurrence at 2 years after excision. (**c**) Radiograph taken for a hard mass at the right pelvis area of 3 months' duration in a 26-year-old man demonstrates a calcifying trabeculated outgrowing mass from the iliac bone (red arrow). (**d**) Pinhole bone scan demonstrates a heterogeneous mild uptake within the mass (red arrow). (**e**) MR images show an exophytic bony mass with high signal of a thin cartilage cap as well as thin outer dark signal on fat-suppressed T2-weighted image (yellow arrow). Post-contrast image reveals a relatively thick enhancement of the peripheral portion of the mass (yellow arrow) as well as subcutaneous tissue suggesting an inflammation by local mechanical irritation (red arrow). (**f**) Radiograph taken for a hard mass of 3 months' duration in a 16-year-old girl reveals a calcifying multilobulated projecting mass in the scapular spine. (**g**) Bone scan demonstrates a moderately increased uptake in the mass (red arrow). (**h**) MR images reveal a pedunculated bony projection continuous with the host medullary cavity of the scapula. T2-weighted image clearly presents a thin cartilage cap of 6–7 mm in thickness with a high signal (yellow arrow). A peripheral thick enhancement may suggest an associated small bursa or inflammatory reaction by mechanical irritation (red arrow)

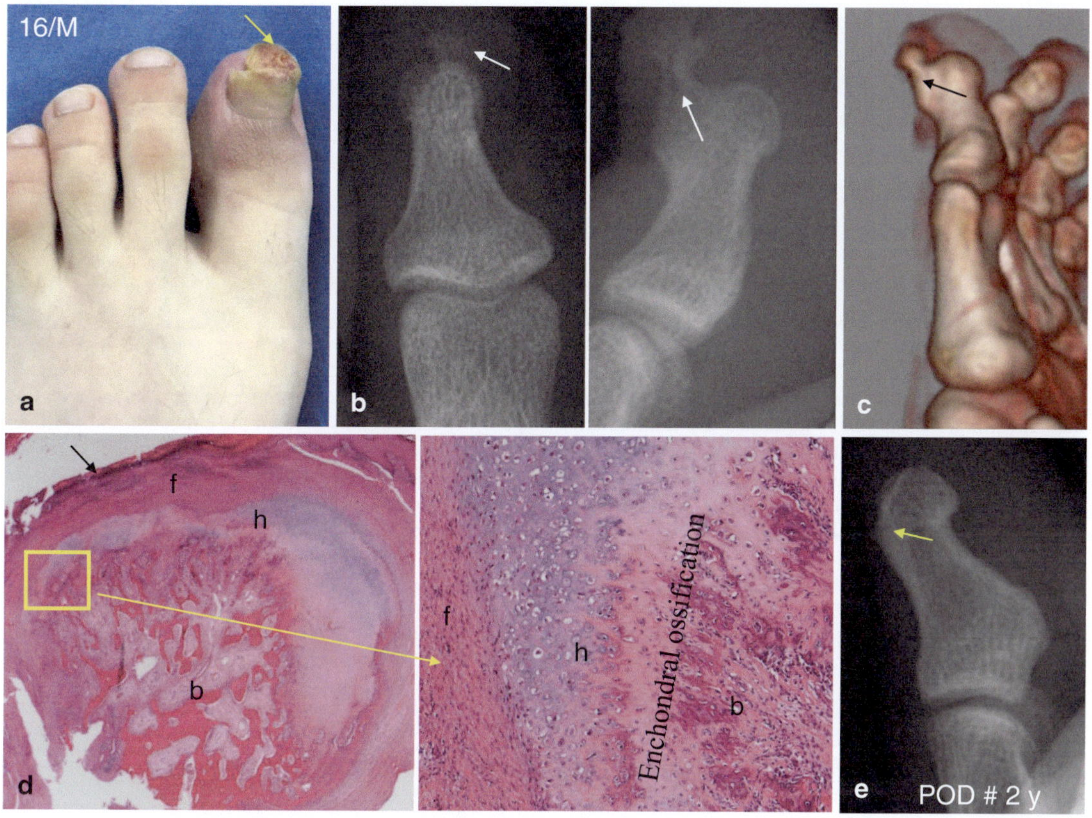

Fig. 13.6 ***Subungual OC***. (**a**) A 16-year-old boy presented with a slowly growing subungual hard mass with nail deformity of 2 years' duration and recently developed superimposed infection (arrow). (**b**) Radiographs reveal a relatively well-defined pedunculated bony mass with clearly discernible cortico-medullary continuity with the host bone, so-called *flaring* appearance (arrows). (**c**) 3D CT also clearly demonstrates the same continuity, favoring a dignosis of subungual OC (SO) over subgungual exostosis (SE) (black wrrow). (**d**) However, microscopic examination reveals features overlapped with those of SE. (Left) Low-power magnification demonstrates a small osteocartilaginous mass surrounded by fibrocartilage blending with a non-neoplastic fibrous tissue (f) underneath the epidermal tissue (black arrow). (Right) Medium-power magnification of yellow box in low-power view notes a focal fibrocartilage between fibrous connective tissue (f) and hyaline cartilage (h) as well as woven bone spicules formed by endochondral ossification as in OC (b). These overlapped radiographic and microscopic findings can make a debate whether SO is the same clinical entity as SE. (**e**) Follow-up radiograph at 2 years after excision reveals no evidence of recurrence with completely restored cortex (yellow arrow)

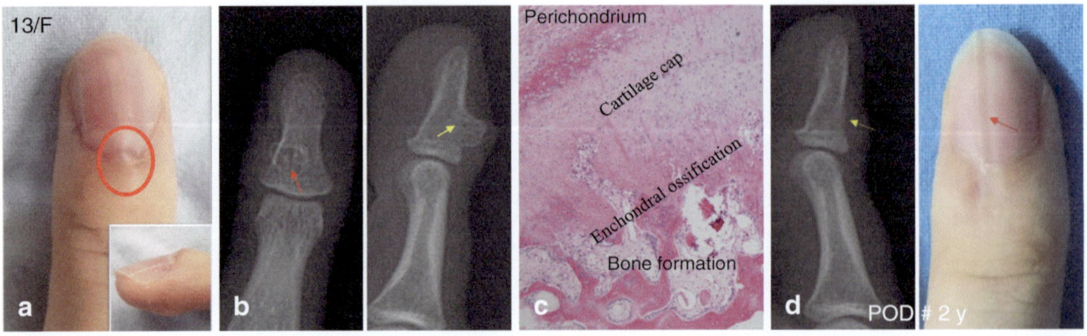

Fig. 13.7 ***Subungual OC***. (**a**) A 13-year-old girl presents with a subungual hard mass with nail deformity in the right ring finger of 2 years' duration. (**b**) Radiographs show a well-defined, small, exophytic from the distal phalanx (red arrow) with a characteristic *flaring* appearance, indicating a cortico-medullary continuity with the host bone (yellow arrow). (**c**) Microscopic examination of the excised mass reveals typical findings of OC including all three layers of perichondrium, hyaline cartilage cap, and spongy bone typically formed via endochondral ossification originating from the base of cartilage cap. (**d**) Follow-up radiograph at 2 years after surgery notes no evidence of recurrence (yellow arrow). However, a longitudinal groove is seen over the nail (red arrow)

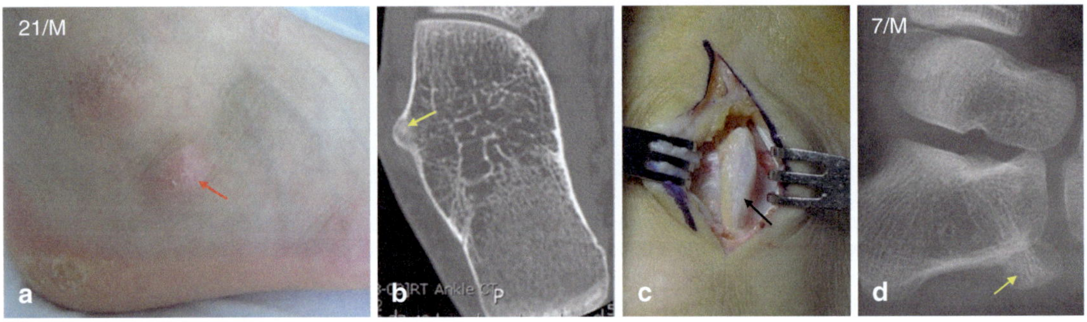

Fig. 13.8 ***Other rare locations***. (**a**) A 21-year-old soldier presents with right foot mass (arrow) of 2 months' duration, which causes pain when wearing army boots. (**b**) CT scan reveals a small bony projection with a thin cartilage cap, which is continuous with the host calcaneus cortex and medulla (arrow). (**c**) A small stony mass with a glistening cap was exposed for surgical excision (black arrow). (**d**) Radiograph taken for heel pain on weight bearing in a 7-year-old boy shows a well-demarcated, exophytic, sclerotic mass from the inferior border of calcaneus (arrow), which was surgically excised and histologically proven as an OC

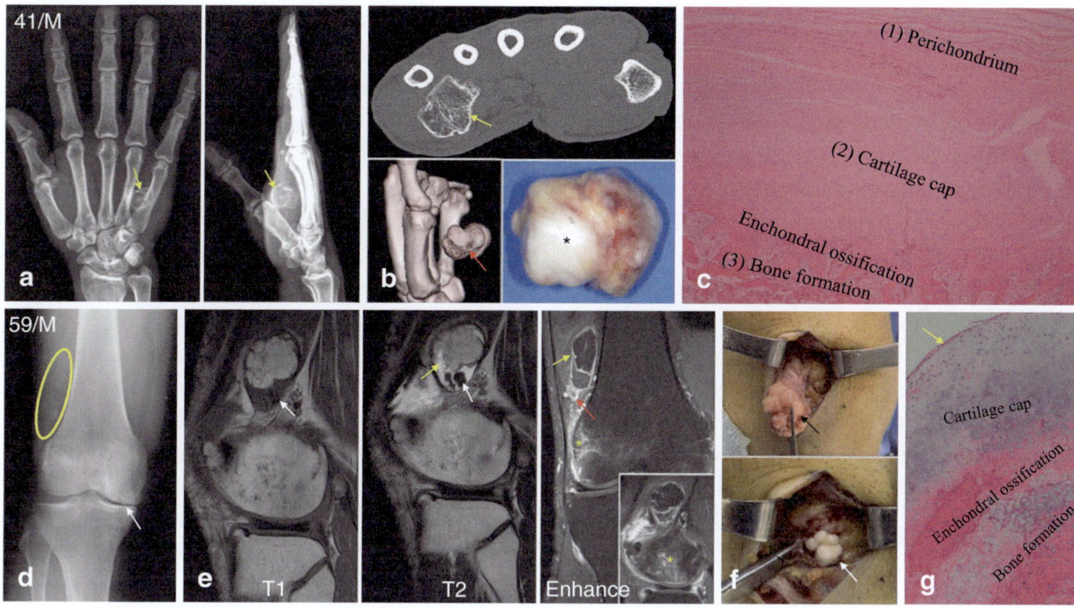

Fig. 13.9 ***Extra-skeletal OC***. (**a**) Radiographs taken for right-hand mass of 3 years' duration in a 41-year-old man show a partially densified mass between the fourth and fifth metacarpal bones. On the lateral view, the mass appears to be attached to the metacarpal bone (yellow arrows). (**b**) However, CT scan reveals a well-defined mass with internal densification (yellow arrow), which is located within the soft tissue between the two metacarpal bones, wihtout any contiuity with the adjacent bones. The mass is also clearly visualized on 3D CT scan (red arrow). Note the excised mass with a white glossy cartilage cap (black asterisk) covered by a perichondrium (red asterisk). (**c**) Microscopic examination shows the typical 3 layers, consisting of perichondrium, cartilage cap, and woven bone spicules formed via endochondral bone ossification originating from the base of the cartilage cap. (**d**) Radiographs taken for right knee mass with medial joint pain of 5 years' duration in a 59-year-old man show a hazy, multilobulated, calcific, soft tissue mass in the lateral aspect of the distal femur (circle) and narrowing of medial joint space (arrow). (**e**) MR images demonstrate a well-defined, multilobulated, *cauliflower-like*, soft tissue mass with intermediate to high SI on both sequences and high signal of thin cartilage cap (yellow arrow) on T2-weighted image. There are several dark signals of several osteochondral loose bodies (white arrows) in the suprapatellar pouch. There is no contiuity between the mass and the femur. The mass lesion (yellow arrow) and loose bodies (red arrow) are peripherally enhanced. The associated focal bone marrow edema is focally enhanced (asterisks). (**f**) The osteochondral mass covered by fibrous tissue (black arrow) and the white glistening loose bodies (white arrow) were excised. (**g**) Microscopic examination of the larger mass reveals a thin perichondrium (yellow arrow), cartilage cap, and woven bone formation via endochondral bone ossification from the base of the cartilage cap, indicating extra-osseous OC

13.6 Clinical Features

Most patients present with a solitary lesion, but the remainder have multiple lesions in the setting of "multiple OCs" or "osteochondromatosis or multiple hereditary exostoses (MHE)" often with other skeletal anomalies and positive family history. Although some patients are asymptomatic and incidentally found on image studies for other reasons, the most frequent presentation is a slowly growing hard mass for a longstanding duration. The mass grows slowly during child patient's growth and growing of the mass generally stops after puberty. Rapid growth of the mass or swelling in adults may herald development of pseudoaneurysm, malignant transformation, or infarction of cartilage cap particularly when pain is accompanied. Symptoms depend on the size and location of a mass. It can be painful due to impingement or irritation on adjacent tendons, nerve irritation or compression, overlying bursitis, fracture of stalk, and rarely malignant transformation. A bursa formed external to the cartilage cap (exostosis bursata) produces symptoms due to inflammation or fluid collection by chronic mechanical irritation of the mass [12–14]. Other symptoms include discomfort or mild pain on squatting or during exercise, limitation of adjacent joint motion, and snapping hip or winged scapula. Rarely, skin dislocation or pulsatile mass can be found in the patient having a pedunculated mass with a sharply pointed end which makes a tear in an adjacent artery to develop a pseudoaneurysm, mostly popliteal artery [15–18] (Fig. 13.13a, b).

13.7 Radiologic Findings

The typical radiographic appearance with metaphyseal location of OC is pathognomonic, particularly in long bones. A bony mass on a narrow-based, pedunculated stalk with a bulbous tip typically points away from the adjacent joint toward the diaphysis, so-called *pedunculated* type (Fig. 13.1a). The shape and size of the mass vary from *globular* to *mushroom or cauliflower-like*. Tiny to small exostosis has a sharp *thorn-like* projection. OC can also present a wide base with a dimension exceeding its length but no stalk, so-called *sessile* type (Fig. 13.1d). Characteristically, the cortex of the host bone flares into the OC mass, and the spongy bone of the mass blends into the medulla of host bone, so-called *flaring* appearance (Fig. 13.10a, b), while parosteal osteosarcoma (POS) is broadly fused to the surface of the intact cortex without continuity to the medulla of the host bone, a characteristic *paste-on* appearance (Fig. 13.10c, d). Any other bone lesions other than OC do not display this kind of *flaring with medullary continuity*, which is pathognomonic and allows diagnosis without biopsy. However, the typical appearance can be obscured by heavily mineralized large OC (Fig. 13.2a). The finding of *flaring* is clearly seen even in subungual OC (Figs. 13.6b, c and 13.7b) in contrast to subungual exostosis (SE) lacking the clear cortico-medullary continuity (refer Figs. 17.1, 17.2, and 17.3 in Chap. 17), which is useful to distinguish both entities. Radiographic finding of *flaring* appearance in association with microscopic finding of typical cap consisting of *hyaline cartilage* rather than fibrocartilage (Figs. 13.6d and 13.7c) can distinguish subungual OC from SE. A cartilage cap does not appear on plain radiographs. Complete or incomplete "U" shaped line can be observed on anteroposterior radiograph when a mass is imaged en face (Figs. 13.1e and 13.12b). If the mass exists for a long duration in the ankle, it can compress the adjacent bone with resultant concave erosion (Fig. 13.3a, f). Radiographic findings such as newly developed lucent area, soft tissue mass formation with extensive chondroid matrix or calcification, destruction of the mass base or host bone, or irregularity of the margin strongly herald a malignant transformation to chondrosarcoma (CSA), particularly when combined with pain and/or continuous growth of the mass after puberty (Figs. 13.14

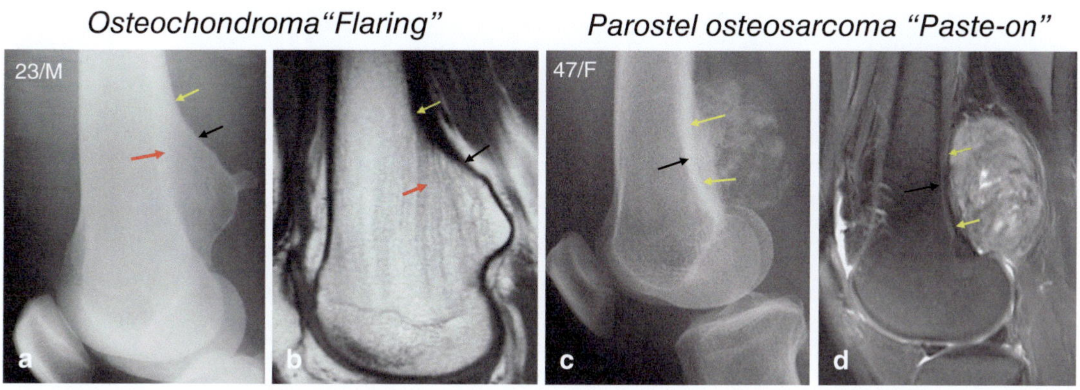

Fig. 13.10 ***Radiographic difference between OC and POS.*** (**a, b**) Radiograph and MR image taken for a mass at the right popliteal fossa since childhood in a 23-year-old man show a direct continuity of the host femur (yellow arrows) with exophytic mass (black arrows) as well as blending of the host medullary bone with spongy bone of the mass, referred to as *flaring* appearance, indicating OC. Notably, there is loss of the underlying host cortex (red arrows). (**c, d**) In contrast, radiograph and MR image taken for a palpable mass at the right popliteal fossa of 2 years' duration in a 47-year-old woman reveal a well-demarcated, lobulated, irregularly dense, oval mass attached to the thickened cortex of the distal femur (black arrow). A thin radiolucent line between the tumor mass and the thickened host cortex (yellow arrows), known as the *string sign*, produces characteristic *paste-on* appearance, indicating parosteal osteosarcoma (POS). Both characteristic radiologic findings of *flaring* for OC and *paste-on* appearance for POS are pathognomonic and allow no biopsy for a diagnosis

and 13.15). **Bone scan** The extent and intensity of isotope uptake correlate directly with the extent and degree of endochondral ossification in the cartilage cap (Figs. 13.1, 13.2, 13.3, 13.4, 13.5, and 13.11). A radionuclide bone scan does not contribute to the preoperative anatomic evaluation of OC and CSA and does not always distinguish benign from malignant lesions [19]. The uptake is strong in growing patients but becomes no more active than normal bone with time. If the uptake is increased in adult patients, complications such as stalk fracture or malignant change should be suspected. Occasionally, similar uptake can also be observed in cases of bursitis or adjacent bone reaction. **CT scan** allows optimal depiction of the pathognomonic medullary continuity between the lesion and the parent bone even in anatomically complex areas such as the pelvis and spine as well as in heavily calcified cases. It can be also useful in accurate measurement of the thickness of the mineralized cartilage cap (Fig. 13.2c). However, it is difficult to accurately measure the thickness of an entirely nonmineralized cartilage cap because it cannot be easily differentiated from surrounding bursa [20]. Hudson et al. [21] reported that CT did not reliably detect the cartilage cap when the actual cartilage thickness was in the range of 1.5–2.5 cm of maximum thickness. Therefore, the authors concluded CT did not solve the difficult problem to distinguish between OC with a thick cartilage cap and exostotic secondary CSA with a relatively thin cap. However, Kenney et al. [22] suggested CT appeared to be effective in differenciating of OC and CSA, including cases where this distinction could not be made with conventional radiographs. The thickness of the cartilage cap was less than 3 cm, with an average of 6 mm in OC and greater than 3 cm in CSA. **MR images** also clearly demonstrate a pathognomonic continuity between the bony mass and the parent bone (Figs. 13.1, 13.2, 13.3, 13.4, and 13.5). MRI is the best to assess cartilage thickness and consequently, to evaluate malignant transformation, the presence of edema in bone or adjacent soft tissues or overlying bursa, and visualizing neurovascular structures in the vicinity. The bony mass exhibits identical SI to that of the host medullary bone, and the signal of the cartilage cap is the same as that of cartilage elsewhere on all sequences. However, mineralized portions of the cartilage cap present low SI on

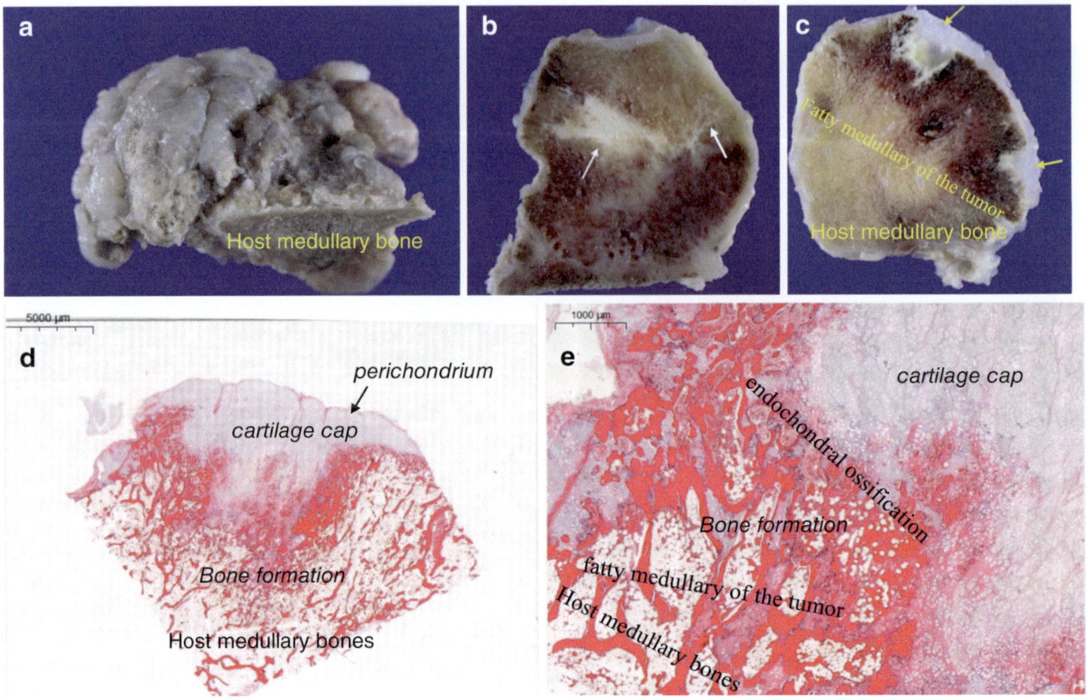

Fig. 13.11 (**a**) ***Gross specimen***. The excised mass exhibits a sessile type with a wide base in *mushroom-like* or *cauliflower-like* shape. The external surface presents a shiny, glistening, and blue-white in color, with a cartilage cap covered by a thin fibrous tissue. (**b**) The gross specimen should be cut perpendicularly to measure the real thickness of the cartilage cap and to evaluate the bone formed under the cartilage cap. At the junction between the cartilage cap and underlying spongy bone, an irregular, wavy, chalk-like zone (black arrow), suggesting an endochondral ossification. (**c**) The cartilage cap is irregularly thin with 3–4 mm in thin area and up to 10–12 mm focally in this case (yellow arrows). The marrow of the tumor can be fatty or hematopoietic and shows contiuity with with the host medullary bone, reflecting a *flaring* with medullary continuity on imaging studies. ***Microscopic examination***: (**d**) Low-power magnification shows typical triapartite architecrue consisting of *perichondrium*, *cartilage cap*, and *bone with marrow cavity*. The outermost layer consists of a thin *perichondrium* of a dense, nonspecific fibrous tissue which is continuous with periosteum of the underlying host bone. (**e**) Middle-power magnification reveals the *cartilage cap* simulates disorganized growth plate that is least cellular at periphery and most cellular in deeper area. Endochondral ossification occurs at the bone-cartilage interface. In the deep area of cartilage cap, hyaline matrices are calcified and some chondrocytes are necrotized. The remaining cartilage matrix could be acting as a scaffold for bone deposition. Newly formed trabecular bone mimics primary spongiosa at the base of normal growth plate. The thickness of the cap is variable depending on the age of the patients. It is thick and active in growing patients but thin or focally resorbed by endochondral ossification at the base of the cap in adults. The lesional bones with focal dystrophic calcification and fatty marrow imperceptibly blend into the host medullary bones

both sequences, and nonmineralized portions show low to intermediate SI on T1-weighted image and high to bright SI on T2-weighted image, reflecting high water content of the cartilage. Thus, T2-weighted image allows the cartilage cap to be most clearly distinctuished from the overlying muscle or bursa and to measure the thickness of the cap best. The cartilage cap is usually less than 2 cm thick, and the thickness decreases with age. The thickness greater than 1.5–2 cm in adults and greater than 3 cm in children have been considered as a herald sign of malignant change, particularly when pain is accompanied. Increased thickness of the cartilage cap in young patients is caused by a response to continued active growth and should not be considered as a finding of malignant transformation. The cartilage cap can be heterogeneously

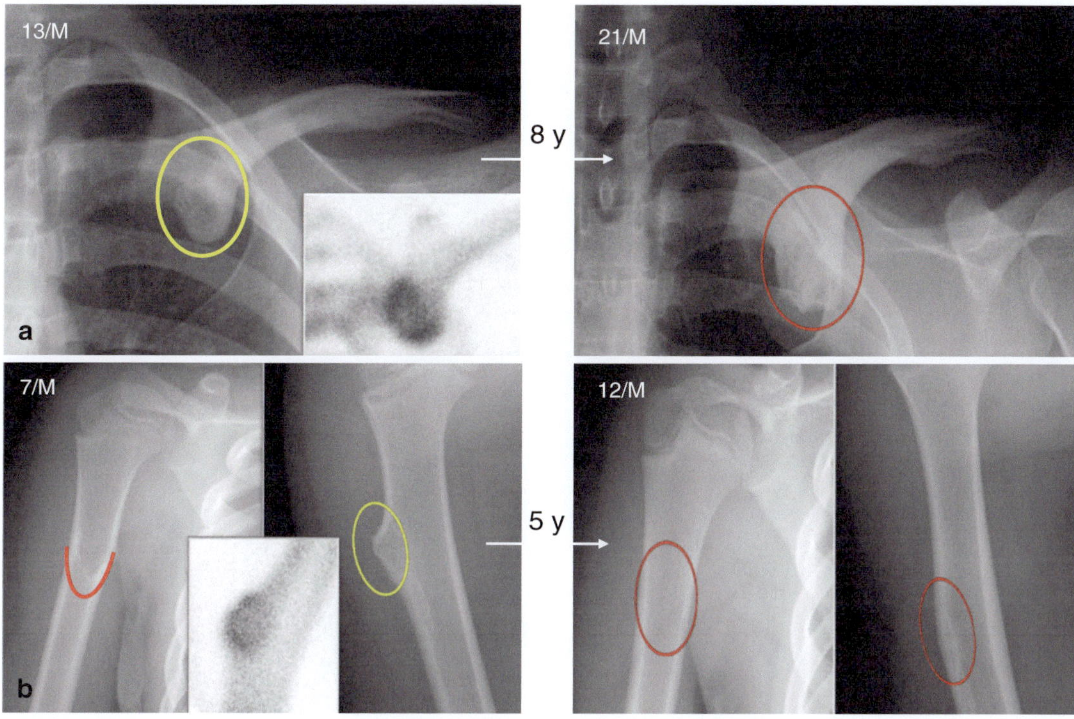

Fig. 13.12 ***Growing OC***. (**a**) OC involving the mid-shaft of the left clavicle (yellow circle) was discovered in a 13-year-old boy, which was not excised because of no pain. Pinhole bone scan shows heterogeneously increased uptake in the protruding mass (inset). The OC grdually increased in size over 8 years. The patient evntually requested surgical excision due to cosmetic concerns (red circle). ***Regressed OC***. (**b**) Anteroposterior radiograph taken for right arm pain after a bicycle accident in a 7-year-old boy incidentally shows a "U"-shaped cortical line, suggesting sessile type OC involving the diaphysis of the proximal humerus (red line). The lesion is clearly presented as a sessile type of OC on lateral view. Pinhole bone scan reveals mildly increased uptake along the periphery of the protruding mass (inset). The mass has spontaneously disappeared with remodeling of the underlying cortex (red circles) on the 5 years' follow-up radiograph

enhanced by contrast medium in septal and peripheral pattern (Figs. 13.1, 13.2, 13.3, 13.4, and 13.5). A thin low signal outside the high signal surrounding the cartilage cap represents a fibro-vascular perichondrium covering the cap, which is peripherally enhanced. Occasionally, a thick peripheral enhancement may be seen if hypertrophy of the perichondrium, small flat bursa, or reactive inflammation of the adjacent soft tissue is associated (Fig. 13.5e). In addition, MRI also offers an assessment of other complications. It is useful to assess displacement and/or impingement on the adjacent nerve and vascular complications such as compression, occlusion, or pseudoaneurysm (Fig. 13.12). Radiograph and MRI features suggesting malignant change include (a) increased size of the previously unchanged OC in a skeletally mature patient, (b) irregular or indistinct margin of the mass, (c) internal focal radiolucent areas, (d) erosion or destruction of the adjacent bone, (e) a significant soft-tissue mass containing scattered or irregular calcification, and (f) a cartilage cap more than 1.5 cm thick in a skeletally mature patient [20] (Figs. 13.13 and 13.14). The cartilage cap thickness is one of the most important criteria for suspicion of harboring malignant transformation. In a separated series, the thickness is reported with a wide range of 0.1–3.0 cm with an average of 0.6–0.8 cm in OC and 1.5–12 cm with an average of 5.5–6.0 cm in CSA [21, 23]. They also reported that 80% of OCs have a cartilage cap of less than 1 cm thick, but about 80% of patients with malignant change have a cap greater than

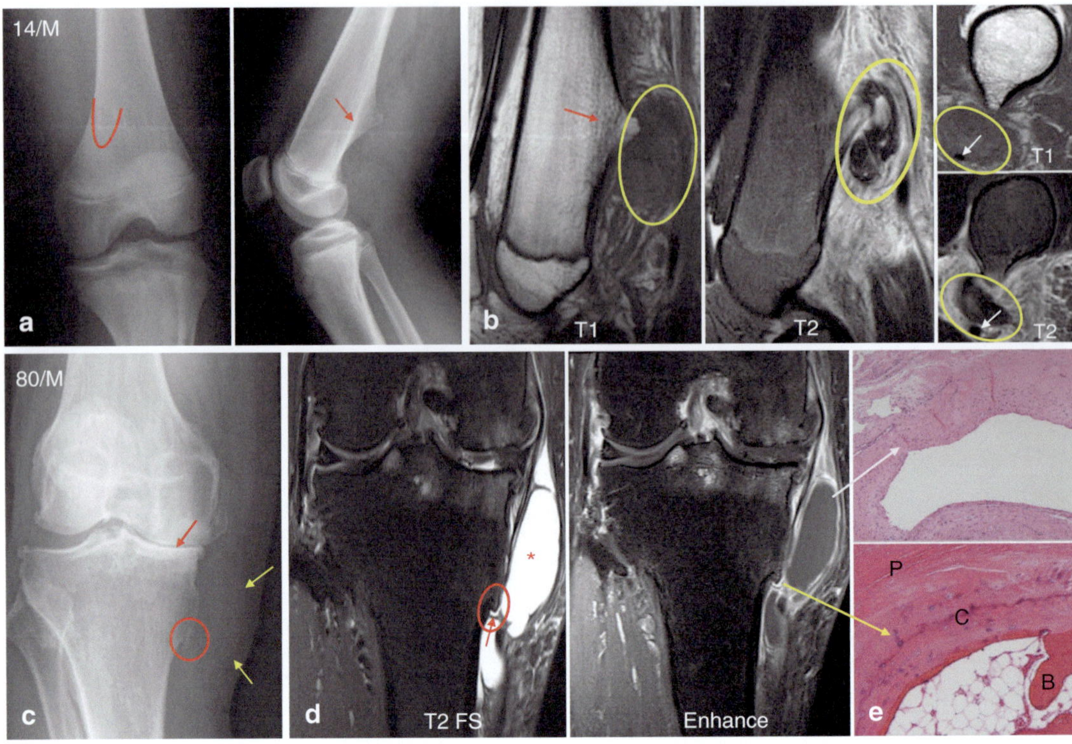

Fig. 13.13 ***Pseudoaneurysm***. (**a**) Radiograph taken for pain in the left popliteal region after slipping during a soccer play in a 14-year-old boy shows an incomplete "U"-shaped cortical line (red line). The lateral view reveals an outgrowing, sharply pointed mass from the posterior aspect of the distal femur with underlying thin cortex, which appears to have no continuity with the host medullary bone (arrow). (**b**) However, MR images show a well-defined, sharply pointed, exophytic mass with a typical *flaring* with cortico-medullary continuity between the exophytic mass and the parent bone (arrow). The SI is identical to that of host bone marrow on both sequences, and the exophytic mass is covered by a high signal of cartilage cap. There is a separate adjacent cystic lesion (yellow circles) cystic mass (yellow circles) adjacent to the exophytic mass, with low SI on T1-weighted image and heterogeneous SI with focal high signal on T2-weighted image. The axial images suggests a probable *pseudoaneurysm* arising from the popliteal artery (white arrows), attributed to mechanical irritation by a sharp *thorn-like* projection. The osteochondral mass was excised along with the removal of organizing hematoma and mutiple layers of pseudocapsule. Then, a vertically oriented defect in the femoral artery was repaired. ***Ganglion cyst formed by marginal osteophytes***: (**c**) Radiograph taken for a palpable mass and joint pain of the right knee in an 80-year-old man shows narrowing of medial joint space (red arrow) with a tiny sharp spur-like projection from the proximal tibia (red circle) as well as a large surrounding soft tissue density (yellow arrows). (**d**) MR images reveal a tiny sharp bony projection with SI identical to tht of the host bone (red circle) on fat-saturated T2-image. This projection is continuous with the host bone and covered by a thin cartilage cap or perichondrium of high signal (red arrow). Note an associated bright signal of a large cyst (red asterisk). The thin cartilage cap or perichondrium covering the tiny projection show thin peripheral enhancement (yellow arrow), and the cystic mass exhibits peripheral rim enhancement by contrast medium (white arrow). (**e**) Microscopic examination demonstrates histolgic features consistent with a ganglion cyst (top) and a degenerative osteophyte (bottom) with perichondrium (P), ossifying cartilage with scanty cellularity (C), and mature trbecular bone with fat cells (B)

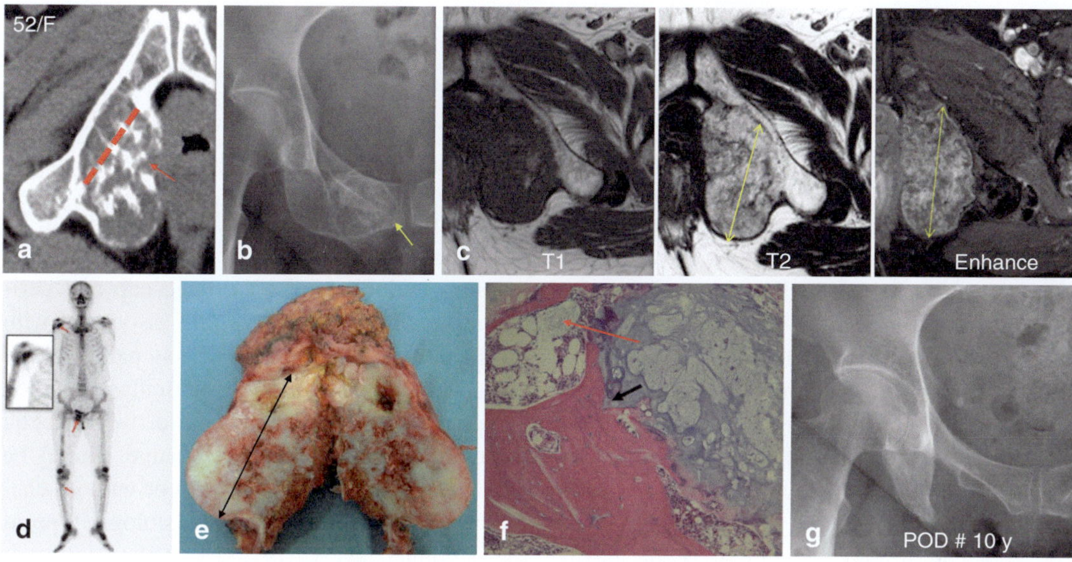

Fig. 13.14 ***Malignant transformation***. (**a**) CT scan taken for a palpable hard mass on vaginal examination in the Department of Gynecology shows a large, well-defined, calcifying, exophytic mass with irregular thin margin and focal destruction, suggesting a possible malignant change of longstanding benign mass (arrow). Note a direct contiuity between the mass and the medullary cavity through a cortical defect (dotted line), indicative of a preexisting OC. On past history taking, she had a palpable hard mass on her right inguinal area for 20 years but did not seek medical attention. (**b**) Radiograph reveals a relatively well-defined sclerotic mass with osteolytic foci in the right pubic ramus (arrow). (**c**) MR images demonstrate a well-defined large exophytic mass with low SI on T1-weighted image and heterogeneous high SI with a markedly thickened cartilage component measuring up to 5 cm in maximum thickness (double-headed arrows) on T2-weighted image. The lesion is heterogeneously enhanced in a *rings and arcs* pattern, consistent with a cartilage component. (**d**) Bone scan shows multiple foci of increased uptake in the right shoulder and scapular area, femur shaft, and pubic bone (arrows), indicating a multifocal bone lesion. (**e**) Wide resection was performed with an imaging diagnosis of malignant change to CSA from a longstanding OC. Note a significantly thickened cartilage component on gross specimen (double-headed arrow). (**f**) Microscopic examination shows that cartilage tumor cells infiltrate the host lamellar bone (black arrow) and focal invasion to marrow cavity through a cortical defect (red arrow), so-called *invasion of marrow fat* pattern of CSA (refer to Chondrosarcoma chapter). The cellularity is low with mild cytologic atypia, consistent with low-grade (Grade 1) CSA. (**g**) Follow-up radiograph at 10 years after en-bloc resection shows no evidence of local recurrence

2 cm thick. Thus, a cartilage cap more than 1.5 cm thick in a skeletally mature patient should raise for possible malignant change [20].

13.8 Histologic Findings

Grossly, the mass presents as sessile or pedunclated, often showing a *mushroom-like* or *cauliflower-like* shape with a shiny, glistening, and blue-white surface (Figs. 13.2f and 13.11a). The external surface shows a multilobulated cartilage cap covered by a fibrous membrane. At the junction between the cartilage cap and underlying spongy bone, a narrow, wavy, chalk-like zone is observed, suggesting an endochondral ossification (Fig. 13.11b). The thickness is usually thin or even absent in adults, measured from 2 mm to 1 cm in thickness, but thicker in actively growing children, often exceeding 1 cm in thickness that shoud not be considered indicative of malignant change. The marrow of the tumor can be fatty or hematopoietic and continuous with the host medullary bone, reflecting a *flaring* with medullary continuity on imaging studies (Fig. 13.11c). Microscopically, most lesions characteristically consist of three layers of perichondrium, cartilage cap, and spongy bone underneath the cap (Fig. 13.11d) (1). The outermost layer is *a perichondrium* of non-neoplastic fibrous tissue blending imperceptibly with the outer layer of hyaline cartilage of the cap (2). Beneath the perichondrium, *a cartilage cap* of variable thickness mimicking disorganized growth plate exists and undergoes endochondral ossification with calcification at the junction with the underlying host cancellous bone. Some chondrocytes show mild atypia with a few binucleated nuclei which should not be interpreted as CSA. Chondrocytes may undergo necrosis in focal areas (Fig. 13.2f). A cartilage cap thickness is one of the most important parameters for differentiation of OC and CSA (3). The innermost layer is *spongy bone* typically formed by endochondral ossification from the base of cartilage cap. The marrow of the tumor can be fatty or hematopoietic and is continuous with the host medullary bone (Fig. 13.11e).

13.9 Management

Asymptomatic, nongrowing, small mass can be observed with periodic follow-up. Complete excision including total cartilage cap and perichondrium is necessary for OC associated with mechanical complications such as pain, limited adjacent joint motion, neurovascular irritation symptoms, fracture of the stalk, or for cosmetic reason. OC with malignant change should be managed by wide resection with or without chemotherapy, depending on the histologic type of the sarcoma (Figs. 13.14 and 13.15).

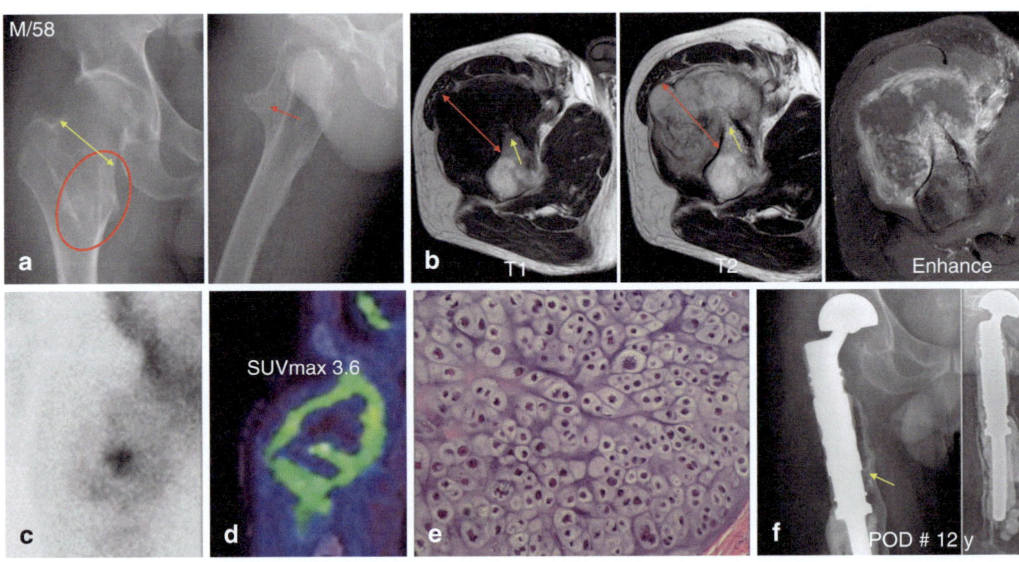

Fig. 13.15 ***Malignant transformation.*** (**a**) Radiograph taken for right hip pain of 6–7 months' duration in a 58-year-old man shows an ill-defined, sclerotic lesion overlapping the underlying lesser trochanter accompanied by marked valgus deformity and widening of the right femoral neck (double-headed arrow). He had a past history of surgical excision of OC in the same area 13 years ago. The lateral view reveals an outgrowing triangular-shaped bony mass, showing medullary continuity with the underlying femur (red arrow), suggesting a probable remained or recurrent OC. (**b**) MR images reveal a large multilobulated cartilaginous mass with low SI on T1-weighted image and high SI on T2-weighted image. There is a narrow bone stalk with an identical signal to the femur, which is continuous with the host medullary cavity (yellow arrows), suggesting previous OC. The cartilage cap is markedly thickened up to about 3 cm in maximum thickness (double-headed arrows), strongly suggesting a malignant change from residual or recurrent mass particularly in the contex of consideration of newly developed pain. The mass is peripherally well enhanced with "*rings and arcs*" pattern of internal enhancement. (**c**) Bone scan shows heterogeneous uptake with a focal hot accumulation. (**d**) PET/CT scan reveals a huge protruding mass with peripheral moderate FDG uptake (SUVmax 3.6) and large central photon defect. (**e**) Microscopic examination demonstrates high cellularity and varying degrees of pleomorphic chondrocytes with bizarre nuclei in size and shape and frequent bi-nucleated chondrocytes along with occasional atypical mitoses, indicating high-grade (Grade 4) CSA. (**f**) Wide resection followed by reconstruction using a tumor prosthesis was performed. Subsequently, multiple surgical procedures including debridement and insertion of anbiotic-impregnated cement beads were performed for infection control. Radiograph at 12 years after initial surgery shows no evidence of local recurrence with reactive bone formation (yellow arrows)

13.10 Clinical Course

The OC mass slowly grows while physeal plate is open and usually ceases at puberty. The mass is usually increased in size as the patient grows (Fig. 13.12a), but it can be rarely regressed or resorbed even during growing period of the patient (Fig. 13.12b). Rarely, vascular complication including arteriovenous fistula, arterial rupture, venous thrombosis, or pseudoaneurysm due to extrinsic compression by exostosis with a sharp *thorn-like* projection (Fig. 13.13a, b), large bursa or ganglion due to chronic friction (Fig. 13.13c, d). More rarely, osteomyelitis may be complicated. The most serious complication is malignant transformation, which is rare in solitary OC (1–2%) [2, 5, 6], but the incidence will be increased in patients with multiple OCs (5–25%) [2, 4, 6, 24]. However, other studies suggest a lower prevalence of approximately 3–5% in patients with HME [25–28]. In a study of pedigree spanning 6 generations of a family with 114 living adult members, 46 of them with multiple exostoses, Kivioja et al. [24] described an overall frequency of malignant transformation of 8.7% for adult patients, representing the highest reported number in recent literature. In a Mayo Clinic series, the incidence was 7.6% for the solitary OC group and 36.3% for the multiple exostoses group with an overall rate of 12% [29]. The malignant tumors arising in the OC are generally low-grade CSA [19, 29, 30]. In a series of 75 patients with CSA arising in solitary OC, Garrison et al. reported that the risk of malignant transformation in a solitary OC is estimated to be only around 1%. They also reported that 64 patients (85%) had grade 1 CSA, the rest having grade 2 and 3 CSA [30]. Other high-grade sarcomas including malignant fibrous histiocytoma and osteosarcoma were also reported in solitary OC [31, 32] and in MHE [33, 34]. A synchronous multiple malignant transformation of MHE was reported in the left pubic bone and the left greater trochanter [35].

13.11 Osteochondromatosis (Multiple hereditary exostoses)

Osteochondromatosis is often referred to as multiple hereditary exostoses (MHE) because more than half of the patients with multiple OCs have a positive family history. It is also known as familial osteochondromatosis or diaphyseal aclasis. MHE is an autosomal dominant hereditary condition transmitted by both sexes with incomplete penetration in females. For example, if one of the parents is affected, half of their children will inherit the disease. When a male member is normal, he will not transmit the disease, but a female member may transmit the disease even if she is phenotypically normal. The number of lesions and associated deformity can lead to early medical consultation and radiologic evaluation with diagnosis of HME, in contrast to the relatively later detection of solitary OC. Most patients are discovered by age 5 years, and virtually all are diagnosed by age 12 years [6, 36] (Fig. 13.16). As for solitary OC, complete excision including cartilage cap and perichondrium is necessary for any growing tumors producing mechanical complications such as pain, disrupting the child's movement, limited range of motion, neurovascular irritation symptoms, or cosmetic reasons. However, excision of exostotic masses itself has little effect on the progression of the deformities. Corrective surgery including such as stapling for epiphysiodesis during skeletal growth, lengthening or shortening of the ulna or fibula, and corrective osteotomy is often necessary. More importantly, patients with multiple lesions have a greater tendency to develop malignant transformation when compared to those with single lesion [4, 37]. Thus, lifelong follow-up with serial radiographs in patients with MHE is mandatory for early detection of the malignant change.

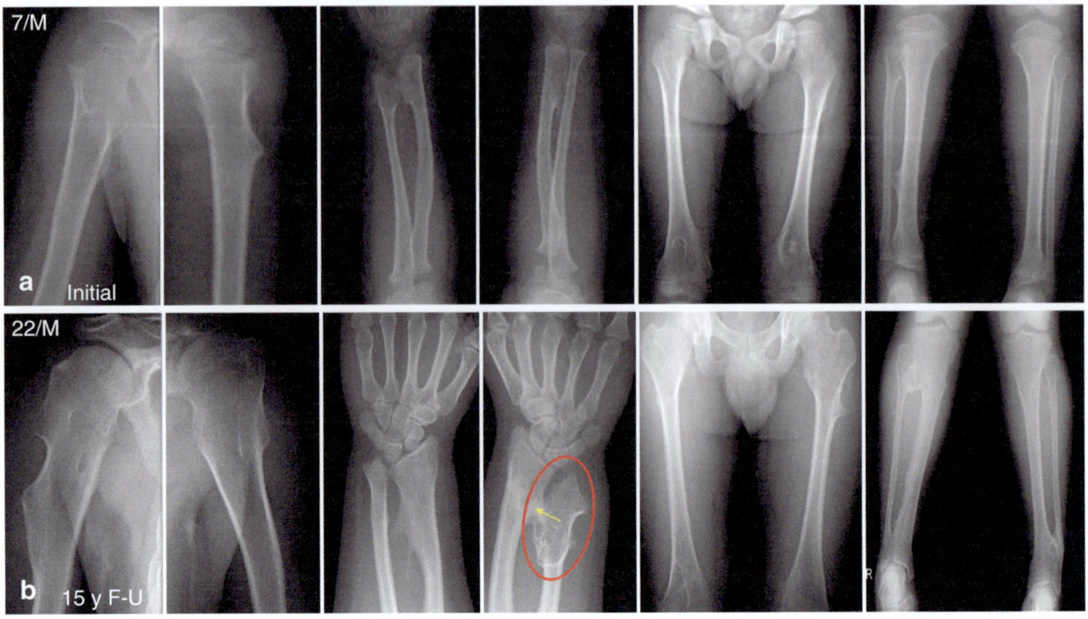

Fig. 13.16 *MHE*. (**a**) Radiographs taken for multiple palpable masses since early childhood in a 7-year-old boy with positive family history of OCs show multiple projecting bony masses from long bones of both upper and lower extremities, indicating MHE. Multiple surgical procedures have been performed to excise the masses from scapular, calcaneus, proximal humerus, distal femur, and proximal fibula because of pain. (**b**) Follow-up radiographs at 15 years after the initial visit reveal a mild to moderate enlargement of the masses as the host bone grows. The mass from the right distal ulna becomes markedly larger and results in growth disturbance producing radio-ulnar synostosis with a mild Madelung's deformity (red circle), but no severe functional deficit of the wrist joint. There is no definite evidence of malignant change during follow-up

References

1. Ahn J, Lüdecke HJ, Lindow S, Horton WA, Lee B, Wagner MJ, et al. Cloning of the putative tumour suppressor gene for hereditary multiple exostoses (EXT1). Nat Genet. 1995;11(2):137–43.
2. Czerniak B. Benign cartilage lesions. In: Dorfman HD, Czerniak B, editors. Dorfman and Czerniak's bone tumors. 2nd ed. (eBook): Elsevier; 2016. p. 356–473.
3. Stickens D, Clines G, Burbee D, Ramos P, Thomas S, Hogue D, et al. The EXT2 multiple exostoses gene defines a family of putative tumour suppressor genes. Nat Genet. 1996;14(1):25–32.
4. Unni KK, Inwards Y. Osteochondroma. In: Dahlin's bone tumors: general aspects and data on 10,165 cases. Philadelphia: Lippincott Williams & Wilkins; 2010. p. 9–21.
5. Mirra JM. Benign cartilaginous exostoses. Osteochondroma and osteochondromatosis. In: Mirra JM, editor. Bone tumors: clinical, radiologic, and pathologic correlations. 2nd ed. Philadelphia: Lea & Febiger; 1989. p. 1626–59.
6. Resnick D, Kyriakos M, Greenway GD. Osteochondroma. In: Resnick D, editor. Diagnosis of bone and joint disorders. 3rd ed. Philadelphia: Saunders; 1995. p. 3725–46.
7. Giudici M, Moser RP Jr, Kransdorf MJ. Cartilaginous bone tumors. Radiol Clin North Am. 1993;31(2):237–59.
8. Scarborough MT, Moreau G. Benign cartilage tumors. Orthop Clin North Am. 1996;27(3):583–9.
9. Bovée JVMG, Bloem JL, Heymann D, Wuyts W. Osteochondroma. In: WHO Classification of Tumours Editorial Board, editor. Soft tissue and bone tumours. 5th ed. Lyon: International Agenchy for Research on Cancer; 2020. p. 356–8.
10. Oliva F, Marconi A, Fratoni S, Maffulli N. Extraosseous osteochondroma-like soft tissue mass of the patello-femoral space. BMC Musculoskelet Disord. 2006;7(1):1–6.
11. Li C, Arger PH, Dalinka MK. Soft tissue osteochondroma. Skeletal Radiol. 1989;18(6):435–7.
12. Borges AM, Huvos AG, Smith J. Bursa formation and synovial chondrometaplasia associated with osteochondromas. Am J Clin Pathol. 1981;75(5):648–53.
13. El-Khoury G, Bassett G. Symptomatic bursa formation with osteochondromas. Am J Roentgenol. 1979;133(5):895–8.
14. Griffiths HJ, Thompson RC, Galloway HR, Everson LI, Suh J-S. Bursitis in association with solitary

osteochondromas presenting as mass lesions. Skeletal Radiol. 1991;20(7):513–6.
15. Ferriter P, Hirschy J, Kesseler H, Scott W, Popliteal pseudoaneurysm. A case report. J Bone Joint Surg. 1983;65(5):695–7.
16. Eschelman DJ, Gardiner GA Jr, Deely DM. Osteochondroma: an unusual cause of vascular disease in young adults. J Vasc Interv Radiol. 1995;6(4):605–13.
17. Lieberman J, Mazzucco J, Kwasnik E, Loyer R, Knight D. Popliteal pseudoaneurysm as a complication of an adjacent osteochondroma. Ann Vasc Surg. 1994;8(2):198–203.
18. Marcove RC, Lindeque BG, Silane MF. Pseudoaneurysm of the popliteal artery with an unusual arteriographic presentation. A case report. Verh Dtsch Ges Pathol. 1988;234:142–4.
19. Hudson T, Chew F, Manaster B. Scintigraphy of benign exostoses and exostotic chondrosarcomas. Am J Roentgenol. 1983;140(3):581–6.
20. Murphey MD, Choi JJ, Kransdorf MJ, Flemming DJ, Gannon FH. Imaging of osteochondroma: variants and complications with radiologic-pathologic correlation. Radiographics. 2000;20(5):1407–34.
21. Hudson T, Springfield D, Spanier S, Enneking W, Hamlin D. Benign exostoses and exostotic chondrosarcomas: evaluation of cartilage thickness by CT. Radiology. 1984;152(3):595–9.
22. Kenney PJ, Gilula L, Murphy WA. The use of computed tomography to distinguish osteochondroma and chondrosarcoma. Radiology. 1981;139(1):129–37.
23. Malghem J, Berg BV, Noël H, Maldague B. Benign osteochondromas and exostotic chondrosarcomas: evaluation of cartilage cap thickness by ultrasound. Skeletal Radiol. 1992;21:33–7.
24. Kivioja A, Ervasti H, Kinnunen J, Kaitila I, Wolf M, Böhling T. Chondrosarcoma in a family with multiple hereditary exostoses. J Bone Joint Surg Br. 2000;82(2):261–6.
25. Bell RS. Musculoskeletal images. Malignant transformation in familial osteochondromatosis? Can J Surg. 1999;42(1):8.
26. Fischgrund JS, Cantor JB, Samberg LC. Malignant degeneration of a vertebral osteochondroma with epidural tumor extension: a report of the case and review of the literature. J Spinal Disord. 1994;7(1):86–90.
27. Young CL, Sim FH, Unni KK, McLeod RA. Chondrosarcoma of bone in children. Cancer. 1990;66(7):1641–8.
28. Willms R, Hartwig C-H, Böhm P, Sell S. Malignant transformation of a multiple cartilaginous exostosis–a case report. Int Orthop. 1997;21(2):133–6.
29. Ahmed AR, Tan T-S, Unni KK, Collins MS, Wenger DE, Sim FH. Secondary chondrosarcoma in osteochondroma: report of 107 patients. Clin Orthop Relat Res. 2003;411:193–206.
30. Garrison RC, Unni KK, McLeod RA, Pritchard DJ, Dahlin DC. Chondrosarcoma arising in osteochondroma. Cancer. 1982;49(9):1890–7.
31. Fennel E. Osteogenic sarcoma from exostosis. Am J Surg. 1938;39(1):121–6.
32. Nojima T, Yamashiro K, Fujita M, Isu K, Ubayama Y, Yamawaki S. A case of osteosarcoma arising in a solitary osteochondroma. Acta Orthop Scand. 1991;62(3):290–2.
33. Matsuno T, Ichioka Y, Yagi T, Ishii S. Spindle-cell sarcoma in patients who have osteochondromatosis. A report of two cases. J Bone Joint Surg. 1988;70(1):137–41.
34. Picci P, Stilli S. Malignant fibrous histiocytoma arising from an exostosis in a patient affected by multiple exostoses. Ital J Orthop Traumatol. 1982;8(2):205–6.
35. Ozaki T, Hillmann A, Blasius S, Link T, Winkelmann W. Multicentric malignant transformation of multiple exostoses. Skeletal Radiol. 1998;27(4):233–6.
36. Carroll KL, Yandow SM, Ward K, Carey JC. Clinical correlation to genetic variations of hereditary multiple exostosis. J Pediatr Orthop. 1999;19(6):785–91.
37. Mirra JM. Malignant cartilaginous exostoses: Chondrosarcomatous transformation of osteochondroma(tosis). In: Mirra JM, editor. Bone tumors: clinical, radiologic, and pathologic correlations. 2nd ed. Philadelphia: Lea & Febiger; 1989. p. 1660–72.

14 Dysplasia Epiphysealis Hemimelica (Trevor's Disease)

14.1 Definition

Dysplasia epiphysealis hemimelica (DEH) is a rare, nonfamilial developmental error characterized by the presence of an osseocartilaginous mass arising from the epiphyses or epiphyseal equivalent, typically localized to one side of the body, particularly in young children [1, 2].

14.2 Synonym

Tarso-epiphyseal aclasia/Trevor's disease/ Epiphyseal osteochondroma/ Tarsomegalie.

14.3 Classification

Azouz et al. [3] subdivided DEH into three forms (1) *Classic form* is characterized by hemimelic distribution involving more than one epiphysis within a single lower extremity (2) *Localized form* unilaterally or bilaterally affects a single epiphysis (3) *Generalized form* involves the whole limb, from the pelvis to the foot.

14.4 Age

Most patients are young children in their early first and early to middle second decade of life (Figs. 14.1, 14.2, and 14.3).

W.-J. Bahk, *Diagnosis and Management of Primary Bone Tumors*,
https://doi.org/10.1007/978-981-96-3484-2_14

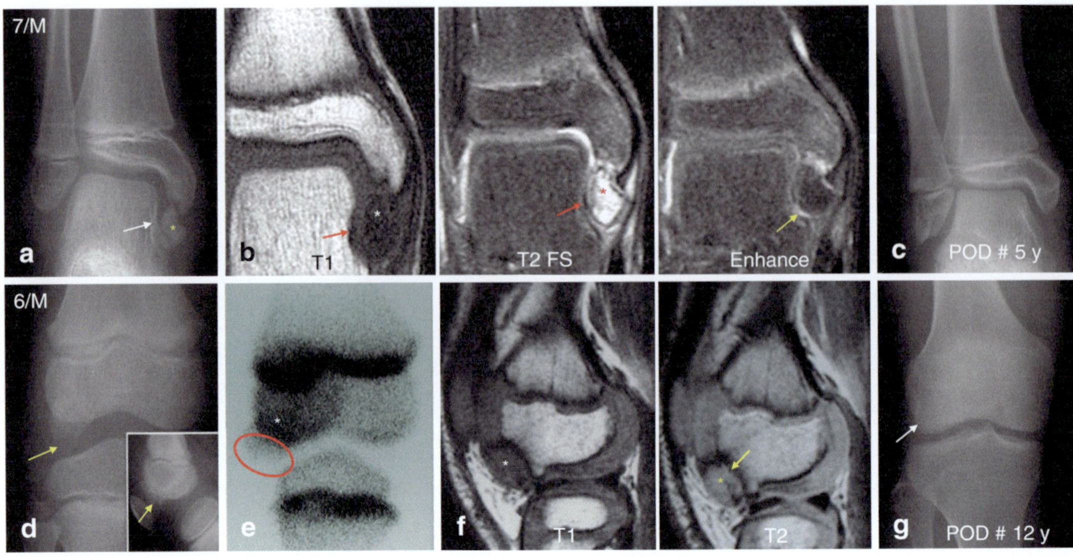

Fig. 14.1 (**a**) Radiograph taken for left ankle mass of 3 months duration in a 7-year-old boy shows a well-defined dense mass arising from the medial malleolus (asterisk) with a mild erosion and sclerotic change at the medial aspect of the opposing talus (arrow). The lateral malleolus is irregularly enlarged with mild deformation. (**b**) MR images reveal a well-demarcated mass arising from medial malleolus (asterisks) with low SI on T1-weighted image and high SI on fat-saturated T2-weighted image. There is an erosive cortical margin of the opposing talus with adjacent soft tissue edema by mechanical irritation (red arrows). The mass presents a thin peripheral enhancement by contrast medium (arrow). (**c**) Follow-up radiograph taken at 5 years after surgical excision notes remodeling of the affected bones with no evidence of local recurrence. (**d**) Radiograph taken for limping gait with different thigh circumference of 3 months duration in a 6-year-old boy shows a well-defined dense mass with stippled calcification arising from the right lateral femoral condyle (yellow arrows). (**e**) Pinhole bone scan shows a mild uptake in the mass area (circle) with a reactive stronger uptake in the epiphysis of the distal femur (asterisk). (**f**) MR images show a well-defined extruding mass arising from the lateral femoral condyle (asterisks) with low SI on T1-weighted image and intermediate to high SI on T2-weighted image. There is a cleavage between the mass and the underlying epiphysis (arrow), which facilitates removal of the mass from the epiphysis. (**g**) Follow-up radiograph at 12 years after complete excision reveals no evidence of recurrence and generative change. He is free of limping gait with a near-normal thigh circumference. Microscopic examination of the excised mass revealed identical findings to those of OC in both cases

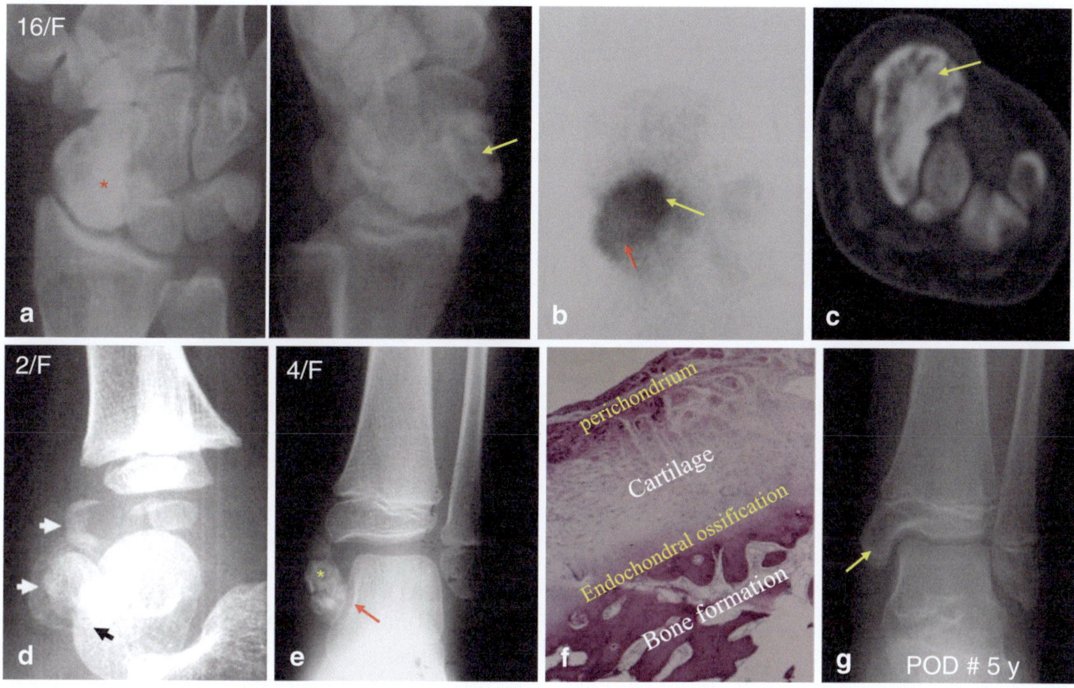

Fig. 14.2 (**a**) Radiograph taken for left wrist mass of 5–6 years duration in a 16-year-old girl shows an ill-defined, densely ossifying mass overlapped with the scaphoid (asterisk). Lateral view reveals a relatively well-demarcated, ovoid bean-shaped, irregularly dense mass arising from the scaphoid (arrow). (**b**) Pinhole bone scan notes a focal hot uptake distally, indicating an avid lesion (yellow arrow) and less active uptake proximally, suggesting a reactive change of underlying scaphoid (red arrow). (**c**) CT scan demonstrates a lobulated densely ossifying mass with a thin cartilage cap (yellow arrow) reflecting the hot uptake area and thick reactive sclerosis within the scaphoid (red arrow) reflecting the less active uptake area on bone scan. There is clear medullary continuity between the lesion and the parent bone (curved line). Microscopic examination of the excised mass revealed identical findings to that of OC. (**d**) Radiograph taken for right ankle swelling of 2 months duration in a 2-year-old infant boy shows a densely ossifying, lobulated mass (white arrows) arising from the talus with no definite radiolucent line between mass and the talus (black arrow). He has no evidence of local recurrence at 4 years after surgical excision. (**e**) Another radiograph taken for left ankle swelling of unknown period in a 4-year-old girl reveals a well-defined multilobulated ossifying mass arising from the medial malleolus (asterisk) with no definite radiolucent line between mass and the talus, which compresses and erodes the opposing talus (arrow). (**f**) Low-power microscopic examination exhibits the same findings recalling those of OC. The outermost layer consists of a perichondrium covering the cartilage cap containing disorganized hyaline cartilage. In the deep area of the cartilage cap, endochondral ossification occurs and bone formation with bone marrow is progressing. (**g**) Follow-up radiograph at 5 years after surgical excision reveals no evidence of recurrence with normal-looking medial malleolus (arrow)

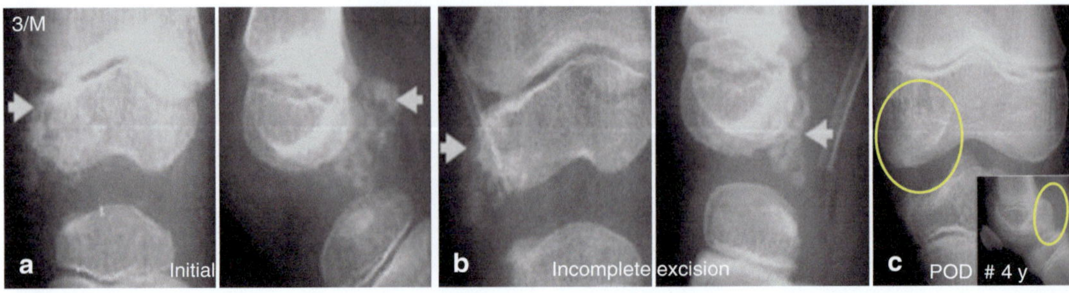

Fig. 14.3 ***Incomplete excision and fate of the remained mass.*** (**a**) Radiographs taken for a limitation of left knee motion with limp of 3–4 months duration in a 3-year-old infant boy show an ill-defined, irregularly mottled calcific mass protruding from the medial epiphysis of the distal femur, typically suggesting DEH (arrows). (**b**) Immediate postoperative radiographs reveal a remaining mass suggesting an incomplete excision by initial surgeon in another hospital (arrows). (**c**) He was transferred to me for a second opinion regarding diagnosis and further management, and I decided to observe without further surgical treatment. Follow-up radiographs at 4 years after surgery show a complete resolution of the residual mass (circles) with normal-looking medial condyle. The patient is doing well with a full range of knee motion

14.5 Location

The lower extremity, particularly about the knee and ankle regions, is affected much more commonly than the upper extremity. The distal end of the long bone is more commonly involved than the proximal end. It occurs most frequently in the distal femoral and distal tibial epiphyses or talus. Medial side of the joint is affected about twice as common as the lateral aspect in a review of the literature [4] (Figs. 14.1a, 14.2e, and 14.3a).

14.6 Clinical Features

The most common presentation is a painless mass or swelling around the affected joints, most frequently the knee and ankle. Other manifestations include pain after physical activities, antalgic gait, limited joint motion, repeated joint locking, deformity such as knock knee, flat foot, limb length discrepancy, and muscle atrophy in the affected area.

14.7 Radiologic findings

Plain radiogrpah often shows characteristic features, although vary depending on the patient's age. The lesion is typified by an irregular, lobulated, ossifying mass with stippled or dense calcification arising from one side, more commonly the medial side of the epiphysis of the long bones and the carpal or tarsal bones (Figs. 14.1, 14.2, and 14.3). Over time, the affected host bone becomes widened, deformed, or irregularly enlarged at one side of the primary ossification center. As the lesion matures, the calcification becomes disorganized and the lesion is irregularly ossified. Subsequently, the ossifying epiphyseal mass becomes incorporated into the adjacent bone and eventually forms exostosis of a lobular ossified mass [5]. However, marrow and cortical continuity with underlying bone may not be as clear as in osteochondroma (OC) [6]. A clear plane of separation between the mass and the normal epiphysis can be observed in rare cases. Parosteal osteosarcoma (OSA) should be differentiated when such a radiolucent cleavage line between the base of mass and the host bone, referred to as *string sign*, is observed [7, 8]. Lesions may remain separated from the host bone, mimicking intra-articular loose bodies when they are multiple [9]. **Bone scan** demonstrates heterogeneously increased uptake in the mass. It is necessary to detect multifocal or whole-limb involvement in a generalized form. Pinhole bone scan more clearly depicts a heterogeneous uptake in the mass itself and surrounding reactive change (Figs. 14.1e and 14.2b). **CT**

scan is useful for the detection of small foci of early calcification or ossification within the cartilaginous mass with a thin cartilage cap as well as reactive sclerotic bone. It can clearly identify cortical and medullary continuity between the lesion and the parent bone (Fig. 14.2c). **MR images** reveal an osteochondral mass with a SI similiar to that of epiphyseal cartilage and bone, being intermediate SI on T1- and high SI on T1-weighted image and high on T2-weighted image. Focal areas of dark signal on both sequences reflects calcification or ossification that increases as the lesion matures and the patient's skeletal maturity progresses [6]. In addition, MRI is also effective to evaluate the status of the involved joint and surrounding soft tissue. It can reveal the extent of the lesion, epiphyseal or joint involvement, and condition of the epiphysis as well as a cleavage of *string sign* between the epiphysis and the mass if presents (Fig. 14.1f). However, marrow and cortical continuity with parent bone may not be as apparent as in OC. In such cases with a *string sign, particularly if involving tarsal bones*, parosteal OSA should be differentiated. However, the characteristic radiographic or MR findings including the locations can exempt a preoperative biopsy in most cases.

14.8 Histologic Findings

Histologic findings are identical to those of OC (Fig. 14.2f). The lesion presents a bony mass with a multilobulated cartilage cap of disorganized hyaline catilage, covered by a perichondrium. There is normal progression of cancellous bone formation beneath the cap via the endochondral ossification. Among other differential features, recent molecular studies for EXT1 and EXT2 gene expression present normal levels, comparable to that of normal growth plate [10–12]. However, the levels of the gene expression are low in development of solitary and multiple forms of OC due to gene mutation [13–15]. These histologic and genetic difference, in conjunction with distinct clinical and radiographic features, enable patholists to distinguish these entities [12].

14.9 Management

Treatment options include observation for early asymptomatic lesions and simple excision for painful extra-articular lesions. If the lesion is intra-articular and associated with deformity, extra-articular osteotomy may be indicated to correct an angular deformity. Kuo et al. [16] reported excellent result following excision of extra-articular lesions, but only fair and poor outcomes after excision of intra-articular lesions. Thus, they did not recommend excision of an articular lesion unless it becomes a loose body. The presence of a cleavage or separation between the mass and the normal cartilage facilitates its removal from the epiphysis (Fig. 14.1f). Arthroscopic resection is indicated for the intra-articular lesion to preserve the integrity of the affected joint as much as possible.

14.10 Clinical Course

Simple complete excision of the extra-articular mass yields favorable results. Even incompletely removed lesions often regress spontaneously and cause no problems [2, 17] (Fig. 14.3), but local recurrence has also been reported [18]. However, intra-articular lesions are less amenable to surgery because simple excision may further damage articular cartilage and increase the risk of degenerative joint disease. Following corrective osteotomy, recurrence of the deformity is common [19]. There has been no reported case of malignant transformation in the literature to date.

References

1. Trevor D. Tarso-epiphyseal aclasis. J Bone Joint Surg. 1950;32-B(2):204–13.
2. Fairbank T. Dysplasia epiphysialis hemimelica. J Bone Joint Surg Br. 1956;38(1):237–57.
3. Azouz E, Slomic A, Marton D, Rigault P, Finidori G. The variable manifestations of dysplasia epiphysealis hemimelica. Pediatr Radiol. 1985;15(1):44–9.
4. Rosero VM, Kiss S, Terebessy T, Köllö K, Szöke G. Dysplasia epiphysealis hemimelica (Trevor's disease): 7 of our own cases and a review of the literature. Acta Orthop. 2007;78(6):856–61.

5. Kettelkamp D, Campbell C, Bonfiglio M. Dysplasia epiphysealis hemimelica: a report of fifteen cases and a review of the literature. J Bone Joint Surg. 1966;48(4):746–66.
6. Murphey MD, Choi JJ, Kransdorf MJ, Flemming DJ, Gannon FH. Imaging of osteochondroma: variants and complications with radiologic-pathologic correlation. Radiographics. 2000;20(5):1407–34.
7. Jee W, Choe B, Ok I, Kim J, Choi Y, Choi K, et al. Recurrent parosteal osteosarcoma of the talus in a 2-year-old child. Skeletal Radiol. 1998;27(3):157–60.
8. Iwasawa T, Aida N, Kobayashi N, Nishimura G. MRI findings of dysplasia epiphysealis hemimelica. Pediatr Radiol. 1996;26(1):65–7.
9. Noyes FR, Kivi LP. Dysplasia epiphysealis hemimelica: a case simulating an intra-articular body. Clin Orthop Relat Res. 1972;86:175–7.
10. Bovée JV, Hameetman L, Kroon HM, Aigner T, Hogendoorn PC. EXT-related pathways are not involved in the pathogenesis of dysplasia epiphysealis hemimelica and metachondromatosis. J Pathol. 2006;209(3):411–9.
11. Legeai-Mallet L, Rossi A, Benoist-Lasselin C, Piazza R, Mallet JF, Delezoide AL, et al. EXT 1 gene mutation induces chondrocyte cytoskeletal abnormalities and defective collagen expression in the exostoses. J Bone Miner Res. 2000;15(8):1489–500.
12. Glick R, Khaldi L, Ptaszynski K, Steiner GC. Dysplasia epiphysealis hemimelica (Trevor disease): a rare developmental disorder of bone mimicking osteochondroma of long bones. Hum Pathol. 2007;38(8):1265–72.
13. Ahn J, Lüdecke H-J, Lindow S, Horton WA, Lee B, Wagner MJ, et al. Cloning of the putative tumour suppressor gene for hereditary multiple exostoses (EXT1). Nat Genet. 1995;11(2):137–43.
14. Czerniak B. Benign cartilage lesions. In: Dorfman HD, Czerniak B, editors. Dorfman and Czerniak's bone tumors. 2nd ed. (eBook): Elsevier; 2016. p. 356–473.
15. Stickens D, Clines G, Burbee D, Ramos P, Thomas S, Hogue D, et al. The EXT2 multiple exostoses gene defines a family of putative tumour suppressor genes. Nat Genet. 1996;14(1):25–32.
16. Kuo R, Bellemore M, Monsell F, Frawley K, Kozlowski K. Dysplasia epiphysealis hemimelica: clinical features and management. J Pediatr Orthop. 1998;18(4):543–8.
17. Bahk W-J, Lee H-Y, Kang Y-K, Park J-M, Chun K-A, Chung Y-G. Dysplasia epiphysealis hemimelica: radiographic and magnetic resonance imaging features and clinical outcome of complete and incomplete resection. Skeletal Radiol. 2010;39:85–90.
18. Rao SB, Roy DR. Dysplasia epiphysealis hemimelica: upper limb involvement with associated osteochondroma. Clin Orthop Relat Res. 1994;307:103–9.
19. Keret D, Spatz DK, Caro PA, Mason DE. Dysplasia epiphysealis hemimelica: diagnosis and treatment. J Pediatr Orthop. 1992;12(3):365–72.

Enchondroma (Central Chondroma)

15

(***en-*** "in" + ***chondros*** "cartilage" + ***ōma*** "forming")

15.1 Definition

Enchondroma (EC) is a common benign cartilage-producing tumor composed of chondrocytes producing a mature cartilagihous cartilage matrix, EC originates from the medullary cavity of long bones, but very rarely grows in exophytic pattern, forming a prominent mass beyond the cortex, so-called *EC protuberans* or *ecchondroma*. The lesion is mostly solitary, but occasionally multifocal affecting one or multiple bones (enchondromatosis).

15.2 Synonym

Chondroma.

15.3 Incidence

EC is the second most common primary bone tumor next to osteochondroma (OC), accounting for 3–10% of all bone tumors and 10–25% of benign bone tumors [1–3]. However, the incidence should be much higher because of many asymptomatic patients who do not seek medical attention.

15.4 Age

Patients present in a wide range of age, but are diagnosed in young aduts, with a peak incidence between the third and fourth decades of life. Over half of the patients are discovered in their age of 10–40 years [3, 4]. EC is rarely discovered in young children and elderly. About 70% of patients with multiple ECs are diagnosed during the first and second decades of life [3].

15.5 Location

EC can arise in any bones formed by endochondral ossification but is not developed in bones made by intramembranous ossification. Most frequently, it involves the short tubular bones of the hands and feet (Figs. 15.1 and 15.2), in which chondrosarcoma (CSA) occurs very rarely, accounting for about half of the cases [1–3], followed by metadiaphysis of the distal femur and proximal humerus (Figs. 15.3, 15.4, 15.5, and 15.6). EC occurs less commonly in other long bones including tibia, fibula, radius, and ulna. The small bones of the hands are several times more commonly affected than those of the feet. However, EC is uncommon in trunk bones such as pelvis, rib, and scapula, in which CSA occurs more frequently [1, 3].

W.-J. Bahk, *Diagnosis and Management of Primary Bone Tumors*,
https://doi.org/10.1007/978-981-96-3484-2_15

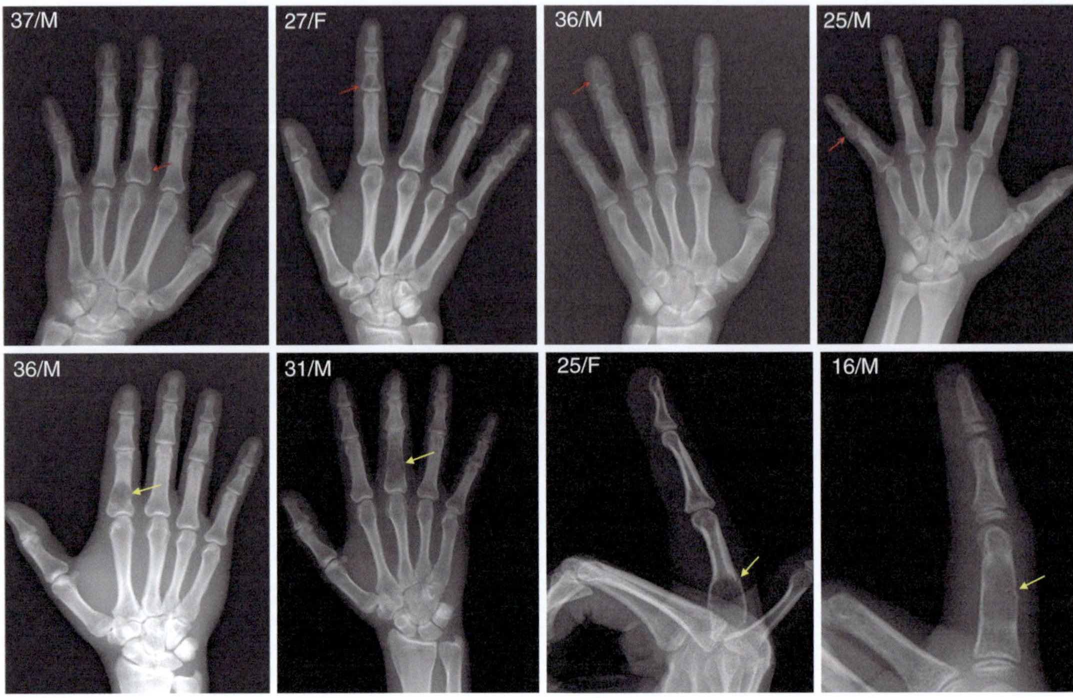

Fig. 15.1 ***Location of the hands***. Radiographs show a well-defined, predominantly lytic lesion with varying degrees of discrete foci of mineralization in a *stippled* or *punctate* pattern. Mineralization is generally in ECs of the digits compared to the long bones. Continuous slow growth of tumors in short tubular bones produce a mild to significant expansion with significant thinning of cortex in *egg-shell* appearance (red arrows). The significantly thinned cortex is easily broken to produce crack or incomplete fracture (yellow arrows), often by trivial events, or even in the absence of any recollected injury. The finding of cortical thinning with moderate to significant expansion in the digits should not be considered as a sign of CSA as in the long bones

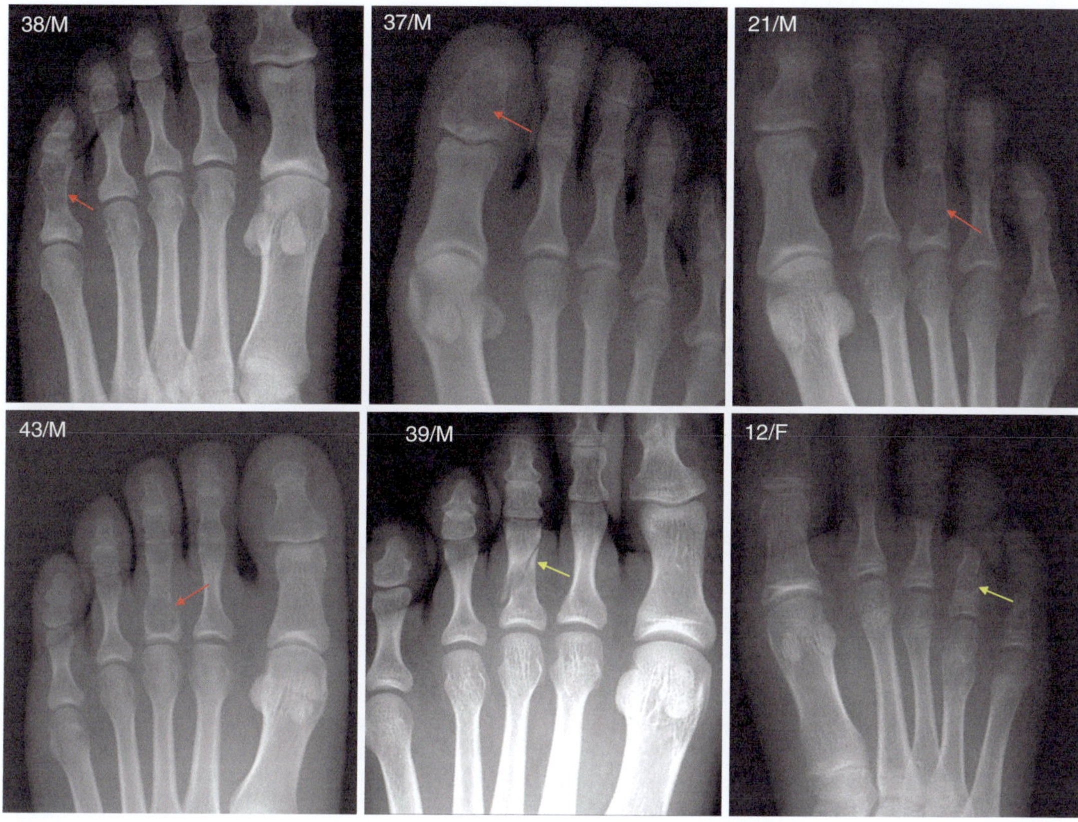

Fig. 15.2 *Location of the feet*. Radiographic features are essentially identical to those observed in the hands (red arrows). Pathologic fracture tends to occur more frequently, and fracture line tend to be more distinct or complete, even accompanied by displacement or angulation, likely due to weight-bearing force (yellow arrows)

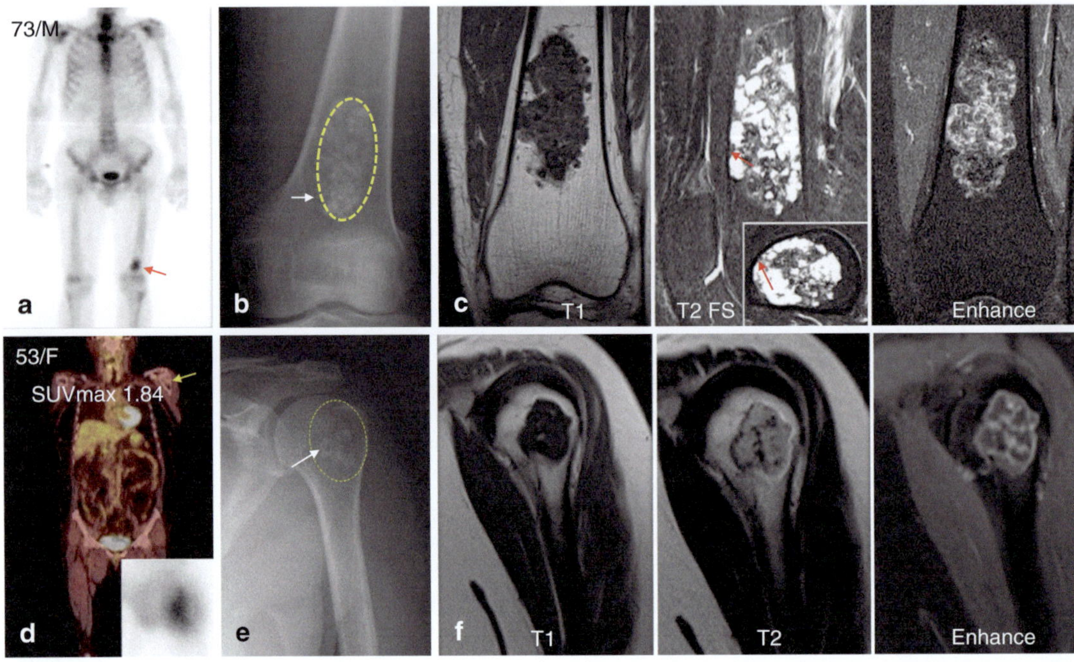

Fig. 15.3 ***Incidentally found EC during evaluation of liver cancer.*** (**a**) Bone scan for staging of hepatocellular carcinoma in a 73-year-old man shows a focal strong uptake in the distal femur (red arrow). (**b**) Radiographs show a relatively well-defined, large, oblong radiolucent lesion with *popcorn-like* dense calcification that is well circumscribed by an imaginary border line (dotted circle). (**c**) MR images demonstrate a large multilobulated mass-like lesion with low SI on T1-weighted image and heterogeneous intermediate and high SI on fat-saturated T2-weighted images with dark signal foci of calcification on both sequences. Superficial mild endosteal scalloping by tumor adjacent to the inner cortex is seen in the range of benignancy (red arrows). The lesion typically presents peripheral and nodular enhancement in a *rings and arcs* pattern. Microscopic examination of incision biopsy confirms a diagnosis of EC. ***Incidentally found EC during medical check-up***: (**d**) PET/CT scan for medical checkup in 53-year-old woman notes a mildly hypermetabolic lesion (SUVmax1.84) in the left proximal humerus (arrow). Pinhole bone scan also shows an inhomogeneous hot uptake in the same area (inset). (**e**) Radiograph reveals an ill-defined radiolucent lesion with internal *popcorn-like* calcification (white arrwow), which is also well circumscribed by an imaginary border (dotted circle). (**f**) MR images note a well-defined mass-like lesion with low SI on T1-weighted image and intermediate to high SI on T2-weighted image with internal dark signal void of calcification on both sequences. The lesion shows *peripheral and septal* enhancement. There is no evidence of adjacent bone marrow abnormality or marked cortical scalloping, findings consistent with EC. The patient is doing very well with no interval change of the lesion on follow-up radiograph at 5 years after the initial visit

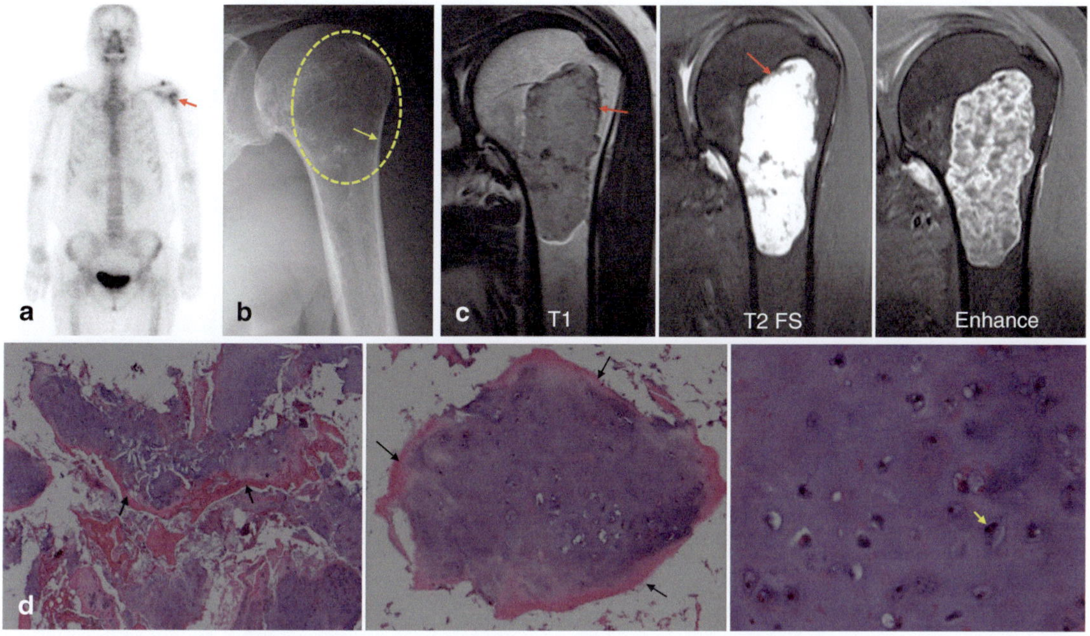

Fig. 15.4 ***Incidentally found EC during evaluation of breast cancer***. (**a**) Bone scan taken for staging of breast cancer in a 53-year-old woman shows mildly increased uptake in the left proximal humerus (red arrow). (**b**) Radiograph reveals an ill-defined, round to oval, predominantly radiolucent lesion with scanty stippled calcification (dotted circle) and superficial cortical erosion (yellow arrow). (**c**) MR images demonstrate a well-defined lobulated lesion with low to intermediate SI on T1-weighted image and high SI on fat-saturated T2-weighted image. There are internal focal dark signals corresponding to scanty calcification and thin surrounding dark signal of sclerotic rim (red arrows) on both sequences. Adjacent bone marrow abnormality and marked cortical scalloping are not observed. Post-contrast image shows a typical peripheral and septal enhancement in a *rings and arcs* pattern. (**d**) Microscopic examination: (Left) Low-power magnification notes several cartilage nodules partially or completely encased by a lamellar bone (black arrows). (Middle) Medium-power magnification reveals a low cellular, bland-looking cartilage nodule with a characteristic *lamellar bone encasement* for EC (arrows). (Right) Higher-power magnification of single nodule show low cellularity with bland to mild atypia and bi-nucleated chondrocytes (arrow)

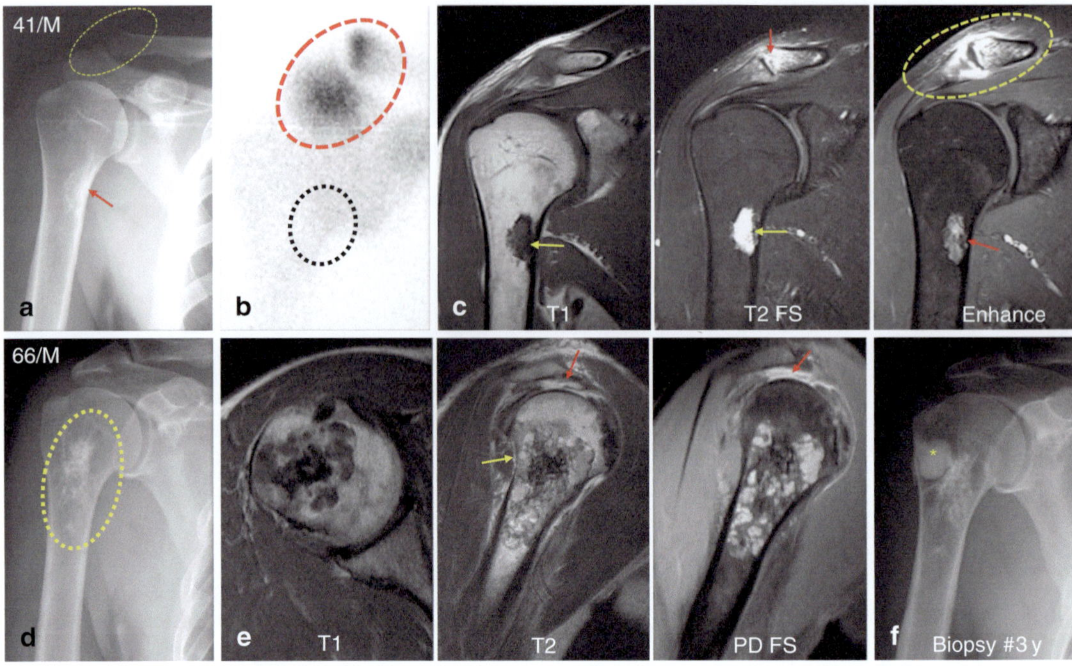

Fig. 15.5 ***Incidentally found ECs during evaluation of shoulder pain.*** (**a**) Radiograph taken for right shoulder after fall in a 41-year-old man incidentally shows a relatively well-defined radiolucent lesion with multiple foci of stippled mineralization in the proximal humerus (black dotted circle). There is no discernible fracture or other abnormal findings in the acromioclavicular (AC) joint (dotted circle). (**b**) Pinhole bone scan reveals no abnormal uptake in the lesion (yellow dotted arrow). However, a moderately increased uptake is seen in the acromion of the right scapula and lateral end of the clavicle (red dotted circle). (**c**) MR image demonstrates an ill-defined medullary and surrounding soft tissue lesion with low SI on T1-weighted image and high SI on T2-weighted image in the acromion tip and distal end of the clavicle (red arrow). The lesion is strongly well enhanced (dotted circle), suggesting a possible microfracture and capsular injury with hemorrhage and edema which is thought to be a pain source. In addition, there is a relatively well-defined small mass-like lesion with low SI on T1-weighted and high SI on T2-weighted image in the proximal humerus (yellow arrows). The lesion is heterogeneously enhanced by contrast medium in the absence of periosteal reation or bone marrow edema (red arrow), indicating incidentally found EC. The pain has subsided by conservative care including local rest and pain killer. (**d**) Radiograph taken for right shoulder pain of 2 years' duration in a 66-year-old man shows an ill-defined radiolucent lesion with *popcorn-like* cacifications in the proximal humerus (dotted circle). There is no discernible abnormality except a mild arthritic change at the AC joint. (**e**) MR images demonstrate a large multilobulated medullary lesion with low to intermediate SI on T1-weighted image and intermediate to high on T2-weighted image with internal dark signals on both sequences. Mild endosteal scalloping with cortical thinning is seen (yellow arrow). However, there is no marrow edema and no definite soft tissue extension. Note another finding of complete thickness tear of supraspinatus tendon (red arrows) with high signal on T2-weighted image and bright signal on fat-suppressed PD image, which is thought to be a cause of the pain. The patient requested a biopsy to exclude the possibility of low-grade CSA, and a histologic diagnosis of EC was rendered. The pain was relieved by conservative management. Pain would be erroneously attributed to EC without MR evaluation. (**f**) Follow-up radiograph 3 years after biopsy reveals no interval change of the EC lesion and the patient is free of pain. The radiodense material (asterisk) is previously inserted bone cement to reduce post-biopsy bleeding

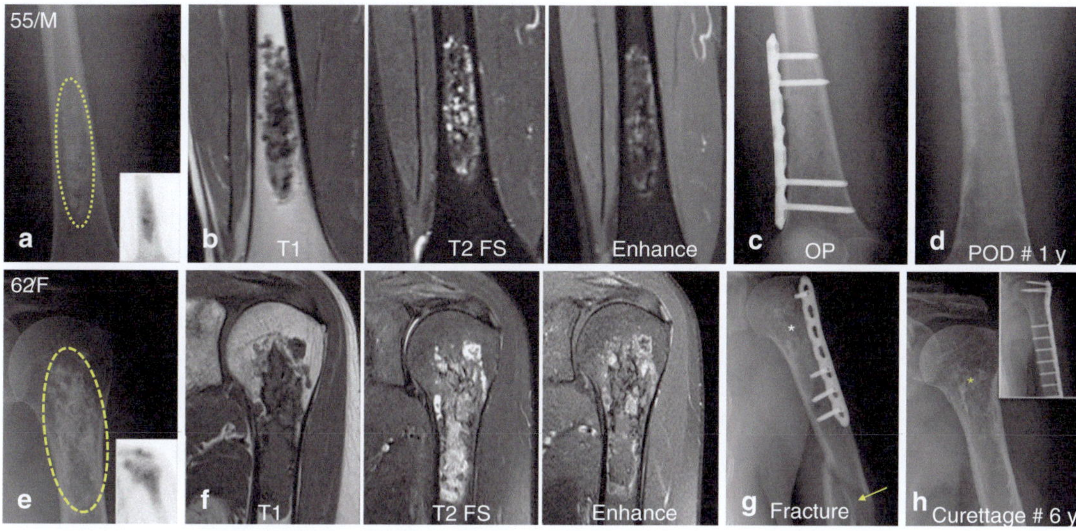

Fig. 15.6 ***Painful EC.*** (**a**) Radiographs taken for left distal thigh pain of 4 months' duration, which became aggravated after playing tennis in a 55-year-old man show a large, oblong, radiolucent lesion popcorn-like calcification that is circumscribed with an imaginary line (dotted circle) in the diaphysis of the distal femur. Bone scan shows a mildly increased uptake with a focal hot uptake (inset). (**b**) MR images demonstrate a relatively well-defined, oblong, medullary lesion with low SI on T1-weighted image and heterogeneous high and bright SI on fat-saturated T2-weighted image, containing internal dark signal of calcification in a typical *rings and arcs* pattern. There is no definite cortical erosion or endosteal scalloping. The lesion is heterogeneously enhanced in a *nodular and peripheral* pattern. (**c**) Curettage followed by allo-chip bone grafting and plate fixation was performed with histologic confirmation of EC by frozen biopsy during surgical procedure. (**d**) Follow-up radiograph at 1 year after surgery notes consolidation without definite evidence of local recurrence. (**e**) Radiograph taken for left shoulder pain of 6 months' duration in a 62-year-old woman reveals an ill-defined large oblong radiolucent lesion with diffuse calcification that is also circumscribed by an imaginary line (dotted circle). Bone scan reveals a mild uptake with a focal hot spot (inset) (**f**) MR images present a relatively ill-defined intramedullary lesion with low SI on T1-weighted image and heterogeneous intermediate and high to bright SI on fat-saturated T2-weighted image, containg focal dark signal void of calcifications on both sequences. There is no definite cortical erosion or endosteal scalloping. The lesion is heterogeneously enhanced in a *nodular and peripheral* pattern. There is no evidence of rotator cuff tear or other soft tissue patholgy, that could explain a cause of the shoulder pain. Thus, the lesion itself was considered the likely cuase of the shoulder pain. Curettage followed by allo-chip bone graft and plate fixation was performed with histologic confirmation of EC by intraoperative frozen section biopsy. (**g**) Radiograph taken for new-onset left upperm pain following a at 1 week after surgery notes a spiral fracture of the humeral shaft distal to the plate (arrow) and previously inserted radiodense allo-chip bones (asterisk). (**h**) The fracture is completely healed by open reduction and exchange of longer plate fixation (inset). Follow-up radiograph at 6 years after curettage demonstrates consolidation of the lesion without a local recurrence (asterisk)

15.6 Clinical Features

Many patients are asymptomatic particularly when involving the long bones, and are often incidentally detected on radiographs or bone scans obained for unrelated reasons (Figs. 15.3, 15.4, and 15.5). According to Mirra, about 40% of patients with single EC complain of some form of pain [2]. About half of the patients have a sudden pain immediately following strenuous physical activity (Fig. 15.6a). The remaining patients may complain of a vague pain of long duration (Fig. 15.6b), which is more ominous to interpret because this nature of pain can be a hallmark of CSA. Swelling or palpable mass with or without pain and pathologic fracture is frequently present in the short tubular bones of the hands and feet due to moderate to severe expansion with significant cortical thinning by the tumor mass. The incidence of pathologic fracture is higher in the feet because of the mechanical stress from weight-bearing forces [5]. The presence of newly developed pain or enlargement of the lesion particularly after cessation of patient's growth may be a significant clinical finding of aggressive biologic behavior. Adjacent shoulder joint pain in patients with EC affecting the proximal humerus is often unrelated to the tumor itself. However, this pain can be erroneously attributed to EC in many instances in the absence of MRI evaluation, which is mandatory to evaluate other reasons for the shoulder pain, including arthritis, rotator cuff tear, microfracture, or capsular injury (Fig. 15.5c, e). The vast majority of cf cases presents as solitary involvement (over 90%), and the remaining few cases involve multiple bones (enchondromatosis, Ollier's disease, Maffucci's syndrome).

15.7 Radiologic Findings

EC is usually central, spherical to oblong, radiolucent lesion with internal foci of discrete mineralization in *stippled or punctate* to *popcorn-like* or *ring and arc* patterns (Figs. 15.3, 15.4, 15.5, and 15.6). Generally, the margin is well-defined with a narrow zone of transition. Large tumors in short tubular bones of the hands and feet can cause a significant bone expansion and thinning of cortex, so-called *egg-shell* appearance, which frequently allows a cortical crack or pathologic fracture even with minor trauma (Figs. 15.1 and 15.2). When affecting the feet, a fracture line tends to be more complete even with displacement or angulation (yellow arrows) due to weight-bearing force [5]. In other small bones such as the rib and fibula, the cortex is usually thinned with mild to moderate expansion. The oblong or spherical lesion could be circumscribed with an imaginary line when a large long bone is affected [2] (Figs. 15.3 and 15.6). Tumors adjacent to the inner cortex or large tumors may produce a superficial endosteal scalloping or superficial erosion, but no expansion in the major long bones. There is no periosteal reaction or naked soft tissue mass. In the long bone, cortical thinning and thickening, cortical destruction with soft tissue extension, bone expansion, and periosteal reaction may herald a malignant transformation. Exceptionally, a well-defined, lobulated, radiolucent intramedullary lesion can be presneted with an exophytic growth pattern. Thus, the lesion is accompanied by an eccentric expansion of one cortex producing exophytic mass beyond the cortex, so-called *EC protuberans* by Caballes [6], which simulates OC or even central CSA with soft tissue mass formation. However, the morphologic differences between these entities are quite obvious and are easily demonstrable [6] (Fig. 15.7). **Bone scan** reveals varying degrees of uptake from mild to strong uptake, or occasionally nouptake at all, depending on the lesion activity (Figs. 15.3, 15.4, 15.5, 15.6, and 15.7). Intense uptake is commonly observed in cases involving short tubular bones with pathological fracture or cortical expansion. **CT scan** typically reveals a relatively well-defined. Nonaggressive osteolytic lesion with varying degrees of internal mineralization. The lesion is sharply demarcated with a narrow zone of transition and often displays superficial endosteal scalloping. Typically, calcification is well present in the *rings and arcs* pattern. There should be no periosteal reaction, cortical destruction, and soft tissue mass in the absence of complication such as pathologic fracture or malignant transformation. **MR images** demonstrate a well-circumscribed, lobulated, mass-like lesion with low to intermediate SI on T1-weighted images and mostly high SI on T2-weighted images. The high to bright signal reflects the high water content of cartilage, while the internal foci of dark signal of calcification appear as signalvoid (dark foci) on fat-saturated T2-weighted image, producing the characteristic *rings and arcs* pattern of a chondroid matrix (Figs. 15.3, 15.4, 15.5, 15.6, and 15.7). The calcified chondroid matrix appear as a dark signal on all sequences. There is usually no marrow edema and never cortical destruction with soft tissue extension if pathologic fracture or malignant change is not associated. Endosteal scalloping and cortical expansion are acceptable for short tubular bones. In a larger long bone, there can be minimal endosteal scalloping but there should not be cortical expansion, periosteal thickening, cortical destruction, or soft tissue mass formation. Variable contrast enhancement can be observed along the periphery of the nodules and internal septa of the lesion in a typical *rings and arcs* pattern (Figs. 15.3, 15.4, 15.5, 15.6, and 15.7).

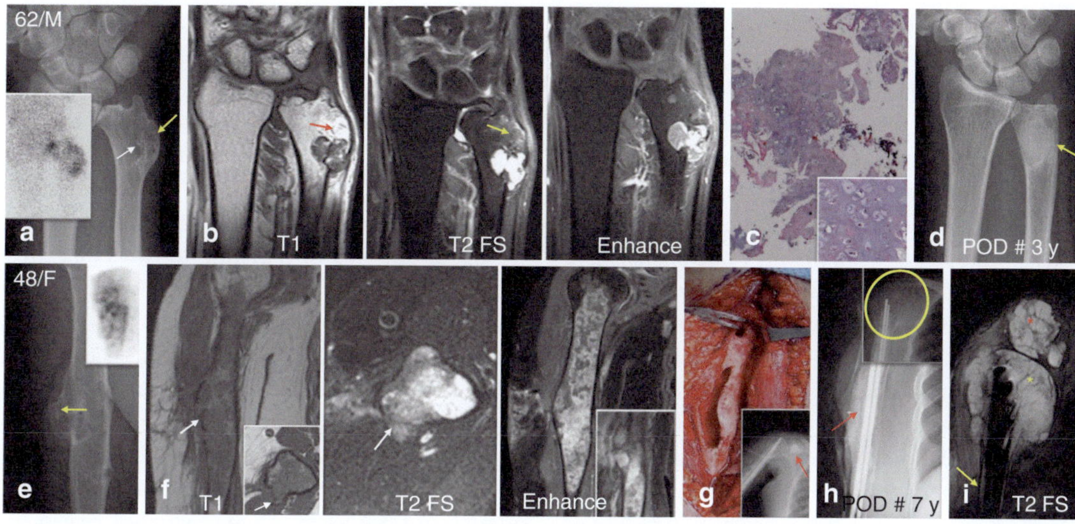

Fig. 15.7 ***EC protuberans***. (**a**) Radiograph taken for right wrist mass of about 30 years' duration and recently developed mild pain in a 62-year-old man shows a relatively ill-defined, lobulated, radiolucent intramedullary lesion with internal stippled calcification in the distal ulna (white arrow). In addition, the lesion eccentrically expands through the medial cortical defect, forming an exophytic mass beyond the cortex (yellow arrow). Bone scan reveals a heterogeneous mild uptake with focal areas of increased uptake (inset). (**b**) MR images delineate a connection between the medullary lesion and the exophytic mass through the cortical defect (red arrow), simulating *flaring* appearance seen in OC. There is, however, no discernible cartilage cap covering the mass unlike OC. Both the intramedullary and exophytic components shows with heterogeneous low and high SI on T1-weighted image and mainly bright and intermediate SI on fat-saturated T2-weighted image, scattered dark spots on all sequences. These imxed signal characteristics likely reflect secondary alterations, including calcification, cystic change, hemorrhage, or fat components. The main lesion is surrounded by a dark signal of incomplete sclerotic rim on both sequences. There is edema in the soft tissue and adjacent tendons, likely due to mechanical irritation from the protruding mass, which is thought to be the cause of recently developed pain. The medullary lesion and exophytic component are heterogeneously and peripherally enhanced by contrast medium. Excision of the exophytic component and curettage of the intramedullary lesion followed by allochip bone graft were perfomed. (**c**) Microscopic examination notes fragmented cartilage nodules with bland-looking, uniform-sized chondrocytes. Higher-power magnification shows moderate cellularity with mild atypica, consistent with EC (inset). There are absence of cartilaginous cap and underlying trabecular bone, which are typically presented in OC. Based on imiging and histologic findings, a diagnosis of *ES protuberans* is rendered. (**d**) Follow-up radiograph at 3 years after resection of the mass with curettage of medullary lesion followed by allo-chip bone graft shows no evidence of recurrence, with consolidation of the graft material (arrow). ***EC protuberans associated with adjacent CSA:*** (**e**) Radiograph taken for right upper arm mass in a 48-year-old woman shows an ill-defined, hazy, mutilobuated, medullary, radiolucent lesion with focal internal sclerosis. In adition, an irregularly contoured exophytic mass is observed extending through a defect in the leateral cortex (yellow arrow). Pinhole bone scan reveals heterogeneously increased uptake with multiple dicrete foci of strong uptake (inset). (**f**) MR images demonstrate a diffuse intramedullary occupying lesion with intermediate SI on T1-weighted image and heterogeneous high SI on fat-saturated T2-weighted image. Note a focal unilateral expansion with a defect in the lateral cortex with an exophytic mass beyond the defect, exhibiting signal characteristic identical to the medullary component (white arrows). Both medullary and exophytic lesions present a typical enhancement with the *rings and arcs* pattern, consistent with cartilage-forming tumor. (**g**) Excision of exophytic cartilage mass and extended curettage of the diffuse medullary EC lesion were performed through a wide cortical window, followed by cementing and flexible nail insertion. Radiologic and histopathologic evaluations confirmed the diagnosis of diffuse EC in association with a focal EC protuberans. In addition, extended curettage with bone cementing was simultaneously done for scapular lesion under a pathologic diagnosis of low-grade CSA (red arrow in inset). (**h**) Follow-up radiograph after 7 years after surgery shows no local recurrence of the EC protuberans and medually EC lesions in the humeral shaft (red arrow). However, there is marked destruction of proximal humerus and distal clavicle (yellow circle), indicating local recurrence and progression of the CSA. (**i**) Corresponding MR image also shows no evidence of recurrence of both medullary EC and EC protubernas (yellow arrow), but significant progression and expansion of the cartilage tumor in the shoulder (red asterisk) and proximal humerus, around the entry of the flexible nails (yellow asterisk). The EC protuberans itself does not recur in the last follow-up

15.8 Histologic Findings

EC consists of multiple lobules of mature hyaline cartilage in a lobular architecture, so-called *islands of cartilage*, which are partially or completely encased by various thicknesses of reactive host lamellar bone at the periphery of cartilaginous lobules, a typical *lamellar bone encasement* pattern [2]. The individual lobules are separated by normal bone marrow spaces with hematopoietic elements (Fig. 15.8a–c). In clinical practice, the specimen is often severely fragmented by curettage procedure, thus the characteristic tissue patterns can be distorted. The cartilaginous lobules undergo endochondral ossification in the periphery beginning to produce premature woven bone (Fig. 15.8d), and finally resulting in the typical mantles of mature lamellar bone encasing the cartilage nodules, which produce a peripheral enhancement of the nodules seen on MRI (Fig. 15.8a–c). Calcification presents a basophilic to deep purple, irregular, dense material producing characteristic discrete foci of densification (Fig. 15.8e). Radiologically, these calcifications present as *stippled* or *punctate* to *rings and arcs* patterns on radiograph and MRI. Generally, the cellularity is low to moderate, and bland-looking chondrocytes are located in lacunar spaces with small dark nuclei and condensed chromatin. A few bi-nucleated chondrocytes and necrosis with empty lacunae lacking nuclei can be also seen, and the findings should not be automatically considered as CSA (Fig. 15.8f). Myxoid matrix is rarely observed, but usually focal if presents.

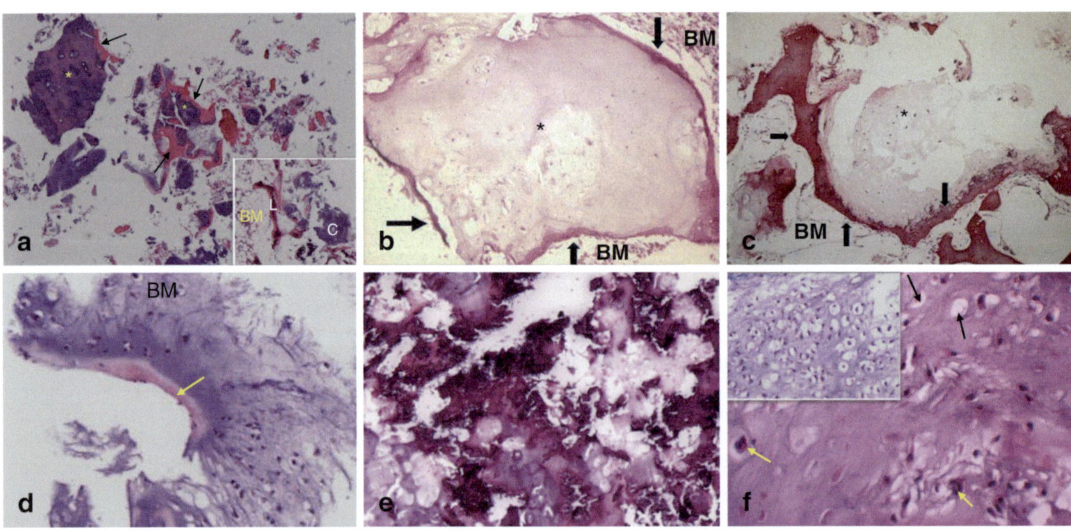

Fig. 15.8 ***Microscopic examination***. (**a**) Low-power magnification usually shows severely fragmented, cartilage nodules of varying size (asterisks), surrounded by lamellar bone plates of variable thickness (black arrows). Thorough curettage during surgery makes the specimen jumble of disorderly arranged cartilage nodules (C), bone marrow (BM), and lamellar bone chips (L) that might be misinterpreted as CSA invasion pattern (inset). (**b**, **c**) Tissue patterns of *islands of cartilage* and *lamellar bone encasement* are diagnostic for EC. Intramedullary nodules consisting of pure hyaline cartilage (asterisks) are separated by the bone marrow components (BM) and encased by thin or thick lamellar bone plates (black arrows). The reactive, host lamellar encasement might be partial or complete. (**d**) The cartilaginous lobule undergoes endochondral ossification in the periphery, initiating the formaiton of premature woven bone (yellow arrow), and eventually giving rise to characteristic mantles of mature lamellar bone encasing the cartilage nodules, as in **b** and **c**. (**e**) Heavily calcified specimen shows a deep purple, irregular, dense stains, which correspond the characteristic discrete foci of mineralization, so-called *popcorn-like*, *stippled*, *ring and arc*, or *punctate* calcification on radiograph, CT, and MRI. (**f**) Higher magnification notes bland chondrocytes typically located within sharp-edged lacuna spaces, with occasional double nuclei (yellow arrows). The cells usually have uniform, small, round, hyperchromatic nuclei and some cells undergo apoptosis with hazy or empty lacunae (black arrows). If short tubular bones of hands and feet are affected, cellularity is often higher with mild to moderate cytologic atypia, which should not be automatically interpreted as CSA (inset)

Extensive myxoid change may, however, raise suspicion for CAS. Some cases of EC particularly involving small bones of hands and feet may show overlapping cytologic features with low-grade CAS in terms of higher cellularity and mild atypia with enlarged nuclei, numbers of chondrocytes, double-nucleated chondrocytes, and mitoses [2, 7]. Thus, it may be impossible to distinguish low-grade CSA from EC by cytology alone. Mirra et al. [8] proposed that the tumors can be distinguished by a histologic approach based on tissue architecture architecture rather than cytologic features alone, including *islands of cartilage* and *lamellar bone encasement* for EN (Figs. 15.4d and 15.8a–c), and "trapping" host lamellar bone, "bands of fibrosis," "infiltration of the Haversian systems or marrow fat," and/or development of a "soft tissue mass" for CSA. The tissue pattern rather than cytologic findings itself is much more likely valuable when correlated with clinical and radiologic features, so-called *diagnostic triangle*. *EC protuberans* which may mimic OC on image studies presents essentially histologic findings identical to those of medullary EC (Fig. 15.7c). However, there is absence of cartilage cap unlike to OC.

15.9 Management

Asymptomatic and small lesions in the long bones require no treatment, but clinical and radiographic monitoring is necessary if it grows or becomes aggressive and painful. Incision biopsy is necessary to exclude CAS when the lesion is moderate to large in size, painful, prominently lytic with deep cortical erosions and marrow edema. The amount of biopsy specimen should be enough to comprehensively evaluate the tissue architecture as well as cytologic features, which are critical in differentiating EC from Low-grade CSA. Curettage with or without bone graft is indicated for painful lesion or pathologic fracture. Resection of exophytic cartilage mass in combination with curettage of intramedullary cartilage lesion is indicated for *EC protuberans* [9] (Fig. 15.7d).

15.10 Clinical Course

Recurrence is usually uncommon even after simple curettage, but it is higher if removal of the lesion is incomplete. Recurrent tumors, particularly those in short tubulat bones, are usually treated by a repeated curettage [10–12]. However, recurrence itself after complete curettcurettage, especially in lesions affecting the lon bones, may raise concern for possible malignancy [13]. Rarely, the recurrent tumor may present increased anaplasia suggesting a malignant change [4]. Although the incidence of malignant transformation has been reported about 1% in solitary EC, the true incidence is unknown because many patients are asymptomatic and the exact frequency of EC is undetermined. In a long-term follow-up study of 44 patients with multiple ENs, Schwartz et al. estimated the incidence of secondary CSA in patients who had Ollier's disease to be approxiamately 25% by the age of 40 years in Ollier's patients and almost a certainty in patients with Maffucci's syndrome in lifetime from life-table analyses [14].

15.11 Enchondromatosis (Multiple Enchondromatosis)

Enchondromatosis or multiple ECs, unlike osteochondromatosis or multiple hereditary exostosis, is a rare, nonhereditary, sporadic disorder in which more than two bones are affected by EC (Fig. 15.9). Occasionally, it can occur in the clinical settings of Ollier's disease (Fig. 15.9c) and Maffucci's syndrome (Fig. 15.10), which are not simply multifocal ECs of bone. The number and distribution of ECs are widely variable from case to case. Originally, Ollier [15] described a nonhereditary condition with proliferating multiple cartilage masses. He introduced a term *dyschondroplasia* to imply a developmentally abnormal growth of cartilage without normal process of endochondral ossification. According to Jaffe, the term Ollier's disease should be reserved for severe cases of multiple enchondromatosis

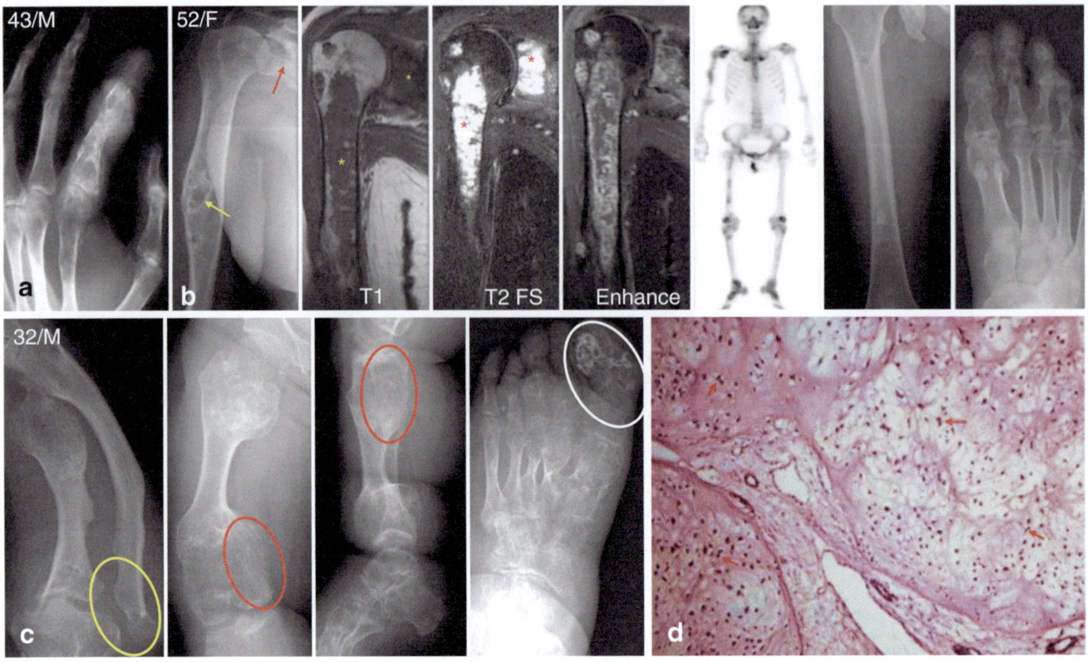

Fig. 15.9 ***Multiple ECs***. (**a**) ***Small number of bone involvement***. Radiograph taken for a gradual enlargement of the fingers in a 43-year-old man shows multiple, bubbly or multilobulated, expansive osteolytic lesions with internal increased densities involving only phalanges and metacarpals. There is no other bony lesion. (**b**) ***Moderate number of bone involvement***. Radiograph taken for painful swelling of the right arm in a 52-year-old woman reveals a bubbly radiolucent lesion with moderate expansion and surrounding sclerosis (yellow arrow) in the right humeral shaft. There is another ill-defined hazy radiolucent lesion in the glenoid of the scapula (red arrow). MR images demonstrate well-defined, lobulated, medullary mass-like lesions with low SI on T1-weighted image and mostly high SI on fat-saturated T2-weighted image in the humerus and scapular glenoid (asterisks). The lesion is typically enhanced in a *ring and arc* pattern, consistent with cartilage-forming tumor. Bone scan shows strong uptake in right shoulder and mild to moderate uptake in right femur and tibia as well as small bones of hands and feet. Additional radiographs reveal similar lesions in the right distal and proximal femur and phalanges of toes, which appear radiologically stable. (**c**) ***Extensive involvement in Ollier's disease***. Plain radiographs reveal severe bowing deformities with shortening of right forearm, thigh, leg, and foot with dislocation of radial head and proximal radioulnar joint, producing grotesque skeletal configuration (circles). As Jaffe originally stated, this case is a typical case of Ollier's disease severely and extensively involving one side of the body. There are multiple thin vertical striations along the long axis of bone (red circles). With progression of the lesion, severe distortion of the parallel arrangement of the vertical striations presents the lesion as a large multilobular mass involving the bone end. (**d**) Histologic examination demonstrates a high cellularity with mild nuclear atypia in size and shape and several double-nucleated chondrocytes (red arrows). This degree of cytologic abnormality can be often observed in Ollier's disease, synovial chondromatosis, or parosteal chondroma, which can be mistaken for low-grade CSA, particularly in the absence of characteristic radiographic findings

with extensive involvement of one side of the body as Ollier originally described. Enchondromatosis has been used as a substitute for *dyschondroplasia*, but it does not explain all of the abnormal deposition of cartilage observed in Ollier's disease. In the strict sense, Ollier's disease and Maffucci's syndrome would not be a pure multiplicity of EC [16]. The true incidence of multiple enchondromatosis including Ollier's disease and Maffucci's syndrome is unknown, but these conditions occupied about 11% of all ECs in a Mayo Clinic series [3]. Although the lesions may present at birth (congenital), they usually become apparent during early childhood when symptoms such as deformities or improper limb growth are more obvious. It has predilection for the appendicular skeleton, most frequently short tubular bones of the hands and feet, followed by femur, tibia, humerus, and forearm bones. The rib, pelvis, and scapula are also occasionally

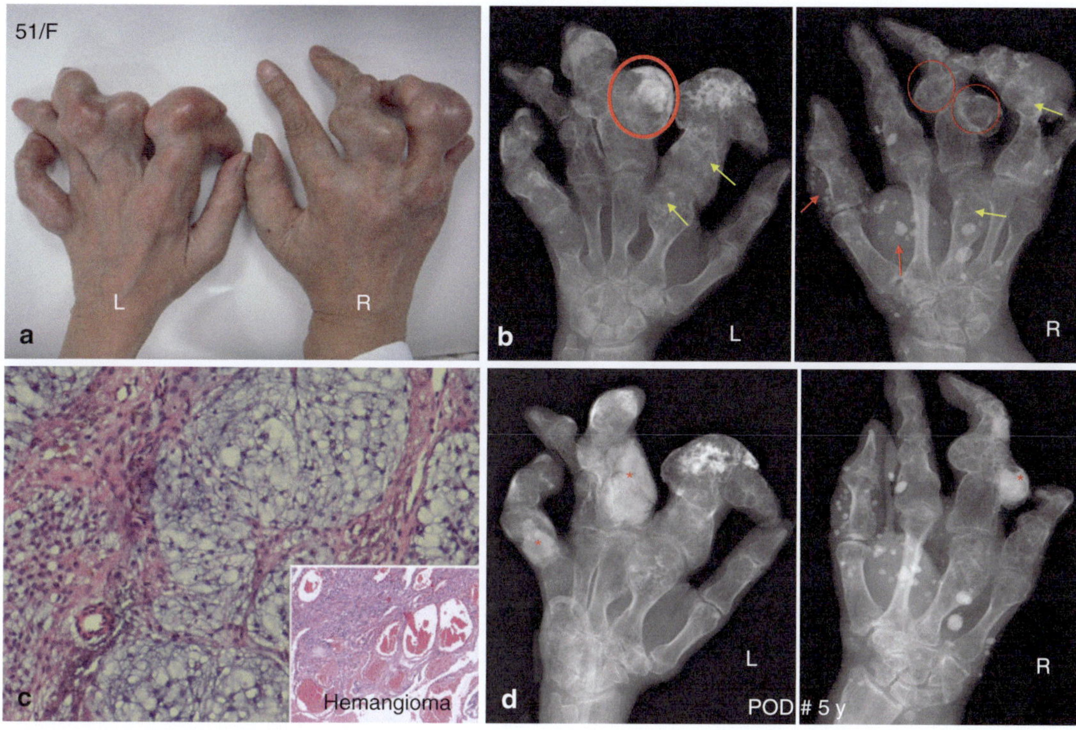

Fig. 15.10 ***Maffucci's syndrome***. (**a**) A 51-year-old female patient presents with gradual enlargement of multiple masses of both hands since childhood, which produce resultant grotesque deformities with limitation of joint motion. (**b**) Radiographs show multiple, expansive, bubbly to trabeculated, lytic and sclerotic lesions with significant cortical thinning in the phalanges and metacarpals of both hands, representing ECs (yellow arrows) with densely calcifying nodules protruding into the adjacent soft tissue (red circles). The lesions result in a severe grotesque deformity, the so-called *dyschondroplasia* originally described by Ollier. Note additional soft tissue masses with multiple phleboliths (red arrows), representing soft tissue hemangiomas with calcifying thrombi. (**c**) Microscopic examination reveals high cellularity and mild to moderate nuclear atypia compared with conventional EC. Note multiple dilated lumens with endothelium which are filled with red blood cells, indicating cavernous hemangioma of the soft tissue (inset). (**d**) Follow-up radiographs at 5 years after curettage with cement packing (red asterisks) and ray amputation of right ring finger for superimposed infection control and intractable pain reveal no further progression of the disease. There was no evidence of malignant change at the last follow-up

affected. However, other axial bones such as skull, spine, clavicle, or sternum only sporadically involved [1, 16]. Although clinical presentations are variable, the initial complaint is often related to gradual enlargement of the digits in mild cases (Fig. 15.9a). Abnormal and/or slow growth of extremities is often observed with mild to moderate deformity and pain during periods of rapid growth. After puberty, the tumor may be stabilized in size or continue to grow (Fig. 15.9b). The pain occurring in adults would raise the concern of pathologic fracture or malignant change. The lesion could be severe enough for growth disturbance, limitation of joint motion, dislocation or subluxation of the joint, grotesque appearance with significant deformity of hands, and length discrepancy of limbs (Fig. 15.9c), which could make the limb useless in some cases. Radiographic features are usually characteristic in most cases, which are basically similar to those seen in solitary EC. However, the severe lesion can be markedly extensive, sometimes bubbly or trabeculated, with expanded underlying bone as well as significant thinning or absence of cortex to produce "naked" cartilage nodules in the adjacent soft tissue, particularly in the small bones of the hands. In long bones, the lesion may form elongated grooves or longitudinal lucent columns along the

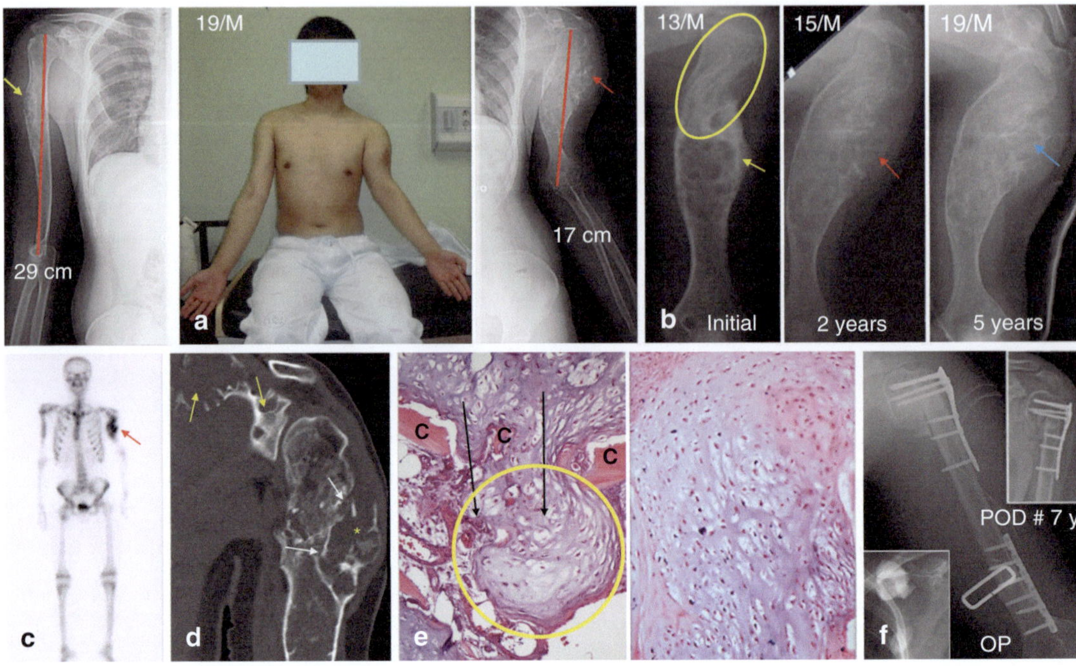

Fig. 15.11 ***Malignant transformation*.** (**a**) Radiographs of a 19-year-old patient with a progressively enlarging mass, deformity, and shortening of the left upperarm since early childhood show a huge, bubbly to trabeculated lesion with cortical destruction and soft tissue extension (red arrow) in the nearly entire left humerus, resulting in 12 cm shortening and bending deformity of the left upper arm. In contrast, there is a relatively mild lesion with superficial cortical erosion (yellow arrow) in the mid-shaft of the right humerus without deformity. (**b**) ***Chronologic radiograph series*.** Initial radiograph shows thickened cortex with no soft tissue extension (yellow arrow). The proximal lesion presents multiple thick elongated grooves and longitudinal lucent columns that obliquely extend from the growth plate downward into the shaft, the so-called *fluted-column* sign (circle). Two years later, radiograph reveals cortical destruction and soft tissue extension (red arrow) with moderate shortening of the left upper arm. Five years later, follow-up radiograph notes soft tissue extension with densifying soft tissue mass (blue arrow) with significant shortening of the left upper arm. Clinically, he presents with newly developed pain in the left upper arm. (**c**) Bone scan shows strong uptake in a large area of the left humerus (red arrow), suggesting a possible malignant transformation, particularly in consideration of newly developed pain. (**d**) CT scan shows a multilobulated radiolucent lesion with internal densification as well as cortical destruction (white arrows) and soft tissue extension (asterisk) in the left humerus. There are also multiple radiolucent lesions in the scapular glenoid and body (yellow arrows). (**e**) Microscopic examination: (Left) Medium-power magnification reveals the cartilage tumor breaks down the host cortex (c) and invade adjacent soft tissue (black arrows), indicating malignant change to CSA. (Right) Higher-power magnification notes a cartilage nodule consisting of high cellularity, moderate atypia with small, dark nucei and condensed chromatin as well as myxoid matrix with calcification, suggesting a moderate-grade CSA. (**f**) Wide resection followed by reconstruction with vascularized fibular graft for the humerus lesion was performed. The scapular lesion was treated by curettage, and cement insertion was performed with a diagnosis of benign EC (Lower inset). He is doing well with no evidence of local recurrence 7 years after surgery (upper inset)

long axis of bone. These represents a parallel arrangement of rows of dysplastic cartilage extending from the growth plate toward the diaphysis, so-called *fluted-column* sign (Fig. 15.11c). With progression of the lesion, the parallel arrangement of the cartilaginous lesion is so distorted that it can present as a large multilobulated mass involving the bone end [1]. In Ollier's disease, significant bowing deformities with shortening of the short and long tubular bones producing grotesque figures are observed (Fig. 15.9c). Histologic findings are identical to those of solitary EN. The cartilage in Ollier's disease has an overall lobular architecture with cartilage lobules or islands encased by plates of reactive host lamellar bone as in EC. However, the individual nodules tend to display increased cellularity, often to a singnificant degree, along with moderate cytologic atypia, or relatively high numbers of double-nucleated chondrocytes, somtimes up to the range noted in low-grade CSA [16] (Fig. 15.9d). When Ollier's disease is accompanied by soft tissue hemangiomas, the lesion is referred to as Maffucci's syndrome. The hemangiomas in the setting of Maffucci's syndrome typically affect the soft tissue or skin but may involve viscera including the lung and liver. Most frequently, the hemangiomas are cavernous type often with phleboliths on plain radiograph (Fig. 15.10). The most serious complication is malignant transformation to CSA that occurs more commonly in severely involved long and flat bones (Fig. 15.11). The transformed CSA usually occurs at an earlier age than in patients with primary conventional CSA. Clinical evidence of rapid growth in one of the affected bones and radiographic findings of newly developed or abruptly enlarged lesion destructing the cortical bone with soft tissue extension may herald malignant transformation. Earlier in 1958, Jaffe [17] described that over half of the patients with Ollier's disease would suffer a malignant change. The estimated incidence has been reported to be about 25–30% in Ollier's disease [14, 18] and much higher in Maffucci's syndrome [14]. They estimated that malignant degeneration is almost a certainty in patients who have Maffucci's syndrome with a predilection to the development not only of secondary CSA but also of other malignant lesions, many of which are life-threatening. In the extensive review [19], 16 cases of CSA were found in 105 patients with Maffucci's syndrome (15%). Sun et al. [20] reported a CSA incidence of 18% in patients with Maffucci's syndrome on the basis of their patients and those reported in the English literature. More recently, sarcoma was reported to arise in 24 of 54 (44%) patients with multiple ECs in the Mayo Clinic series [3].

References

1. Czerniak B. Benign cartilage lesions. In: Dorfman HD, Czerniak B, editors. Dorfman and Czerniak's bone tumors. 2nd ed. (eBook): Elsevier; 2016. p. 356–473.
2. Mirra JM, Eckardt J. Enchondroma versus chondrosarcoma. In: Mirra JM, editor. Bone tumors: clinical, radiologic, and pathologic correlations. 2nd ed. Philadelphia: Lea & Febiger; 1989. p. 476–535.
3. Unni KK, Inwards CY. Chondroma. In: Unni KK, Inwards CY, editors. Dahlin's bone tumors: general aspects and data on 10,165 cases. 6th ed. Philadelphia: Lippincott William & Wilkins; 2010. p. 22–40.
4. Schajowicz F. Cartilage-forming tumors. In: Schajowicz F, editor. Tumors and tumorlike lesions of bone and joints. Pathology, radiology, and treatment. 2nd ed. Berlin Heidelberg: Springer-Verlag; 1994. p. 141–256.
5. Bahk WJ, Kim NH, Park KS, Kim JY. Clinical and radiographic outcomes of simple curettage and graft using allogenic bone or bone substitute for enchondroma involving short tubular bone of the hand and foot. J Korean Orthop Assoc. 2016;51(1):85–90.
6. Caballes RL. Enchondroma protuberans masquerading as osteochondroma. Hum Pathol. 1982;13(8):734–9.
7. Schajowicz F, McGuire MH. Diagnostic difficulties in skeletal pathology. Clin Orthop Relat Res. 1989;240:281–310.
8. Mirra JM, Gold R, Downs J, Eckardt JJ. A new histologic approach to the differentiation of enchondroma and chondrosarcoma of the bones. A clinicopathologic analysis of 51 cases. Clin Orthop Relat Res. 1985;201:214–37.
9. Crim JR, Mirra J. Enchondroma protuberans. Skeletal Radiol. 1990;19(6):431–4.
10. Kuur E, Hansen S, Lindequist S. Treatment of solitary enchondromas in fingers. J Hand Surg Eur. 1989;14(1):109–12.
11. Noble J, Lamb D. Enchondromata of bones of the hand. A review of 40 cases. Hand. 1974;6(3):275–84.
12. Takigawa K. Chondroma of the bones of the hand: a review of 110 cases. J Bone Joint Surg. 1971;53(8):1591–600.
13. Ryzewicz M, Manaster B, Naar E, Bennie Lindeque M. Low-grade cartilage tumors: diagnosis and treatment. Orthopedics. 2007;30(1):35.
14. Schwartz HS, Zimmerman N, Simon M, Wroble R, Millar E, Bonfiglio M. The malignant potential of enchondromatosis. J Bone Joint Surg Am. 1987;69(2):269–74.
15. Ollier M. De la dyschondroplasia. Bull Soc Chir Lyon. 1899;3:22–3.
16. Mirra JM. Multiple cartilageneous dysplasia (Ollier's disese and Maffucci's syndrome). In: Mirra JM, editor. Bone tumors: clinical, radiologic, and pathologic

correlations. 2nd ed. Philadelphia: Lea & Febiger; 1989. p. 449–76.
17. Jaffe H. Tumors and tumorous conditions of the bones and joints. Philadelphia: Lea & Febiger; 1958.
18. Liu J, Hudkins PG, Swee RG, Unni KK. Bone sarcomas associated with Ollier's disease. Cancer. 1987;59(7):1376–85.
19. Lewis RJKA. Maffucci's syndrome: functional and neoplastic significance: case report and review of the literature. J Bone Joint Surg. 1973;55(7):1465–79.
20. Sun TC, Swee R, Shives T, Unni K. Chondrosarcoma in Maffucci's syndrome. J Bone Joint Surg. 1985;67(8):1214–9.

16 Periosteal Chondroma

(***Peri***- "near or around" + ***osteal***- "bone" + ***chondros*** "cartilage" + ***ōma*** "forming")

16.1 Definition

Periosteal chondroma (PC) is a rare, slow-growing, benign cartilage tumor located on the cortical surface of bone, arising from the periosteal tissue. It is the periosteal counterpart of enchondroma, which occurs within the medullary cavity.

16.2 Synonym

Juxtacortical/parosteal/subperiosteal chondroma.

16.3 Incidence

PC occupies approximately 1–2% of all chondromas [1–4] and 0.5% of biopsy-proven primary bone tumors [5].

16.4 Age

The lesion may occur in patients of all ages, but it is most frequently observed in adolescents and young adults in their second and third decades of life [4, 6] (Figs. 16.1 and 16.2). Approximately 75% of the patients are younger than the age of 30 years [5]. Very rarely, it can be found in a quiet old patient (Fig. 16.3).

W.-J. Bahk, *Diagnosis and Management of Primary Bone Tumors*,
https://doi.org/10.1007/978-981-96-3484-2_16

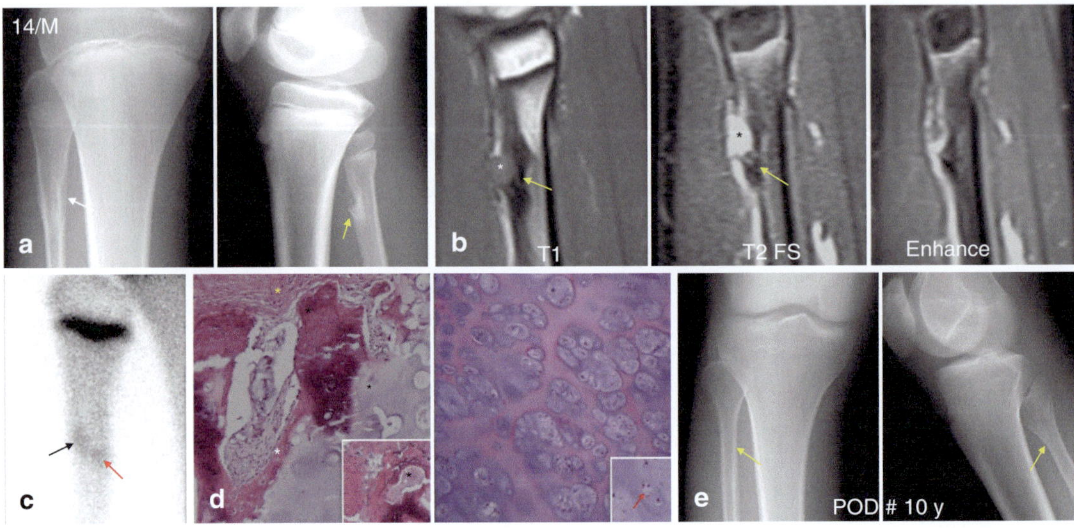

Fig. 16.1 (**a**) Radiograph taken for right knee pain of 3 months' duration in a 14-year-old boy shows an ill-defined hazy predominantly lytic lesion in the proximal fibula (white arrow). Lateral view clearly reveals a radiolucent small mass lesion with scanty internal punctuated calcification on the surface of the proximal fibula, which results in well-demarcated cortical erion with periosteal solid buttress, producing a typical *saucer-shaped* defect (yellow arrow). (**b**) MR images reveal a well-defined periosteal small mass measuring 2 cm in diameter (asterisks) with intermediate SI on T1-weighted image and high SI on T2-weighted image. The mass is covered by an elevated periosteum. Note erosion of underlying cortical surface as well as periosteal solid buttress and irregular thick rim of reactive bone with low SI on both sequences (yellow arrows). The cortex remains intact, with no bone marrow invasion and reactive marrow edema. The lesion is focally enhanced by contrast medium. (**c**) Pinhole bone scan notes a mild uptake at the site of "*saucer-shaped*" defect and mass, with possible mild reactive uptake in the proximal fibula (black arrow). (**d**) Microscopic examination shows a hyaline cartilage matrix with bland chondrocytes, which is bordered by reactive bone (white asterisk) beneath the periosteum (yellow asterisk). Small satellite nodules of cellular hyaline cartilage are seen within the peripheral sclerotic bone (black asterisk in inset) by tangential cut of marginal irregularity, which should not be interpreted as local invasiveness. Higher-power magnification reveals high cellularity with nuclear enlargement and prominent nucleoli as well as bi-nucleation (red arrow in inset). (**e**) Follow-up radiograph at 10 years after complete marginal excision reveals no evidence of recurrence with complete remodeling of the affected bone (arrows)

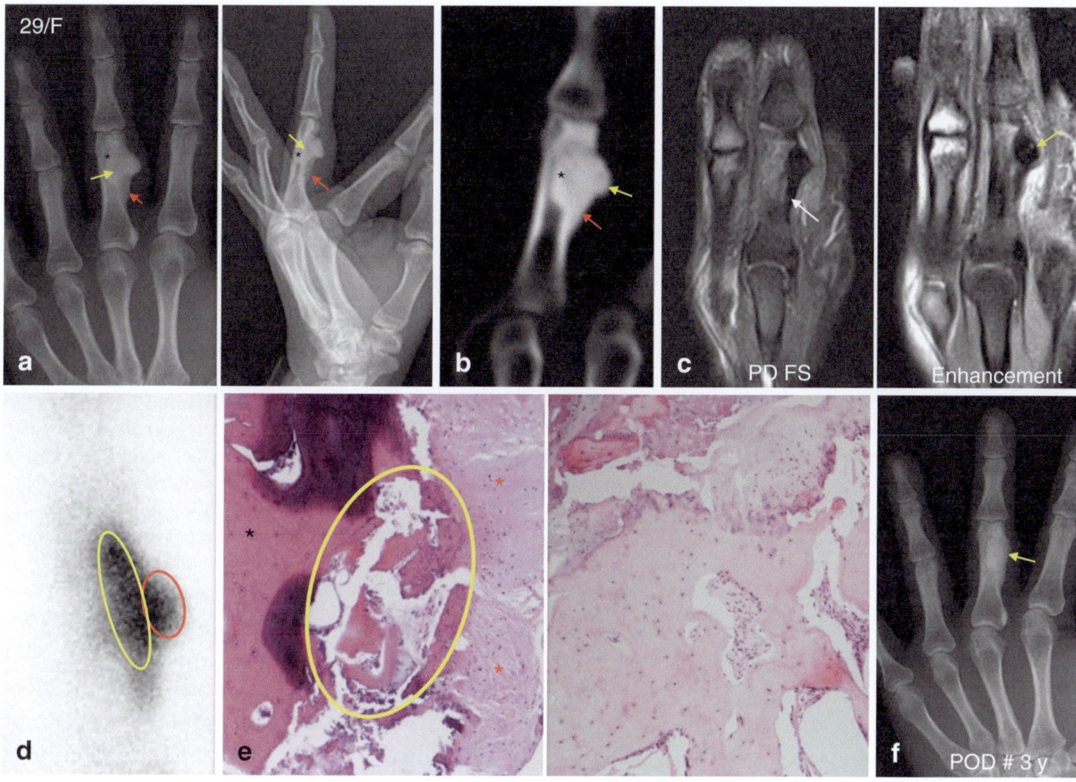

Fig. 16.2 (**a**) Radiographs taken for mass with mild pain at the left middle finger of 6 months' duration in a 31-year-old young lady show a well-defined, small, juta-cortical, outgrowing, densely mineralized mass arising from th eproximal aphlanx. The lesion is associated with sclerotic hyperostosis of medullary cavity (black asterisks), suggesting incidentally found melorheostosis of the underlying host bone. There is a linear radiolucency resembling "*saucer-like*" defect between the ecophytic mass and sclerotic medullary cavity (yellow arrows), indicating PC. Additionally, a periosteal thick solid buttress of reactive bone is noted (red arrows). (**b**) CT scan confirms the same findings observed on plain radiographs. (**c**) MR image demonstrates a well-defined outgrowing small mass on the thick sclerotic cortex (white arrow) with dark SI and tiny dots of high signal on fat suppression Proton density image. The lesion presents a tiny focal enhancement (yellow arrow). (**d**) Pinhole bone scan demonstrates a localized hot uptake in the protruding mass (red circle) and in the sclerotic medullary lesion (yellow circle). (**e**) Microscopic examination: (Left) Lower-power magnification shows several hyaline cartilage nodules with bland chondrocytes (red asterisks), which erode the underlying thickened host lamellar bone (black asterisk). There are several distorted pieces of lamellar bone by curettage procedure due to unclear cleavage between the tumor and underlying host cortex (yellow circle). (Right) Higher-power magnification reveals a cartilage nodule with low cellularity and bland chondrocytes. (**f**) Follow-up radiograph at 3 years after surgery reveals no evidence of recurrence and no interval change of concurrent sclerotic medullary lesion of melorheostosis (arrow)

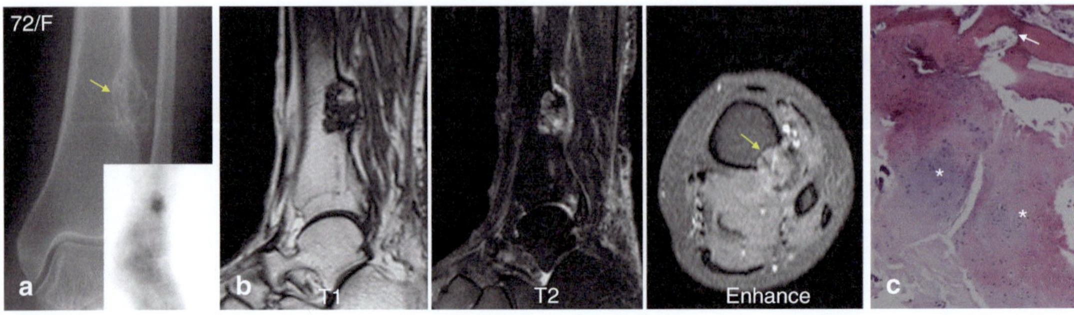

Fig. 16.3 *Quiet old patient.* (**a**) Radiograph taken for swelling with intermittent mild pain of left ankle of 1 year's duration in a 72-year-old woman shows a well-defined, eccentric, juxta-cortical, lytic mass with internal trabeculation and punctate calcification, with underlying cortical sclerosis forming a *crater-like* excavator (arrow). Bone scan reveals a focal increased uptake (inset). (**b**) MR images demonstrate a well-circumscribed, eccentric, juxta-cortical mass with an irregular sclerotic outer margin in the distal tibia. The mass presents low SI with focal high signal on T1-weighted image and intermediate to high SI with internal dark signal of calcification on T2-weighted image. The mass is covered by an elevated periosteum. Post-contrast image portrays heterogeneously enhanced mass overhanging the intact underlying cortex (yellow arrow). (**c**) Microscopic examination shows hyaline cartilage nodules with bland chondrocytes (asterisks) surrounded by reactive lamellar bones at the periphery (arrow) and pieces of host lamellar bone which are fragmented and distorted by curettage

16.5 Location

Lesions are most commonly located adjacent to the metaphysis in the long bones (55%), followed by short tubular bones of hand and foot (40%) [5]. The proximal humerus is the single most common site, representing about half of the cases [4]. Rarely, other bones such as pelvis, spine, or rib can be also involved.

16.6 Clinical Features

The most common presentation is a palpable hard mass or bump with or without mild pain, often of long duration. The presence of pain in adult patients may suggest aggressive biologic bahavior, as seen in other cartilaginous tumors. Rarely, PC can be discovered incidentally on radiographs taken for unrelated reasons.

16.7 Radiologic Findings

Plain radiograph PC is a well-defined, eccentric, predominantly radiolucent lesion located on the cortical surface of bone beneath the periosteum, in the so-called *periosteal* or *juxtacortical* area, often with punctuate to heavy calcification. However, some lesions can be purely lytic without calcification. And, a discernible soft tissue mass may be seen in some cases. Smaller lesion tends to be roud to oval in shape while lager ones are oblong or elongated, parallel to the long axis of the affected bone. The size of the lesion has been reported to range from 1 cm to 6.5 cm a mean diameter of 2.6 cm in one series [1]. The lesion typically exhibits a thin cortical shell and/or internal calcifications in a *ring and arcs* or *popcorn-like* pattern, indicating a cartilage tumor. Typically, the underlying host cortex is sharply eroded and sclerotic, with elevated edge formed by a thick solid buttress of reactive bone producing a crater-like excavator, referred to as *saucer-shaped* defect, result from a chronic compression and stimulation by the longstanding mass (Figs. 16.1a and 16.3a). The excavated cortex is usually not destroyed without medullary extension, which clearly delineate the mass from the medullary cavity (Fig. 16.2a). A rim of subcortical sclerosis beneath the lesion is often seen. **Bone scan** shows heterogeneous mild to strong uptake in most cases (Figs. 16.1, 16.2, and 16.3). **CT scan** more clearly demonstrates an extra-skeletal mass with a cartilaginous matrix or focal scattered calcification and intact underlying host cortex with no intramedullary extension. **MR Findings** The lesion appears as a well-defined, multilobulated, soft tissue mass abutting the cortex with low to intermediate SI on T1-weighted images and high to bright SI on T2-weighted images, with internal dark signals of calcification on both sequences, and better demonstrate a pressure erosion of neighboring bone. A typical *crater-like* excavation or *saucer-shaped* defect with intact cortical bone is clearly visualized. In general, the mass is covered by an elevated periosteum (Figs. 16.1, 16.2, and 16.3). Edema in marrow cavity or adjacent soft tissue may be rarely observed, and it can be mistaken for tumor extension if presents. The lesion is heterogeneously and peripherally enhanced, or only focally enhanced in certain cases.

16.8 Histologic Findings

Low-magnification shows a lobular arrangement consisting of hyaline to myxoid cartilage, surrounded by dense fibrous tissue and/or reactive lamellar bone. The mass is well-demarcated from the underlying sclerotic cortex which is focally scalloped and eroded. However, the typical arrangement of periosteum, cartilage tumor mass, and host lamella bones may be severely fragmented and distorted by curettage procedure. The periosteum and underlying host cortex are frequently not visible in curetted specimens. The tumor never permeates the eroded cortex, but some tumor cartilage can be microscopically seen to bulge into the underlying medullary cavity, separated by a border of intervening lamellar bone. Small satellite nodules of cellular hyaline cartilage can be seen in the peripheral sclerotic border due to tangential cut of marginal irregularity, which should not be interpreted as local invasiveness [4] (Fig. 16.1d). The lesion typically consists of lobules of hyaline cartilage surrounded by a partial to complete lamellar bone suggesting benignancy (Figs. 16.2e and 16.3c). Often, the cartilage component is arranged in a lobular pattern surrounded by a fibroperiosteal tissue [5]. Cellularity varies from low to very high. The individual chondrocytes are mostly bland-looking as other chondromas, but occasionally show focal mild atypia with high cellularity, nuclear plumpness, prominent nucleoli, and bi-nucleation [1, 5]. However, the nuclei never exhibit features of unequivocal anaplasia, including abnormal mitotic figures.

16.9 Management

Asymptomatic lesion can be observed with periodic monitoring following histologic confirmation if necessary. Thorough curettage or complete excision of cartilaginous mass with reasonable margin of healthy tissue is the preferred method of management for symptomatic lesion. En-bloc excision with marginal or wide margin guarantees healing. However, intralesional removal is enough for a high success rate if removal is complete [7].

16.10 Clinical Course

Recurrence is very rare regardless of the surgery type if the surgical removal is complete [1, 2, 7] (Figs. 16.1 and 16.3). However, recurrence may occur following incomplete removal, and a recurrence rate of 3.6% (6 of 165 cases) was reported in a literature review [2].

References

1. Bauer TW, Dorfman HD, Latham JT Jr. Periosteal chondroma. A clinicopathologic study of 23 cases. Am J Surg Pathol. 1982;6(7):631–7.
2. Lewis MM, Kenan S, Yabut SM, Norman A, Steiner G. Periosteal chondroma: a report of ten cases and review of the literature. Clin Orthop Relat Res. 1990;256:185–92.
3. Nojima T, Unni KK, McLeod RA, Pritchard DJ. Periosteal chondroma and periosteal chondrosarcoma. Am J Surg Pathol. 1985;9(9):666–77.

4. Czerniak B. Benign cartilage lesions. In: Dorfman HD, Czerniak B, editors. Dorfman and Czerniak's bone tumors. 2nd ed. eBook: Elsevier; 2016. p. 356–473.
5. Mirra JM. Parosteal chondroma. In: Mirra JM, editor. Bone tumors: clinical, radiologic, and pathologic correlations. 2nd ed. Philadelphia: Lea & Febiger; 1989. p. 1673–83.
6. Boriani S, Bacchini P, Bertoni F, Campanacci M. Periosteal chondroma. A review of twenty cases. J Bone Joint Surg. 1983;65(2):205–12.
7. Campanacci M. Periosteal chondroma. In: Campanacci M, editor. Bone and soft tissue tumors. Wien New York: Springer-Verlag; 1999. p. 229–33.

Subungual Exostosis

17

(***sub***- "under" + ***ungual*** "pertaining to unguis (nail)" + ***ex***- "out of" + ***ostosis*** "osteogenesis")

17.1 Definition

Subungual exostosis (SE) is a rare, benign, outgrowing, osteocartilaginous tumor that is firmly attached to the tip of the distal phalanx underneath the nail bed.

17.2 Synonym

Dupuytren exostosis.

17.3 Incidence

The incidence is relatively rare, accounting for less than 1% of all bone tumors in the Mayo Clinic series [1].

17.4 Age

Most patients are adolescents and young adults with a peak incidence in the second and third decades of life [1]. An extensive review of 13 studies comprising 10 or more patients reported that about half of the patients were younger than 18 years of age with average age of 25.7 years [2].

17.5 Location

SE can develop from the distal phalanx of any finger or toe beneath the nail bed. In the toes, it most frequently affects the great toe representing 80% of reported cases, followed by the second toe (6%), third toe (7%), fourth toe (5%), and fifth toe (2%) [2]. In another literature review, only 21 of 203 cases (10%) occurred in the fingers [3].

17.6 Clinical Features

Although the etiology is unknown, it probably results from spindle cell metaplasia, likely induced by mechanical irritations and/or inflammatory stimuli such as ingrown nail or microtrauma. Patients with SE often give a history of trauma, repeated or chronic infection at the site of subungual lump [1]. Painful mass or swelling with inflammation, caused by pressure on the nail bed or plate, is the most common clinical presentation. Frequently, nail deformity and/or nail bed ulceration with erythema, discharge, or bleeding is observed, especially in longstanding cases (Figs. 17.1, 17.2, and 17.3), which may result in a deleterious impact on quality of life. In addition, the condition is reported to be misdiagnosed as

W.-J. Bahk, *Diagnosis and Management of Primary Bone Tumors*,
https://doi.org/10.1007/978-981-96-3484-2_17

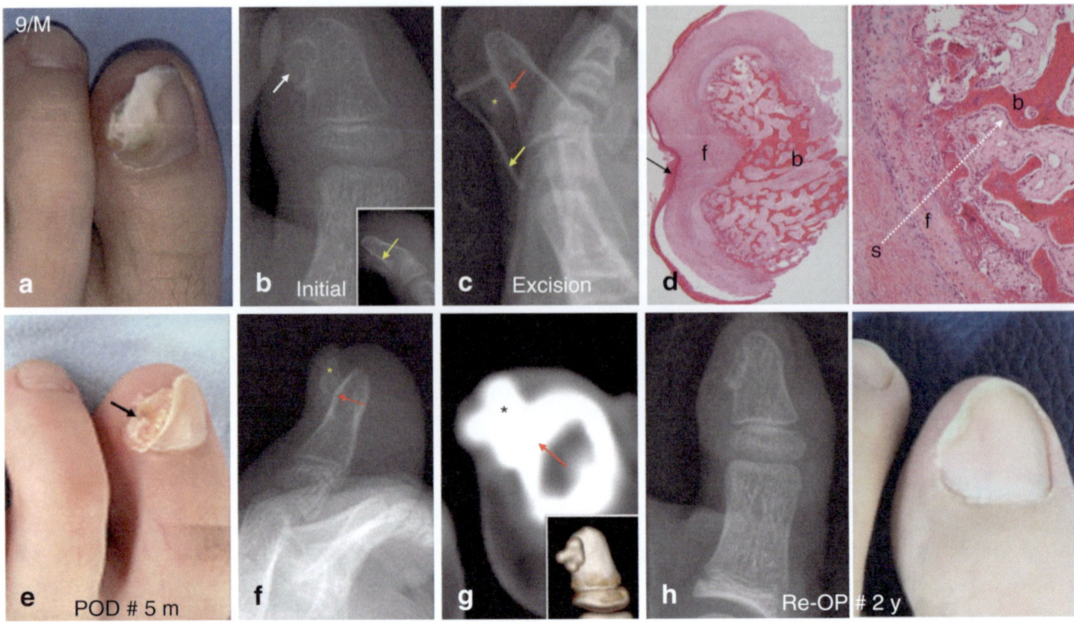

Fig. 17.1 (**a**) A 9-year-old boy presented with a slowly growing subungual mass with deformity and whitish discoloration of 1 year's duration affecting the left great toe. (**b**) Radiograph shows a well-defined, broad-based, outgrowing mass attached to the distal phalanx (white arrow). The underlying cortex is intact, and there is contiuity with the host cortical and medullary bone, referred to as "*flaring*" appearance, that is pathognomonic for SO (yellow arrow in inset). (**c**) Immediate postoperative radiograph reveals a hazy mass shadow (asterisk), indicating incomplete excision. Note the clearly visible intact host cortex with no communication with medullary cavity (red arrow). You can see the inserted silastic drain as well (yellow arrow). (**d**) Microscopic examination: (Left) Low-power magnification shows a small mass consisting of callus-like bony trabeculae (b), which is covered by a fibrocartilage cap (f) with epidermal tissue in the outermost layer of the mass (black arrow). (Right) Medium-power magnification reveals a transformation of peripheral spindle cells (s) directly to fibrocartilage (f) and then to trabecular bone spicules (b) with prominent osteoblastic rimming (dotted long arrow) and loosely arranged, bland-looking spindle cells in the intertrabecular spaces. (**e**) The patient presents a recurrent mass at 5 months after surgery (black arrow). (**f**) Radiograph and (**g**) CT scan demonstrate a recurrent mass (asterisks) with intact underlying cortex but no continuity to medullary cavity (arrows). (**h**) Follow-up radiograph at 2 years after re-excision shows no recurrent mass and the nail is nearly normal-looking as well

ordinary verrucae, mycoses, or pyogenic disease in about 80% of the cases [4], which might delay a correct diagnosis. There has been debate whether subungual osteochondroma (SO) is the same clinical entity as SE because the histologic and radiologic findings are different in some cases (Figs. 17.1 and 17.2) but similar and overlapping in other cases (Fig. 17.3) (refer Chap. 13, Fig. 13.9).

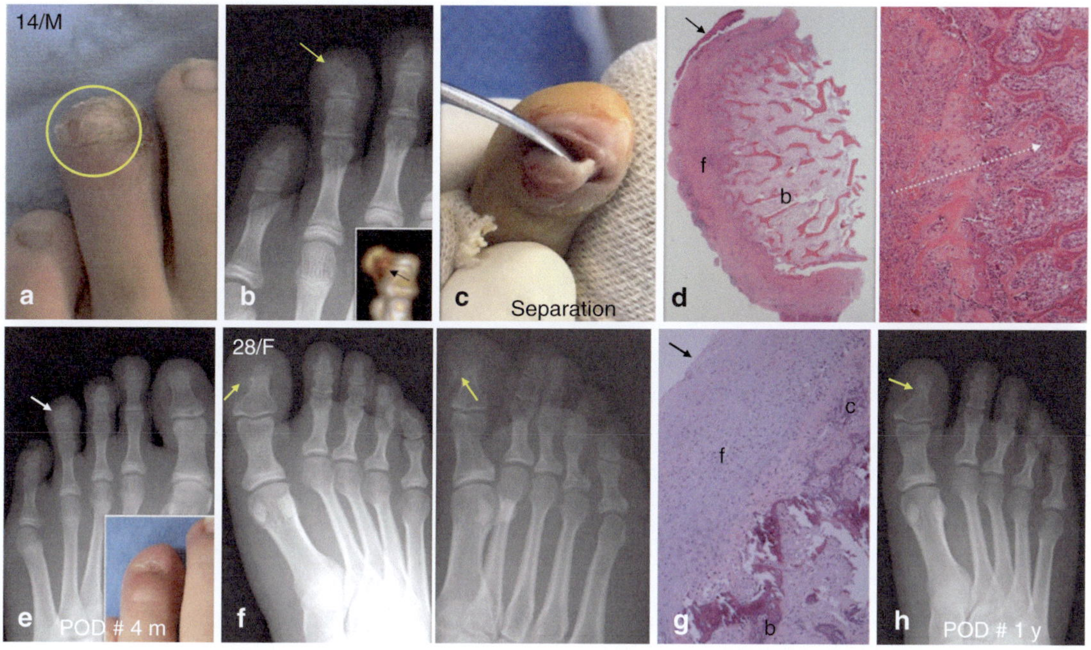

Fig. 17.2 (**a**) A 14-year-old boy presented with a subungual hard mass and nail deformity of 4 months' duration and recently developed superimposed infection with pus discharge in the left fourth toe (circle). (**b**) Radiograph shows a broad-based dense mass projecting from the lateral aspect of the distal phalanx (yellow arrow). The mass has no clear continuation with the medullary cavity of underlying bone on CT scan (inset). (**c**) The infected mass with pus is carefully separated from the nail bed and completely excised using a small elevator after nail extraction. (**d**) Microscopic examination: (Left) Low-power magnification reveals a well-defined osseo-cartilaginous mass consisting of fibrocartilage cap (f) and callus-like trabecular bone (b) underneath the cap. The epidermal tissue is nearly detached with a focal residual tissue (black arrow). (Right) Medium-power magnification shows a transformation of hypercellular peripheral spindle cells to fibrocartilage and then to trabecular bone spicules (dotted long arrow). (**e**) Follow-up radiograph at 4 months after surgery shows a tiny residual mass (arrow). However, the nail looks near normal with control of superimposed infection (inset), and the patient is doing well without pain. (**f**) Radiograph taken for subungual painful hard mass of right great toe for 2 months in a 28-year-old lady shows an ill-defined hazy exophytic mass with intact host cortex without a cortico-medullary continuity in the distal phalanx (arrows). (**g**) Microscopic examination reveals a small OC-like mass covered with a fibrocartilage cap (f) formed directly from the fibrous tissue (black arrow). The fibrocartilage gradually undergoes calcification (c) and produces callus-like trabecular bone spicules (b). (**h**) Follow-up radiograph at 1 year after surgery notes no local recurrence (arrow)

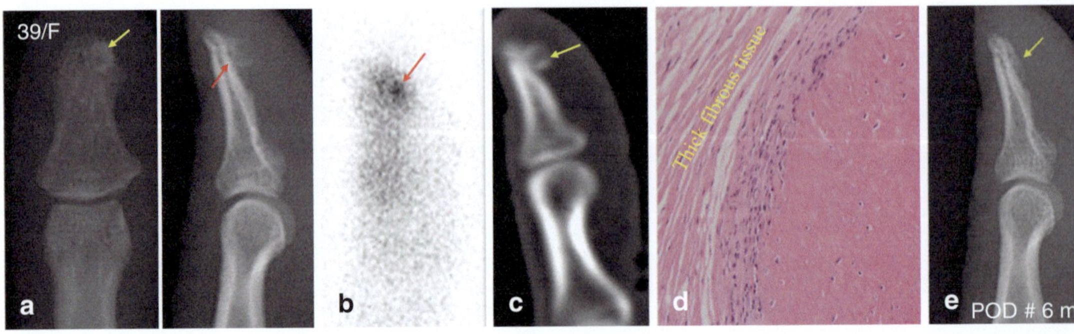

Fig. 17.3 (**a**) Radiographs taken for pain of right thumb on touch or pressure in a 39-year-old lady show a tiny outgrowing bony mass from volo-ulna aspect of distal phalanx (yellow arrow). The underlying cortex is intact, and there is no continuity with medullary cavity (red arrow). (**b**) Pinhole bone scan reveals focal uptake in the tip of the distal phalanx. (**c**) CT scan reveals a tiny projecting bony mass attached to the intact cortex without definite continuity with marrow cavity and cartilage cap (yellow arrow). (**d**) Histologic examination of excised mass demonstrates a fibrocartilage cap produced directly from proliferating fibrous tissue of the nail bed, favoring a diagnosis of SE rather than SO, considering the finding of "*paste-on*" appearance on plain radiograph and CT scan. (**e**) Follow-up radiograph at 6 months after surgery shows no evidence of recurrence

17.7 Radiologic Findings

A well-circumscribed, broad-based, pedunculated dense mass is almost invariably connected to the intact distal phalanx. However, there is usually no clear continuity between the mass and the medullary cavity, so-called "flaring" appearance, that is pathognomonic for SO (Figs. 17.1, 17.2, and 17.3).

17.8 Histologic Findings

SE consists of a bony stalk covered by a fibrocartilage cap associated with or without hyaline cartilage, and the bone spicules are made directly from the fibrous tissue of the nail bed (Figs. 17.1d, 17.2, and 17.3d). The cap is surrounded by proliferating fibrous connective tissue rather than a periosteum. The callus-like trabecular bone is formed directly from fibrous tissue or through endochondral ossification, and is usually not continuous with the medullary cavity of the bone it arises from. The trabecular bone can be formed by an endochondral mechanism similar to that of SO in some cases, although more often the mechanism is of the intramembranous or mixed type [3]. In contrast, SO consists of pure hyaline cartilage and trabecular bones derived from endochondral ossification, which is characteristically continuous with the medullary cavity of the host bone. Medium-power magnification reveals a gradual transformation of peripheral fibrous connective tissue to cartilage and then to trabecular bone. The cartilage gradually undergoes calcification at the basal layer. The thickness of the cartilaginous cap is determined by the age of the lesion. In the early stage, immature SE usually shows a thick cellular cartilaginous tissue with proliferating fibrous tissue from the nail bed. However, an interconnecting network of irregular trabecular bone with a prominent osteoblastic rimming dominates the mass with a thinned or even absent cartilage cap in later stage. Higher-power magnification of the cartilage cap may demonstrate high cellularity with nuclear plumpness, bi-nucleated chondrocytes, and occasional mitoses, which may simulate malignancy. An inadequate biopsy sample taken from the peripheral area of the mass, showing only a small portion of the cartilage component with such atypical findings can make a misdiagnosis of chondrosarcoma. However, definite features of anaplasia, including abnormal mitoses, is never observed.

17.9 Management

Surgical treatment consists of careful separation of the mass from the nail bed and complete excision, followed by meticulous wound closure to minimize postoperative onycholysis or nail deformity. Nail extraction may be necessary in severely deformed and infected cases (Fig. 17.2c).

17.10 Clinical Course

SE is usually curative by complete surgical excision. Recurrence is more likely to occur more likely after incomplete surgical excision (Fig. 17.1e), which can be cured by second excision (Fig. 17.1h). In a Mayo Clinic series of 44 patients, 5 patients (11%) had local recurrence [5].

References

1. Unni KK, Inwards CY. Subungual exostoses. In: Unni KK, Inwards CY, editors. Dahlin's bone tumors: general aspects and data on 10,165 cases. 6th ed. Philadelphia: Lippincott William & Wilkins; 2010. p. 17–8.
2. DaCambra MP, Gupta SK, Ferri-de-Barros F. Subungual exostosis of the toes: a systematic review. Clin Orthop Relat Res. 2014;472(4):1251–9.
3. Hoehn JG, Coletta C. Subungual exostosis of the fingers. J Hand Surg. 1992;17(3):468–71.
4. Ippolito E, Falez F, Tudisco C, Balus L, Fazio M, Morrone A, Subungual exostosis. Histological and clinical considerations on 30 cases. Ital J Orthop Traumatol. 1987;13(1):81–7.
5. Landon G, Johnson K, Dahlin D. Subungual exostoses. J Bone Joint Surg Am. 1979;61(2):256–9.

18 Bizarre Parosteal Osteochondromatous Proliferation (Nora's Lesion)

18.1 Definition

Bizarre parosteal osteochondromatous proliferation (BPOP) is a benign but locally aggressive exophytic reactive lesion typically on the bone surface beneath the periosteum, which may simulate a bone tumor. In 1983, Nora et al. [1] first reported BPOP of the hands and feet, which are radiologically and histologically resembling osteochondroma (OC) but distinctive.

18.2 Synonym

Nora's disease or lesion.

18.3 Incidence

BPOP is very uncommon, and the incidence is not exactly known.

18.4 Location

In the original article by Nora et al. [1], the lesions exclusively affect the short tubular bones of the hands and feet. The lesion is much more frequent in the hands than feet. Later studies in the same Clinic reported that it most commonly involved phalanges of the hand (55%) and foot (15%), and the rest affected mostly the long bones (26%) [2, 3].

18.5 Age

BPOP can occur in various age groups, but it is most often seen in adolescents and young adults between the second and fourth decades of life [2, 4, 5].

18.6 Clinical Features

Occasionally, BPOP can be asymptomatic and incidentally found. Most patients present with swelling or small mass with or without mild pain that slowly grows over months to years. However, the mass may grow rapidly in some cases. Range of motion of the adjacent joints can be limited. The lesion is often mistaken for a malignant tumor because of aggressive clinical features of occasional rapid growth potential and high recurrence rate as well as atypical histologic appearance. In general, patients do not recall a traumatic episode.

W.-J. Bahk, *Diagnosis and Management of Primary Bone Tumors*,
https://doi.org/10.1007/978-981-96-3484-2_18

18.7 Radiologic Findings

Plain radiograph The findings are usually characteristic to distinguish BPOP from many of its mimickers without biopsy [6, 7]. The lesion is a well-delineated, irregular, round to mushroom-shaped, densely calcified, small nodular mass attached to the surface of the bone with a broad base. The mass outgrows into the soft tissues without breaching the cortex. Typically, there is no continuity with medullary cavity, so-called *paste-on* appearance (Figs. 18.1, 18.2, and 18.3), which is critically different from OC. Sometimes, a radiolucent plane of separation is clearly visible between the lesion and bone, which allows the *paste-on* appearance more distinct (Figs. 18.2A and 18.3A). **Bone scan** may show a focal hot uptake (Fig. 18.1C). **CT scan** can more clearly demnostrate a well-defined, oval to mushroom-shaped, small mass with no medullary or cortical

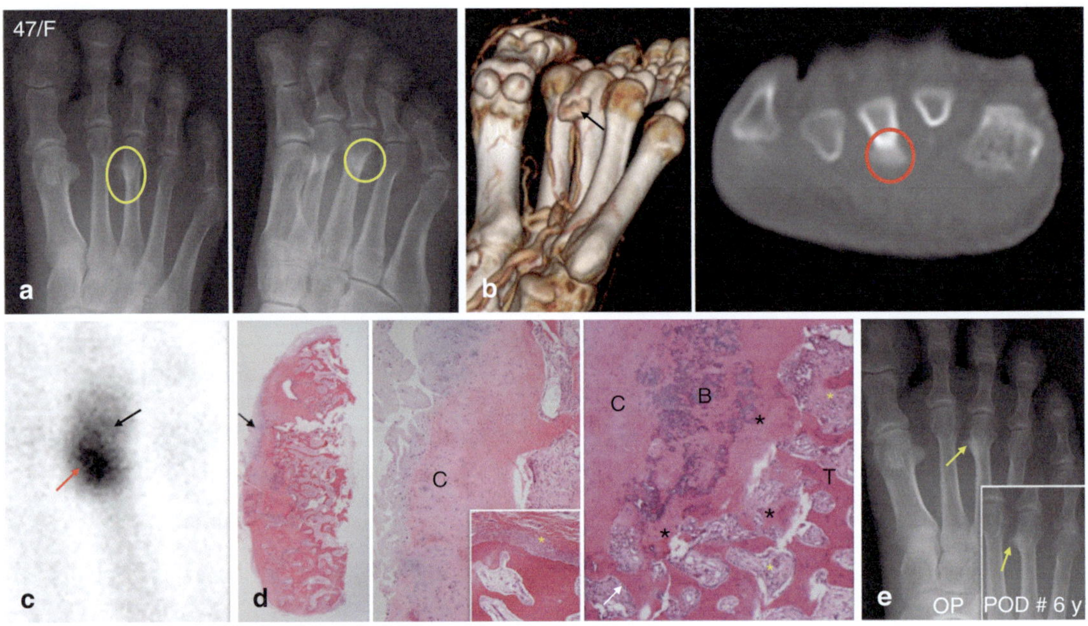

Fig. 18.1 (**A**) Radiographs taken for right forefoot pain on weight bearing of 7–8 years' duration in a 47-year-old woman show an ill-defined, irregular, hazy, dense mass attached to the third metatarsal neck (yellow circles). (**B**) 3D CT scan reveals a well-defined, round to oval, sclerotic mass projecting from the plantar surface of the third metacarpal neck (arrow). There is no cortical and medullary continuation between the mass and the underlying host bone, so-called *paste-on* the cortex appearance (red circle). (**C**) Pinhole bone scan reveals a hot uptake in the mass (red arrow) as well as surrounding milder reactive uptake (black arrow). (**D**) Microscopic examination: (Left) The scan view demonstrates a small nodular mass consisting of an irregular thin cartilage cap (black arrow) and trabecular bone spicules with interposed spindle cell proliferation mimicking OC. (Middle) Medium-power magnification reveals a hyaline cartilage cap with moderate cellularity of chondrocytes (C), which are arranged in a more disorganized fashion. Another field shows bland-looking fibrous tissue (asterisk) and woven bone spicules but no cartilage component (inset). (Right) The stalk under a cartilage cap consists of trabecular bones rimmed by prominent osteoblasts (T). The intertrabecular spaces are filled with abundant reactive fibrous tissue, fat, and vessels (asterisks). There is a peculiar deep blue to purple-colored bones (B), so-called *blue bone*, between the cartilage cap and the bone stalk, which is focal in this case. (**E**) Immediate postoperative radiograph reveals a tiny residual mass (arrow) due to incomplete excision. However, follow-up radiograph at 6 years after surgery shows no interval growth of the residual mass (arrow in inset), and she is free of symptom

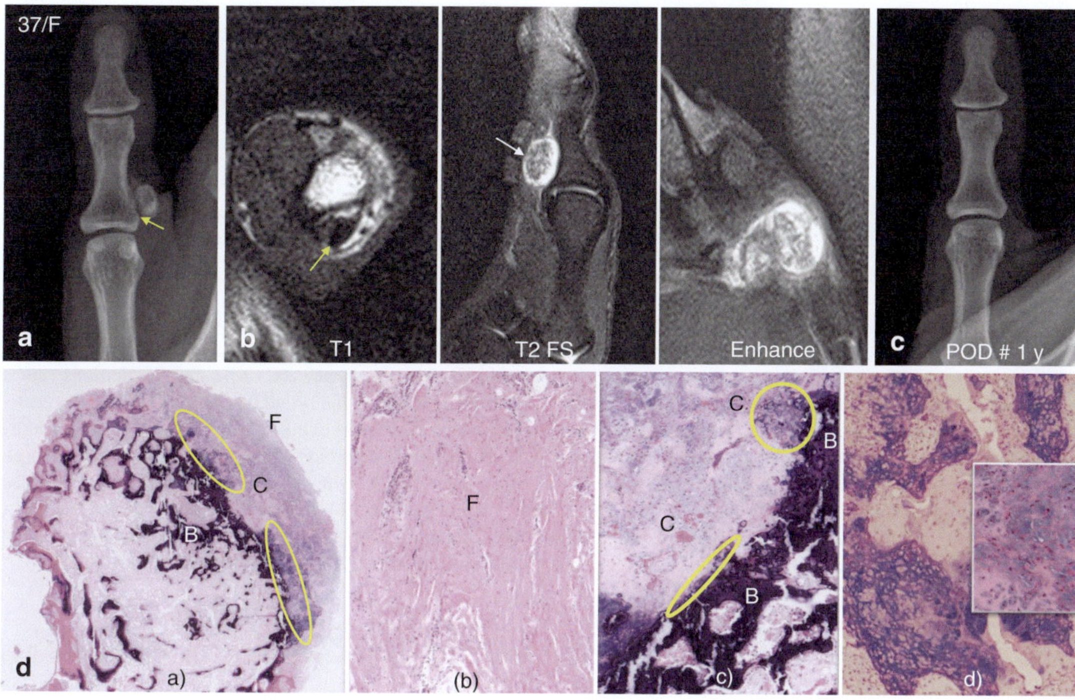

Fig. 18.2 (**A**) Radiographs taken for slowly growing mass of left thumb for 2 years' duration in a 37-year-old woman show a well-demarcated, small, round to oval, densely ossified, nodular mass attached to the proximal phalanx. A clearly visible radiolucent plane of separation between the lesion and the underlying cortex allows the *paste-on* appearance more distinct (arrow). (**B**) MR images reveal a well-defined small nodular mass (arrows) with low SI on T1-weighted image and heterogeneous intermediate and high SI surrounded by a thin bright signal of caftilage cap (white arrow) on fat-saturated T2-weighted image. There are multiple dots of dark signal on both sequences. The mass is heterogeneously enhanced by contrast medium. (**C**) Follow-up radiograph at 1 year after complete excision notes no evidence of local recurrence. (**D**) Microscopic examination: **a**) Low-power magnification shows a well-defined small nodular mass composed of a thin outermost layer of fibrous tissue (F), hyaline cartilage cap (C), and trabecular bone spicules (B) with a prominent fibrous matrix between the trabeculae. The bone component is located within the basal and central area, and the cartilage forms an irregular cap-like structure at the periphery of the lesion, producing a peculiar zonal architecture. There is a characteristic light blue to purple-colored tissue, so-called *blue bone* (circles), between the cartilage cap (C) and the deep purple trabecular bone spicules (B). **b**) The fibrous tissue layer (F) is hypocellular, and the cells are arranged in short intersecting fascicles. **c**) The cartilage cap (C) contains a higher number of chondrocytes arranged in a disorganized pattern. The cartilage of deeper base area undergoes endochondral ossification to form irregularly distributed trabeculae of woven bone. Note the early stage of blue bone formation (circles) between cartilage (C) and he poorly decalcified, deeply basophilic underlying bone spicules (B). **d**) Higher-power magnification following appropriate re-decalcification reveals a mixture of abundant *blue bone* and cartilage with high cellularity and mild cytolgic atypia (inset)

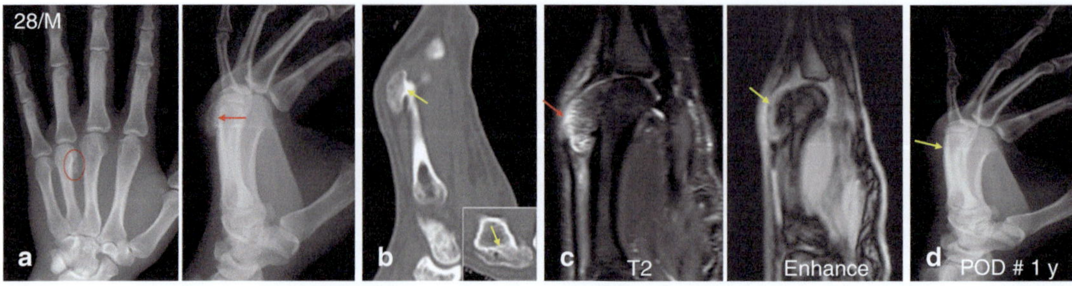

Fig. 18.3 (**A**) Radiograph taken for a mass over the right fourth knuckle of 3 years' duration in a 28-year-old man shows an ill-defined irregular, round to oval, dense nodular mass attached to the fourth metacarpal head (red circle). Lateral view reveals a well-defined, bean-shaped, dense mass with intact underlying host cortex and clearly visible radiolucent cleavage plane between the lesion and the naive bone (red arrow). (**B**) CT scan better delineates a well-defined, small, mushroom-shaped, dense mass attached to the dorsal surface of the underlying intact bone without continuation with the medullary cavity (arrows), thereby producing a "paste-on" (keep Italic & double quotation mark) appearance. (**C**) MR images demonstrate a protruding mass with a broad base attachment to the cortical surface. The mass exhibits heterogeneously intermediate and high SI covered with a thin cartilage cap of high bright signal on T2-weighted image (red arrow). The mass is peripherally well-enhanced by the contrast medium (yellow arrow). (**D**) Follow-up radiograph at 1 year after complete excision reveals no evidence of recurrence

continuity between the lesion and underlying host bone (Figs. 18.1B and 18.3B). **MR images** also present clearly a typical *paste-on* appearance of the mass with low to intermediate SI on T1-weighted image and heterogeneous signal in the deeper area with bright SI of a thin cartilage cap on T2-weighted image (Figs. 18.2B and 18.3C). There can be mild soft tissue edema around the lesion. The mass is heterogeneously enhanced by contrast medium.

18.8 Histologic Findings

The lesion is a well-circumscribed mass composed of varying proportion of fibrous tissue, cartilage cap, and bone stalk, simulating OC (Figs. 18.1D and 18.2D). However, there is a characteristic "*blue bone*" between cartilage cap and bone stalk, which is not observed in OC. The mass is usually smaller than 3 cm in diameter and often presents in a more disorganized pattern than OC. Reactive fibrous tissue may cover the outer layer of the cartilage cap. The fibroblastic cells are usually hypercellular and arranged in short intersecting fascicles, but the fibrous layer can be often absent. Cartilage cap consists of variably calcified hyaline cartilage with an irregular cartilage-bone interface. The cartilage is also usually hypercellular and matures into trabecular bones via endochondral ossification. The matrix between cartilage cap and bone stalk presents a peculiar deep blue to purple tinctorial appearance of *blue bone*, even after adequate decalcification (Figs. 18.1D and 18.2D). Cocks et al. [4] yielded a ratio of bone, cartilage, and fibrous tissue as well as *blue bone* in each case by histomorphometric quantification using Adobe Photoshop. Bone and/or cartilage components can be not seen in some cases. The portion of bone varied widely among specimens, ranging from 0% to 75% with a mean of 21%. Cartilage tissue was similarly variable, ranging from 0% to 55% with mean of 23%. Amount of fibrous tissue spanned from 15% to 70% with a mean of 35%. The percentage of *blue bone* ranged from 5% to 30% of cases with a mean of 20%. They concluded BPOP exhibited a highly heterogeneous tissue composition, and the presence of *blue bone* as well as a significant fibrous component may be useful to diagnose BPOP. However, it is not pathognomonic because a similar matrix has been described in other entities. A similar "blue reticulated chondroid-like material" was described in aneurysmal bone cysts [8], and "spiculate blue bone" was observed in osteoblastoma [9, 10].

Frequently, chondrocytes exhibit moderately atypical appearance with plump nucleus, hyperchromatism, distinct nucleoli. and frequent binucleation (*bizarre* proliferation) that can be mistaken for chondrosarcoma (CSA). However, significant atypism and abnormal mitoses are never seen. Hypervascular tissues with bland-looking spindle cell proliferation but no marrow component fill the spaces between trabeculae. Due to such bizarre proliferation, clinical-radiologic-pathologic correlation is essential for a correct diagnosis of BPOP.

18.9 Management

Complete excision is recommended to reduce local recurrence as well as to obtain an adequate specimen for histologic confirmation.

18.10 Clinical Course

Recurrence rate has been reported from 25% [11] to over 50% [1, 2]. About 20% had more than one recurrence [3]. In spite of the high rate of recurrence and a disturbing histologic appearance including marked proliferative activity, enlarged or bi-nucleated chondrocytes mimicking CSA, behavior as a malignant tumor is either exceedingly rare or nonexistent [1].

References

1. Nora FE, Dahlin DC, Beabout JW. Bizarre parosteal osteochondromatous proliferations of the hands and feet. Am J Surg Pathol. 1983;7(3):245–50.
2. Meneses MF, Unni KK, Swee RG. Bizarre parosteal osteochondromatous proliferation of bone (Nora's lesion). Am J Surg Pathol. 1993;17(7):691–7.
3. Unni KK, Inwards CY. Bizarre parosteal osteochondromatous proliferation. In: Unni KK, Inwards CY, editors. Dahlin's bone tumors: general aspects and data on 10,165 Cases. 6th ed. Philadelphia: Lippincott William & Wilkins; 2010. p. 18–21.
4. Cocks M, Helmke E, Meyers CA, Fayad L, McCarthy E, James AW. Bizarre parosteal osteochondromatous proliferation: 16 Cases with a focus on histologic variability. J Orthop. 2018;15(1):138–42.
5. Flint JH, McKay PL. Bizarre parosteal osteochondromatous proliferation and periosteal chondroma: a comparative report and review of the literature. J Hand Surg Am. 2007;32(6):893–8.
6. Dhondt E, Oudenhoven L, Khan S, Kroon H, Nieborg A, Bloem J, et al. Nora's lesion, a distinct radiological entity? Skeletal Radiol. 2006;35(7):497–502.
7. Torreggiani WC, Munk PL, Al-Ismail K, O'Connell JX, Nicolaou S, Lee MJ, et al. MR imaging features of bizarre parosteal osteochondromatous proliferation of bone (Nora's lesion). Eur J Radiol. 2001;40(3):224–31.
8. Bahk WJ, Mirra JM. Differential diagnostic value of "blue reticulated chondroid-like material" in aneurysmal bone cysts: a classic histopathologic analysis of 215 cases. Am J Clin Pathol. 2015;143(6):823–9.
9. Lucas DR, Unni KK, McLeod RA, O'Connor MI, Sim FH. Osteoblastoma: clinicopathologic study of 306 cases. Hum Pathol. 1994;25(2):117–34.
10. Mendonça BB, de Camargo OP, Pinto EM, Nascimento SAB, Maria do Rosario D, Zerbini MCN. Classical osteoblastoma, atypical osteoblastoma, and osteosarcoma. A comparative study based on clinical, histological, and biological parameters. Clinics (Sao Paulo). 2007;62(2):167–74.
11. Berber O, Dawson-Bowling S, Jalgaonkar A, Miles J, Pollock R, Skinner J, et al. Bizarre parosteal osteochondromatous proliferation of bone: clinical management of a series of 22 cases. J Bone Joint Surg Br. 2011;93(8):1118–21.

Chondromyxoid Fibroma

19

(***chondros*** "cartilage" + ***myx(o)*** "mucus" + ***oid, eidos*** "to form" + ***fibra*** "fiber" + ***oma*** "forming")

19.1 Definition

Chondromyxoid fibroma (CMF) is a rare benign cartilaginous tumor characterized by pseudolobular architecture, consisting of stellate or spindle-shaped cells embedded in variable amounts of chondroid and fibro-myxoid matrix.

19.2 Incidence

CMF is very rare, accounting for less than 1% of all primary bone tumors [1–4] and less than 2% of all benign tumors [4].

19.3 Ages

The lesion most frequently occurs in older children and young adults during the second and third decades of life [4, 5], representing about 60% of all patients in the Mayo Clinic files [4]. Mirra reported about 75% of the patients were before 30 years of age, most being between 10 and 20 years [6].

19.4 Location

CMF is most frequently located in the metaphyseal area of long bones of lower extremity, mostly proximal tibia and distal femur around the knee joint. The bones of the upper extremities are rarely affected. Localization in the skeleton of the lower limb and foot is 5–6 times more common than in the upper limb and hand [3]. Occasionally, the lesion moves toward the diaphysis during skeletal growth as other benign bone tumors do. Rarely, the lesion extends to the epiphysis (Figs. 19.1a and 19.3a). Very rarely, it can occur purely in the epiphysis of a long bone (Fig. 19.3d), a presentation that has been sporadically reported in the literature [7–10]. Flat bones, mainly ilium, and small bones of feet including calcaneus are the next frequently affected sites. Overall, the knee area, the small bones of the feet, and the ilium are the three most frequent sites of involvement [5]. Less frequently, CMF may involve the ribs, spine, short tubular bones of the hand as well as, and craniofacial bones. More rarely, it arises from the cortex (cortical, subperiosteal, periosteal, parosteal), collectively referred to as *juxtacortical* CMF, which usually occurs in older patients than those with intramedullary CMF. It is not easy to determine where the precise origin of such surface region is, and the term "*juxtacortical*" is used to encompass this group (Fig. 19.4). Baker et al. [11] reported *juxtacortical* CMF occupied 7.7% of all CMF in their 259 CMF series, and it occurred over a wide age range from 12 to 82 years with a median age of 40 years. The proximal tibial metaphysis was the most common location.

W.-J. Bahk, *Diagnosis and Management of Primary Bone Tumors*,
https://doi.org/10.1007/978-981-96-3484-2_19

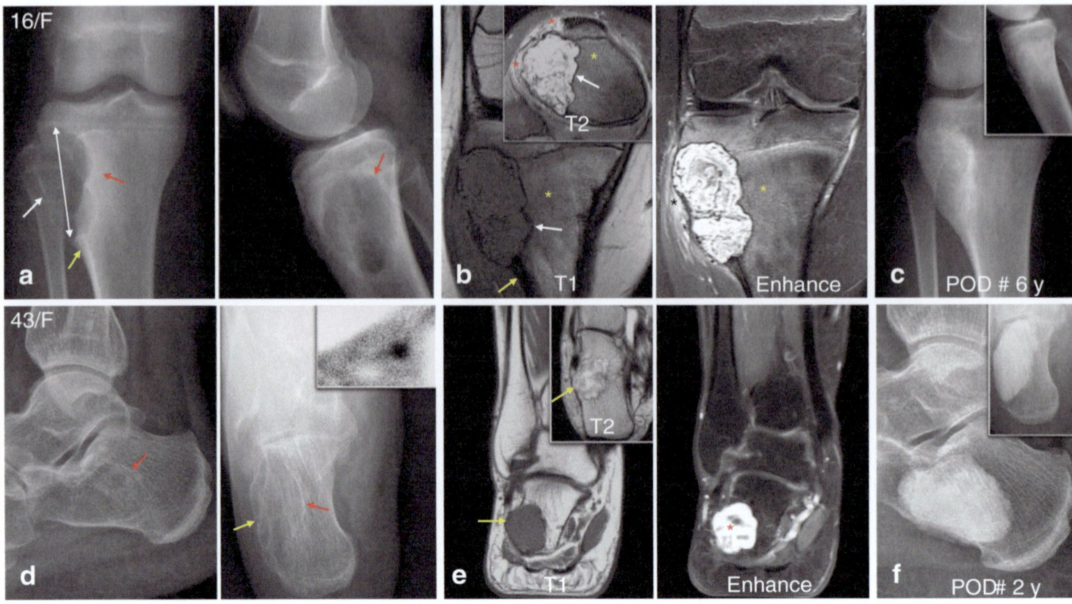

Fig. 19.1 (**a**) Radiographs taken for slowly growing mass with mild pain of 1 year's duration in a 16-year-old girl show a sharply defined, eccentric, multilobulated, geographic destruction with an internal thin rim of sclerosis (red arrows) mainly in the metaphysis and focal extension into the epiphysis. The lesion is unilaterally expanded with complete loss of the cortex and focal extension of the tumor into soft tissue with an outer thin sclerotic rim in a typical *bubbling out* pattern (white arrow). The long axis of the lesion is parallel to the long axis of the diaphysis (double-headed arrow). Note a thick *periosteal buttress* which is similar to that of periosteal chondroma (yellow arrow). There is an internal focal tiny calcification but no periosteal reaction. (**b**) MR images reveal a well-defined, eccentric, bubbling-out, intramedullary lesion with low SI on T1-weighted image and high SI on T2-weighted image, with tiny foci of dark signal representing calcification on both sequences. There are internal irregular septa with low signal and a thin sclerotic surrounding rim of dark signal on both sequences (white arrows). Note a thick periosteal buttress (yellow arrow), and peritumoral bone marrow and surrounding soft tissue edema (asterisks). The lesion itself is enhanced in peripheral and nodular pattern, and edemas are diffusely enhanced (asterisks). (**c**) After histologic confirmation of CMF, extended curettage using high-speed bur and allogenic chip bone graft was performed. Radiograph at 6 years after surgery shows good consolidation of the lesion with no evidence of recurrence. (**d**) Radiographs taken for right heel pain of 5 years' duration in a 43-year-old woman show an ill-defined, lobulated, radiolucent lesion with a thin surrounding sclerosis in the calcaneus (red arrows). Axial view more clearly reveals an eccentric, multilobulated, radiolucent lesion with thin internal septa and unilateral *bubbling-out* expansion (yellow arrow). Bone scan reveals a strongly increased uptake in the lesion (inset). (**e**) MR images demonstrate a well-defined mass-like lesion with low SI on T1-weighted image and heterogeneous intermediate and high SI on T2-weighted image with a focal extension into the soft tissue surrounded by a thin sclerosis of dark signal (arrows). The lesion is diffusely well enhanced with focal nonenhancing areas of calcification (asterisk). (**f**) After histologic confirmation, extended curettage using high-speed bur followed by adjuvant therapy with anhydrous ethanol and cement filling of the defect was performed. Radiograph at 2 years after surgery shows no evidence of recurrence

19.5 Clinical Features

Pain is the most common presentation that is usually mild and often longstanding for several months to years due to slow growth of the tumor. Local swelling is commonly noted if the small bones of hands and feet are affected. Rarely, CMF can be incidentally identified on radiographs taken for unrelated reasons.

19.6 Radiologic Findings

Plain radiograph The lesion is characterized by a sharply demarcated, eccentric, ovoid to elliptical, geographic destruction with a sclerotic margin in the metaphyseal area of the long bone at a variable distance from the epiphyseal line. The lesion is often lobulated with internal septa that produces a characteristic *soap-bubble* appearance, and unilaterally expanded into the adjacent soft tissue in a *bubbling-out* fashion, often with complete loss of the cortex (Figs. 19.1, 19.2, and 19.3). The outer margin of *bubbling-out* focal expansion is usually surrounded by a thin rim of periosteal new bone formation, which corresponds to the intramedaullary rim of sclerosis seen in other benign bone tumors. The long axis of the lesion is typically aligned parallel to that of the diaphysis. A thin and incomplete rim of the new cortex often seen with periosteal *buttress* or *collarette* which is similar to that seen in periosteal chondroma (Fig. 19.1a). Internal matrix calcification is rarely observed, and periosteal reaction is uncommon unless pathologic fracture is complicated. In short tubular bones, the lesion is frequently centrally located with fusiform expansion of the bone. CMF involving flat bone such as pelvis or calcaneus can be larger in size and irregular in outline with prominent intrale-

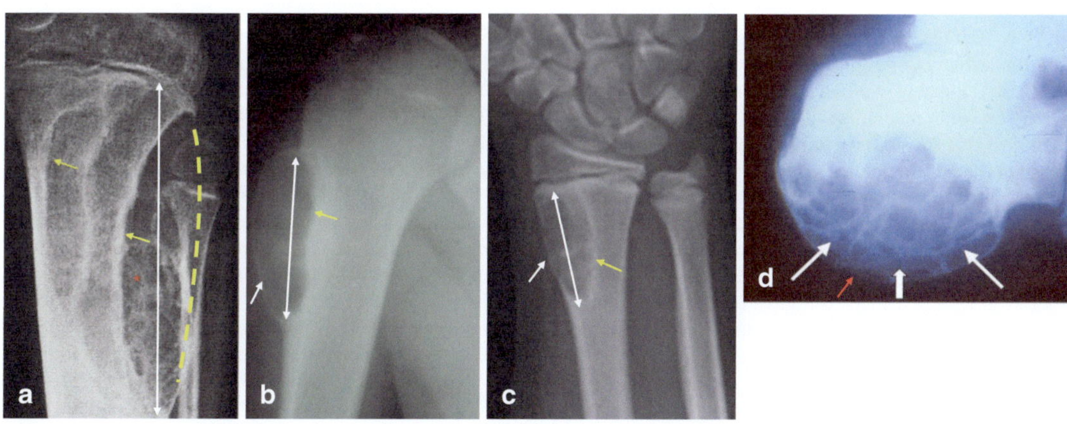

Fig. 19.2 (**a**) Radiograph shows large multilobulated, oblong, eccentric, radiolucent lesions surrounded and separated by rims of reactive sclerotic bone (yellow arrows) in the meta-diaphysis of the proximal tibia. The lesion is eccentrically expanded in a *bubbling-out* fashion with complete loss of the cortex and a thin outer rim of periosteal new bone formation (yellow dotted line). Note a characteristic *soap-bubble* appearance (asterisk) with a long axis parallel to that of the tibial diaphysis (double-headed arrow). (**b**) Radiograph reveals an eccentric radiolucent lesion with unilateral cortical expansion in a typical *bubbling-out* fashion with complete loss of the cortex covered by internal (yellow arrow) and external (white arrow) thin rims of reactive sclerosis in the meta-diaphyseal area of the proximal humerus. The lesion shows a long axis paralleling to that of the tibial diaphysis (double-headed arrow). (**c**) Radiograph demonstrates an eccentric radiolucent lesion with a mild *bubbling-out* expansion and internal (yellow arrow) and external (whiste arrow) thin rims of new bone formation in the meta-diaphysis of the distal radius. All three lesions of long bones share the following characteristic features of (1) an eccentricity with varying degrees of expansion in a *bubbling-out* fashion, (2) intramedullary and outer thin sclerotic rims of reactive sclerosis, and (3) a long axis of the lesion parallel to that of the affected bone. (**d**) Radiograph of the calcaneus shows a typical *soap-bubble* appearance with multiple variable-sized rounds to oval lesions separated by thin internal septations (white arrows). Note a diffuse cortical expansion covered with a thin rim of periosteal new bone, producig a volar convexity in *bubbling-out* fashion (red arrow)

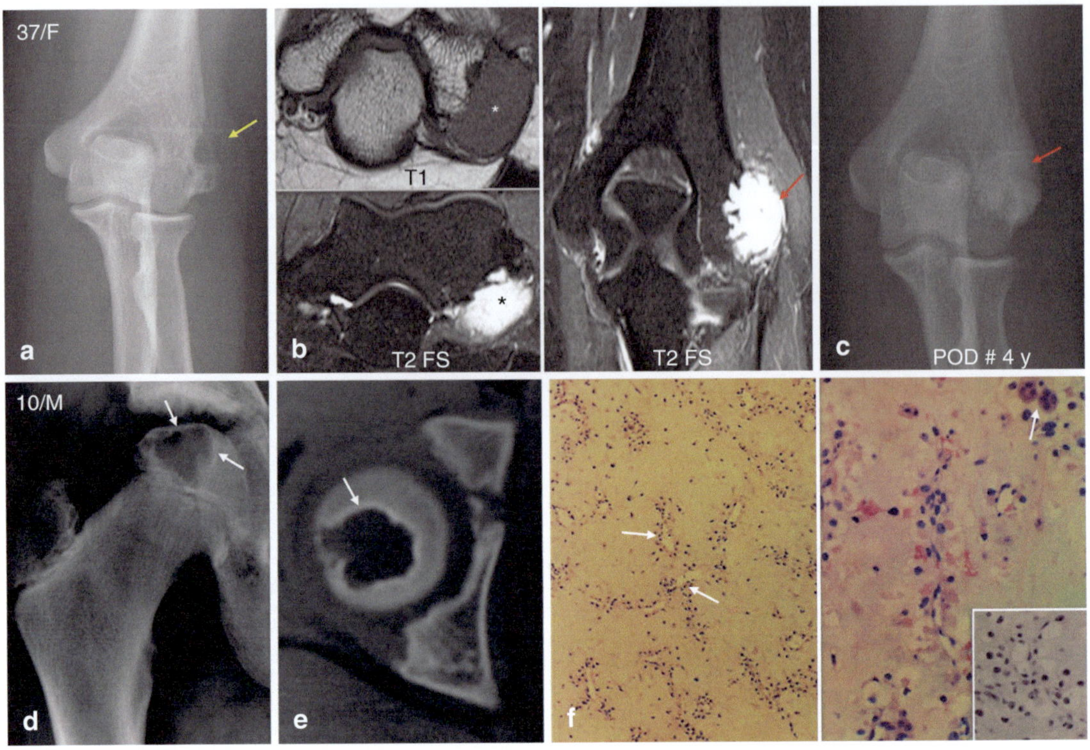

Fig. 19.3 ***Rare location of distal humerus***. (**a**) Radiograph taken for left elbow swelling of 7–8 years' duration with recently developed pain of 2 months' duration in a 37-year-old lady shows an eccentric, radiolucent lesion with cortical destruction and soft tissue extension (yellow arrow) in the lateral condyle of the left humerus. There is no discernible internal matrix or periosteal reaction. (**b**) MR images reveal a well-defined, infiltrating, multilobulated medullary mass-like lesion (asterisks) in a *bubbling-out* fashion (arrow), with intermediate SI on T1-weighted image and bright SI on fat-saturated T2-weighted image. (**c**) Follow-up radiograph at 4 years after thorough curettage and cementation reveals no evidence of local recurrence (arrow). ***Rare location of femoral epiphysis***: (**d**) Radiograph taken for right hip pain with limping gait of several months' duration in a 10-year-old boy shows a well-defined eccentric lytic lesion with flattening of subchondral surface (yellow arrow). The lesion is surrounded by a thin sclerotic rim (white arrow) and confined to the epiphysis of the femoral head that is a fairly classical location for chondroblastoma (CB) or less likely for epiphyseal enchondroma. (**e**) CT scan also reveals a well-defined geographic destruction, surrounded by a thin rim of sclerosis (arrow) without internal calcifying densities. (**f**) Microscopic examination does not correlate with the above-mentioned radiologic differential diagnosis. The lesion exhibits a cartilage tumor with a lobular growth pattern. (Left) The lesion consists of a light bluish, loose cartilage-like chondromyxoid stroma admixed with clusters of ovoid cells mainly distributed around capillaries (arrows). Fibroid area is not observed. (Right) Higher-power magnification shows foci of a few spindle cells with deeply stained round to oval nuclei and a couple of multinucleated giant cells embedded in myxoid to chondromyxoid matrix (arrow). The cells hug small blood vessels, reminiscent of a CMF. There are no evidence of bone production, polygonal chondroblasts, and chicken wire calcification. This case was consulted to Dr. Mirra and he confirmed the diagnosis of CMF, consisting of two of three components, chondromyxoid without fibroid elements, which is confined to epiphysis

sional loculation, producing a characteristic *soap-bubble* appearance (Fig. 19.2d). **Bone scan** The lesion may show peripherally increased uptake with central void uptake, so-called *dough-nut* sign, as in various other bone lesions such as chondrosarcoma (CSA), telangiectatic osteosarcoma, giant cell tumor, or cystic lesions. **MR images** are not particularly specific but typically show a well-demarcated metaphyseal lesion with low to intermediate SI on T1-weighted image and intermediate to high SI on T2-weitghted image. The lesion is usually enhanced in peripheral and nodular pattern as seen in other cartilage tumors (Fig. 19.1b), but can be diffusely enhanced throughout the lesion in some cases (Fig. 19.1e).

19.7 Histologic Findings

The lesion typically exhibits a lobular growth pattern with an overall pseudolobulated architecture with pinkish chondroid and bluish myxoid elements, separated by fibrous bands or condensed zones of elongated to stellated spindle cells (Fig. 19.6a, b). However, frank areas of hyaline cartilage are unusual in CMF, which were found in only about 20% of cases of a large series [3]. A large number of cases exhibit a worrisome appearance with significantly high cellularity and other cytologic atypia in the active stage. However, both the number and size of cells are reduced, and the cells become quite bland in the maturation stage of chondroid elements [6]. Typically, the lesion demonstrates *biphasic* pattern consisting of a central *light* area of lower cellularity with chondroid matrix and another peripheral *dark* area of high cellularity with fibro-myxoid matrix (Figs. 19.4c and 19.6a, c). Generally, the lesion consists of a mixture of chondroid, myxoid, and fibroid elements in varyingproportion, but many cases are composed predominantly of only two elements. It may often contain only chondromyxoid without fibroid elements (Fig. 19.3f). Most lesions exhibit peripheral condensation of fibroid tissue with high cellularity around the periphery of the chondroid lobules. Varying sizes of prominent vasculatures

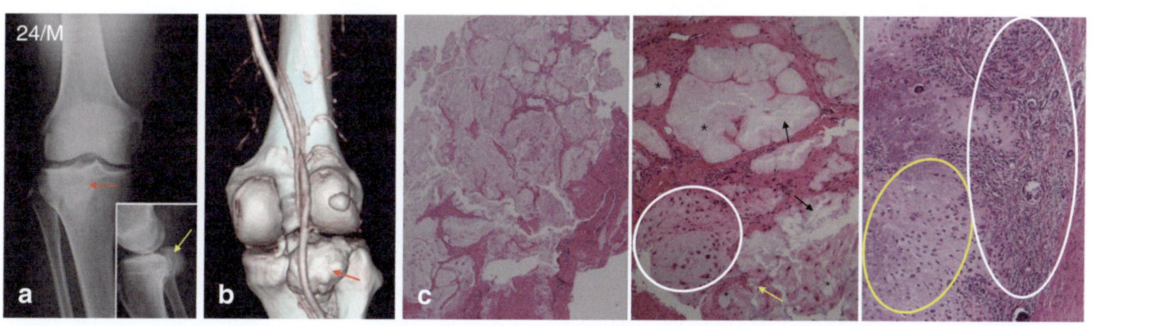

Fig. 19.4 ***Juxtacortical CMF***. (**a**) Radiograph taken for a protruding hard mass of right knee with intermittent pain of 4–5 years' duration in a 24-year-old young man shows a hazy, irreugular, radiodense mass (red arrow) in the proximal tibia. Lateral view reveals a sharply demarcated, round to oval, dense mass attached to the surface of the proximal tibia (yellow arrow in inset). (**b**) 3D CT scan reveals a well-defined dense mass attached to the proximal tibia (arrow), indicating a juxta-cortical benign tumor. (**c**) Microscopic examination: (Left) Lower-power magnification exhibits a lobular growth pattern of the lesion with an overall pseudolobulated architecture. (Middle) Medium-power magnification shows lobules of varying sizes, separated by thick bands of fibroid septa. Each lobule cotains varying numbers, ranging from sparse to moderate, of benign-looking spindle cells. As it matures, the chondroid element becomes pinkish with a lower cellularity and quite bland-looking cells (circle). There are prominent vasculatures of varying sizes (black arrows), which are usually absent in other cartilage tumors. There are multiple minute microcysts (yellow arrow) that gradually coalesce to become much looser and bigger macrocystic cavities (black asterisks). (Right) The lesion typically shows a *biphasic appearance* consisting of a central *light* area of low cellularity with chondroid matrix (yellow circle) and a peripheral *dark* area of high cellularity with fibro-myxoid matrix (white circle). A few multinucleated giant cells are also scattered throughout the lesion

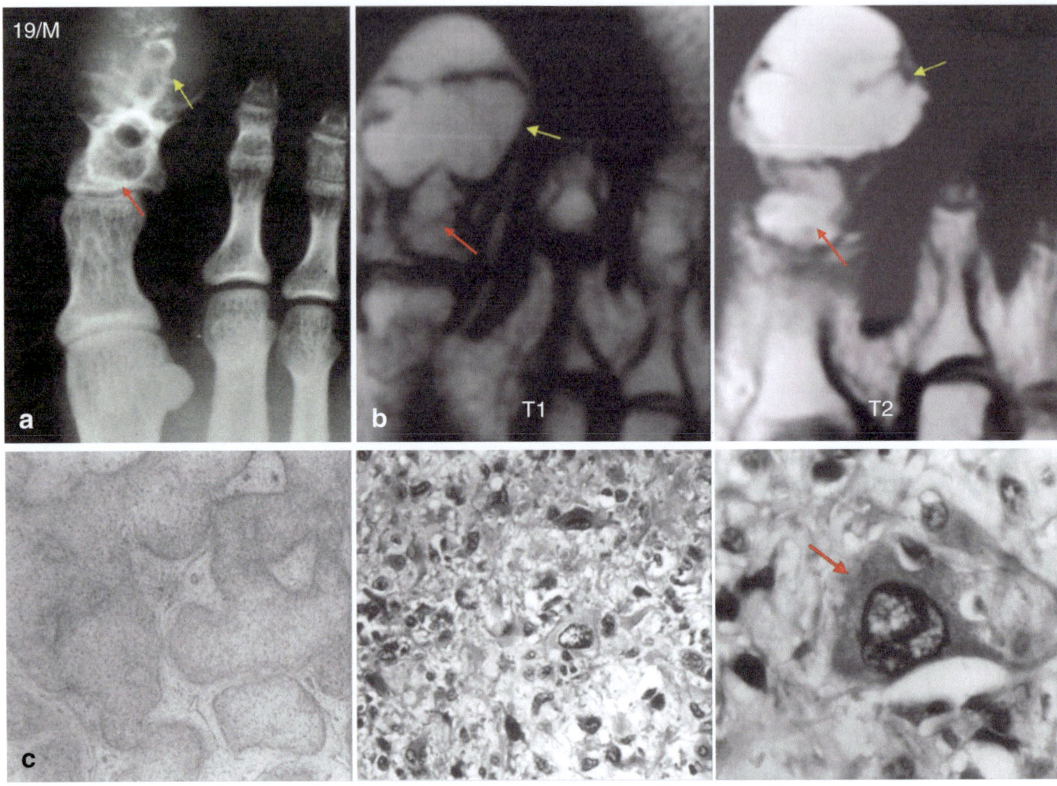

Fig. 19.5 ***Pseudoanaplastic*** **CMF**. (**a**) Radiograph taken for a slowly growing, painless mass of 10 years' duration in a 19-year-old young man shows a multilobulated, expansile mass-like lesion distally (yellow arrow) and a lytic lesion with a thick rim of sclerosis proximally (red arrow) in the distal phalanx of great toe. (**b**) MR images reveal a well-defined multilobulated intramedullary mass-like lesion involving the entire distal phalanx (arrows) with intermediate to high SI on T1-weighted image and bright SI on T2-weighted image. The distal portion of the lesion is markedly expanded and ballooned out, with a well-defined margin surrounded by a reactive bone (yellow arrows), possibly suggesting a benignancy despite its locally agressive appearance. (**c**) Microscopic examination: (Left) Low-power magnification exhibits a multilobulated lesion with a *biphasic* pattern of low and high cellularity within chondroid and myxoid elements separated by bands of high cellularity of spindle cells with fibroid elements. (Middle) Medium-power magnification demonstrates significantly bizarre and pleomorphic-looking stromal cells. Some cells had a stellate configuration, abundant pink cytoplasm and large, dark blue nuclei with irregular chromatin condensation. (Right) Higher-power magnification reveals an extremely bizarre-shaped cell containing a markedly enlarged, hyperchromatic, vacuolated nucleus (red arrow), mimicking anaplasia. However, there is no frank abnormal mitotic figures. The lesion was initially mistaken for CSA due to the significant nuclear aberrations by a general pathologist, and the patient was managed by great toe amputation. However, the disgnosis was ultimately revised to *pseudoanaplastic* CMF by Dr. Mirra, based on a diagnostic triangle: the *clinical history* of slow growth of the mass for such a long duration, the *radiographic finding* of rind of sclerosis, and the *pathologic finding* of no abnormal mitoses. He is doing well without local recurrence at 20 years after surgery without chemotherapy, which clinically proves a total benignancy of the lesion

can be often seen in *staghorn* pattern, reminiscent of hemangiopericytoma (Fig. 19.6a, d). Such vasculatures usually do not exist in most other cartilage tumors. The myxoid elements may undergo a degenerative microcystic change, which terms as *microcystic myxoid elements* by Mirra [6]. The cells in this area are usually sparse to small in number and appear quite bland. The microcysts may be fused to form macrocystic cavities in some cases (Figs. 19.4c and 19.6d). Frequently, multinucleated giant cells are scattered with hemosiderin and inflammatory cells in the high cellular peripheral areas (Fig. 19.6e). High-power magnification reveals elongate to stellate (multipolar) or

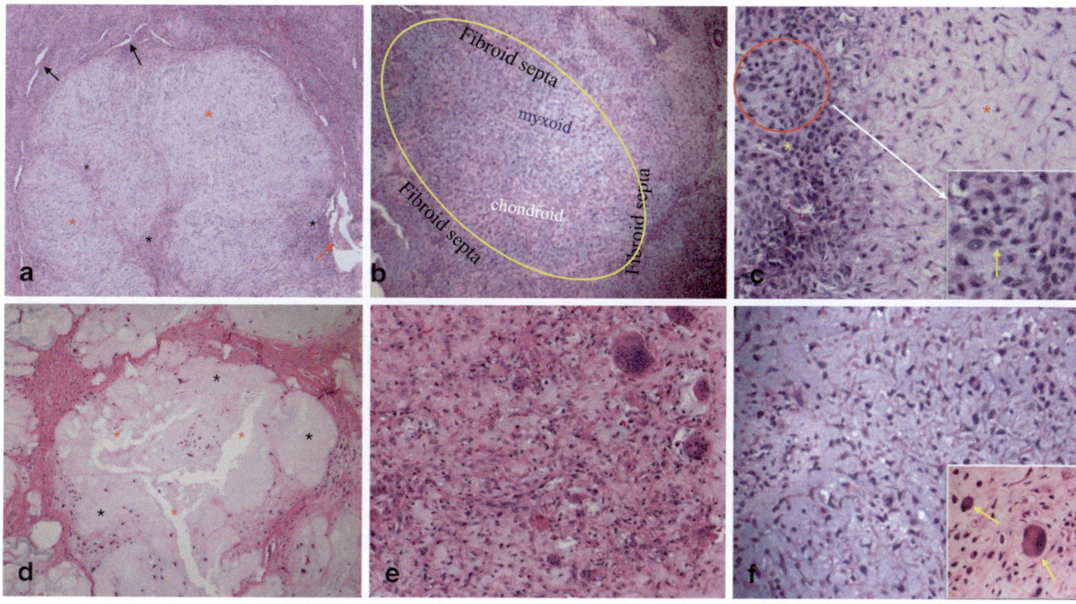

Fig. 19.6 ***Microscopic examination***. (**a**) Low-power magnification shows a typical lobular growth pattern with fibroblast-like spindle cells embedded in a chondromyxoid matrix, which is compartmentalized into several lobules by fibrous septa. The lesion exhibits a typical *biphasic* appearance with *lower* cellularity (*light* area) in the center of the lobules (red asterisks), a morphological feature resembling a hyaline cartilage tumor, and *higher* cellularity (*dark* area) in the periphery and fibrous septa (black asterisks). Note prominent vasculatures of varying sizes (black arrows), and some are markedly dilated in *staghorn* pattern (red arrow). Such a vascular pattern is not typically seen in most other cartilage tumors. (**b**) Each lobule typically consists of pinkish chondroid and light purple to bluish myxoid background, which is surrounded by dense fibrous bands containing elongated to stellated spindle cells. (**c**) Higher-power magnification reveals a lower cellular chondroid area with round to oval, spindle-shaped, or stellate-shaped cells in the center (red asterisk) and higher cellular myxo-fibroid area of sheets with polygonal cells at the periphery (yellow asterisk). Note occasional cells with central longitudinal nuclear groove, so-called *coffee bean* nucleus, resembling those seen in CB and LCH (inset). (**d**) Chondroid or myxoid elements may undergo microcystic change, in which cells are usually very sparse, and the microcysts fuse to make large macrocystic cavities with myxoid material (black asterisks). Note multiple empty spaces of dilated capillaries in *staghorn* pattern, reminiscent of hemangiopericytoma (red asterisks). (**e**) Several multinucleated giant cells are also scattered throughout the hypercellular area. (**f**) High-power magnification demonstrates show stellate or plump spindle cells embedded in myxoid to chondroid matrix. The individual cells show a moderate degree of nuclear atypia with enlarged, irregular, hyperchromatic, vacuolated, bizarre-shaped nuclei, which are considered degerative changes. Even striking bizarre pleomorphism of the cells in terms of size and shape is occasionally seen (inset), which can be easily mistaken for CSA, particularly if the typical radiographic and clinical findings are not considered. Most importantly, there should be no definite abnormal mitosis for a diagnosis of *pseudoanaplastic* CMF

plump spindle cells embedded in myxoid to chondroid matrix. Cytoplasm of the cell is eosinophilic and the nucleus is deeply stained, rounded to elongated, triangular to stellate (Fig. 19.6f). The tumor cells may be fairly atypical and pleomorphic in size and shape with enlarged, irregular, hyperchromatic, vacuolated, or bizarre-shaped nuclei, which does not indicate malignancy but is considered to be degenerative change [12]. Occasional tumor cells exhibit central longitudinal nuclear groove, so-called *coffee bean* nucleus, being equivalent to those seen chondroblastoma (CB) and Langerhans cell histiocytoma (LCH) (Fig. 19.6c). Occasionally, hyaline cartilage with focal or extensive calcification can be observed. Microscopic foci of calcification are observed in about one-third of the cases, and spontaneous necrosis is found in about 12% of cases in Mayo Clinic series [4]. Pleomorphic cells with enlarged, hyperchromatic, bizarre nuclei are rarely observed in about 20% of cases [3]. Even more striking pleomorphism with extreme bizarre cells but no atypical mitosis, so-called *pseudoanaplastic* CMF, can be observed in extremely rare cases [13] (Fig. 19.5). Mitoses are relatively rare in most cases.

19.8 Management

Through extended curettage and bone graft with or without adjuvant therapy such as phenol or anhydrous ethanol is the standard option for management (Fig. 19.1c, f). For a large defect after curettage, cement filling may be necessary to provide immediate postoperative biomechanical stability. En-bloc resection can be rarely required in cases with multiple recurrences, more extensive lesions, or expendable bones [12].

19.9 Clinical Course

Simple curettage alone was reported to have poor results with high recurrence rate of 20–40% in most large series [2, 3, 14, 15]. Schajowicz and Gallardo [2] reported a reduction in a recurrence rate down to 4% by a higher proportion of wide en-bloc excisions in their series. A high rate of recurrence up to 80% with curettage alone but significantly low rate to 7% with thorough curettage and bone graft or cementing was reported with overall recurrence of 27% in a Rizzoli Institute series [1]. Recurrence typically occurs within the bone at the site of curettage, but rarely in the adjacent soft tissue, or both [16–19]. Heydemann et al. [16] suggested that soft tissue recurrence may may result from spillage of tumor during surgical procedure, supporting the possibility of an iatrogenic origin. Exceptionally rare cases of malignant transformation have been reported in the absence of prior radiation therapy [3, 20]. However, the issue of sarcomatous transformation still remains a subjective of ongoing patholgic debate [4, 5].

References

1. Gherlinzoni F, Rock M, Picci P, Chondromyxoid fibroma. The experience at the Istituto Ortopedico Rizzoli. J Bone Joint Surg. 1983;65(2):198–204.
2. Schajowicz F, Gallardo H. Chondromyxoid fibroma (fibromyxoid chondroma) of bone: a clinico-pathological study of thirty-two cases. J Bone Joint Surg Br. 1971;53(2):198–216.
3. Wu CT, Inwards CY, O'laughlin S, Rock MG, Beabout JW, Unni KK. Chondromyxoid fibroma of bone: a clinicopathologic review of 278 cases. Hum Pathol. 1998;29(5):438–46.
4. Unni KK, Inwards CY. Chondromyxoid fibroma. In: Unni KK, Inwards CY, editors. Dahlin's bone tumors: general aspects and data on 10,165 cases. 6th ed. Philadelphia: Lippincott William & Wilkins; 2010. p. 50–9.
5. Czerniak B. Benign cartilage lesions. In: Dorfman HD, Czerniak B, editors. Dorfman and Czerniak's bone tumors. 2nd ed (eBook). Elsevier; 2016. p. 356–473.
6. Mirra JM. Chondromyxoid fibroma. In: Mirra JM, editor. Bone tumors: clinical, radiologic, and pathologic correlations. 2nd ed. Philadelphia: Lea & Febiger; 1989. p. 623–48.
7. Choi YS, Kim B-S, Joo J-E, Park Y-K, Lee SH, Song BY. A rare case of epiphyseal chondromyxoid fibroma of the proximal tibia. Korean J Radiol. 2011;12(6):761–4.
8. Fotiadis E, Akritopoulos P, Samoladas E, Akritopoulou K, Kenanidis E. Chondromyxoid fibroma: a rare tumor with an unusual location. Arch Orthop Trauma Surg. 2008;128:371–5.
9. Gardner DJ, Michel AE. Solitary lucent epiphyseal lesions in children. Skeletal Radiol. 1988;17:497–504.
10. Wilson A, Kyriakos M, Ackerman L. Chondromyxoid fibroma: radiographic appearance in 38 cases and in a review of the literature. Radiology. 1991;179(2):513–8.
11. Baker AC, Rezeanu L, O'Laughlin S, Unni K, Klein MJ, Siegal GP. Juxtacortical chondromyxoid fibroma of bone: a unique variant: a case study of 20 patients. Am J Surg Pathol. 2007;31(11):1662–8.
12. Campanacci M. Chondromyxoid fibroma. In: Campanacci M, editor. Bone and soft tissue tumors. Wien/New York: Springer-Verlag; 1999. p. 265–77.

13. Bahk WJ, Mirra JM, Sohn KR, Shin DS. Pseudoanaplastic chondromyxoid fibroma. Ann Diagn Pathol. 1998;2(4):241–6.
14. Rahimi A, Beabout JW, Ivins JC, Dahlin DC. Chondromyxoid fibroma: a clinicopathologic study of 76 cases. Cancer. 1972;30(3):726–36.
15. Zillmer DA, Dorfman HD. Chondromyxoid fibroma of bone: thirty-six cases with clinicopathologic correlation. Hum Pathol. 1989;20(10):952–64.
16. Heydemann J, Gillespie R, Mancer K. Soft tissue recurrence of chondromyxoid fibroma. J Pediatr Orthop. 1985;5(6):725–7.
17. Kyriakos M. Soft tissue implantation of chondromyxoid fibroma. Am J Pathol. 1979;3(4):363–72.
18. Mikulowski P, Östberg G. Recurrent chondromyxoid fibroma. Acta Orthop Scand. 1971;42(5):385–90.
19. Troncoso A, Ro JY, Edeiken J, Carrasco CH, Murray JA, Ayala AG. Case report 798: recurrent chondromyxoid fibroma in connective tissue of leg. Skeletal Radiol. 1993;22(6):445–8.
20. Sehayik S, Rosman M. Malignant degeneration of a chondromyxoid fibroma in a child. Can J Surg. 1975;18(4):354–357 360. PMID: 1148963.

20 Chondroblastoma

(***chondros*** *"cartilage"* + ***blastos*** *"germ"* + ***ōma*** *"forming"*)

20.1 Definition

Chondroblastoma (CB) is a benign but locally aggressive cartilage-matrix forming tumor, typically consisting of chondroblasts and islands of chondroid matrix with a strong predilection for the epiphysis or apophysis of a long bone, predominantly in skeletally immature patients.

20.2 Synonym

Calcifying giant cell tumor/epiphyseal chondromatous giant cell tumor/Codman tumor.

20.3 Incidence

CB is relatively rare, accounting for approximately 5% of all benign bone tumors [1], and about 1–1.5% of all bone tumors in major series [1–7].

20.4 Ages

The lesion mostly occurs in growth spurt period of children, adolescents, or young adults, typically younger than 25 years of age, either before or immediately after epiphyseal closure, while giant cell tumor (GCT) typically occurs in adults between 20 and 40 years after epiphyseal closure. More than 50–60% of CB cases occur in skeletally immature patients in their second decade of life [1, 4]. It is very rare in young children and elderly patients. The youngest patient was 11 years old and the eldest, 69 years in our series (Fig. 20.6).

20.5 Locations

The lesion most frequently affects epiphysis or epi-metaphysis of the long bones, particularly proximal and distal femur, proximal tibia, and proximal humerus (Figs. 20.1 and 20.2). Apophyses including greater trochanter of the femur and greater tuberosity of the humerus are also frequently involved (Figs. 20.1e and 20.2d). Flat bones such as pelvic bones, talus, calcaneus, and patella are other classic sites of involvement (Figs. 20.2e and 20.3a, d). The vast majority of cases in long bones are confined to the medullary cavity, but very rare cases can occur in the intracortical or juxtacortical location. A pure metaphyseal or diaphyseal location is very rare, occupying only about 2% in a large series of 390 CBs along with a review of pertinent large series in the literature, and it frequently presents a diagnostic dilemma [8]. Furthermore, an intracortical lesion in the metaphysis or diaphysis is exceptionally rare [9–12] (Fig. 20.5).

W.-J. Bahk, *Diagnosis and Management of Primary Bone Tumors*,
https://doi.org/10.1007/978-981-96-3484-2_20

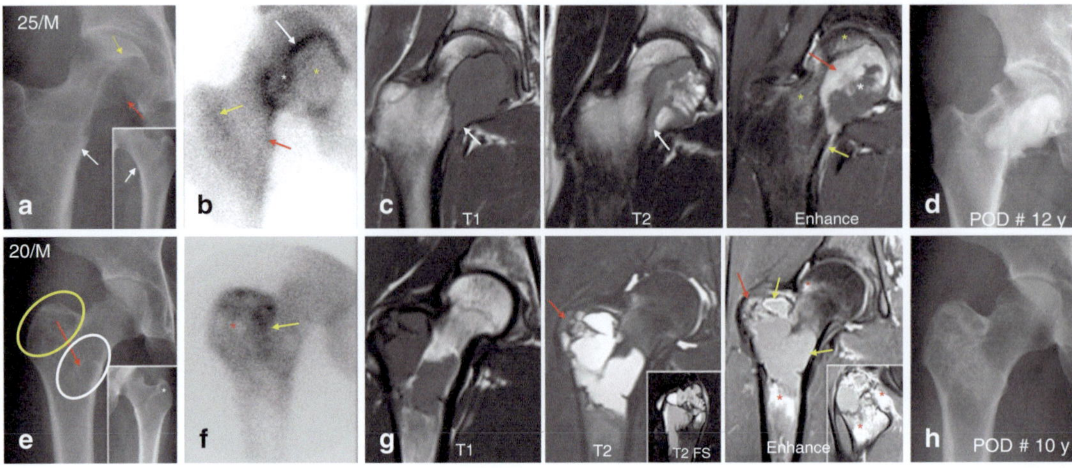

Fig. 20.1 ***Proximal femur***. (**a**) Radiograph taken for right hip pain of 1 year's duration in a 25-year-old man shows a well-defined, eccentric, round to oval, lytic lesion surrounded by a thin rind of sclerosis (yellow arrow) in medial half of the femoral head and neck. There is mild external expansion with a possible cortical breakage (red arrow). Note a marked thickening of the medial cortex with distinctive thick, solid periosteal reaction distal to the lesion (white arrow) when compared to the contralateral normal medial cortex (inset). (**b**) Pinhole bone scan reveals a curvilinear strong uptake along the peripheral reactive bone (white arrow) and focal uptake in the peripheral lesion (white asterisk) with a central photon defect (yellow asterisk). There is mild uptake in the thickened medial cortex (red arrow). There is also mild uptake in the trochanteric area adjacent to the lesion (yellow arrow), suggesting mild reactive change. (**c**) MR images demonstrate a well-defined medullary mass-like lesion with mild expansion and cortical breach (white arrows). The SI is intermediate SI on T1-weighted image and intermediate SI with high signals on T2-weighted image, with a thin dark signal of surrounding sclerosis on both sequences. The lesion is thickly enhanced along the peripheral area by contrast medium (red arrow) but only focally enhanced in the center (white asterisk). Moderate enhancement is also noted in the adjacent bone marrow (yellow asterisks), suggesting perilesional edema. Note well-enhanced solid periosteal reaction along the medial cortex (yellow arrow). (**d**) Follow-up radiograph at 12 years after curettage and bone cementing with histologic confirmation of conventional CB shows no evidence of recurrence. **Apophysis (great trochanter):** (**e**) Radiograph taken for right hip pain after a slip while playing football in a 20-year-old young man incidentally shows an ill-defined, multilobulated, hazy radiolucent lesion with somewhat bubbly appearance in the apophyseal greater trochanter (yellow circle), which extends into the intertrochanteric area of the femur (white circle). Note moderate expansion of the greater trochanter when compared to the controlateral normal greater trochanter (inset). (**f**) Pinhole bone scan reveals moderate uptake with irregular focal areas of hot uptake along the periphery of the lesion (arrow) and internal photon defect (asterisk). (**g**) MR images demonstrate mostly a well-defined multilobulated cystic lesion of low to intermediate SI on T1-weighted image and mostly bright SI with focal solid areas of heterogeneous intermediate signal on T2-weighted image (red arrow). Note multiple *fluid-fluid* levels in the cystic lesion on fat-saturated T2-weighted image, indicating secondary ABC in the underlying solid tumor (inset). The focal solid lesion is heterogeneously enhanced (red arrow) and the cystic lesion is peripherally enhanced (yellow arrows). The adjacent bone marrow edema is extensive and is well enahnced by contrast medium (red asterisks in inset). (**h**) Follow-up radiograph at 10 years after extended curettage using high-speed bur and allo-chip bone graft with histologic histologic confirmation of CB with prominent secondary ABC shows consolidation of the lesion with no evidence of recurrence.

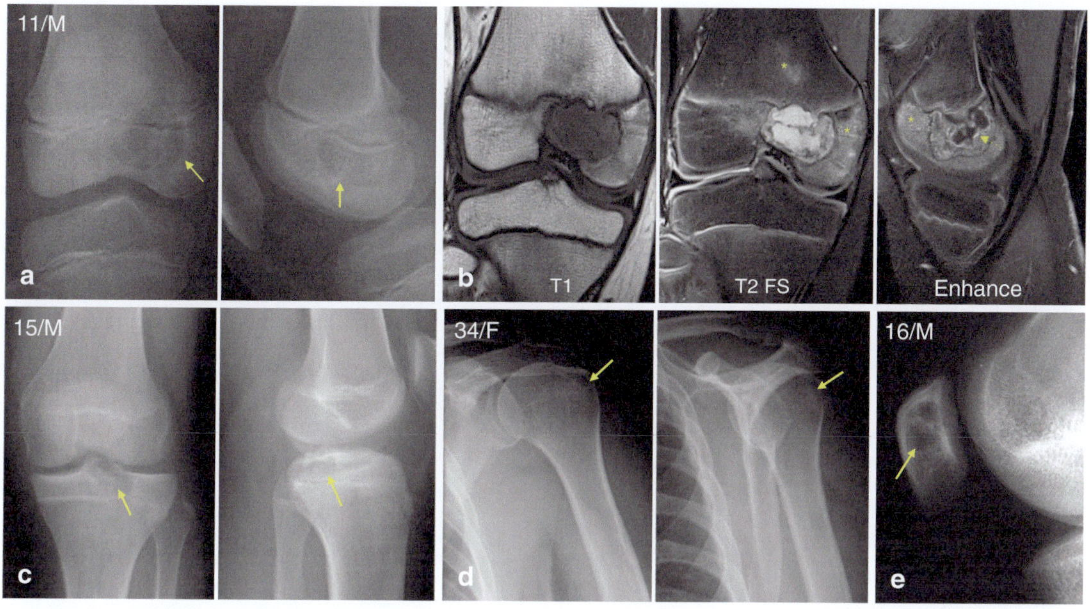

Fig. 20.2 ***Distal femur*.** (**a**) Radiographs taken for right knee pain of 4 months' duration in a 11-year-old boy show a well-defined, round to oval, osteolytic lesion surrounded by a thin rim of sclerosis with internal stippled calcifications, which occupies less than half of the epiphysis of the distal femur (arrows). (**b**) MR images reveal a well-defined lesion purely confined to epiphysis with low SI on T1-wighted image and heterogenous high to bright SI on fat saturated T2-weighted image, with a thin dark signal of surrounding sclerosis on both sequences. Note prominent edema in the adjacent bone marrow (asterisks). The lesion is enhanced in a septal and peripheral pattern (arrow), and the bone marrow edema is diffusely enhanced by contrast medium (asterisk). **Other classic locations:** Radiographs demonstrate a well-defined, non-aggressive looking, small radiolucent lesions occupying less than half of the epiphysis in the proximal tibia (**c**), the greater tuberosity of the humerus (**d**), and the patella (**e**)

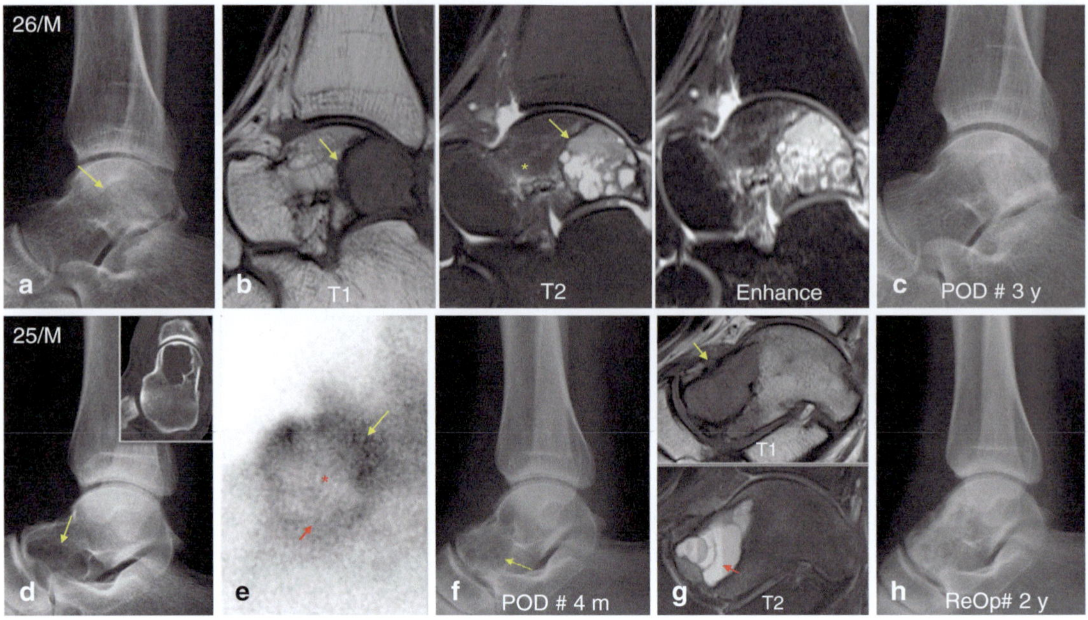

Fig. 20.3 ***Talus***. (**a**) Radiograph taken for right ankle pain of 1 year's duration in a 26-year-old man shows a hazy osteolytic lesion surrounded by a thin rim of sclerosis (arrow) in the posterior aspect of the talus body. (**b**) MR images reveal a well-defined mass-like lesion with low SI on T1-weighted image and intermediate SI with focal high signals on T2-weighted image, which is surrounded by an irregular sclerotic rim of dark signal (arrows). There is adjacent bone marrow edema (asterisk). The lesion, as well as bone marrow edema, is heterogeneously well enhanced. (**c**) Follow-up radiograph at 3 years after curettage and allo-chip bone graft with a pathologic diagnosis of CB notes no evidence of recurrence. (**d**) Radiograph taken for right ankle pain of 9 months' duration in a 25-year-old man shows a well-defined multilobulated osteolytic lesion with an incomplete thin rim of sclerosis (arrow) in the anterior aspect of the talus body. CT scan more clearly reveals a well-defined lytic lesion bordered by a thin complete sclerotic rim with no internal mineralization or trabeculations (inset). (**e**) Pinhole bone scan reveals a heterogeneously increased uptake along the posterior periphery of the lesion (yellow arrow) and lesser uptake in the anterior periphery (red arrow). However, the central portion shows little to isoactive uptake (asterisk). (**f**) Follow-up radiograph taken for recurrent ankle pain at 4 months after curettage and bone graft demonstrates variably sized, multiple, round or oval, radiolucent holes in the hazy lesion, suggesting a possible local recurrence. (**g**) MR images present a recurrent lesion with a focal cortical perforation (yellow arrow) showing low SI on T1-weighted image. Note multiple lobulations with *fluid-fluid* levels (red arrow) on T2-weighted image, indicating a local recurrence with a newly developed ABC. On microscopic examination, there were findings of CB with secondary ABC that were not seen on initial evaluation, but no evidence of aggressive or malignant change. (**h**) Radiograph taken 2 years after re-operation shows no evidence of local recurrence with consolidation of the lesion.

20.6 Clinical Features

Gradually increasing localized pain of long duration is the most common presenting symptom. The pain is often referred to the adjacent joint and is usually mild to moderate, due to the epipyseal location that can affect the articular cartilage or irritate the synovium, leading to joint effusion. Other symptome, such as swelling, limping gait, joint effusion or stiffness, muscle atrophy, and a soft tissue mass are less commonly presented. Rarely, CB can may be found incidentally on radiographs taken for unrelated reasons (Figs. 20.1e and 20.5a).

20.7 Radiologic Findings

Plain radiograph CB typically presents a well-defined, round to oval, lytic lesion often surrounded by a thin rim of sclerotic bone. The lesion is usually small and occupies less than half of the epiphysis of long bones, with still open, in the process of closing, or just closed growth plate (Figs. 20.1 and 20.2). Scattered minute punctate or stippled calcification can be often seen in the lesion. However, the densities are usually difficult to identify on standard radiographs due to minute size of the calcification and poor radiographic exposure, which explains the significant discrepancies in the reported incidence of punctate or stippled calcification [6]. Mineralization is radiologically absent in about two-thirds of the cases in Mayo Clinic series [1]. However, the calcification was observed in about 75% of the cases on microscopic examination By Mirra [6]. Generally, the lesion is eccentrically located and confined to the epiphysis or apophysis (Fig. 20.2), but a large lesion may extend into the metaphysis as in GCT (Fig. 20.1). Kurt et al. [13] reported the lesion was completely confined to the epiphysis in 37% of long bone lesions, and it affected the epiphysis and extended into the adjacent metaphysis in 60% in their series. The authors also reported about 25% of the long bone lesions affected apophyses, either the greater trochanter of the femur or the greater tuberosity of the humerus (Figs. 20.1e and 20.2d). The overall bone contour, including growth plate, is usually not changed by the lesion, but a large lesion may expand the bone contour, particularly in the flat bones or short tubular bones (Fig. 20.4a), or even in apophysis of a long bone (Fig. 20.1e). Cortical breakage with soft tissue mass formation is very rare in contrast to GCT. Periosteal reaction is also rare and typically focal if exists. However, Brower et al. [14] described a distinctive thick, solid periosteal reaction distal to the lesion in 47% of all cases and 57% of CB in long bones (Fig. 20.1a), while such periosteal reaction was not observed in any of the other lesions centered in the epiphysis. Thus, they concluded the presence of this unique periosteal response may help distinguish CB from other epiphyseally centered lesions. Occasionally, widening of the adjacent joint space can be seen, suggesting coexistent effusion. Extensive bony expansion may suggest secondary ABC change. In contrast, GCT is located in the eipphysis, usually extending to subchondral bone plate and meta-diaphysis of the long bones with a closed growth plates. The lesion is typically larger, with incomplete or absent sclerotic rim and no internal calcification. Furthermore, the cortex can be eroded, scalloped, and often expanded with focal destruction suggesting at least locally aggressive lesion or even significant destruction with a naked soft tissue mass mimicking a malignant tumor. Typically, clear cell chondrosarcoma (CC-CSA) also affects the end of the long bone with similar imaging features which can make it difficult to radiologically differentiate from CB. However, CC-CSA usually occurs in adult patients with completely closed growth plate (fourth and fifth decades of life), being one to two decades older than those with CB. **Bone scan** typically shows increased uptake in the lesion, as well as in the adjacent uninvolved bone(s) to a lesser degree (Figs. 20.1, 20.3, 20.4 and 20.5). This suggests that radionuclide uptake in CB is a function of the blood supply to the tumor rather than primary matrix extraction [15]. The increased activity in the

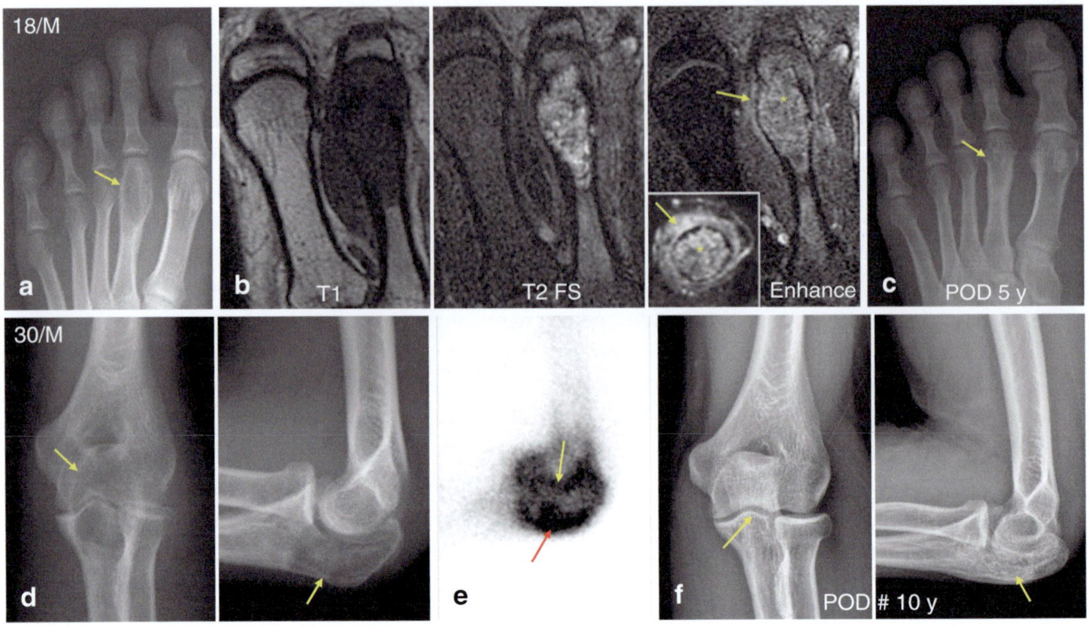

Fig. 20.4 ***Rare location of Metatarsal bone***. (**a**) Radiograph taken for left foot pain of 3 months' duration in a 18-year-old male adolescent shows a well-defined, eccentrically ballooned, oval, osteolytic lesion with a thin rim of sclerosis (arrow) in the distal half of the second metatarsal bone. (**b**) MR images reveal a well-defined, mildly expanding, mass-like lesion mainly in the meta-diaphysis of the second metatarsal bone. The SI is low on T1-weighted image and heterogeneous high SI with focal internal dark signals of calcification on fat saturated T2-weighted image. The bone lesion (asterisks) as well as surrounding soft tissue edema (arrow) is heterogeneously enhanced. (**c**) Follow-up radiograph at 5 years after curettage and allo-chip bone graft notes complete healing of the lesion with contour remodeling of the affected bone (arrow). **Rare location of ulnar**: (**d**) Radiograph taken for left elbow pain of 5 months' duration in a 30-year-old man shows a well-defined radiolucent lesion with internal sclerotic areas, which is surrounded by a thin rim of sclerosis (arrows) in the ulnar olecranon process. (**e**) Bone scan notes a heterogeneous strong uptake in the CB itself of the olecranon (red arrow) with similiar uptake in the unaffected opposing distal humerus (yellow arrow). (**f**) Follow-up radiographs taken at 10 years after curettage and bone graft with a histologic confirmation of CB demonstrate complete healing of the lesion without evidence of local recurrence (arrows)

adjacent uninvolved bone can be as strong as in the CB itself (Fig. 20.4e) or even more extensive than the CB itself, simulating a pattern of uptake in inflammatory lesions and aggressive neoplasms [14]. **CT scan** more celarly delinetes the lesion's relationship to the growth plate and articular surface. Cortical erosion and scalloping, internal calcification, or completeness of a sclerotic rim which is not seen on plain radiographs can be more clearly assessed (Fig. 20.3d). **MR images** typically reveal a well-circumscribed lobular mass-like lesion confined to the epiphysis, often extending into the metaphysis, with low to intermediate SI on T1-weighted image and heterogeneous high SI with areas of low signal on T2-weighted image (Figs. 20.1, 20.2, 20.3, 20.4, and 20.5). The signal on T2-wieghted image is heterogeneous and variable, depending on the

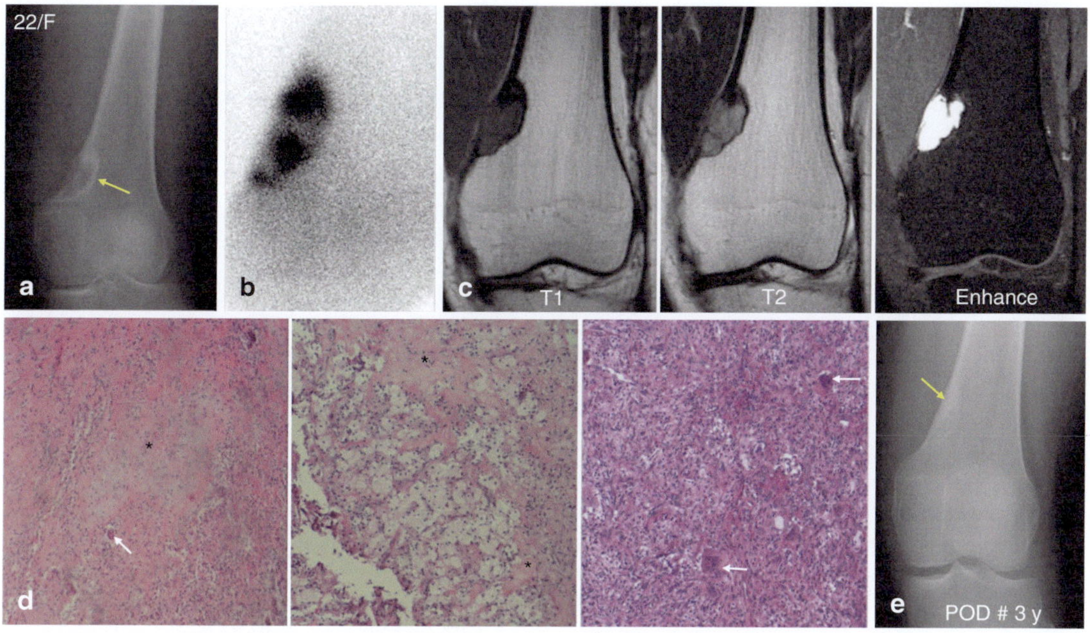

Fig. 20.5 ***Purely metaphyseal and cortical location*****.** (**a**) Radiograph taken for right knee pain after passenger traffic accident in a 22-year-old lady incidentally shows an eccentric, cortex-based, radiolucent lesion surrounded by a thin rim of sclerosis (arrow) purely in the metaphysis rather than the epiphysis of the distal femur, which is very unusual location for CB. (**b**) Pinhole bone scan reveals a heterogeneous strong uptake associated with focal internal void areas. (**c**) MR images demonstrate a well-defined lobulated cortex-based lesion with low SI on T1-weighted image and intermediate to high SI on T2-weighted image, with a peripheral dark signal of sclerotic rim on both sequences. The lesion is purely located in the metaphysis without epiphyseal involvement. Periosteal reaction, peritumoral, or adjacent soft tissue edema is not observed. The lesion is intensely enhanced by contrast medium. (**d**) Microscopic examination shows typical features of CB. Note sheets of uniformly arranged chondroblasts embedded in a pinkish chondroid matrix (asterisks) and randomly distributed multinucleated giant cells (arrows). (**e**) Follow-up radiograph at 3 years after curettage and bone graft demonstrates complete healing of the lesion (arrow).

histologic components, and low SI is most strongly associated with an abundance of immature chondroid matrix, hypercellularity, calcifications, and hemosiderin pigmentation [16]. The lesion is usually surrounded by a thin dark signal of sclerotic rim on both sequences. Edema in the perilesional bone marrow and surrounding soft tissue, joint effusion, or periosteal reaction is often observed, and it can be extensive enough to simulate an accompanied inflammatory lesion or locally more aggressive tumor in some cases. However, CC-CSA is usually larger in size generally with minimal to absent perilesional edema and high signal intensity. The imaging finding can easily differentiate CC-CSA from CB, particularly when considering the typical patient's age. Occasionally, *fluid-fluid levels* (Figs. 20.1g and 20.3g) are associated with moderate to significant expansion, suggesting a secondary aneurysmal bone cyst (ABC). The lesion usually

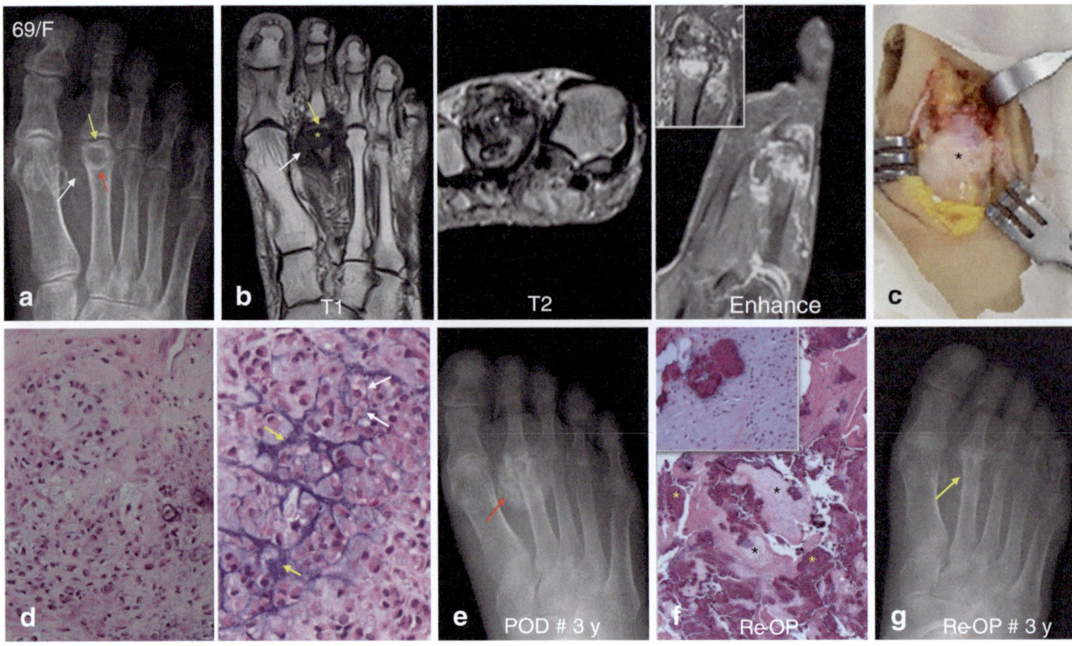

Fig. 20.6 ***The oldest patients in our series.*** (**a**) Radiograph taken for right second toe pain on weight bearing of 10 months' duration in a 69-year-old woman shows a well-defined, round to oval, radiolucent lesion surrounded by a rind of sclerotic bone (red arrow) with a hazy soft tissue mass density (white arrow). Note flattening of the metatarsal head, suggestive of concomittent Freiberg's disease (yellow arrow). (**b**) MR images demonstrate a well-demarcated medullary lesion (asterisks) and soft tissue mass (white arrow) with low SI on T1-weighted image and heterogeneous low and high SI on T2-weighted image. The second metatarsal head is flattened (yellow arrow). The tumor lesion is heterogeneously enhanced by contrast medium. Peri-tumoral and surrounding soft tissue edema is also noted with enhancement. (**c**) A glossy white to yellow soft tissue mass is initially seen on surgical exposure, consistent with a cartilage-rich tumor matrix (asterisk). (**d**) Microscopic examination: (Left) Lower-power magnification reveals proliferation of ovoid to polygonal cells representing chondroblasts arranged in a sheet-like fashion, which are embedded within variably sized nodules of pinkish to light purple chondroid to cartilage-like matrix. (Right) Higher-power magnification reveals fine, linear, thin streaks of calcification surrounding the individual tumor cells, a pathognomonic *chicken-wire* calcification (white arrows). Such fine deposits gradually become confluent and thicker (yellow arrows). Bone necrosis with scattered inflammatory cells is also found, suggesting infarction of the metatarsal head, so-called Freiberg's disease (not shown here). (**e**) Follow-up radiograph taken for aggravating pain on weight bearing at 3 years after curettage and excision of the soft tissue mass notes a recurrent heavily densified large mass (red arrow). (**f**) Microscopic examination of the re-excised specimen shows characteristic multiple chondroid nodules with proliferation of bland-looking ovoid to polygonal cells (black asterisks). In addition, there are numerous foci of coarse, granular, heavy calcification accounting for the heavily densifiedmass on radiograph (yellow asterisks). (**g**) Follow-up radiograph at 3 years after the second surgery reveals no evidence of recurrence of the lesion and she is free of pain.

reveals heterogeneous, lobular, marginal, or septal enhancement (Figs. 20.1, 20.2, 20.3, 20.4, 20.5, and 20.6).

20.8 Histologic Findings

CB is typified by a proliferation of the basic tumor cells representing chondroblasts with areas of chondroid matrix and other foci of varying degrees of spindle cells mixed with scattered multi-nucleated giant cells which are thought to be reactive (Fig. 20.7a, b). Other secondary elements including mature cartilage, calcification, focal hemorrhage or necrosis, foam cells, and/or cholesterol cleft may be observed. The basic tumor cells are uniformly small to intermediate in size, round to polygonal in shape, and are typcially arranged in a sheet-like fashion. Typically, the chondroid matrix is an amorphous pinkish substance deposited as variable-sized nodules which are usually small (Fig. 20.7b). The individual cells have round to oval nucleus, occasionally showing central longitudinal grooves or indentations, producing a so-called *reniform* or *coffee bean* appearance (Fig. 20.7c), similiar to that of Langerhans cells in Langerhans cell histiocytosis. The cytoplasm is clear to mildly basophilic and its border is clearly

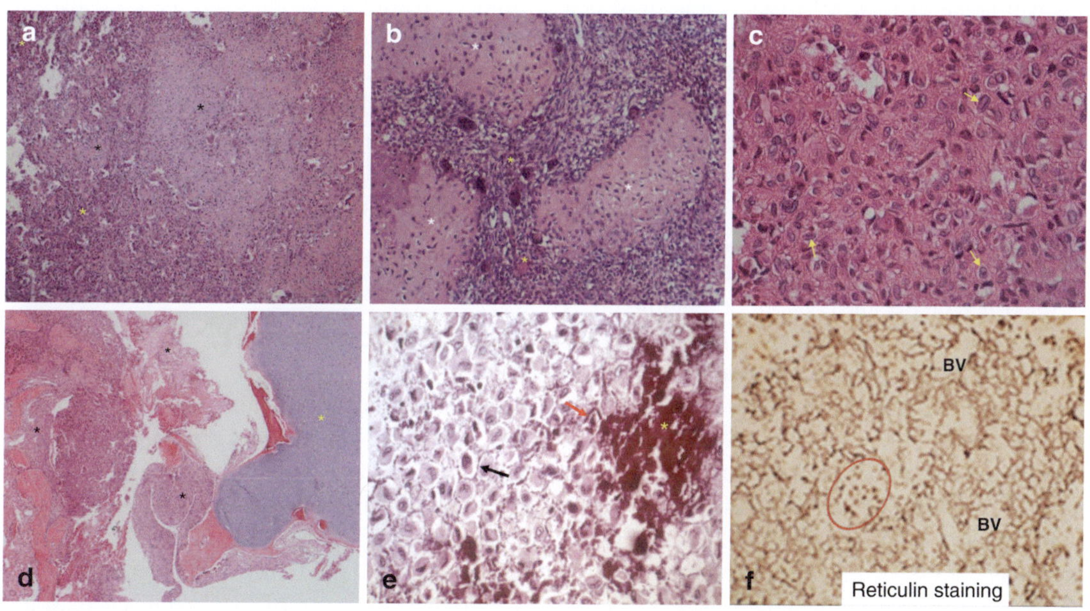

Fig. 20.7 ***Microscopic examination*.** (**a**) Low-power magnification shows uniformly small- to intermediate-sized tumor cells (chondroblasts) arranged in a sheet-like pattern, which are embedded within a pinkish chondroid matrix forming lobular architectures (black asterisks) and other foci of spindle cell proliferation lacking a chondroid matrix (yellow asterisk). (**b**) Medium-power magnification reveals mononuclear chondroblasts embedded within small nodules of pinkish chondroid matrix (white asterisks) and areas of significant proliferation of spindle cells admixed with scattered multinucleated giant cells resembling those those seen in GCT (yellow asterisks). (**c**) Higher-power magnification notes uniformly oval to polygonal chondroblasts with a distinct cytoplasmic margin. Note characteristic nuclear groove and indentation on the nuclei of a few cells, so-called "*reniform* or *coffee bean*" nuclei (yellow arrows), which resemble those in Langerhans cells. (**d**) Rarely, mature cartilage structure rather than chondroid is seen (yellow asterisk). Secondary ABC is also associated in this field (black asterisks). (**e**) A honeycomb pattern of reticulin fibers encompassing the individual chondroblasts is usually not visible without calcification. When lacy calcification proceeds on the fine fibers (black arrow), they can be well visualized in a *honeycomb* or *chicken-wire* pattern. As gradually become confluent and larger (red arrow), they interfere with nutrient supply to the cells which eventually undergo degeneration and necrosis. Finally, this process stimulates the formation of irregular heavy calcific clumps (asterisk). (**f**) Reticulin staining clearly shows an exquisite honeycomb pattern of reticulin fibers encompassing the individual chondroblasts. However, there is no honeycomb pattern in the areas containing multinucleated giant cells (red circle) and blood vessels (BV).

defined. Mitoses can be often observed, but atypical mitosis is never found. Microscopic foci of blood-filled cystic spaces resembling secondary ABC are found in more than one-third of cases, but they usually do not obscure the underlying CB [1]. However, a significant amount of ABC component, which my dominate and nearly obliterate the underlying solid lesion even on radiograph or MRI, is rarely seen presented (Fig. 20.1g). The prominent larger cyst-like spaces filled with blood, indicative of secondary ABC component (Fig. 20.7d), have been found in about 10–20% of cases [4, 6, 17, 18]. Schajowicz and Gallardo [17] described areas with moderate vascularization, frequent hemorrhage, and multiloculated cystic space in 17% of their 69 cases, some of which were lined by tumor cells, often indistinguishable from ABC. They named the lesions with this special pattern *cystic CB*. Dahlin and Ivins [3] also described this type of cystic change can occasionally present as a cystic lesion with serous fluid rather than blood, distinguishing it from secondary ABC. Such cystic change resembling an SBC have also been reported [19]. Fine granular calcium can be deposited on the fine network of reticulin fibers surrounding individual chondroblasts chondroblasts, producing a peculiar *honeycomb* or *chicken-wire* calcification that is pathognomonic if presents (Fig. 20.7e), and found in about two-thirds of the cases [6]. Such pericellular microcalcification can result in degeneration and necrosis of cells, which leads to more calcium deposition. Such deposits gradually become confluent and larger to form clumps, accounting for the minute speck of densification that can be seen even on radiographs. Less frequently, the tumor can be heavily calcified, with numerous foci of coarse granular calcification.

20.9 Special Stains

Reticulin stain clearly exhibits an exquisite "*honeycomb*" or "*chicken-wire*" pattern of reticulin fibers encompassing the individual chondroblasts (Fig. 20.7f). S100 stain is positive in most CBs but negative in GCT, chondromyxoid tumor, and ABC.

20.10 Management

Thorough curettage followed by filling with bone graft or bone substitutes is the standard option for treatment of CB with or without secondary ABC. Local adjuvant therapy, such as liquid nitrogen, phenol, argon-beam coagulation, or ethanol can be added to extend killing of residual tumor cells and to reduce recurrence. Most local recurrences can be healed by a second curettage (Figs. 20.3 and 20.6). Percutaneous radiofrequency heat ablation can be considered for a non-aggressive, localized lesion, with satisfactory results [20, 21]. En-bloc resection with reconstruction using tumor prosthesis or allograft is indicated in selected cases of tumor invading large areas of the metaphysis, soft tissue, and even joint cavity with little residual structural bone. In addition, lung nodules resulting from tumor implantation are simply managed by wedge pulmonary resection, including the implanted nodule.

20.11 Clinical Course

Local recurrence rate after curettage and bone graft with local adjuvant ranges from 5% to 15% [7, 17, 18, 22, 23]. The lesion may recur within the bone or as implantation in the soft tissue. Inadequate surgery including incomplete removal and spreading of the tumor to adjacent soft tissue is an important cause of local recurrence. Some authors reported an increased recurrence rate if ABC is complicated, but the recurrence rate was not higher in CB with secondary ABC in Mayo Clinic series [1]. Similar to GCT, CB is truly benign but rarely disseminates to the lungs in less than 3% of patients [1, 6]. The lung spreading of the tumor probably represents self-limited "transplants," "implants," or "benign metastases" [5, 6]. The nodules are appropriately referred to as *benign lung implantation* rather than as a lung metastasis because they do not result in the development of disseminated, clinically malignant pulmonary disease [4]. The term *aggressive CB* is sometimes used in reference to a lesion that is typically CB on histologic examination, but presents aggressive radiographic features, such as cortical erosion or destruction and soft tissue extension, and larger size than conventional CB at the time of diagnosis [6, 24]. However, Kyriakos et al. [25] reported a unique case of fatal metastatic CB which developed before any surgical manipulation of the primary tumor, unlike previously published cases of metastatic CB. The histologic characteristics of the primary, metastatic, and locally recurrent tumors were identical to conventional CB. Although most metastatic CB may result from surgical manipulation of the primary tumor and are clinically benign, rare cases of benign CB can pursue a malignant course, which were designated as *malignant CB* by the authors. CBs involving the pelvic bone, particularly triradiate cartilage, tend to be radiologically and clinically more aggressive than those in long tubular bones [25, 26]. The lung implantation was also reported concomitantly with local recurrence in sporadic cases [3, 23, 24, 27–33]. The single common feature of all these reported cases was that the metastases were followed by a previous surgical management with local recurrence of the primary tumor. Late malignant changes to a high-grade sarcoma without previous radiation therapy were exceedingly rare [34, 35].

References

1. Unni KK, Inwards CY. Benign chondrobastoma. In: Unni KK, Inwards CY, editors. Dahlin's bone tumors: general aspects and data on 10,165 cases. 6th ed. Philadelphia: Lippincott William & Wilkins; 2010. p. 41–9.
2. Bloem JL, Mulder JD. Chondroblastoma: a clinical and radiological study of 104 cases. Skeletal Radiol. 1985;14(1):1–9.
3. Dahlin DC, Ivins JC. Benign chondroblastoma. A study of 125 cases. Cancer. 1972;30(2):401–13.
4. Czerniak B. Benign cartilage lesions. In: Dorfman HD, Czerniak B, editors. Dorfman and Czerniak's bone tumors. 2nd ed (eBook). Elsevier; 2016. p. 356–473.
5. Huvos AG, Marcove RC. Chondroblastoma of bone a critical review. Clin Orthop Relat Res. 1973;95:300–12.
6. Mirra JM. Chondroblastoma. In: Mirra JM, editor. Bone tumors: clinical, radiologic, and pathologic correlations. 2nd ed. Philadelphia: Lea & Febiger; 1989. p. 589–623.
7. Springfield D, Capanna R, Gherlinzoni F, Picci P, Campanacci M. Chondroblastoma. A review of seventy cases. J Bone Joint Surg Am. 1985;67(5):748–55.
8. Maheshwari AV, Jelinek JS, Song AJ, Nelson KJ, Murphey MD, Henshaw RM. Metaphyseal and diaphyseal chondroblastomas. Skeletal Radiol. 2011;40(12):1563–73.
9. Demertzis JL, Kyriakos M, Connolly S, McDonald DJ. Surface-based chondroblastoma of the tibia: a unique presentation. Skeletal Radiol. 2015;44(7):1045–50.
10. Hameed MR, Blacksin M, Das K, Patterson F, Benevenia J, Aisner S. Cortical chondroblastoma: report of a case and literature review of this lesion reported in unusual locations. Skeletal Radiol. 2006;35(5):295–7.
11. Yang J, Tian W, Zhu X, Wang J. Chondroblastoma in the long bone diaphysis: a report of two cases with literature review. Chin J Cancer. 2012;31(5):257–64.
12. Sauer MA, Stegelmeier P, Crim JR, Layfield LJ, Evenski A. A report of an intracortical chondroblastoma of the diaphysis in a skeletally mature patient. Skeletal Radiol. 2022;51(12):2341–6.
13. Kurt A-M, Unni KK, Sim FH, McLeod RA. Chondroblastoma of bone. Hum Pathol. 1989;20(10):965–76.
14. Brower AC, Moser R, Kransdorf M. The frequency and diagnostic significance of periostitis in chondroblastoma. Am J Roentgenol. 1990;154(2):309–14.
15. Humphry A, Gilday DL, Brown RG. Bone scintigraphy in chondroblastoma. Radiology. 1980;137(2):497–9.
16. Jee WH, Park YK, McCauley TR, Choi KH, Ryu KN, Suh JS, et al. J Comput Assist Tomogr. 1999;23(5):721–6.
17. Schajowicz F, Gallardo H. Epiphysial chondroblastoma of bone: a climco-pathological study of sixty-nine cases. J Bone Joint Surg Br. 1970;52(2):205–26.
18. Suneja R, Grimer R, Belthur M, Jeys L, Carter S, Tillman R, et al. Chondroblastoma of bone: long-term results and functional outcome after intralesional curettage. J Bone Joint Surg (Br). 2005;87(7):974–8.
19. Ippolito E, Tudisco C, Mariani P. Rare forms of chondroblastoma. Cystic and diaphyseal types. Ital J Orthop Traumatol. 1986;12(4):455–60.
20. Erickson JK, Rosenthal DI, Zaleske DJ, Gebhardt MC, Cates JM. Primary treatment of chondroblastoma with percutaneous radio-frequency heat ablation: report of three cases. Radiology. 2001;221(2):463–8.
21. Rybak LD, Rosenthal DI, Wittig JC. Chondroblastoma: radiofrequency ablation-alternative to surgical resection in selected cases. Radiology. 2009;251(2):599–604.
22. Lin PP, Thenappan A, Deavers MT, Lewis VO, Yasko AW. Treatment and prognosis of chondroblastoma. Clin Orthop Relat Res. 2005;438:103–9.

23. Ramappa AJ, Lee FY, Tang P, Carlson JR, Gebhardt MC, Mankin HJ. Chondroblastoma of bone. J Bone Joint Surg. 2000;82(8):1140–5.
24. Huvos A, Higinbotham N, Marcove R, Oleary P. Aggressive chondroblastoma: review of the literature on aggressive behavior and metastases with a report of one new case. Clin Orthop Relat Res. 1977;126:266–72.
25. Kyriakos M, Land VJ, Penning HL, Parker SG. Metastatic chondroblastoma. Report of a fatal case with a review of the literature on atypical, aggressive, and malignant chondroblastoma. Cancer. 1985;55(8):1770–89.
26. Matsuno T, Hasegawa I, Masuda T. Chondroblastoma arising in the triradiate cartilage: report of two cases with review of the literature. Skeletal Radiol. 1987;16:216–22.
27. Green P, Whittaker R. Benign chondroblastoma. Case report with pulmonary metastasis. J Bone Joint Surg. 1975;57(3):418–20.
28. Riddell R, Bromberger N, Louis C. Pulmonary metastases from chondroblastoma of the tibia: report of a case. J Bone Joint Surg (Br). 1973;55(4):848–53.
29. Kunze E, Graewe T, Peitsch E. Histology and biology of metastatic chondroblastoma: report of a case with a review of the literature. Pathol Res Pract. 1987;182(1):113–20.
30. Elek EM, Grimer RJ, Mangham DC, Davies AM, Carter SR, Tillman RM. Malignant chondroblastoma of the os calcis. Sarcoma. 1998;2(1):45–8.
31. Kahn L, Wood F, Ackerman L. Malignant chondroblastoma. Report of two cases and reviw of the literature. Arch Pathol. 1969;88(4):371–6.
32. Wellmann KF. Chondroblastoma of the scapula. A case report with ultrastructural observations. Cancer. 1969;24(2):408–16.
33. Wirman JA, Crissman JD, Aron BF. Metastatic chondroblastoma. Report of an unusual case treated with radiotherapy. Cancer. 1979;44(1):87–93.
34. Sirsat M, Doctor VM. Benign chondroblastoma of bone: report of a case of malignant transformation. J Bone Joint Surg (Br). 1970;52(4):741–5.
35. Reyes CV, Kathuria S. Recurrent and aggressive chondroblastoma of the pelvis with late malignant neoplastic changes. Am J Surg Pathol. 1979;3(5):449–56.

Central Low-Grade/Atypical Cartilaginous Tumor and High-Grade Conventional Chondrosarcoma

21

(***chondros*** "cartilage" + ***sarkos*** "*flesh*" + ***ōma*** "*forming*")

21.1 Definition

Central chondrosarcoma (CSA) is a locally aggressive (low-grade) or malignant (intermediate to high grade) bone tumor producing a cartilaginous matrix that is uniformly and entirely chondroid in nature, arising in the medulla of the bone with diverse morphological features and clinical behavior. Grade 1 or atypical cartilage tumor (ACT) is low-grade, grade 2 is intermediate-grade, and grade 3 is a high-grade malignant tumor. Primary central CSA arises de novo in normal bone without a preexisting benign bone tumor (Figs. 21.1, 21.2, 21.3, 21.4, 21.5, 21.6, 21.7, 21.8, 21.9, 21.10, 21.11, 21.12, and 21.13). Secondary CSA may arise centrally in enchondroma(s) (EC) (Figs. 21.14 and 21.15) or peripherally in osteochondroma(s) (OC) (Figs. 21.16, 21.17, 21.18, and 21.19), especially in multiple lesions of both entities. It can also develop in (polyostotic) fibrous dysplasia, synovial chondromatosis, Paget's disease, and after irradiation.

W.-J. Bahk, *Diagnosis and Management of Primary Bone Tumors*,
https://doi.org/10.1007/978-981-96-3484-2_21

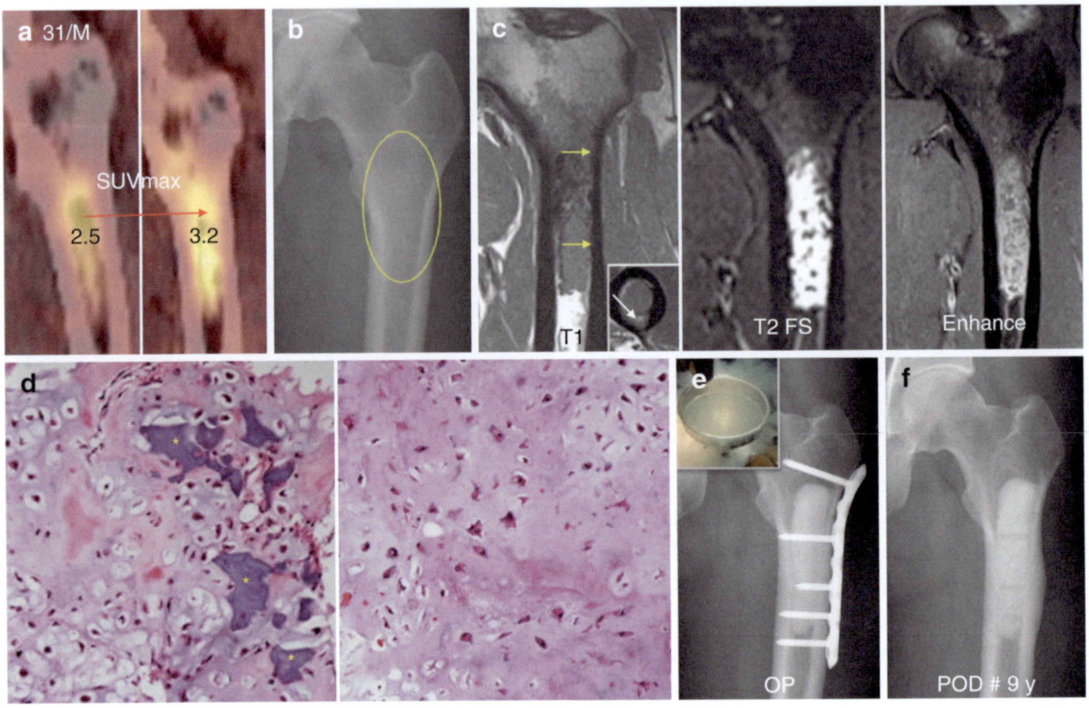

Fig. 21.1 ***ACT/Grade 1 (low-grade) CAS. Incidentally found CSA***. (**a**) A 31-year-old man, previously treated with orchiectomy and chemotherapy for testicular seminoma, was transferred to our department because of increased SUVmax from 2.5 to 3.2 in the left proximal femur on follow-up PET/CT scan which was found after orchiectomy followed by chemotherapy for testicular seminoma of the testis. The lesion was incidentally found and the patient reminaed asymptomatic. (**b**) Radiograph notes no definite abnormal findings in the corresponding area (circle). (**c**) However, MR images reveals a relatively well-defined intramedullary lesion with iso SI on T1-weighted image and bright SI with focal dark signal on T2-weighted image in the diaphysis of the proximal femur. Note irregular endosteal scalloping about two-thirds of lesion extent (between arrows) and greater than two-thirds of the cortical thickness at its most prominent area, suggesting CSA rather than EC (white arrow in inset). The lesion shows a characteristic peripheral and septal enhancement in *rings and arcs* pattern. (**d**) Microscopic examination: (Left) Medium-power magnification shows chondroid to cartilage matrix undergoing osseous metaplasia via endochondral ossification, which finally produces purple islands of bone deeply buried within the cartilage matrix (asterisks). This should not be misinterpreted as a *permeation* or *entrapment* pattern of the host lamellar bone. (Right) On higher-power magnification, the cellularity is moderate and chondrocytes exhibit mild to moderate atypia in size and shape, indicating Grade 1 CSA in consideration of longer cortical endosteal scalloping and deeper cortical invasion on MRI. (**e**) Extended curettage using high-speed burr and adjuvant therapy with cryosurgery using liquid nitrogen (inset), followed by cement filling and plating to prevent perioperative fracture. (**f**) Follow-up radiograph at 9 years after surgery notes no evidence of recurrence, which can clinically support the lesion would be low-grade CSA rather than higher-grade CSA

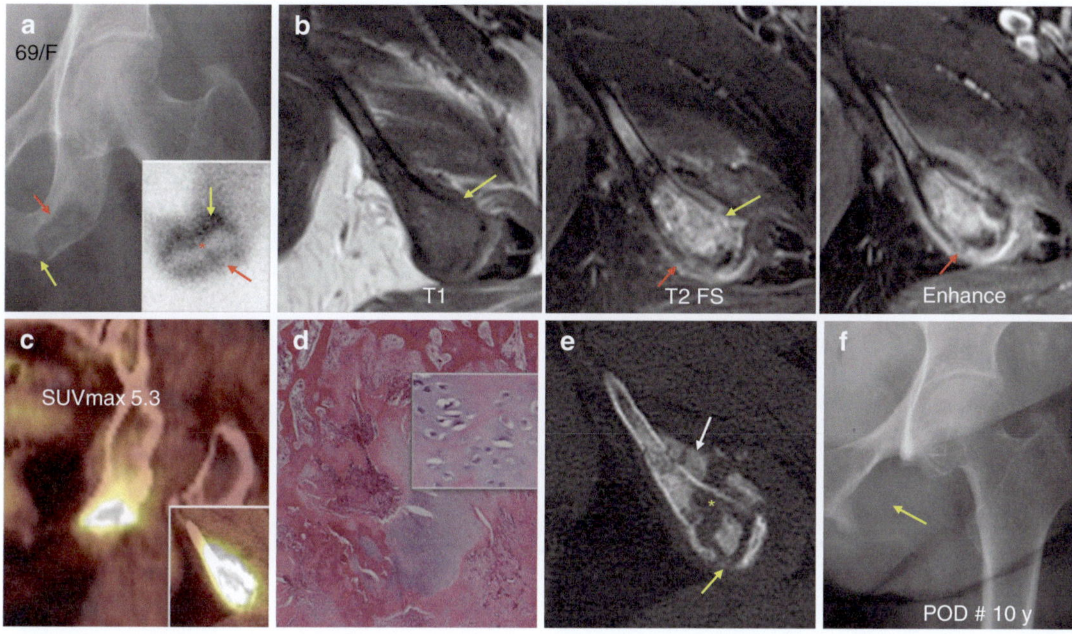

Fig. 21.2 *ACT/Grade 1 (low-grade) CAS*. (**a**) Radiograph taken for left buttock pain of 6 months' duration in a 69-year-old woman shows a relatively well-defined radiolucent lesion with a wispy "windblown" density (red arrow) and cortical breakage (yellow arrow) in the ischial tuberosity. Pinhole bone scan reveals strong uptake along the upper margin of lesion (yellow arrow) and mild uptake in the lower margin (red arrow) with an activity-free inner portion (red asterisk). (**b**) MR images demonstrate an intramedullary mass-like lesion with low and intermediate SI on T1-weighted image and high SI with focal bright signals on fat-saturated T2-weighted image with focal cortical breakage and soft tissue extension (yellow arrows). There is also soft tissue edema or hemorrhage (red arrow). Both the osseous and soft tissue lesions as well as adjacent soft tissue edema or hemorrhage are well enhanced by contrast medium. (**c**) PET/CT scan reveals a destructive lesion with cortical breakage and soft tissue mass in the ischial tuberosity with a high FDG uptake (SUVmax 5.3). (**d**) Microscopic examination notes an infiltrative growth of cartilage matrix with *permeation* of host bone spicules by tumor cartilge, as well as areas of focal necrosis and calcification. Higher-power magnification shows low to moderate cellularity with only mild atypism, indicating Grade 1 CSA (inset). (**e**) CT scan after incision biopsy shows a relatively well-defined radiolucent lesion (yellow asterisk) with cortical breakage (yellow arrow) and internal calcification, as well as callus formation (white arrow). (**f**) Follow-up radiograph at 10 years after wide resection reveals no evidence of local recurrence (red arrow)

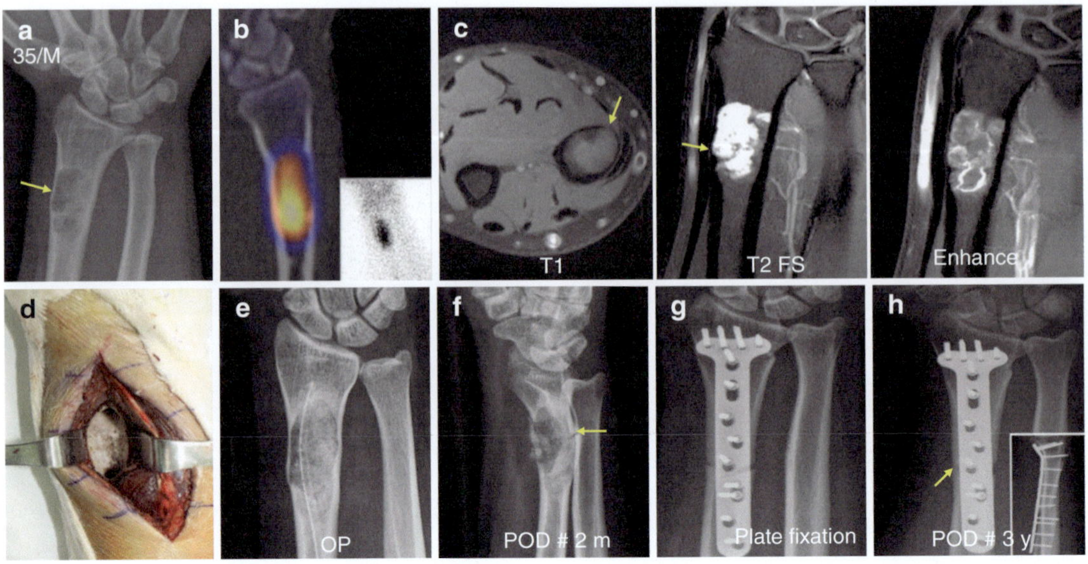

Fig. 21.3 *ACT/Grade 1 (low-grade) CAS.* (**a**) Radiograph taken for right wrist pain of several months in a 35-year-old man shows a multilobulated, mildly expanding, radiolucent lesion with internal sclerotic density in the distal diaphysis of the radius. Note significant scalloping longer and deeper than tow-thirds of the involved cortex, producing marked cortical thinning (arrow). (**b**) Bone SPECT and bone scan reveal an intense focal uptake. (**c**) MR images demonstrate a multilobulated mass-like lesion with intermediate SI with focal low signal on T1-weighted image and bright SI on fat-suppressed T2-weighted image. Note that the lesion is invading the cortex and eroding more than two-thirds of cortical thickness with suspicious breaching (yellow arrows), strongly suggesting a malignancy. The lesion presents a thin enhancement characteristically in *peripheral and nodular* pattern. (**d**) With histologic confirmation of Grade 1 CSA, extended curettage using high-speed bur followed by adjuvant therapy using anhydrous ethanol with electric cauterization and allogenic chip bone graft was performed. (**e**) Immediate postoperative radiograph shows allogenic chip bone filling the defect. (**f**) Follow-up radiograph taken for severe right wrist pain at 2 months after surgery reveals a pathologic fracture (arrow). (**g**) Plate fixation was performed. (**h**) Follow-up radiograph at 3 years after surgery shows no evidence of local recurrence with healing of fracture (red arrow)

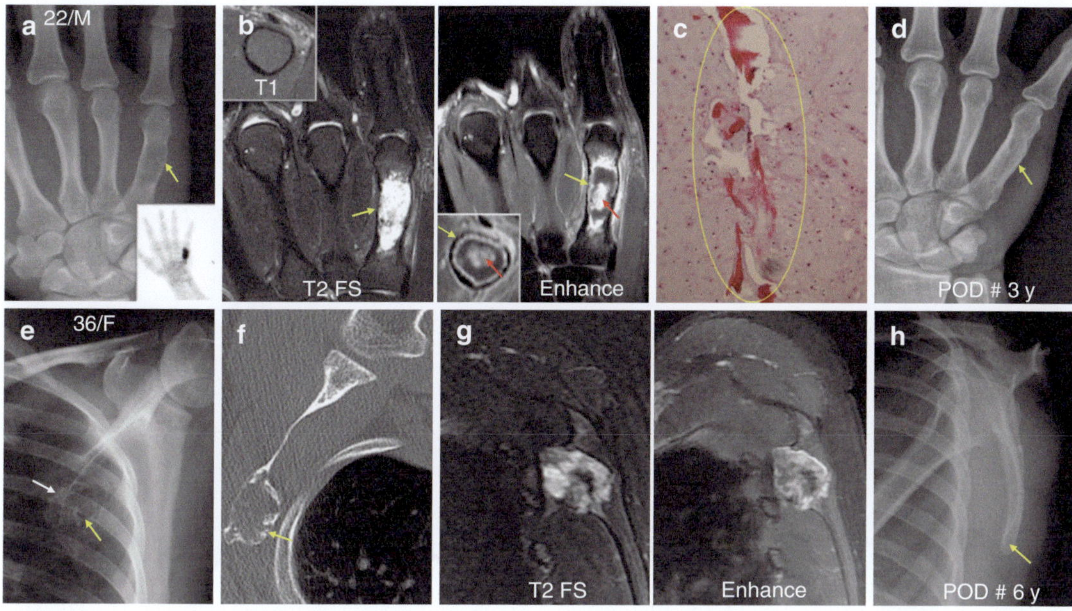

Fig. 21.4 ***ACT/Grade 1 (low-grade) CAS. Rare location of the hand***. (**a**) Radiograph taken for right hand pain of 2 months' duration in a 22-year-old young man shows a relatively ill-defined fusiform osteolytic lesion with hazy tiny stippled calcifications in the right fifth metacarpal. There is a mild expansion with "egg shell-like" cortical thinning (arrow). Bone scan reveals a strong focal uptake (inset). (**b**) MR images reveal a relatively ill-demarcated medullary lesion involving the entire diaphysis with minimal ballooning, cortical thinning, and longer and deeper scalloping greater than two-thirds of the cortex thickness (yellow arrow). SI is iso to muscle on T1-weighted image and diffusely bright with focal dark signals stippled calcification on fat suppressed T2-weighted image. The lesion is enhanced typically in peripheral (yellow arrows) and central nodular pattern (red arrows). (**c**) Microscopic examination typically notes *permeation* and *entrapment* tissue pattern of host bone spicules by tumor cartilage indicative of CAS of any grade (circle). The cytologic features are moderately cellular with mild atypia with a few bi-nucleated chondrocytes but no mitosis, indicating Grade 1 CSA. (**d**) Follow-up radiograph at 3 years after thorough curettage and allogenic bone graft reveals consolidation of the graft and remodeled cortex without evidence of local recurrence. **Incidentally found CSA**: (**e**) Chest radiograph taken for routine medical check-up in a 36-year-old lady incidentally shows a relatively ill-defined, mildly expanding lesion with multiple stippled calcification in inferior body of the scapula (white arrow) and soft tissue mass with irregular sclerotic rim and internal calcification as well (yellow arrow). (**f**) CT scan reveals a markedly expanding, osteolytic lesion with ballooning of the contour and focal cortical destruction (arrows). (**g**) MR images reveal an expansile mass with heterogeneous intermediate and high SI with internal dark signal of calcification on fat-saturated T2-weighted image. The lesion is heterogeneously enhanced in *peripheral and nodular* pattern. (**h**) Follow-up radiograph at 6 years after wide resection under histologic diagnosis of Grade 1 CSA with a *CSA Permeation* tissue pattern notes consolidation of the lesion with no local recurrence (arrow)

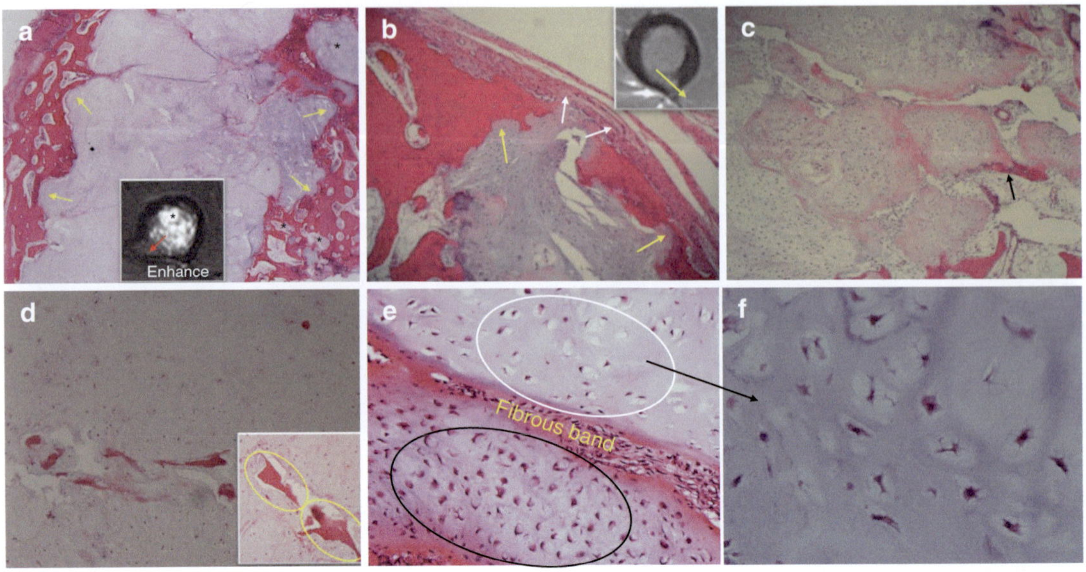

Fig. 21.5 ***ACT/Grade 1 (low-grade) CAS. Microscopic examination***. (**a**) Low-power magnification shows a lobulated architecture with irregular-shaped and variable-sized cartilage lobules separated by thin fibrous bands, which erode the cortices (arrows) and infiltrate host lamellar bone trabeculae (asterisks). The lobular growth pattern represents a deep cortical scalloping (red arrow) and *peripheral and nodular* enhancement (black asterisk) on MR image (inset). (**b**) Medium-power magnification reveals cartilage nodules with bland-looking tumor cells of low cellularity deeply infiltrating the host cortex (yellow arrows). Cortical destruction with extension of the tumor cells into the subperiosteal space can produce a periosteal lifting (white arrows) and soft tissue mass, which is represented as deep erosion and cortical breakage with soft tissue extension on MRI (inset). (**c**) Higher-power magnification presents variable-sized hyaline cartilage lobules with moderate to high cellularity, myxoid change, dystrophic calcification, and progressed surrounding osseous metaplasia via endochondral ossification (black arrow) which represent an enhancement in *rings and arcs pattern* on MRI. A varying degree of myxoid change in the hyaline cartilage matrix can be another criterion for differentiation of CSA from EC. (**d**) Several residual lamellar bone trabeculae of host bone surrounded by tumor cells on all sides are found with low to moderate cellularity, hyperchromatic, and plump nuclei that are considered as the same or slightly higher grade to EC. However, this *permeation* or *entrapment* pattern is the most valuable hallmark of CSA, no matter how the cytologic features are bland or innocent. (**e**) Note hyaline nodules are separated by *fibro-vascular band* consisting of collagen layers of fibroblast-like cells with microvasculature. The interlobular cartilage bands are another diagnostic tissue pattern for CAS. Cytological features include slightly increased cellularity with mild nuclear atypia indicating Grade 1 CSA (white circle). Another lower area with greater degree of cellularity and mild to moderate atypism makes an overall diagnosis of Grade 2 CSA (black circle). (**f**) Higher-power magnification of the upper field (white circle) reveals a low cellularity with hyperchromatic and plump nuclei that would be within range of EC. However, Grade 1 CSA can be rendered by the tissue pattern of *band of fibrosis*. If a biopsy specimen includes only the upper part of the tumor, a differential diagnosis between Grade 1 CSA and EC should be extremely difficult. Or, it would be diagnosed as Grade 1 CSA when the biopsy specimen only includes the area with low-grade component and other tissue patterns of CSA (Fig. 21.9d). Biopsy material should be enough to thoroughly evaluate the cytologic features and tissue patterns in as many field as possible. Thus, proper incision biopsy is strongly recommended rather than needle or trocar biopsy particularly in cartilaginous tumors which are not radiographically high-grade

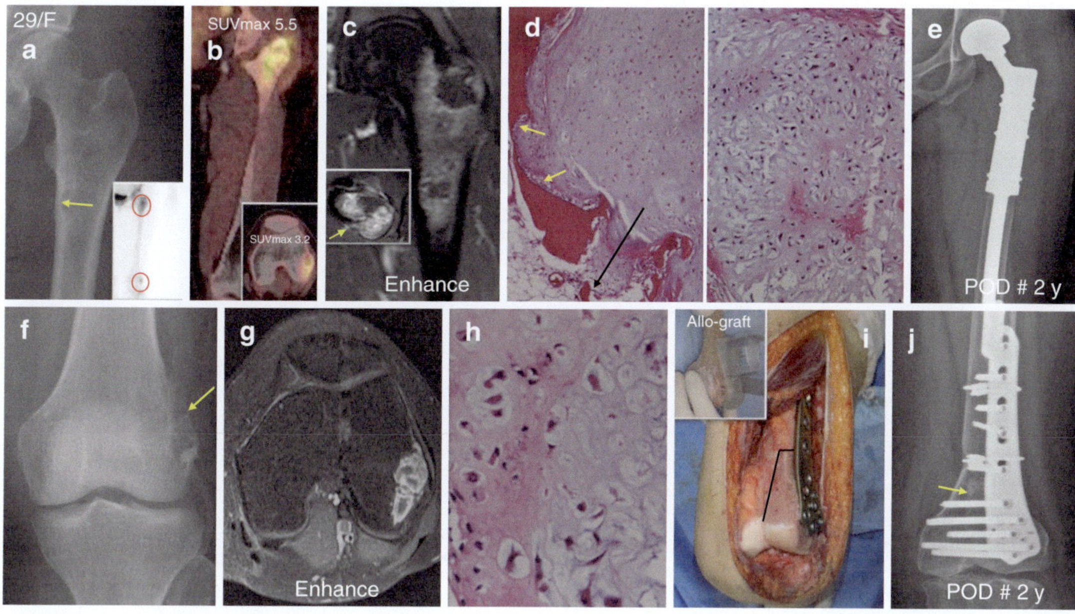

Fig. 21.6 ***Grade 2 (intermediate-grade) CAS.*** (**a**) Radiograph taken for left hip pain of 3 months' duration in a 29-year-old young lady shows a fuzzy, ill-defined, multilobulated radiolucent lesion with mild expansion and moderate cortical scalloping (arrows) in the proximal femur. The grade of endosteal scalloping is only grade 1 in extent and depth. Bone scan reveals heterogeneously increased uptake in the proximal femur and incidental finding of another focal uptake in the lateral condyle of distal femur (red circles). (**b**) PET/CT scan reveals increased FDG uptake in the proximal femur (SUVmax 5.5) and the lateral condyle (SUVmax 3,2), suggesting a possible skip lesion. (**c**) MR image presents an ill-defined medullary lesion with a heterogeneous enhancement, which extends into the adjacent soft tissue through a cortical breakage on axial image (inset). However, the grade of endosteal scalloping is also grade 1 in extent and depth as seen on plain radiograph. (**d**) Microscopic examination: (Left) Lower-power magnification notes permeation of host lamellar bones by tumor cells embedded in cartilaginous stroma (yellow arrows). Note that the tumor entraps the host lamellar bone and extends to the adjacent soft tissue through the bone destruction, indicating CSA (black arrow). (Right) Higher-power magnification notes high cellularity with moderate nuclear atypia in size and shape, which is consistent with Grade 2 CSA. (**e**) Radiograph at 2 years after wide resection and reconstruction with a tumor prosthesis notes good maintenance of the prosthesis without local recurrence. (**f**) Additional radiograph shows an ill-defined, eccentric, radiolucent lesion with hazy internal densities and severe cortical thinning and possible cortical destruction involving the lateral condyle of the ipsilateral femur (arrow). (**g**) Contrast enhancing MR image reveals a well-defined, eccentric medullary lesion with SI similiar to that of the proximal proximal lesion and a typical *peripheral and nodular* enhancement, indicating a very rare skip lesion. (**h**) Microscopic examination reveals histologic findings identical to those observed in (D), indicating a skip lesopn of Grade 2 CSA. (**i**) Wide resection of lateral condyle followed by reconstruction with hemicondylar allogenic femur (black line) designed by 3D printed cutting guide (inset) and plate fixation was performed. (**j**) Follow-up radiograph at 2 years after surgery also reveals no evidence of local recurrence with complete union of the graft (arrow)

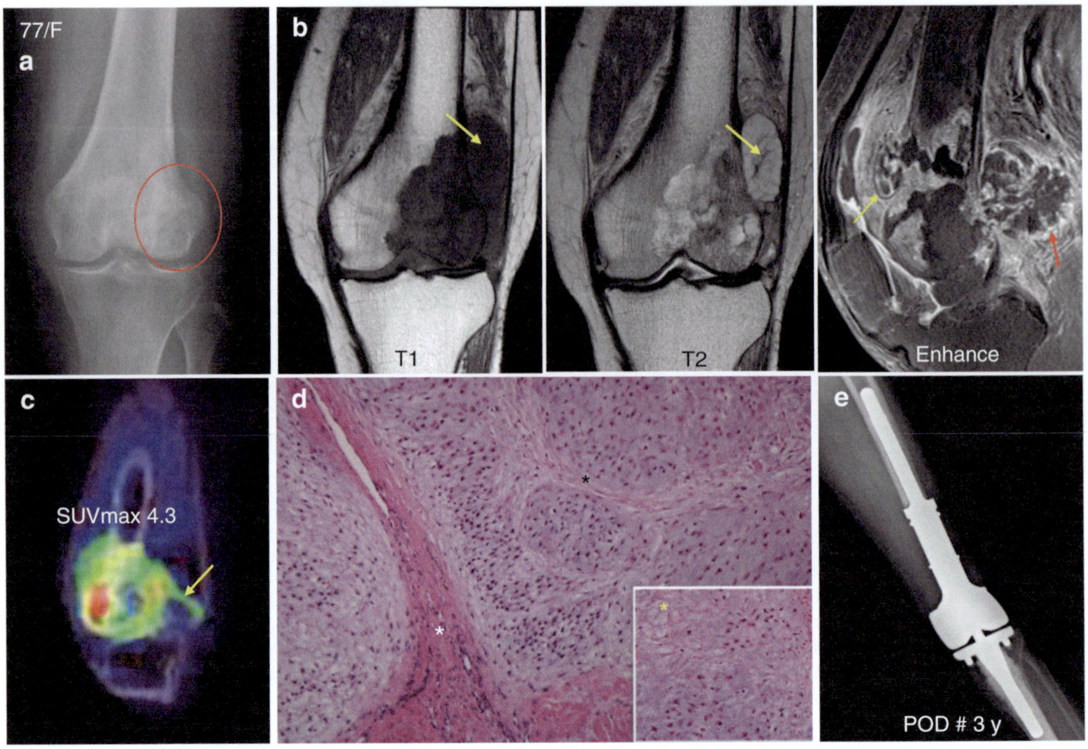

Fig. 21.7 ***Grade 2 (intermediate-grade) CAS***. (**a**) Radiograph taken for left knee pain of 3 months' duration in a 77-year-old woman shows an ill-defined, eccentric, intramedullary osteolytic lesion with internal opacities in the lateral condyle of the distal femur (red circle). (**b**) MR images present a well-defined, eccentric, intramedullary mass-like lesion with cortical destruction and naked soft tissue mass (yellow arrows). The SI is low on T1-weighted image and heterogeneous intermediate and high on T2-weighted image. The medullary lesion (yellow arrow) and soft tissue mass (red arrow) are well enhanced in a typical *peripheral and nodular* pattern. (**c**) PET/CT scan demonstrates increased FDG uptake (SUVmax 4.3) in the distal femur and soft tissue mass as well as additional mild uptake in the previous biopsy tract (arrow). (**d**) Microscopic examination: Lower-power magnification notes irregular and variable-sized cartilage lobules separated by fibrous bands of variable thickness (asterisks). The individual nodules exhibit high cellularity with moderate nuclear atypism, suggesting Grade 2 CSA. Note a thick fibrous band consisting of several fibroblast-like cell lining collagen layers and microvasculature, so-called *bands of fibrosis* pattern (white asterisk), which is one of the diagnostic tissue patterns for CAS. There is a focal field of necrosis with myxoid change (asterisk in inset). (**e**) Follow-up radiograph shows at 3 years after wide resection and reconstruction with a tumor prosthesis reveals good maintenance of the tumor prosthesis without local recurrence

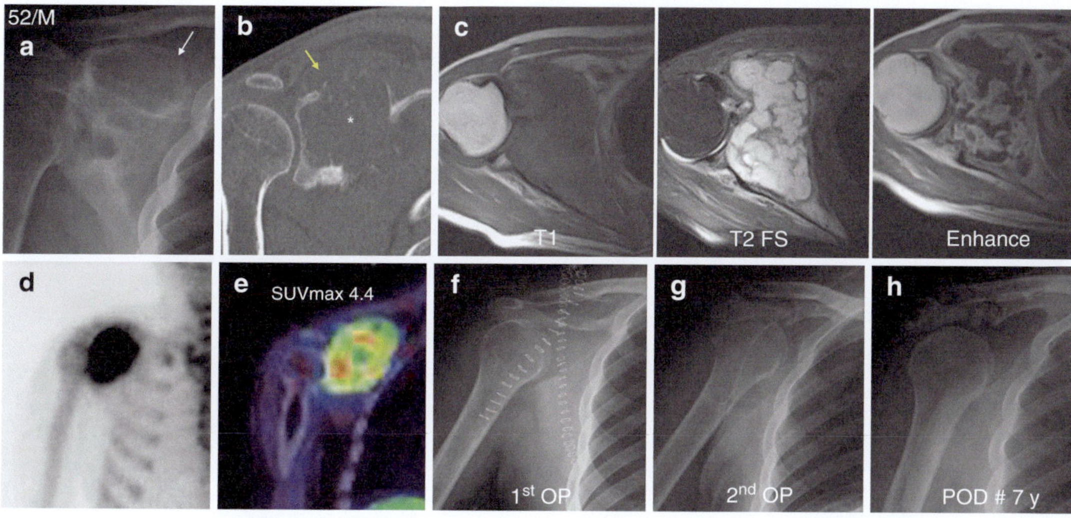

Fig. 21.8 ***Grade 2 (intermediate-grade) CAS***. (**a**) Radiograph taken for right shoulder swelling of 2 years' duration in a 52-year-old man shows a relatively well-defined, expansile, multilobulated predominantly osteolytic lesion with flocculent internal calcification and possible cortical breaches (arrow) in the glenoid and body of the right scapula. (**b**) CT scan more clearly reveals an expanding radiolucent lesion with flocculent internal calcification (asterisk) and soft tissue extension through the severely destructed cortex which is not clearly discernible on radiograph (arrow). (**c**) MR images also demonstrate an expansile, mutilobulated multilobulated mass-like lesion with cortical destruction and soft tissue mass. The SI is low to intermediate SI on T1-weighted image and bright SI surrounded by intermediate signal in a nodular fashion on fat-saturated T2-weighted image. The lesion is heterogeneously enhanced in a typical *peripheral and nodular* pattern. (**d**) Bone scan notes a homogeneous intense uptake in the right scapula. (**e**) PET/CT scan demonstrates large heterogeneous FDG uptake (SUVmax 4.4). (**f**) A partial scapulectomy with adequate margin followed by extra-skeletal musculotendinous unit reconstruction was performed under a histologic diagnosis of Grade 2 CSA. (**g**) Second wide excision of the recurrent tumor mass and biceps short head tendon with reconstruction using palmaris longus tendon was performed based on MR findings of local recurrence in the soft tissue around the biceps tendon. Microscopic examination confirmed a diagnosis of recurrent Grade 2 CSA. (**h**) Follow-up radiograph and MRI at 7 years after first surgery show no evidence of local recurrence

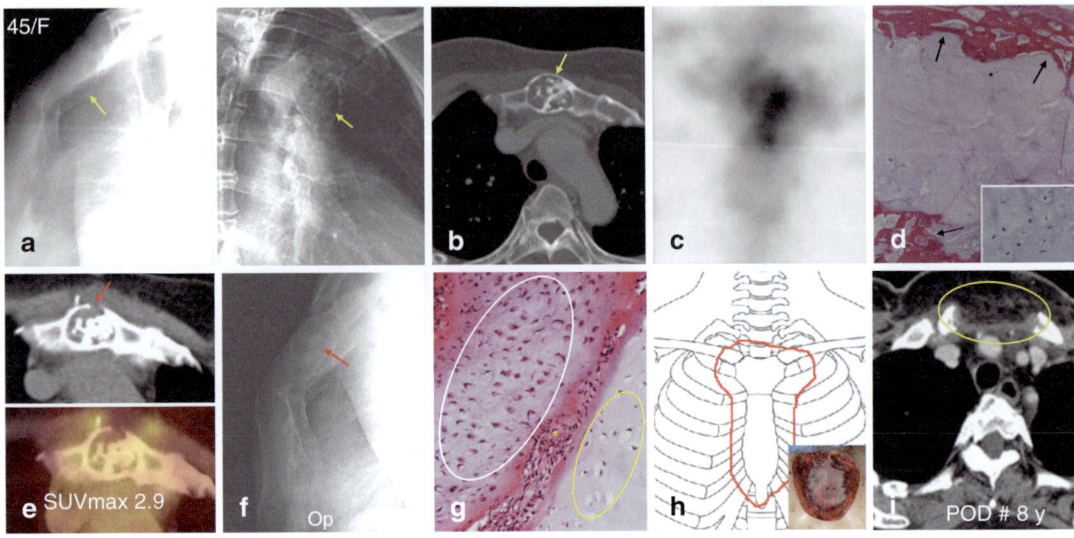

Fig. 21.9 ***Grade 2 (intermediate-grade) CAS***. (**a**) Radiograph taken for sternal mass of 5 months' duration in a 45-year-old woman shows a well-defined, expansile, osteolytic lesion with internal stippled calcification and cortical thinning without an equivocal cortical breakage in the sternal manubrium (arrows). (**b**) CT scan notes a well-defined, ballooning, radiolucent lesion with irregular flecks of calcification and intact cortex (arrow). (**c**) Pinhole bone scan reveals strong uptake with a focal mild uptake in the sternal manubrium. (**d**) Low-power microscopic examination shows lobulated cartilaginous tumor nodules infiltrating the host lamellar bones (arrows). High-power examination notes a low cellularity with normal to mild nuclear atypia within range of EC, indicative of Grade 1 CSA in consideration of the infiltrating pattern (inset). (**e**) PET/CT scan shows cortical perforation persistent with the site of previous incision biopsy (red arrow) with moderately increased FDG uptake (SUVmax 2.9). (**f**) Thorough curettage followed by allogenic chip bone grafting was performed. (**g**) However, microscopic examination of curetted specimen reveals an area of significantly increased cellularity with greater degree of atypism indicating Grade 2 CSA (black circle) and another area of less cellular with mild nuclear atypia indicating Grade 1 CSA (yellow circle), which are divided by *fibro-vascular band* consisting of collagen layers of fibroblast-like cells with microvasculature (asterisk). (**h**) En-bloc resection including sternum, costal cartilage of ribs, and clavicle head (red schematic line) was subsequently performed due to the revised diagnosis of Grade 2 CSA. The resulting defect was reconstructed with double-layered mesh and musculocutaneous pedicle flap (inset). This case emphasizes the importance of obtaining an adequate and representative biopsy sample to ensure an accurate diagnosis. (**i**) Follow-up CT scan at 8 years after en-bloc resection shows no evidence of local recurrence (yellow circle). However, she has intermittent pain over the keloid surgical scar

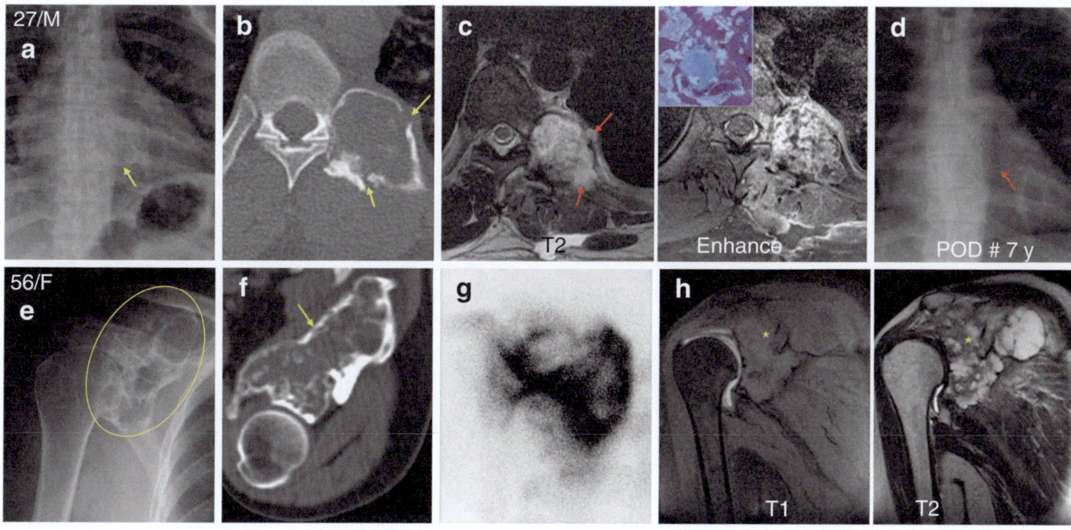

Fig. 21.10 ***Grade 2 (intermediate-grade) CAS*****.** (**a**) Radiograph taken for midback pain of 2 years' duration in a 27-year-old man shows a well-defined ballooning osteolytic lesion with subtle internal density in the left costovertebral junction area of T10 vertebra (arrow). (**b**) CT scan reveals a well-circumscribed, significantly expanding, osteolytic lesion with focal internal calcifications and cortical disruption (arrows). (**c**) MR images demonstrate an expansile lesion mainly affecting the posterior arch of the rib and a part of T10 vertebra with low SI on T1-weighted image and heterogeneous high SI on T2-weighted image. There are focal cortical breakages with small soft tissue masses (arrows). The lesion is heterogeneously enhanced in a *peripheral and nodular* pattern. Incision biopsy confirms a diagnosis of Grade 2 CSA (inset). (**d**) Follow-up radiograph at 7 years after wide resection and posterior fusion of vertebrae shows no evidence of local recurrence. (**e**) Radiograph taken for right shoulder pain of 1 year's duration and recently developed swelling in a 56-year-old woman shows a multilobulated, large, expansile, osteolytic lesion with internal opacities in the glenoid and body of scapula (circle). (**f**) CT scan more clearly reveals a significantly expansile mass with internal flecks of calcification and irregularly thinned and thickened cortex (arrow). (**g**) Pinhole bone scan shows homogeneous strong uptake with multiple focal void areas. (**h**) MR arthrogram reveals a huge expansile mass-like lesion (asterisks) with intermediate (iso SI to surrounding muscle) on T1-weighted image and hetero geneous intermediate and high SI on fat-saturated T2-weighted image. Histologic examination reveals lobular tumor growth with a *permeation* tissue pattern with moderate cellularity and nuclear pleomorphism, consistent with Grade 2 CSA.

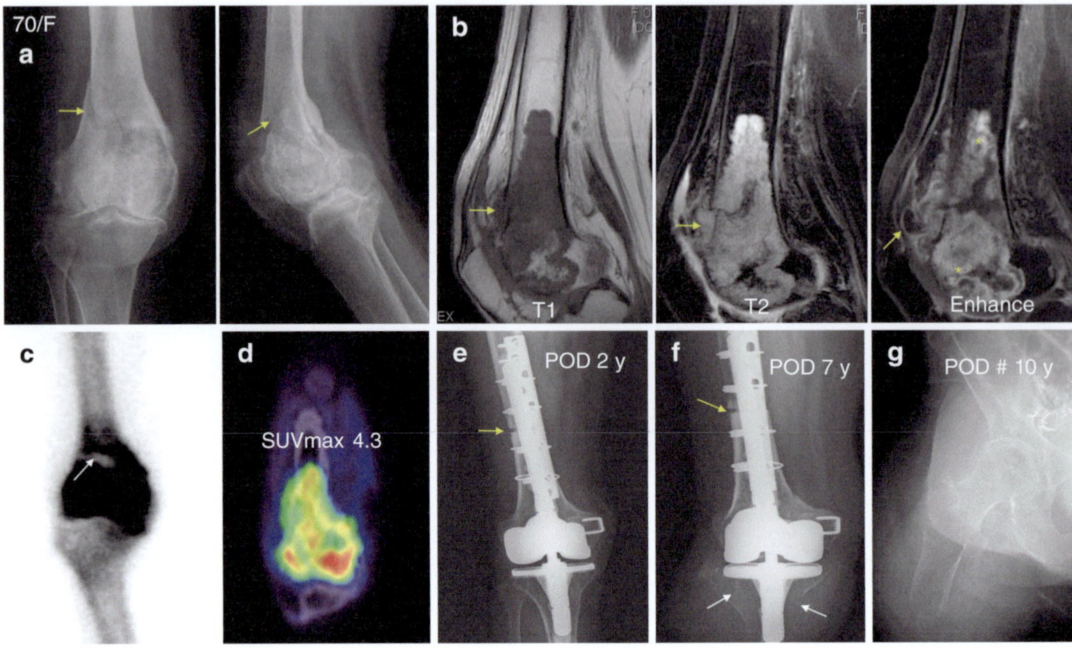

Fig. 21.11 *Grade 3 (high-grade) CAS*. (**a**) Radiograph taken for right knee pain after slip in a 70-year-old woman incidentally shows an ill-defined osteolytic lesion with internal mineralization showing *windblown* and *ring-and-arc* pattern in the distal femur, along with a pathologic fracture (arrows). (**b**) MR images reveal a well-defined intramedullary multilobulated lesion with low to intermediate SI on T1-weighted image and high SI with internal dark signal on T2-weighted image. Note tumor spillage with soft tissue extension through the fracture gap (arrows). The main medullary (asterisks) and soft tissue lesions (arrow) are heterogeneously well enhanced with a characteristic *peripheral and nodular* pattern. (**c**) Bone scan notes a homogeneous strong uptake in the lesion with a focal linear photopenic area, suggesting post-fracture necrosis (arrow). (**d**) PET/CT scan also shows a large heterogenous FDG uptake (SUVmax 4.3). Microscopic examination reveals a typical tissue pattern of CSA permeation with a significant cellular pleomorphism including bizarre nuclei in size and shape, more frequent bi-nucleated chondrocytes, and abnormal mitotic figures, indicating Grade 3 CSA (Fig. 21.13e). (**e**) Radiograph at 2 years after wide resection and reconstruction with allograft-prosthesis composite shows a visible gap at host bone-allograft junction site (arrow) but no evidence of local recurrence. (**f**) Follow-up radiograph at 7 years after surgery still reveals sustained visible gap (yellow arrow), and destructive change with cortical thinning and perforation in the proximal tibia, indicating a local recurrence (white arrows). Above-knee amputation has been performed. (**g**) Follow-up radiograph at 10 years after initial surgery notes no definite evidence of local recurrence or distant metastasis

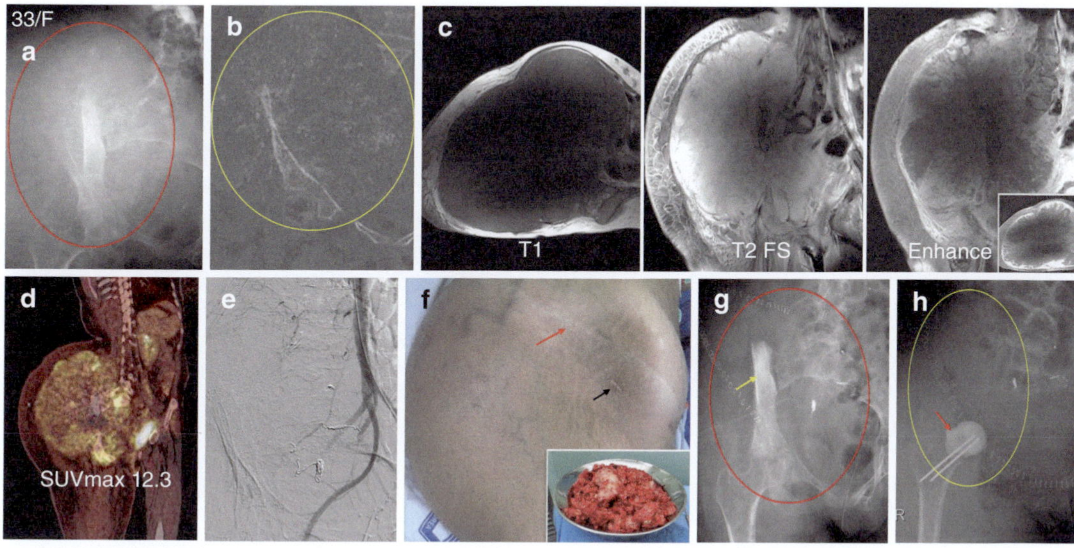

Fig. 21.12 ***Grade 3 (high-grade) CAS***. (**a**) Radiograph taken for a rapidly growing huge pelvic mass with foot drop during pregnancy of 26 weeks after prior surgery with a diagnosis of CSA in a 33-year-old foreigner shows an ill-defined, significantly expansile, huge destruction with an extensive soft tissue mass and radiating speculations in the pelvic bone (red circle). (**b**) CT scan more clearly reveals a relatively well-defined huge mass with widespread irregular punctuated mineralization and diffusely involved pelvic bone lesion of identical pattern with multiple cortical perforation (circle). (**c**) MR images shows a significantly extensive lesion affecting right sided pelvic bones and surrounding soft tissue with low SI on T1-weighted image and heterogeneous bright SI on fat-saturated T2-weighted image. The lesion is mostly enhanced in a *peripheral* pattern with central non-enahncement suggestive of massive necrosis. (**d**) PET/CT scan notes an extensively huge increased FDG uptake (SUVmax 12.3) in right pelvic bone, sacrum, and L4-5 vertebrae. Histologic diagnosis of Grade 3 CSA was rendered by incision biopsy. (**e**) On the day before surgery, following Cesarean section at 34 weeks of gestation, preoperative embolization was performed to reduce perioperative bleeding. (**f**) She was positioned in the lateral decubitus position for intralesional excision and sciatic nerve neurolysis. Note significantly huge mass with the prior incision scar (red arrow) and biopsy scar (black arrow), and huge bulk of excised tumor tissues (inset). (**g**) Postoperative radiograph shows no gross evidence of soft tissue mass and radiating speculations (red circle). A part of sclerotic pelvic bone remains after en-bloc resection and curettage (arrow). (**h**) Skin necrosis with infection was managed by multiple surgical procedures including resection of the remaining pelvic bone. A cement head was inserted to prevent further proximal migration (arrow). She was transferred to her home country

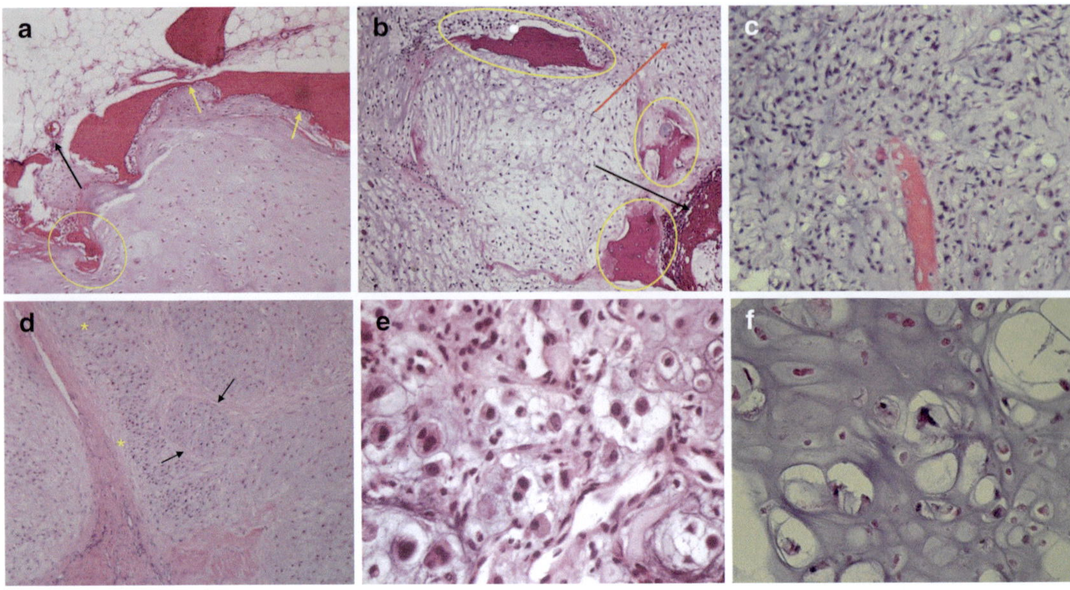

Fig. 21.13 ***Microscopic examination***. (**a**) Low-power magnification shows a lobular tumor mass infiltrates and permeates the host lamellar bone (yellow arrows). The chondrocytes are mildly increased in number with mild to moderate atypia. (**b**) In a more progressed case with higher cellularity and more significant atypia, lamellar bone spicules are surrounded on all sides by tumor cartilage, producing a characteristic *CSA permeation* pattern (circles). The tumor cells at the periphery of cartilage lobules invade the marrow fat cells (black arrow), so-called *invasion of marrow fat* pattern, and eventually obliterate them (red arrow). (**c**) CSA with high cellularity with nuclear atypia completely replaces the fatty marrow and totally encompasses a residual preexisting lamellar bone trabecula. The chondrocytes are moderately to severely increased in number with moderate atypia, suggesting an intermediate Grade 2 CSA. (**d**) Multiple confluent hyaline cartilage nodules of varying size, coposed of moderate cellularity and atypia, are surrounded by thin, delicate delicate fibrovascular bands with focal myxoid change (arrows). There is a thick interlobular band of fibrous tissue consisting of multiple layers of bland fibroblast-like cells, collagen layers as well as microvasculature (asterisks), so-called *band of fibrosis* pattern, is another feature highly suggestive of CSA. (**e**) High-power magnification reveals significantly bizarre-looking cells with prominent nucleoli, frequent bi-nucleated chondrocytes and atypical mitotic figures, indicating a Grade 3 CSA. (**f**) Higher-power magnification of another case shows a lower cellular area but with significantly bizarre and pleomorphic cells in size and shape

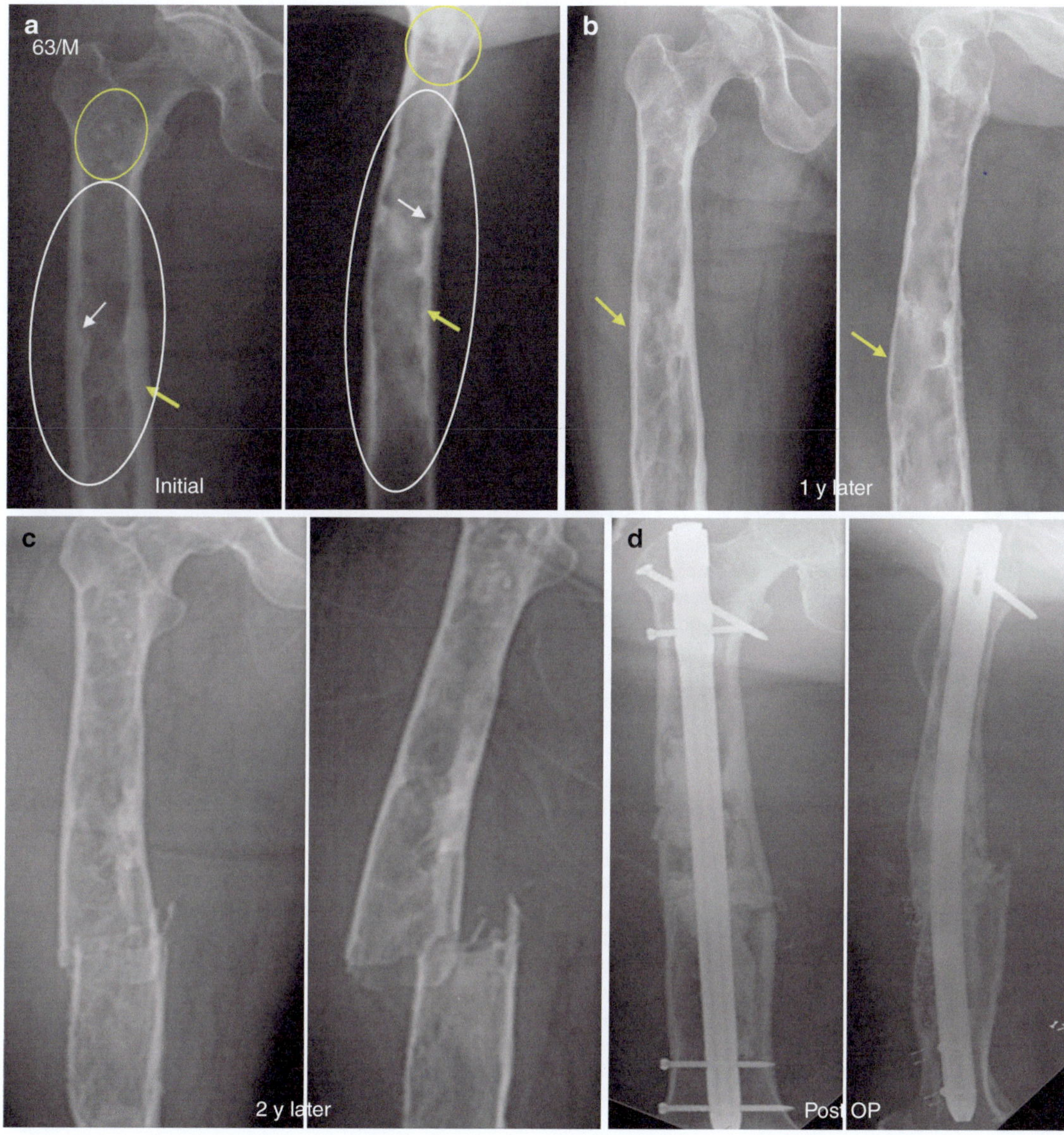

Fig. 21.14 **Secondary central CSA.** ***Grade 1 CSA***. (**a**) Radiograph taken for right hip pain after slip in a 63-year-old man incidentally shows a huge osteolytic lesion with intralesional windblown densities and thickening of cortex (yellow arrows) with deep, elongated endosteal scalloping (white arrows) in the diaphysis of the femur. The femur shaft reveals a moderate expansion with mild bowing (white circle). Note another radiolucent lesion with popcorn-like densities, suggestive of preexisting EC in the trochanteric area (yellow circle). These findings indicate a possible malignant change from the preexisting EC. However, the patient refused biopsy because of the absence of thigh pain at this visit. (**b**) Follow-up radiograph 1 year later notes further expansion of the femur with thinning of cortex (arrows) compared to the initial thickness. The patient continued to decline biopsy and surgical management. (**c**) Radiograph taken for right thigh pain following a slip 2 years later reveals a further progression of the lesion with a displaced pathologic fracture. (**d**) A histologic diagnosis of Grade 1 CSA arising from preexisting EC in the trochanteric area was rendered, based on the characteristic *CSA permeation* pattern with moderate cellularity, along with an adjacent focus of conventional EC. Thorough curettage through the fracture site was performed, followed by bone cementing and intramedullary nailing. The patient was subsequently lost for follow-up

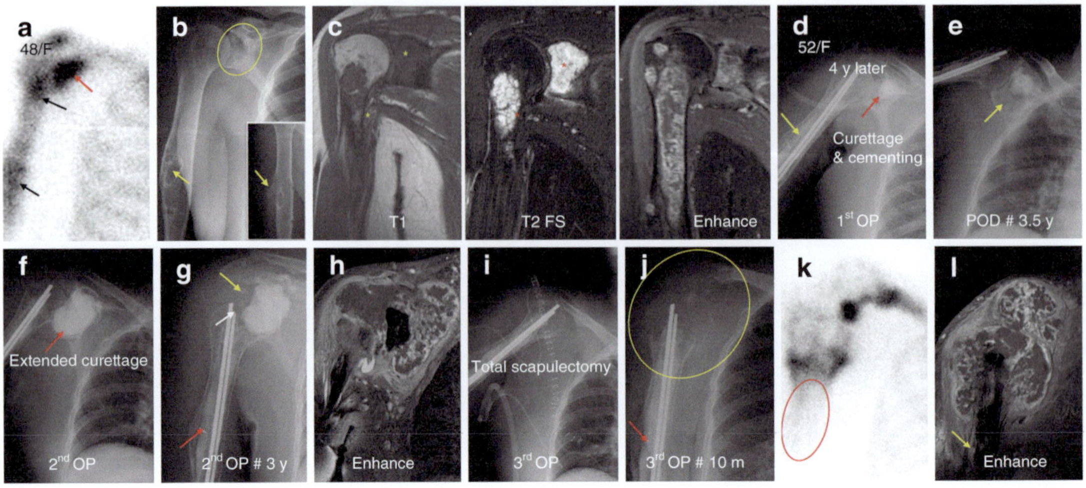

Fig. 21.15 **Secondary central CSA.** ***Grade 1 CSA with local recurrence***. (**a**) Bone scan taken for evaluation of right pelvic mass in the same patient as in Figs. 21.16 and 21.17 shows intense uptake in the scapula (red arrow) and moderate uptake in the humeral shaft and neck (black arrows). (**b**) Radiographs reveal an ill-defined, multilobulated osteolytic lesion with internal opacities in the glenoid and neck of scapular (circle), and another lesion with an irregular outgrowing mass lesion through a cortical defect in the humeral shaft (arrows), consistent with an EC protuberance (Fig. 15.7e in Chap. 15). (**c**) MR images present a multilobulated, intramedullary lesion (asterisks) with low SI on T1-weighted image and heterogeneous high SI on fat saturated T2-weighted image in both the scapula and humerus. The lesions are heterogeneously enhanced in a *nodular and septal* pattern. The patient did not want any further evaluation and management due to the absence of pain at that time. (**d**) Four years later, she complained of slowly aggravated pain of right scapular area and requested an incision biopsy to exclude malignancy. A histologic diagnosis of malignant transformation to Grade 1 CSA from EC in the scapula was rendered. Extended curettage with cementing was performed for the scapular lesion (red arrow). Excision for EC protuberance and thorough curettage followed by cementing and flexible nail insertion were simultaneously performed for the humerus lesion (yellow arrow). (**e**) Follow-up radiograph at 3.5 years after surgery reveals a progression of the radiolucent area in the scapula, indicating local recurrence (yellow arrow). Histologic diagnosis remained Grade 1 CSA. (**f**) Repeated extended curettage with cementing was performed. (**g**) Radiograph at 3 years after second surgery shows a progression of the scapular lesion with soft tissue mass formation (yellow arrow) and destruction around the nail insert site (white arrow). However, the shaft area diagnosed as EC protuberance remains stable (red arrow). (**h**) Enhanced MR image demonstrates a significant progression of the scapular lesion with heterogeneous enhancement in *peripheral and nodular* pattern. (**i**) Total scapulectomy was performed. Microscopic examination revealed significantly increased cellularity with prominent atypia and frequent mitoses, indicating a progression from Grade 1 to 3 CSA. (**j**) Radiograph taken for severe pain at 10 months after the third surgery of total scapulectomy reveals a severe destruction of the proximal humerus and distal clavicle (yellow circle) indicating a local recurrence. However, the shaft area of EC protuberance appears to remain stable (red arrow). (**k**) Follow-up pinhole bone scan shows stronger uptake foci in the proximal destructive areas but no uptake in the shaft area suggesting a stable lesion (circle). (**l**) Enhanced MR image demonstrate extensive destruction and huge soft tissue mass in the scapula and proximal humerus with heterogeneous enhancement in a *peripheral and nodular* pattern. However, the shaft area of EC protuberance is still stable (arrow). She refused any further management and died of disease progression at 13 years after initial diagnosis

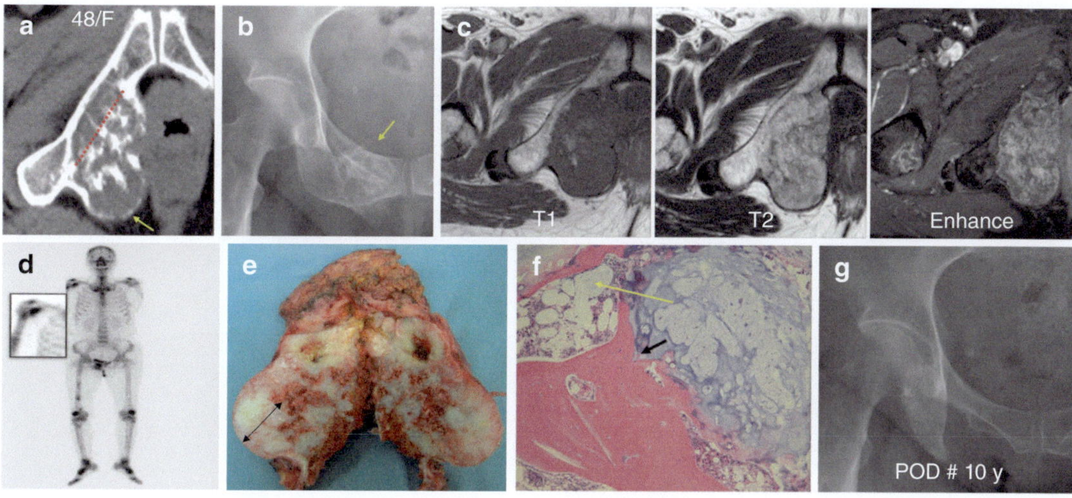

Fig. 21.16 **Secondary peripheral CSA.** ***Grade 1 CSA.*** (**a**) CT scan taken for a hard, large, pelvic mass palpable on vaginal examination in the Department of Gynecology in a 48-year-old woman shows a large, well-defined outgrowing calcifying mass with irregular thin margin in its inferior aspect (yellow arrow). Note a direct continuation of the mass with the medullary cavity through a cortical defect (dotted line), suggesting a possible malignant change of preexisting OC. The patient had a history of a past history of palpable hard mass on her right inguinal area for 20 years but did not seek medical attention. (**b**) Radiograph reveals a well-defined sclerotic mass with osteolytic areas in the right inferior pubic ramus (arrow). (**c**) MR images demonstrate a large well-defined, exophytic, sclerotic mass with low SI on T1-weighted image and intermediate and high SI with focal dark signals of mineralization on T2-weighted image, suggesting cartilage-dominant lesion. The lesion is heterogeneously enhanced in a typical *peripheral and nodular* pattern. (**d**) Bone scan shows multiple areas of increased uptake in the right shoulder and scapular area, right femur shaft, right pubic bone, and tarsal bones of both feet, suggesting multiple bone lesions. Radiographs corresponding to increased uptake reveal another OC in the proximal fibula and ECs in the humerus, scapula, femur, and small bones of the foot (red arrows), indicating simultaneous multiple OCs and ECs. (**e**) Wide resection was performed based on imaging findings suggestive of low-grade CSA. The cut surface of gross specimen shows markedly thickened cartilage cap with varible-sized multiple cartilage nodules, suggesting a malignant change from longstanding OC. (**f**) Microscopic examination shows erosion and infiltration of host lamellar bone (black arrow) and focal invasion into the marrow fat through the cortical breakage by the tumor cells (yellow arrow), so-called *invasion of marrow fat* pattern, with mild cellularity and atypia, indicating Grade 1 CSA. (**g**) Follow-up radiograph at 10 years after en-bloc resection shows no evidence of local recurrence

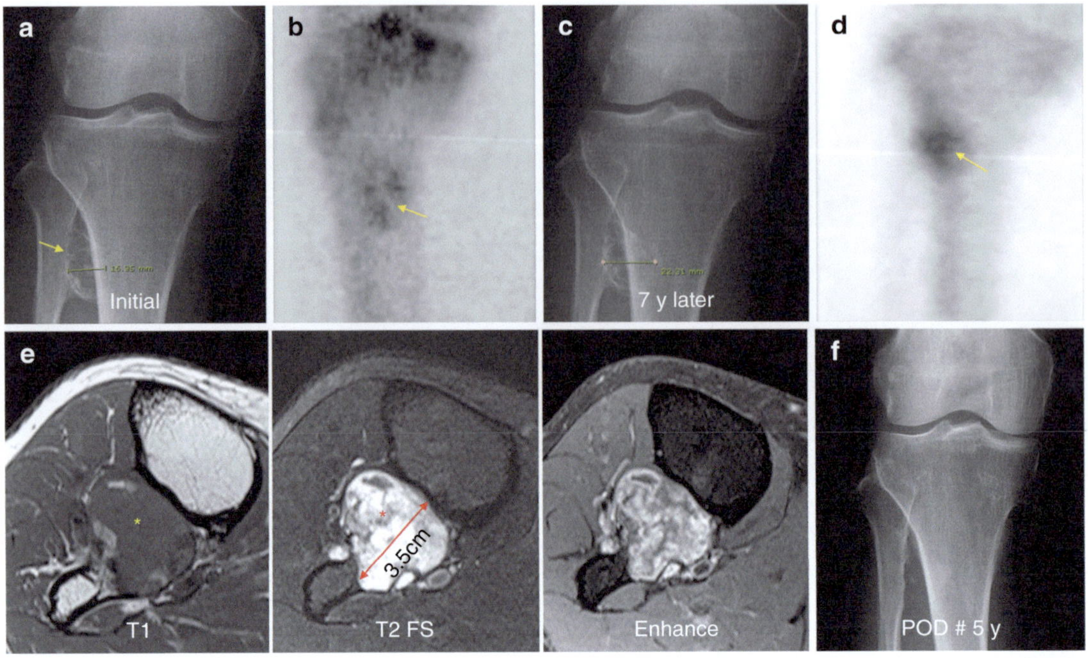

Fig. 21.17 **Secondary peripheral CSA.** ***Another grade 1 CSA in the same patient*.** (**a**) Radiograph of right knee with no pain in the same patient shows a well-defined, outwardly growing, hazy bony mass with internal densification in the proximal fibula. There is subtle medullary continuity between the mass and the proximal fibula (arrow). (**b**) Bone scan reveals only heterogeneous mild uptake in the mass (arrow), suggesting a benignancy particularly in consideration of the absence of pain. (**c**) Seven years later, a radiograph taken for newly developed pain over the mass notes mildly increased diameter by about 5–6 mm. (**d**) Follow-up bone scan reveals a mildly increased uptake compared to the initial bone scan (arrow). (**e**) MR images demonstrate a pedunculated mass arising from the medial aspect of the proximal fibula with a discernible medullary continuity to the cancellous bone of the fibula, suggesting a preexisting OC (asterisks). SI is low on T1-weighted image and bright with small dark signal foci of calcification on fat-saturated T2-weighted image. The lesion mainly consists of cartilage component with a maximum thickness of 3.5 cm, strongly indicating a malignant transformation, particularly in light of new onset of pain over the mass. The mass is heterogeneously enhanced in *rings and arcs* pattern. (**f**) Follow-up radiograph at 5 years after limited wide resection with a histologic diagnosis of malignant transformation of OC to a Grade 1 CSA shows no evidence of local recurrence

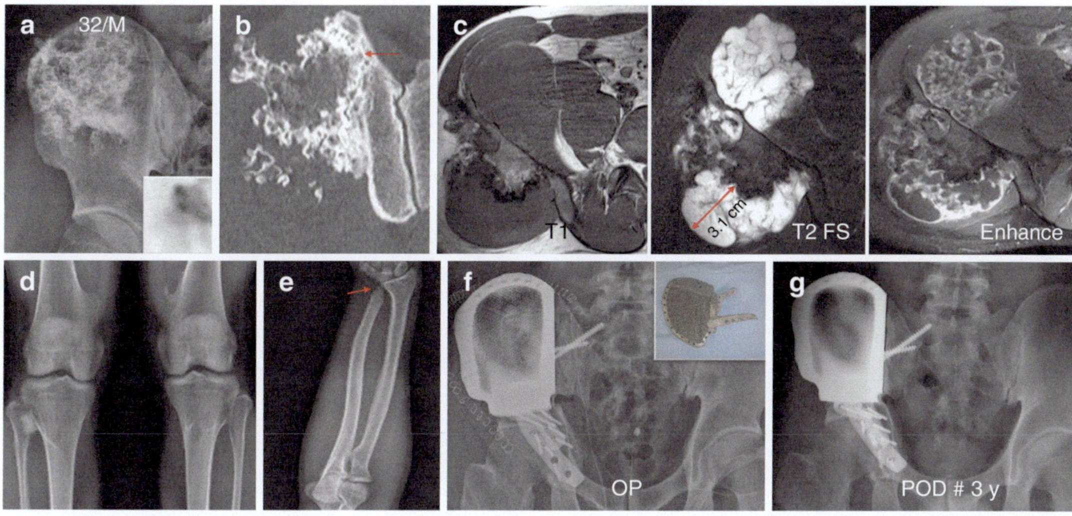

Fig. 21.18 Secondary peripheral CSA. ***Grade 1 CSA.*** (**a**) Radiograph taken for a palpable mass over right iliac crest of several years' duration in a 32-year-old man shows a huge heavily calcifying mass in the iliac wing. The patient had a history of multiple OCs since childhood, and one: in the wrist was excised 10 years ago. Bone scan reveals heterogeneously increased uptake in the right iliac wing and acetabulum with central photon defect (inset) as well as subtle uptake in the distal femurs and the proximal tibias (not shown here), suggesting multiple bone lesions. (**b**) CT scan reveals an outwardly growing heavily calcifying mass from the right ilium with partial invasion into the underlying medullary cavity (red arrow). (**c**) MR images note a large, multilobulated, exophytic mass with intermediate SI on T1-weighted image and bright SI on T2-weighted image. Note a markedly thickened cartilage cap (measuring 3.1 cm), heralding a malignant change. The lesion is typically enhanced in a typical *peripheral and nodular* pattern. (**d**) Radiographs corresponding to increased uptake areas on bone scan note multiple OCs in the distal femurs and the proximal tibias. (**e**) Radiograph of previously excised area shows an absent ulnar head with ulnar deviation deformity (red arrow). (**f**) Wide excision and reconstruction with 3D-printed prosthesis was performed with a pathologic diagnosis of malignant transformation of OC to Grade 1 CSA. (**g**) Follow-up radiograph at 3 years after surgery demonstrates no evidence of local recurrence

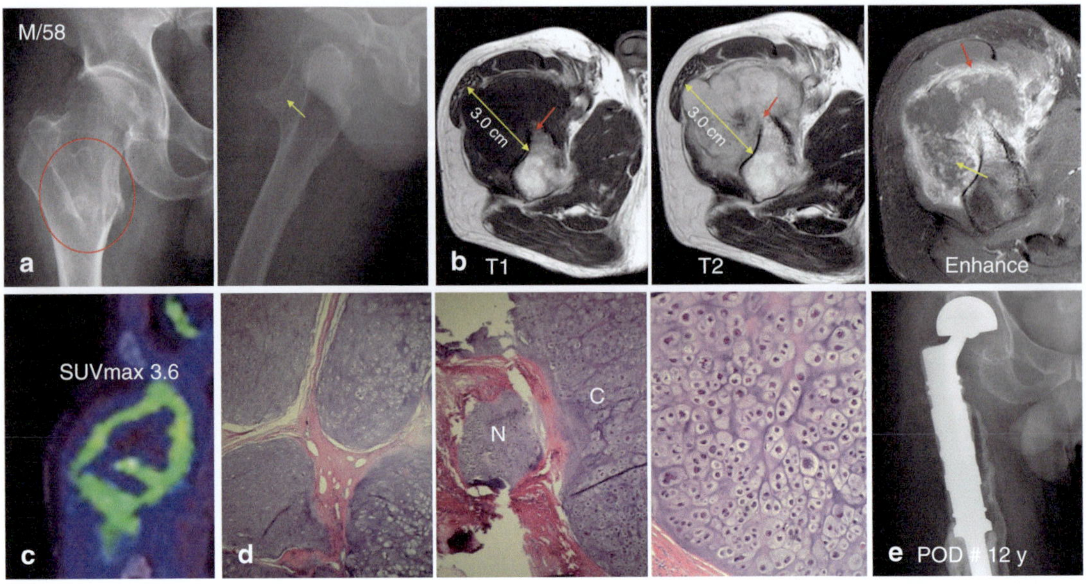

Fig. 21.19 **Secondary peripheral CSA.** ***Rare Grade 3 CSA in recurred or residual EC.*** (**a**) Radiograph taken for right hip pain of 7 month's duration in a 58-year-old man shows an ill-defined, multilobulated, densifying mass overlapping the lesser trochanter (circle), accompanied by widening of femoral neck and valgus deformity. Lateral view reveals a well-defined, outwardly growing, triangular-shaped bony mass with continuity to medullary cavity of the underlying femur (arrow). He had a history of surgical excision of OC involving right proximal femur 13 years ago. (**b**) MR images reveal a well-defined, large, lobulated, exophytic mass continuous with the host medullary bone (arrows), with low SI on T1-weighted image and high SI with focal dark signal on T2-weighted image, suggesting a possible recurrent or residual OC. Note markedly thickened cartilage cap (measuring 3.0 cm), heralding a possible malignant change of the OC, pafticularly particularly in consideration of newly developed pain. The mass is peripherally enhanced (red arrow) with internal nodular enhancement (yellow arrow), so-called "peripheral and nodular" pattern. (**c**) PET/CT scan reveals a peripheral moderate FDG uptake (SUVmax 3.6) and central photon defect in the exophytic mass. (**d**) Microscopic examination: (Left) Low-power magnification notes discrete several cartilage nodules separated by fibrous septa in a *bands of fibrosis* pattern. (Middle) In another area, a bland-looking isolated cartilaginous nodule (N) partially surrounded by normal lamellar bone, so-called *lamellar bone encasement* pattern, indicates a preexisting EC, and a juxtapoed nodule with pleomorphic cells separated by mutiple fibrous bands (C) suggests malignant with pleomorphic cells separated by multiple fibrous bands (C), indicating malignant transformation of OC to high-grade CSA. (Right) Higher-power magni fication shows an increased number of pleomorphic chondrocytes with significantly bizarre nuclei, frequent bi-nucleated chondrocytes, and occasional abnormal mitoses, indicating Grade 3 CSA. This case may suggest that the bland nodules of EC remain probably due to incomplete excision of the cartilage cap and slowly grow, resulting in malignant transformation. (**e**) Follow-up radiograph at 12 years after wide resection with reconstruction using a tumor prosthesis, followed by multiple surgical procedures for infection control shows irregular bone formation around the tumor prosthesis without evidence of local recurrence

21.2 Subtypes of CSA

Non-conventional CSA is subclassified into myxoid, periosteal or juxtacortical, clear-cell, mesenchymal, and dedifferentiated CSA, which are presented in each individual chapter.

21.3 Incidence

Primary CSA is the third most frequent primary malignant bone tumor following bone myeloma and osteosarcoma, representing 3.5% of all biopsy-proven primary bone tumors [1] and about 20–30% of all primary malignant bone tumor in major series [2–6]. An analysis of SEER data showed that CSA accounted for 25% of all primary sarcomas of bone, and 74% of them were conventional CSA [7]. Secondary CSAs are rare, accounting for arrpoximately 1% of all malignant bone tumors and less than 25% of all CSAs in a Mayo Clinic series [8–10]. They occur most commonly in OCs, occupying approximately 80% in major series [1, 4, 11].

21.4 Ages

The incidence of primary CSA shows a gradual age-related increase, occurring most commonly in adulthood and older age between the fourth and seventh decades of life, with a peak incidence during the sixth and seventh decades of life [1, 7, 9] and a mean age of 50 years [1, 12]. It is extremely rare in patients younger than 20 years, and chondroblastic osteosarcoma should be excluded in this age group. Patients with secondary CSA are 10–20 years younger than those with primary CSA having a mean age of 35 years [11].

21.5 Location

The lesion can be found in any bone formed by endochondral ossification. In an analysis of 2890 cases from the SEER Database, tumor location was not uniformly described in the database, and thus, the location was classified as appendicular if it was the arm or leg and as axial if it was the pelvis, spine, or scapula [12]. The tumor was located most commonly in appendicular bones (45%), followed by axial bones (31%), and then by soft tissue (10%). Another study reported that CSA has a predilection for the trunk bones, occupying up to 40% of all cases, including pelvic bones (20%) and ribs (20%). The ilium is the most commonly affected (20%), followed by the femur (15%) and the proximal humerus (10%) [7]. In the long bones, the metaphysis or diaphysis is usually affected. However, it can be unusually located in the epiphysis, accounting for only 16% of cases [13]. Short tubular bones of hands and feet can also be rarely involved. It is extremely rare in the spine and skull bones.

21.6 Clinical Features

Patients usually complain of increasing pain with or without localized swelling of long duration, ranging from months to years. Pain strongly suggests active growth of a central cartilage tumor [1, 9]. The nature of pain is usually insidious, vague, and longstanding. In general, the duration, nature, and cause of pain in EC and CSA are substantially different. Patients with acute sharp pain after strenuous physical activity are more likely to have EC rather than CSA by statistical probability [1]. Newly developed pain over the preexisting painless cartilage tumor may herald a possible malignant transformation. On occasion, primary and secondary CSA can be found incidentally during image studies for other reasons (Figs. 21.1a, 21.4e, 21.11a, and 21.14a). Pathologic fracture infrequently occurs in the long bones due to weakened bone (Figs. 21.11a and 21.14c). Sciatica, weakness, numbness, or urinary incontinence can occur if the spine is affected.

21.7 Radiographic Findings

Plain radiograph vary depending on the different subtypes. However, some general features are nearly always useful and often provide pathognomonic clues. In general, the size of CSA tends to be larger than that of EC. Although the pathologic appearance varies among subtypes, CSA commonly grows with a lobular type architecture, and these hyaline cartilage nodules demonstrate high water content and peripheral endochondral ossification, which is directly reflected on radiograph as typical *ring-and-arc* pattern of matrix mineralization as seen in EC, but the pattern is more irregular, amorphous, and hazy compared to that of calcified EC in addition to the locally aggressive features. Typically, the lesion shows an ill-defined mixed lytic and sclerotic appearance with more irregularly distributed punctate or flocculent opacities or *windblown* densification. The amount of calcification varies from minimal or absent, making the lesion predominantly lytic without a cartilaginous component to heavy and extensive often simulating an osteogenic bone tumor. Even long bones can be somewhat expanded, often with significantly thinned and/or thickened cortices as a result of slow but continuous growth of a relatively low-grade tumor. *Lower-grade CSA* often shows a well-defined border with larger areas of calcification, superficial endosteal scalloping, minimal thinning or thickening of cortex, or mild bone expansion usually without cortical destruction. However, it may present as only spherical or ovoid radiolucent lesion with discrete foci of mineralization but no scalloping or expansion as in EC. However, *higher-grade CSA* reveals a less well-marginated, lobulated deeper endosteal scalloping, more prominent radiolucent area frequently with expanded bone contour, and even soft tissue extension through a destructed cortex. Murphy et al. [13] classified endosteal scalloping by extent and depth with no scalloping present as grade 0. Extent of endosteal scalloping was graded as grade 1, involving less than 1/3 of the lesion extent; grade 2, affecting between 1/3 and 2/3 of the extent; and grade 3, involving greater than 2/3 of the lesion. Depth of endosteal scalloping was graded as grade 1, representing less than 1/3 of cortical thickness; grade 2, between 1/3 and 2/3; grade 3, greater than 2/3; and grade 4, cortical penetration with or without associated soft-tissue mass. Endosteal scalloping greater than 2/3 of the cortical thickness (deeper) with a greater extent of the lesion is strong evidence of CSA rather than EC (Fig. 21.1c). The authors also suggested radiographic features favoring CSA included the above-mentioned degree of endosteal scalloping, extent of matrix mineralization less than 2/3 of the lesion on radiograph, presence of cortical remodeling or destruction and thickening, periosteal reaction, pathologic fracture, and soft-tissue mass. The depth of endosteal scalloping at its most prominent focus is the best distinguishing feature between EC and CSA [11, 12]. However, it can be grade 1 in extent and depth even in some cases with intermediate-grade CSA (Fig. 21.6). Secondary central CSA has the above-mentioned common features in addition to variable-sized areas with well-defined margin containing *popcorn-like* calcification suggesting a preexisting EC. More aggressive pattern of moth-eaten and/or permeative destruction is seen in higher-grade conventional CSA. Such aggressive patterns of destruction are much more commonly demonstrated in mesenchymal and dedifferentiated CSA. **Bone scan** usually shows moderately to significantly increased uptake in all grades of CSA (Figs. 21.2, 21.3, 21.4, 21.6, 21.8, 21.9, 21.10, and 21.11). **PET/CT scan** usually shows a heterogeneously intense FDG uptake in the lesion, suggesting a diagnosis of malignant tumor (Figs. 21.1, 21.2, 21.3, 21.6, 21.7, 21.8, 21.9, 21.11, 21.12, and 21.19). 18F-FDG PET/CT reveals excellent accuracy in the diagnosis of CSA, assisting clinical clinical decision-making [14]. However, SUVmax alone had a limited ability to differentiate benign cartilaginous lesions and CSA as well as between lower-grade and higher-grade CSA. Feldman et al. [15] postulated the SUVmax values might increase with the tumor grade and that PET/CT scan accurately discriminated lower-grade CSA from higher-grade CSA. The maximum standard uptake with cut-off value of 2.0, based on their prior experience with various neoplasms studied, was reported to distinguish benign from malignant cartilaginous tumors with 90.9% overall sensitivity, 100% specificity, and 96.6% accuracy. However, there was significant overlap in

SUVmax values between grade 2 and 3 CSA. Despite some limitations of PET/CT scan for differential diagnosis and staging, SUVmax may be useful as a predictor of biologic behavior and in guiding management of cartilage tumors. Firstly, PET/CT scan identifies tumor aggressiveness and extent visually and quantitatively, providing aid in deciding if biopsy is needed or directing the biopsy sampling [16]. Secondly, SUVmax serves as a useful tool for decision of biopsy location by providing an adequate area with highest SUVmax. Thirdly, 18F-FDG can accurately predict and localize dedifferentiation by its ability to conecentrate in biologically aggressive areas [17]. Lastly, alteration of FDG avidity may indicate a local recurrence or a sarcomatous transformation of preexisting benign cartilaginous neoplasms. In addition, PET/CT scan can also depict very rare skip lesions in CSA (Fig. 21.6b). **CT scan** more clearly reveals a degree of cortical destruction with soft tissue extension and allows optimal detection and characterization of mineralization, particularly when it is subtle or not clearly visble on radiograph (Figs. 21.8, 21.9, and 21.10) or if the lesion is in a complex area of anatomy such as scapula, sternum, spine, or pelvis (Figs. 21.8, 21.9, 21.10, 21.12, and 21.18). Endosteal scalloping depth and identification of soft tissue extension [8–10], which are among the best differentiating features between EC and CSA, can be evaluated more clearly [13]. **MR images** are useful to determine an exact extent of marrow involvement, degree of cortical breakage, and soft tissue extension. Characteristically, MR images show a lobulated medullary mass-like lesion with a low to intermediate SI on T1- and heterogeneous high to bright SI reflecting the high-water content of nonmineralized hyaline cartilage on T2-weighted image with dark signal foci of calcification on all sequences (Figs. 21.1, 21.2, 21.3, 21.4, 21.6, 21.7, 21.8, 21.9, 21.10, and 21.11). The depth and extent of endosteal scalloping are well depicted by MR imaging, particularly with proton density-weighted sequences. CT and MR imaging are superior to radiography for evaluating endosteal scalloping, cortical destruction, or soft tissue mass formation because the entire cortical circumference can be seen on the axial view. CSA revealed endosteal scalloping greater than 2/3 of cortical thickness in 75% of cases on plain radiograph, 90% on CT, and 86% on MR imaging [13]. MRI is the best tool to detect soft tissue extension through cortical destruction, which shows identical signals to those of the intraosseous component. With intravenous injection of contrast medium, the lesion shows a heterogeneous enhancement or thin peripheral rim-like or nodular and septal enhancement in typical *rings and arcs* or *peripheral and nodular* pattern, corresponding to fibro-vascular septations between lobules of hyaline cartilage and peripheral endochondral ossification as in other cartilaginous tumors (Figs. 21.1, 21.2, 21.3, 21.4, 21.5, 21.6, 21.7, 21.8, 21.9, 21.10, 21.11, and 21.12). Findings heralding a malignant change of preexisting benign cartilage tumor include newly developed radiolucent areas with indistinct and fuzzy surface margin, destruction of the base of the mass or host bone, thickness of cartilage cap greater than 2 cm in adults and 3 cm in children with OC, cortical thinning and/or thickening, cortical destruction with soft tissue extension, internal *windblown* densification, bone expansion, and periosteal reaction in patients with preexisting EC.

21.8 Histologic Findings

CSA ranges from locally aggressive nonmetastasizing low-grade tumor to intermediate and high-grade with a marked metastatic potential. Thus, these groups should be separated by the use of histopathologic criteria [18]. However, it has been well known that low-grade CSA is difficult to diagnose by histology alone because of a high variability between inter-observers. All CSA presents a lobulated architecture being uniformly cartilaginous with varying degrees of calcification or peripheral osseous metaplasia by endochondral ossification. The individual lobules are variable in size and shape, and separated by fibrovascular bands with varying degrees of myxoid change. Differentiation of ACT/grade 1 CSA from the cellular EC by cytology alone is very difficult. The importance of a multidisciplinary approach on the basis of clinical setting including adequate biopsy by experienced orthopedic oncologist, radiographic interpretation by musculoskeletal radiologist, and histologic interpretation by musculoskeletal pathologist should be emphasized for a correct diagnosis and adequate treatment of these heterogeneous cartilage tumors. According to JM Mirra, the histologic findings of grade 1 CSA overlap those of EC at least in at least 25% of the cases [1]. He and his colleagues described a new histologic approach based on tissue patterns for differentiation of EC and grade 1 CSA [1, 19]. **Cytologic features** of moderate to high cellularity, higher number of double-nucleated chondrocytes, abnormal mitoses, open chromatin, sometimes with foci of myxoid matrix and *tissue patterns* of "permeation" or "entrapment" of host lamellar bone, "infiltration of Haversian systems," "soft tissue mass," "band of fibrosis," or "invasion of marrow fat" can surely confirm a diagnosis of CSA (Figs. 21.5 and 21.13). The "*permeation* or *entrapment*" pattern is the most important hallmark of CSA no matter how the cytologic features are low-grade or innocent. At least three bone trabeculae should be surrounded on all sides by tumor cartilage within at least one medium-power field for "*CSA Permeation pattern*" (*CPP*) by Mirra [1]. *Entrapment* is defined as the presence of the tumor around three sides of normal spicules of the host lamellar bone by the World Health Organization [20]. However, the CPP pattern may not be observed in samples from a part of the soft tissue mass beyond the cortex or a part of CSA where the medullary bone is totally destructed. The low-grade CSA with such slow growth does not permeate marrow space and never permits the *CPP* to produce, which makes a differential diagnosis of CSA from EC more difficult [1]. In such cases, the diagnosis should depend on other tissue patterns for CSA in correlation with clinical and radiologic findings. Chondroid to cartilage matrix can undergo osseous metaplasia by endochondral ossification, which finally results in islands of bone deeply buried within the cartilage matrix. It should not be misinterpreted as "*permeation* or *entrapment*" of the host lamellar bone (Fig. 21.1d). Cytologic grading is the most important factor in predicting its behavior and prognosis. The grading is based primarily on nuclear atypia in terms of size and shape, hyperchromatism, cellularity, number of bi-nucleated chondrocytes, and mitotic activity including abnormal mitoses. Background stroma consists of an abundant hyaline cartilage matrix with varying degrees of myxoid change. CSAs of different grades represent pathogenetically distinct conditions with different biologic potential and clinical behavior. The most widely accepted method of histologic grading is based on a three-tier system [7, 21]. **Grade 1 CSA/ACT** (Figs. 21.1, 21.2, 21.3, 21.4, and 21.5) is almost similar to EC, with the same degree or mildly to moderately increased cellularity, slightly plumper nuclei with different size, and more occasional bi-nucleated chondrocytes than EC (2-3 per high-power field). However, there is no discernible abnormal mitosis. The distinction between the low-grade CSA and EC remains subjective, with high inter-observer variability. The cartilage lobules are not encased by lamellar bone unlike EC, and rather separated by bands of fibrous tissue, the "*band of fibrosis*" pattern, which is one of the CSA tissue patterns. Typically, the lesion shows an infiltrative growth pattern with endosteal erosion or scalloping and engulfment of the medullary bone (Fig. 21.5). Cytologic findings and some tissue patterns for grade 1 CSA/ACT are summarized in Fig. 21.5. **Grade 2 CSA** (Figs. 21.6, 21.7, 21.8, 21.9, and 21.10) exhibits higher cellularity with larger and hyperchromatic nuclei, higher degree of nuclear pleomorphism in size and shape, hyperchromatism, and frequent bi-nucleated chondrocytes. On occasion, even some multinucleated giant cells may have highly atypical nuclei. Foci of myxoid change are frequently present, and abnormal mitoses can be observed. Approximately 10–15% of Grade 2 CSA metastasize commonly to lungs, regional lymph nodes, and liver. **Grade 3 CSA** (Figs. 21.11 and 21.12) is rare, accounting for 5–10% of all CSAs. It is characterized by significantly increased cellularity with more prominent pleomorphism in nuclear size and shape, more frequent bi-nucleated chondrocytes, and common abnormal mitoses. Occasionally, some cells have tri-nucleated or more nuclei. Cytologic findings and tissue patterns for Grade 2 and 3 CSA are summarized in Fig. 21.13. More than half of Grade 3 CSA eventually metastasize to distant organs. Areas of necrosis, calcification, and endochondral or reactive ossification can be seen in any grade. Despite the new histologic approach based on the tissue patterns [1], the reliability of the histologic grading of cartilaginous lesions remains limited even among specialized and experienced pathologists and radiologists [22]. Accordingly, needle or core biopsy is generally not recommanded because an adequate amount of representative tissue from appropreate location is required to examine the tissue patterns as well as cytologic features for a correct diagnosis of CSA.

21.9 Management

For low-grade CSA, wide resection with various options of reconstruction has traditionally been advocated. However, more recently with improved imaging modalities and a better understanding of the natural behavior of low-grade CSA, a paradigm shift has moved toward less aggressive intralesional surgery, achieving: good functional results, excellent local control, and survival [23–31]. Extended curettage using high-speed high speed bur, with or without local adjuvants such as phenol, ethanol, anhydrous ethanol, and liquid nitrogen has been widely adopted. However, wide excision with adequate margins followed by reconstruction using autologous bone graft (recycled bone and vascularized fibula), allograft, endoprosthesis or tumor prosthesis, or allograft-prosthesis composite (APC), remains the standard option for Grade 2/3 CSA and even Grade 1 CSA with local recurrence or affecting pelvic bones, due to frequent local recurrence with difficulty to treat in this region. Amputation is indicated in limited cases with uncontrollable infection or (multiple) local recurrence with poor bone stalk (Fig. 21.11g). Tumors affecting the pelvis or spine are particularly difficult to manage due to their large size and deep location with a relationship to important adjacent organs such as the bladder or spinal cord. Chemotherapy or radiotherapy plays a limited role because its growth is mainly driven by cartilage matrix production but not so much to DNA replication [32, 33].

21.10 Clinical Course

Prognosis varies depending on various parameters, including histologic grade, location and size of the lesion, extra-compartment spread, surgical margin, patient's age, local recurrence, and metastasis. Parameters of higher histologic grade, soft tissue extension, tumor size greater than 10 cm, inadequate surgical margin, pelvic location, patient's age over 50 years, local recurrence, existence of distant metastasis, and pelvic location may be worse in respect to overall survival. However, independent risk factors have been reported differencially in each study. In an analysis of 2890 cases from the SEER Database between 1973 and 2003, histologic grade and stage were the only independent prognostic factors for survival on multivariate analysis [12]. In addition, the only prognostic factor that was shown to significantly impact the survival of each non-conventional CSA subtype was a metastatic disease at diagnosis. Earlier, MD Anderson Cancer Center group reported that the 5-year survival rates of Grade 1, 2, 3 were 90%, 81%, and 43% respectively, while the corresponding 10-year survival rates were 83%, 64%, and 29% [18]. They also reported the overall survival rate of 77% at 5 years, 67% at 10 years. In Grade 1 CSA treated with extended curettage and local adjuvant therapy, local recurrence was not reported in some studies [23, 25, 30], but occurred in 4.3–13% of patients in other studies [34–37], and even reached 40% in another series [18]. Furthermore, progression to higher grade was reported in recurrent cases [35, 36, 38] (Fig. 21.19). In a large series, the recurrence rate was 6% in adequately treated patients, but 69% in inadequately treated patients, with 5-year survival rates of 81% and 53%, respectively [2]. The authors reported overall 5-year and 10-year survival rates of 94% and 87% in patients with Grade 1 CSA, 61% and 41% in patients with Grade 2 CSA, and 44% and 27% in patients with

Grade 3 CSA, respectively. Recurrence is regarded as a sign of an aggressive phenotype and should be treated accordingly. Therefore, wide resection should be performed in recurrent cases due to the risk of diese progression. Distant metastasis is frequently seen in Grade 3 CSA (more than 50%) and occasionally in Grade 2 CSA (10–15%), but not in Grade 1 CSA [7, 18]. CSA metastasizes most frequently to lung and to lymph node more often than other bone sarcomas. Large-scale studies of all CSAs using SEER database reported five survival rates of 70–75% [12, 39]. Notably, survival rates did not change over the three periods analyzed (1985–1988, 1989–1993, 1994–1998), 74.7%, 76.5%, and 74%, respectively [34]. Another study also concluded that current treatment algorithms have not improved the survival rates of patients with CSA over the past 30 years [12]. The relative 5-year survival rates for conventional, myxoid, juxtacortical, and mesenchymal CSA were reported as 70%, 71%, 87%, and 52%, respectively, in the study by Damron et al. [39], compared with 70%, 71%, 93%, and 48%, respectively, in the study by Giuffrida et al. [12]. The latter study additionally reported the survival rates of 100% and 0% in the clear cell and dedifferentiated types, respectively. More recently, Amer et al. [40] reported 5-year survival rates of 68%, 62%, 49%, 38%, and 11% for periosteal, clear cell, myxoid, mesenchymal, and dedifferentiated subtypes, respectively, in SEER database analysis of patients with CSA subtypes from1973 to 2013, compared with 100%, 93%, 71%, 48%, and 0% in previous analysis of SEER database from 1973 to 2003 by Giuffrida et al. [12]. The inclusion of a larger dataset in the latter analysis may have improved the accuracy of the analyses when compared with older studies on this topic. The highest median survival was found in the juxtacortical subtype (97 months), followed by clear cell (79 months), myxoid (60 months), mesenchymal (33.5 months), and lowest in dedifferentiated (11 months). In more recent analysis, the presence of metastasis on presentation was the only factor with significant value, showing marked differences between subtypes. The metastatic rate is about 2% in periosteal, 6% in clear cell, 8% in myxoid, 11% in mesenchymal, and the highest in dedifferentiated CSA (20%), which is clearly correlated with the survial rate of each subtypes [40].

References

1. Mirra JM, Picci P. Enchondroma versus chondrosarcoma. In: Mirra JM, editor. Bone tumors: clinical, radiologic, and pathologic correlations. 2nd ed. Philadelphia: Lea & Febiger; 1989. p. 476–535.
2. Gitelis S, Bertoni F, Picci P, Campanacci M. Chondrosarcoma of bone. The experience at the Istituto Ortopedico Rizzoli. J Bone Joint Surg Am. 1981;63(8):1248–57.
3. Hudson TH, Moser RP Jr, Gilkey FW, Aoki J. Chondrosarcoma. In: Moser Jr RP, editor. Cartilaginous tumors of the skeleton. Philadelphia: Hanley & Belfus; 1990. p. 155–205.
4. Huvos AG. Chondrosarcoma including spindle cell (dedifferentiated) and myxoid chondrosarcoma: mesenchymal chondrosarcoma. In: Mitchell J, editor. Bone tumors: diagnosis, treatment, and prognosis. 2nd ed. Philadelphia: Saunders; 1991. p. 343–93.
5. Resnick D, Kyriakos M, Greenway GD. Tumors and tumor-like lesions of bone: imaging and pathology of specific lesions. In: Resnick D, editor. Diagnosis of bone and joint disorders. 4th ed. Philadelphia: Saunders; 2002. p. 3897–920.
6. Rosenthal D, Schiller A, Mankin H. Chondrosarcoma: correlation of radiological and histological grade. Radiology. 1984;150(1):21–6.
7. Czerniak B. Malignant cartilage lesions. In: Dorfman HD, Czerniak B, editors. Dorfman and Czerniak's bone tumors. 2nd ed (eBook). Elsevier; 2016. p. 474–569.
8. Garrison RC, Unni KK, McLeod RA, Pritchard DJ, Dahlin DC. Chondrosarcoma arising in osteochondroma. Cancer. 1982;49(9):1890–7.
9. Unni KK, Inwards CY. Chondrsarcoma (primary, secondary, dedifferentiated, and clear cell). In: Unni KK, Inwards CY, editors. Dahlin's bone tumors: general aspects and data on 10,165 cases. 6th ed. Philadelphia: Lippincott William & Wilkins; 2010. p. 60–91.
10. Dahlin DC, Henderson ED. Chondrosarcoma, a surgical and pathological problem: review of 212 cases. J Bone Joint Surg. 1956;38(5):1025–125.
11. Ahmed AR, Tan T-S, Unni KK, Collins MS, Wenger DE, Sim FH. Secondary chondrosarcoma in osteochondroma: report of 107 patients. Clin Orthop Relat Res. 2003;411:193–206.
12. Giuffrida AY, Burgueno JE, Koniaris LG, Gutierrez JC, Duncan R, Scully SP. Chondrosarcoma in the United States (1973 to 2003): an analysis of 2890 cases from the SEER database. J Bone Joint Surg. 2009;91(5):1063–72.
13. Murphey MD, Flemming DJ, Boyea SR, Bojescul JA, Sweet DE, Temple HT. Enchondroma versus chondrosarcoma in the appendicular skeleton: differentiating features. Radiographics. 1998;18(5):1213–37.
14. Zhang Q, Xi Y, Li D, Yuan Z, Dong J. The utility of 18F-FDG PET and PET/CT in the diagnosis and staging of chondrosarcoma: a meta-analysis. J Orthop Surg Res. 2020;15(1):1–11.

15. Feldman F, Van Heertum R, Saxena C, Parisien M. 18FDG-PET applications for cartilage neoplasms. Skeletal Radiol. 2005;34(7):367–74.
16. Purandare NC, Kulkarni AV, Kulkarni SS, Roy D, Agrawal A, Shah S, et al. 18F-FDG PET/CT-directed biopsy: does it offer incremental benefit? Nucl Med Commun. 2013;34(3):203–10.
17. Annovazzi A, Anelli V, Zoccali C, Rumi N, Persichetti A, Novello M, et al. 18 F-FDG PET/CT in the evaluation of cartilaginous bone neoplasms: the added value of tumor grading. Ann Nucl Med. 2019;33:813–21.
18. Evans HL, Ayala AG, Romsdahl MM. Prognostic factors in chondrosarcoma of bone. A clinicopathologic analysis with emphasis on histologic grading. Cancer. 1977;40(2):818–31.
19. Mirra JM, Gold R, Downs J, Eckardt JJ. A new histologic approach to the differentiation of enchondroma and chondrosarcoma of the bones. A clinicopathologic analysis of 51 cases. Clin Orthop Relat Res. 1985;201:214–37.
20. Bovée J, AM F, Lazar A, Nielsen G, Yoshida A. TMN staging of tumors of bone. 5th ed; 2020.
21. Campanacci M. Central chondrosarcoma. In: Campanacci M, editor. Bone and soft tissue tumors. Wien/New York: Springer-Verlag; 1999. p. 283–318.
22. Skeletal Lesions Interobserver Correlation among Expert Diagnosticians (SLICED) Study Group. Reliability of histopathologic and radiologic grading of cartilaginous neoplasms in long bones. J Bone Joint Surg 2007;89(10):2113-2123.
23. Van Der Geest I, De Valk M, De Rooy J, Pruszczynski M, Veth R, Schreuder H. Oncological and functional results of cryosurgical therapy of enchondromas and chondrosarcomas grade 1. J Surg Oncol. 2008;98(6):421–6.
24. Hickey M, Farrokhyar F, Deheshi B, Turcotte R, Ghert M. A systematic review and meta-analysis of intralesional versus wide resection for intramedullary grade I chondrosarcoma of the extremities. Ann Surg Oncol. 2011;18(6):1705–9.
25. Dierselhuis EF, Gerbers JG, Ploegmakers JJ, Stevens M, Suurmeijer AJ, Jutte PC. Local treatment with adjuvant therapy for central atypical cartilaginous tumors in the long bones: analysis of outcome and complications in one hundred and eight patients with a minimum follow-up of two years. J Bone Joint Surg. 2016;98(4):303–13.
26. Souna BS, Belot N, Duval H, Langlais F, Thomazeau H. No recurrences in selected patients after curettage with cryotherapy for grade I chondrosarcomas. Clin Orthop Relat Res. 2010;468(7):1956–62.
27. Hanna S, Whittingham-Jones P, Sewell M, Pollock R, Skinner J, Saifuddin A, et al. Outcome of intralesional curettage for low-grade chondrosarcoma of long bones. Eur J Surg Oncol. 2009;35(12):1343–7.
28. Mohler DG, Chiu R, McCall DA, Avedian RS. Curettage and cryosurgery for low-grade cartilage tumors is associated with low recurrence and high function. Clin Orthop Relat Res. 2010;468(10):2765–73.
29. Verdegaal SH, Brouwers HF, Van Zwet EW, Hogendoorn PC, Taminiau AH. Low-grade chondrosarcoma of long bones treated with intralesional curettage followed by application of phenol, ethanol, and bone-grafting. J Bone Joint Surg. 2012;94(13):1201–7.
30. Leerapun T, Hugate RR, Inwards CY, Scully SP, Sim FH. Surgical management of conventional grade I chondrosarcoma of long bones. Clin Orthop Relat Res. 2007;463:166–72.
31. Ahlmann ER, Menendez LR, Fedenko AN, Learch T. Influence of cryosurgery on treatment outcome of low-grade chondrosarcoma. Clin Orthop Relat Res. 2006;451:201–7.
32. Eriksson A, Schiller A, Mankin H. The management of chondrosarcoma of bone. Clin Orthop Relat Res. 1980;153:44–66.
33. Lee FY, Mankin HJ, Fondren G, Gebhardt MC, Springfield DS, Rosenberg AE, et al. Chondrosarcoma of bone: an assessment of outcome. J Bone Joint Surg. 1999;81(3):326–38.
34. Angelini A, Guerra G, Mavrogenis AF, Pala E, Picci P, Ruggieri P. Clinical outcome of central conventional chondrosarcoma. J Surg Oncol. 2012;106(8):929–37.
35. Errani C, Tsukamoto S, Ciani G, Akahane M, Cevolani L, Tanzi P, et al. Risk factors for local recurrence from atypical cartilaginous tumour and enchondroma of the long bones. Eur J Orthop Surg Traumatol. 2017;27(6):805–11.
36. Schwab JH, Wenger D, Unni K, Sim FH. Does local recurrence impact survival in low-grade chondrosarcoma of the long bones? Clin Orthop Relat Res. 2007;462:175–80. Angelini A, Guerra G, Mavrogenis AF, Pala E, Picci P, Ruggieri P. Clinical outcome of central conventional chondrosarcoma. J Surg Oncol. 2012;106(8):929–37.
37. Brown M, Gikas P, Bhamra J, Skinner J, Aston W, Pollock R, et al. How safe is curettage of low-grade cartilaginous neoplasms diagnosed by imaging with or without pre-operative needle biopsy? Bone Joint J. 2014;96(8):1098–105.
38. Kristensen IB, Sunde LM, Jensen OM. Chondrosarcoma: increasing grade of malignancy in local recurrence. Acta Pathol Microbiol Scand A. 1986;94(1–6):73–7. Schwab JH, Wenger D, Unni K, Sim FH. Does local recurrence impact survival in low-grade chondrosarcoma of the long bones? Clin Orthop Relat Res. 2007;462:175–80.
39. Damron TA, Ward WG, Stewart A. Osteosarcoma, chondrosarcoma, and Ewing's sarcoma: national cancer data base report. Clin Orthop Relat Res. 2007;459:40–7.
40. Amer KM, Munn M, Congiusta D, Abraham JA, Basu Mallick A. Survival and prognosis of chondrosarcoma subtypes: SEER database analysis. J Orthop Res. 2020;38(2):311–9.

22 Periosteal Chondrosarcoma

(***Peri*** "around" + ***osteon*** "bone" + ***chondros*** "cartilage" + ***sarkos*** "*flesh*" + ***ōma*** "*forming*")

22.1 Definition

Periosteal chondrosarcoma (PCSA) is a very rare lower-grade subtype of CSA occurring on the bone surface in close association with the periosteum. It is considered the malignant counterpart of periosteal chondroma.

22.2 Synonym

Parosteal or Juxtacortical CSA.

22.3 Incidence

PCSA is the rarest form among all CSAs, accounting only for about 0.1% of biopsy-analyzed, primary bone tumors [1], and 1–2% of all CSAs [2–6]. A more recent SEER database analysis reported 47 cases of PCSA (3.8%) among 1,235 cases of CSAs [7].

22.4 Age

Most patients are typically diagnosed in young adults between the third and fourth decades of life [3]. About 80% of the patients are older than 20 years with an average of 32 years [1].

22.5 Location

The most common site is the metaphyseal area of the long bones, most commonly the distal femur, followed by the proximal humerus, and proximal tibia [1, 3, 6, 8] (Fig. 22.1). Extremely, it may occur in the small bones of the hand [9, 10] (Fig. 22.2).

W.-J. Bahk, *Diagnosis and Management of Primary Bone Tumors*,
https://doi.org/10.1007/978-981-96-3484-2_22

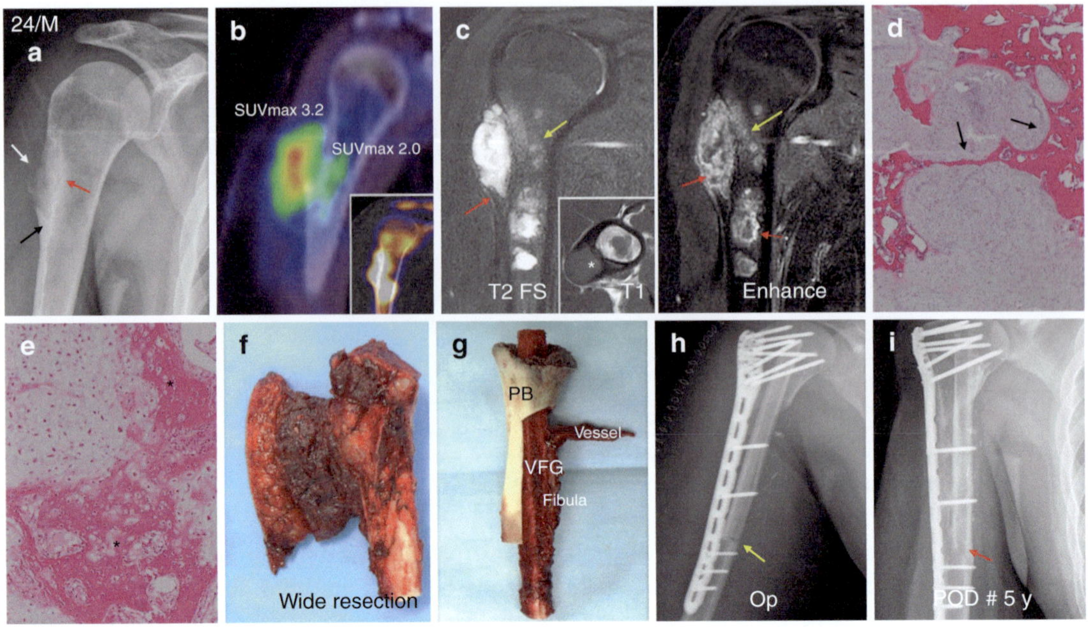

Fig. 22.1 ***Common location of proximal humerus*****.** (**a**) Radiograph taken for right upper arm pain of 8–9 months' duration in a 24-year-old young man shows an ill-defined, ovoid, radiolucent mass-like lesion with internal opacification on the bone surface of the proximal humerus (white arrow). The underlying cortex is deeply eroded and irregularly thinned by the periosteal mass (red arrow). The lesion is bordered by a periosteal solid buttress of reactive periosteal bone at the periphery of the tumor (black arrow), producing a typical *saucer-shaped* defect. There is no definitely discernible intramedullary lesion. (**b**) PET/CT scan reveals an increased FDG uptake in the juxtacortical area (SUVmax 3.2) and milder FDG uptake in the medullary cavity (SUVmax 2.0). Bone SPECT also reveals moderately increased uptake in the same areas (inset). (**c**) MR images demonstrate a well-defined, large, oval, mass lesion on the bone surface, in close association with the periosteum, accompanied by buttress periosteal bone formation (red arrow). The SI is intermediate on T1-weighted image (white asterisk in inset) and bright SI with linear low signal of septa on fat-saturated T2-weighted image. There is patch-like bone marrow edema (yellow arrow) as well as two other mass-like lesions in the medullary cavity (red asterisks) with the same signal as the periosteal main mass, indicating a very rare medullary invasion which is not visible on radiograph. The periosteal mass lesion and medullary invasion lesion are heterogeneously enhanced typically in *peripheral and nodular* pattern (red arrows), and the perilesional bone marrow edema is diffusely enhanced (yellow arrow). (**d**) Low-power microscopic examination notes that the chondrogenic tumor infiltrates the host lamellar bone with a permeative growth pattern as in conventional CSA (arrows). (**e**) Higher-power magnification shows low cellularity with mild nuclear atypia, being consistent with Grade 1 CSA. At the periphery of the cartilage nodule, abundant metaplastic bone formation (black asterisk) is seen. It can be mistaken for periosteal osteosarcoma if the metaplastic bone would be considered as bone production directly from the tumor cells. The final diagnosis of PCSA was rendered in consideration of radiologic periosteal location. (**f**) Wide resection of the proximal humerus including main tumor mass and extending medullary lesions was performed. (**g**) The attached muscles and soft tissues, including the main periosteal mass as well as lesions extending into the bone marrow, are thoroughly removed removed and the resected huemrus was treated with low heat. The pasteurized bone (PB) augmented by vascularized fibula graft (VFG) is prepared for reconstruction. (**h**) The large defect followed by wide resection was reconstructed by the prepared PB augmented with VFG and fixation by a large and strong plate. There is a visible gap at the junction between the host bone and PB (arrow). (**i**) Follow-up radiograph at 5 years after surgery reveals remodeling of the grafted bone with complete union of the junction (arrow) without evidence of local recurrence

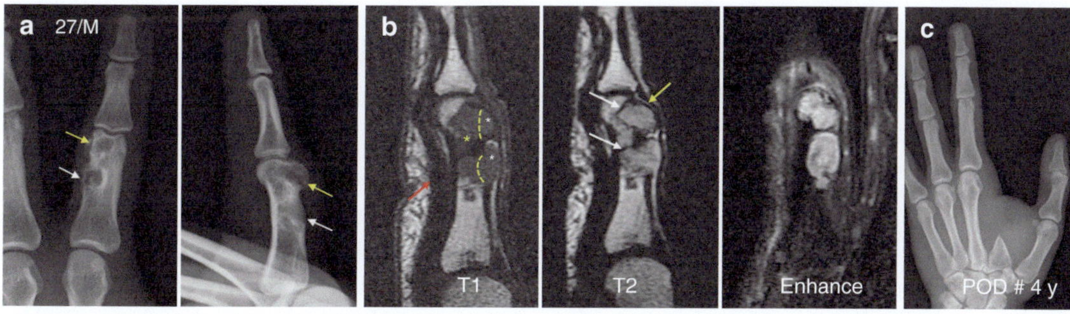

Fig. 22.2 ***Rare location of hand.*** (**a**) Radiograph taken for painful swelling of the right index finger of 2 weeks' duration in a 27-year-old man shows two discrete, eccentric, small, round to oval, radiolucent lesions with sclerotic border and internal calcifications in the proximal phalanx of the index finger. In addition, there are periosteal sclerotic lesions (yellow arrows) and cortical ballooning out (white arrows). Lateral view clearly reveals a periosteal radiolucent exophytic mass with internal punctate calcifications (yellow arrow) and another intracortical to periosteal radiolucent lesion with cortical thickening and medullary extension (white arrow). (**b**) MR images reveal a multilobulated mass-like lesion on the bone surface beyond the cortex (white asterisks) and intramedullary extension (yellow asterisk) with low SI T1-weighted image and intermediate to high SI on T2-weighted image. The exophytic mass lesion is surrounded by a dark signal of thin rim (yellow arrow) and the medullary lesion is also defined by identical rims (white arrows), suggesting the periosteal exophytic mass extending into the medullary cavity. The lesion is heterogeneously enhanced in a *peripheral and nodular* pattern. Microscopic findings were consistent with Grade 1–2 CSA, and the final diagnosis of PCSA was rendered based on its radiologic location. (**c**) Follow-up radiograph taken at 4 years after ray amputation notes no evidence of local recurrence

22.6 Clinical Features

Most patients present with a slowly growing, hard to firm, bulky mass with or without pain, discomfort, or tenderness over the affected area usually persisting for a long period. Knee flexion can be limited when the lesion invovles the posterior distal femur, similiar to parosteal osteosarcoma.

22.7 Radiologic Findings

Plain radiograph The lesion usually appears as a lobulated, round to oval, radiolucent mass, on the surface, with *punctate*, *popcorn,* or *ring-and-arc* calcifications indicating a typical cartilage tumor. The mass is separated from the medullary cavity by a rim of cortical bone and is covered by a periosteal new bone shell. The underlying cortex may be thinned or thickened, deeply eroded or scalloped, often with sclerotic borders. A chronic periosteal reaction may result in periosteal buttressing at the periphery of the tumor, resulting in *saucer-shaped* defect with thickening and sclerosis of the underlying cortex as in periosteal chondroma (Figs. 22.1 and 22.2). Codman triangles are occasionally seen at the lesion margins and elevation of the periosteum with multilayered periosteal new bone formation can also be present. However, perpendicular strations ("hair-on-end") with hazy interface between the mass and underlying cortex, typically seen in periosteal osteosrcoma, are absent in PCSA [3]. **Bone scan** notes variably increased uptake and **PET/CT scan** shows a heterogeneously increased FDG uptake. PET/CT scan with a maximum standardized uptake value (SUVmax) cut-off of 2.0 or 2.3 may distinguish PCSA from periosteal chondroma, even where differentiation of the conditions is challenging on the basis of size and radiographic findings [11] (Fig. 22.1b). **MR images** demonstrate a sharply defined, round or ovoid mass on the bone surface with low to intermediate SI on T1-weighted image and heterogenous intermediate and high SI with lobulated structure by hypointense linear septa on T2-weighted image. Dark signal voids representing mineralization are often seen within the lesion on both sequences. The lesion shows a characteristic enhancement by contrast medium in a *peripheral and septal* pattern as in other cartilage tumors. PCSA frequently erodes or invades the underlying cortex but intramedullary extension or edema rarely occurs [12]. Hatano et al. [13] reported a unique case of medullary invasion. MRI is superior to all other imaging modalities including CT for detecting intramedullary edema or extension (Figs. 22.1c and 22.2b) because of its superior contrast discrimination between the tumor and normal marrow fat [14, 15].

22.8 Histologic Findings

PCSA is histologically identical to conventional CSA with a variable degree of endochondral bone formation (Fig. 22.3). It is typified by solid lobules of hyaline cartilage which permeate the host lamellar bone with focal or extensive myxoid stroma. There can be foci of dystrophic calcification or metaplastic bone formation at the periphery of the cartilage lobules (Fig. 22.1e). However, they should not produce osteoid or woven bone directly from the tumor cells. Individual lobules consist of chondrocytes with moderate cellularity and varying degrees of pleomorphism. The degree of anaplasia varies, but the lesions are almost always corresponding to Grade 1 or 2 CSA. Rarely, the lesion can be Grade 3 and it should be differentiated from periosteal osteosaromca, which predomnantly consists of a cartilage component in the form of irregular poorly marginated lobules separated by fibrous bands mimicking CSA, but with foci of osteoid or primitive woven bone production directly from the undifferentiated spindle cells. Tumor nodules often erode and invade the underlying host cortex, and rarely extend into the medullary cavity resulting in host bone entrapment, as well as invade surrounding soft tissues. Histologically and radiologically, particularly low-grade PCSA is quite similar to periosteal chondroma. Lesion size is often the best finding to distinguish both entities; periosteal chondromas are almost invariably much smaller (2-3 cm in size, average 2 cm) than PCSAs (3-14 cm in size, average 5 cm) [16, 17].

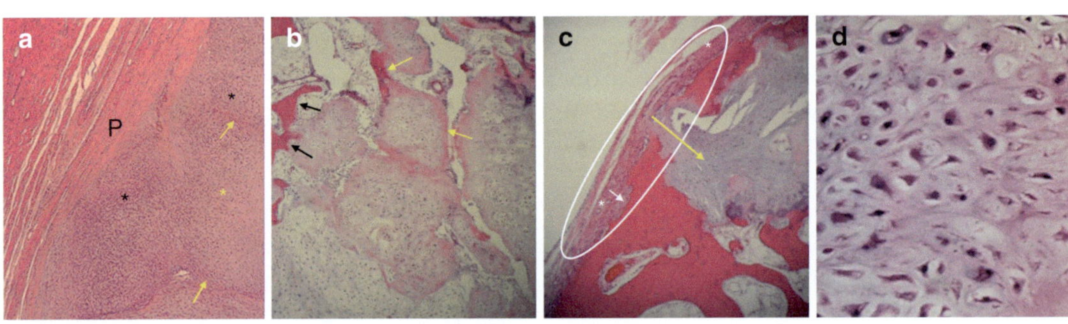

Fig. 22.3 ***Microscopic examination***. (**a**) Low-power magnification shows multiple micro-lobules of chondroid matrix with moderate (yellow asterisk) to high (black asterisk) cellularity, which appear to arise from the periosteum (P). The individual lobules are separated by fibrous bands of varying thickness (arrows). (**b**) The tumor nodules infiltrate the underlying cortex and extend into the medullary cavity resulting in host bone entrapment (black arrows). Formation of metaplastic bone is also observed on the edges of the cartilage nodules (yellow arrows). (**c**) This histologic figure can be interpreted as a tumor perforating the cortex and invading the periosteum. However, the opposite scenario is more likely: a small, thin, periosteally located tumor (circle and asterisks) erodes the underlying host cortex (white arrow), and subsequently invades into the medullary bone through the disrupted cortex (yellow arrow), as suggested by the periosteal or juxtacortical lesion observed on MRI (Fig. 22.2b). (**d**) Higher-power magnification reveals moderate cytologic atypia of the chondrocytes, consistent with Grade 2 CSA

22.9 Management

Wide resection followed by reconstruction is a standard option whenever feasible (Fig. 22.1). Medullary or soft tissue extension should be carefully evaluated before surgery, and the tumor should be treated as a central CSA if such extension is present. Amputation may be indicated for very large, unesectable, or recurrent tumors, particularly those involving the finger (Fig. 22.2).

22.10 Clinical Course

Low rate of local recurrence has been reported if the resected margin is adequate. Distant metastasis is rare and the lung is a common site. The prognosis of PCSA is excellent compared with that of central CSA of the same histologic grade [13, 18]. In the Mayo Clinic series, the 5-year local recurrence-free survival was reported to be only 25% in patients treated with intralesional or marginal excisions, but 93% for the patients treated with wide resection and reconstruction. Six of 24 patients (25%) died of pulmonary metastases. The 5-year metastasis-free survival was reported to be 94% for grade 1 CSA and 50% for grade 2 CSA, with an overall rate of 83% [6]. A more recent SEER database analysis reported 68% of 5-year-survival with median survival of 97 months, which is the highest survival among all CSA subtypes [7]. Metastasis to the lung was reported to be rare in PCSA [2, 5, 18]. The presence of metastasis on presentation was only 2.7% of cases, which is the lowest among all CSA subtypes [7]. Regional metastasis to the adjacent lymph node was also reported during the long clinical course of 32 years [19]. Dedifferentiation has been reported in extremely rare case of primary PCSA [20, 21] with a high risk of metastatic disease and a poor prognosis [20].

References

1. Mirra JM, Picci P. Parsteal chondrosarcoma. In: Mirra JM, editor. Bone tumors: clinical, radiologic, and pathologic correlations. 2nd ed. Philadelphia: Lea & Febiger; 1989. p. 1726–34.
2. Unni KK, Inwards CY. Chondrsarcoma (primary, secondary, dedifferentiated, and clear cell). In: Unni KK, Inwards CY, editors. Dahlin's bone tumors: general aspects and data on 10,165 cases. 6th ed. Philadelphia: Lippincott William & Wilkins; 2010. p. 60–91.
3. Czerniak B. Malignant cartilage lesions. In: Dorfman HD, Czerniak B, editors. Dorfman and Czerniak's bone tumors. 2nd ed (eBook). Elsevier; 2016. p. 474–569.
4. Fechner RE, Mills SE. Juxtacortical chondrosarcoma. In: Rosai J, editor. Tumors of the bones and joints. Washington, DC: Armed Forces Institute of Pathology; 1993. p. 121–3.
5. Goedhart L, Ploegmakers J, Kroon H, Zwartkruis E, Jutte P. The presentation, treatment and outcome of periosteal chondrosarcoma in the Netherlands. Bone Joint J. 2014;96(6):823–8.
6. Papagelopoulos PJ, Galanis EC, Mavrogenis AF, Savvidou OD, Bond JR, Unni KK, et al. Survivorship analysis in patients with periosteal chondrosarcoma. Clin Orthop Relat Res. 2006;448:199–207.
7. Amer KM, Munn M, Congiusta D, Abraham JA, Basu Mallick A. Survival and prognosis of chondrosarcoma subtypes: SEER database analysis. J Orthop Res. 2020;38(2):311–9.
8. Campanacci M. Periosteal chondrosarcoma. (Parosteal or juxtacortical chondrosarcoma). In: Campanacci M, editor. Bone and soft tissue tumors. Wien/New York: Springer-Verlag; 1999. p. 363–7.
9. Kavitha K, MC S, Ramani K, Puthoor D. Periosteal chondrosarcoma of metacarpal bone: report of a rare entity. Aust J Med Sci. 2012;5(11):589–92.
10. Wu KK, Kelly AP. Periosteal (juxtacortical) chondrosarcoma: report of a case occurring in the hand. J Hand Surg Am. 1977;2(4):314–5.
11. Morimoto S, Futani H, Tsuchiyama K, Fukunaga S, Tsukamoto Y, Yoshiya S. Usefulness of PET/CT for diagnosis of periosteal chondrosarcoma of the femur: a case report. Oncol Lett. 2014;7(6):1826–8.
12. Chaabane S, Bouaziz MC, Drissi C, Abid L, Ladeb MF. Periosteal chondrosarcoma. AJR Am J Roentgenol. 2009;192(1):W1–6.

13. Hatano H, Ogose A, Hotta T, Otsuka H, Takahashi HE. Periosteal chondrosarcoma invading the medullary cavity. Skeletal Radiol. 1997;26(6):375–8.
14. McLeod RA, Berquist TH. Bone tumor imaging: contribution of CT and MRI. In: Unni KK, editor. Bone tumors. New York/Edinburgh: Churchill Livingstone; 1988. p. 1–33.
15. Cohen EK, Kressel HY, Frank TS, Fallon M, Burk D Jr, Dalinka M, et al. Hyaline cartilage-origin bone and soft-tissue neoplasms: MR appearance and histologic correlation. Radiology. 1988;167(2):477–81.
16. Bauer TW, Dorfman HD, Latham JT Jr. Periosteal chondroma. A clinicopathologic study of 23 cases. Am J Surg Pathol. 1982;6(7):631–7.
17. Robinson P, White L, Sundaram M, Kandel R, Wunder J, McDonald D, et al. Periosteal chondroid tumors: radiologic evaluation with pathologic correlation. Am J Roentgenol. 2001;177(5):1183–8.
18. Schajowicz F. Juxtacortical chondrosarcoma. J Bone Joint Surg Br. 1977;59(4):473–80.
19. Matsumoto K, Hukuda S, Ishizawa M, Saruhashi Y, Okabe H, Asano Y. Parosteal (juxtacortical) chondrosarcoma of the humerus associated with regional lymph node metastasis. A case report. Clin Orthop Relat Res. 1993;290:168–73.
20. Mitchell A, Rudan JR, Fenton PV. Juxtacortical dedifferentiated chondrosarcoma from a primary periosteal chondrosarcoma. Mod Pathol. 1996;9(3):279–83.
21. Kumta S, Griffith J, Chow LT, Leung PC. Primary juxtacortical chondrosarcoma dedifferentiating after 20 years. Skeletal Radiol. 1998;27(10):569–73.

23 Clear Cell Chondrosarcoma

23.1 Definition

Clear cell chondrosarcoma (CC CSA) is a rare low-grade subtype of CSA, which is characterized by a proliferation of lare chondrocytes with a clear cytoplasm due to the presence of a significant amount of glycogen.

23.2 Incidence

It is very rare, accounting for only 0.2% of biopsy-analyzed bone tumors [1], and approximately 2–5% of all CSAs [1–6].

23.3 Age

Although it has been reported to occur with a wide range of age from the second to ninth decades of life, most tumors arise during adulthood with a peak age between the fourth and fifth decades of life [1, 6, 7]. More than half of patients are in this age group [6]. It is extremely rare in children and the elderly.

23.4 Location

CC CSA shows a significant predilection for the ends (epiphysis or apophysis) of long tubular bones, often extending to the articular cartilage, similar to chondroblastoma (CB) and giant cell tumor. About 60–70% of cases affect the proximal femur and proximal humerus [1, 6, 8]. The rest may occur in flat bones such as ribs, pelvic bones, vertebrae, and short tubular bones, as well as distal femur and proximal tibia.

23.5 Clinical Features

Pain or discomfort is the most frequent presentation with a variable duration, which is usually long due to due to slow growth of the tumor. In the Mayo Clinic series, it was longer than 1 year in about 50% of the patients and over 5 years in about 20% of patients [9]. Rarely, a limitation of motion in the involved joint can be presented. Pathologic fracture of the femoral neck is not infrequent, and underlying CC CSA may often be initially unrecognized (Figs. 23.3 and 23.4).

23.6 Radiologic Finding

Plain radiograph Typically, CC CSA mainly affects the epiphysis of the long tubular bone, extending extending to the articular cartilage and often the metaphysis (Figs. 23.1, 23.2, 23.3, and 23.4), in contrast to conventional CSA, which usually affects the meta-diaphyseal area. In general, the lesion presenrs as a well-circumscribed, geographic destruction, predominantly lucent,

W.-J. Bahk, *Diagnosis and Management of Primary Bone Tumors*,
https://doi.org/10.1007/978-981-96-3484-2_23

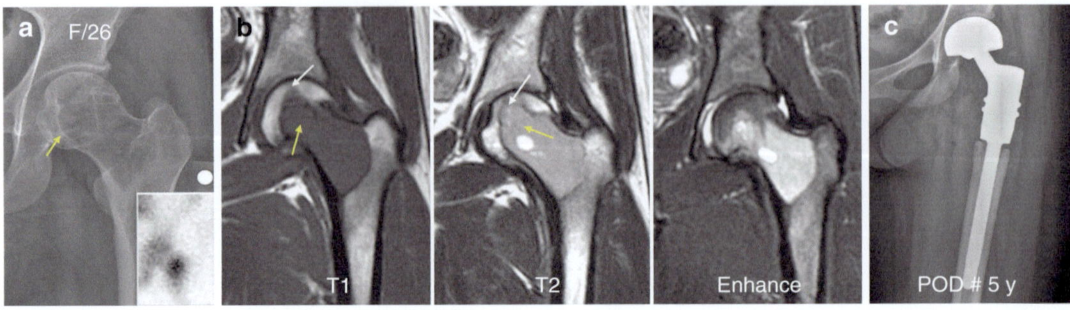

Fig. 23.1 (**a**) Radiograph taken for left hip pain of 5 months' duration in a 26-year-old young lady shows a relatively well-defined, predominantly osteolytic lesion surrounded by a thin sclerosis (arrow) in the femoral head and neck. The femoral neck is mildly expanded. Bone scan reveals a focal hot uptake (inset). (**b**) MR images demonstrate a well-demarcated medullary lesion with low SI on T1-weighted image and intermediate to high SI with internal focal bright signal on T2-weighted image, with a thin dark signal of reactive sclerosis on both sequences. The lesion occupies the epiphysis, extending to the articular cartilage (white arrows) as well as to the neck and trochanteric area (yellow arrows). The lesion is diffusely enhanced by contrast medium. A histologic diagnosis of CC CSA was rendered. (**c**) Follow-up radiograph at 5 years after wide resection and reconstruction using a tumor prosthesis reveals good maintenance of the prosthesis without local recurrence

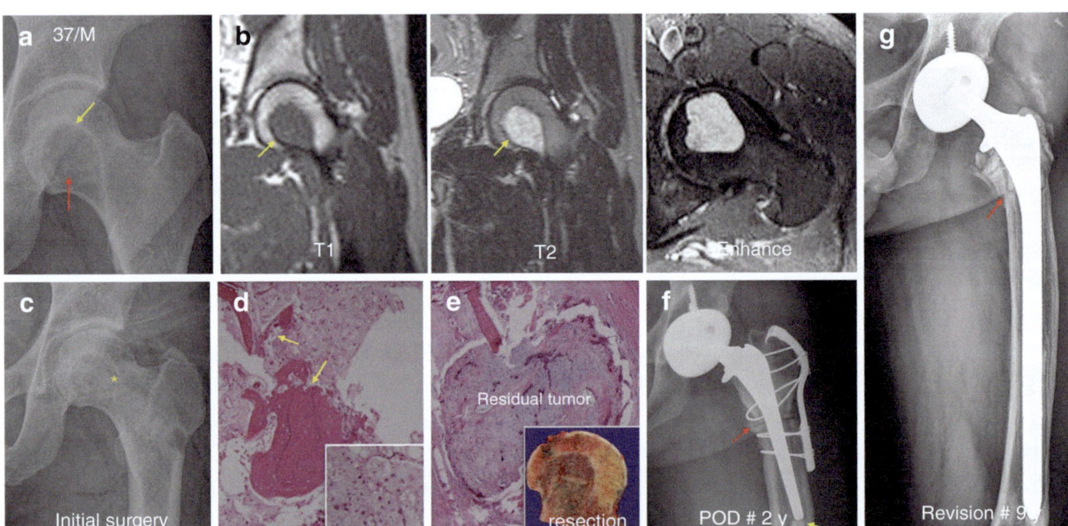

Fig. 23.2 ***Initially mistaken for CB***. (**a**) Radiograph taken for left hip pain on weight bearing of 4 month's duration in a 37-year-old man shows a well-defined, osteolytic osteolytic lesion with some punctate calcifications, surrounded by a thin rim of sclerosis (yellow arrow) in the femoral head and neck, which is quite similar to that of CB (see Fig. 20.1a in Chap. 20). Note lager size, dense sclerotic or trabeculated patterns within the lesion (red arrow). (**b**) MR images reveal a well-defined mass lesion with low SI on T1-weighted image and high SI on T2-weighted image, with a dark signal of thin sclerosis on both sequences (arrows), mimicking CB. The lesion is homogeneously and diffusely enhanced by contrast medium. (**c**) Thorough curettage with allogenic chip bone grafting (asterisk) was performed under a radiologic impression of CB without a biopsy in a private clinic. (**d**) However, microscopic examination of curetted specimen reveals that swollen large chondrocytes with abundant pale to clear cytoplasm embedded in a loose cartilaginous stroma infiltrate and encase the preexisting lamellar bone spicules (arrows), and the patient was transferred to our hospital. (**e**) En-bloc resection of the femoral head and neck followed by reconstruction using an allo-prosthesis composite was performed. Microscopic examination of the resected specimen shows a residual CC CSA with production of metaplastic woven bone spicules. (**f**) Follow-up radiograph at 2 years after surgery shows a nonunion of host bone-allograft junction (red arrow) with loosening of the tumor prosthesis (yellow arrow). (**g**) Follow-up radiograph at 9 years after revision using a long stem reveals union of allogenic graft to host bone (arrow) with no evidence of local recurrence.

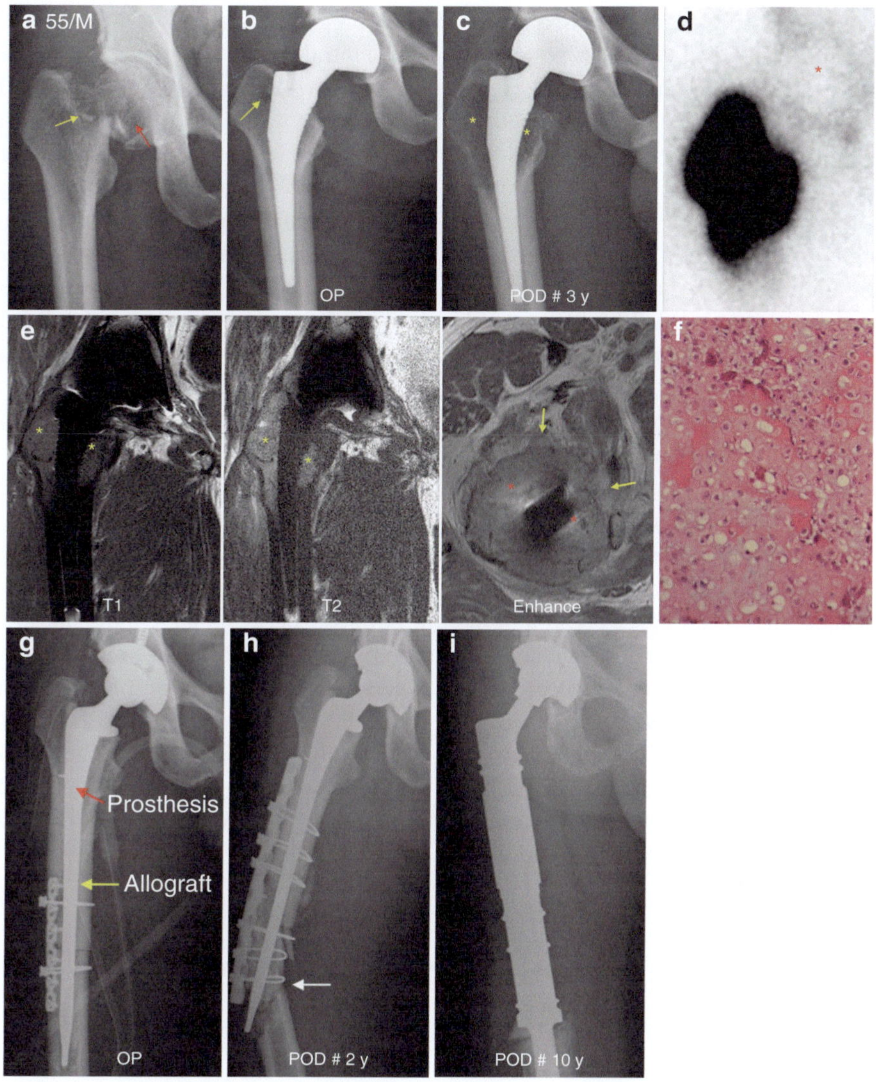

Fig. 23.3 ***Femoral neck fracture with unrecognized CSA***. (**a**) Radiograph taken for right hip pain after slip in a 55-year-old man shows a femoral neck fracture. Several comminuted fragments (yellow arrow) cuased only by a trivial slip rather than a high-speed inury in a middle-aged man and radiolucent areas in the femoral head and neck (red arrows) can be a clue for a pathologic fracture with a preexisting bone lesion. However, the underlying lesion was initially neglected because the hip surgeon considered it disuse osteoporosis due to his right hemiparesis after brain tumor surgery. (**b**) Bipolar hemi-arthroplasty was performed without further study such as CT scan or MRI. Immediate postoperative radiograph notes a peri-prosthetic mottled radiolucency (arrow) which was also not recognized at that time by the hip surgeon. (**c**) However, radiograph taken for right proximal thigh pain at 3 years after surgery demonstrates a significantly progressed radiolucency with expansion and cortical breaches around the proximal part of prosthesis (asterisks), indicating progression of the residual tumor or local recurrence. (**d**) Pinhole bone scan shows a homogeneous intense uptake in the proximal periprosthetic area with photon defect in the prosthetic head (asterisk). (**e**) MR images with changed parameters to minimize the metallic artifacts reveal an intramedullary mass-like lesion in the proximal periprosthetic area (asterisks) with intermediate SI on T1-weighted image and high SI on T2-weighted image. The periprosthetic lesion is heterogeneously enhanced (red asterisks), and the lesions extending to surrounding muscles though the cortical breakages are also diffusely enhanced (yellow arrows). (**f**) Microscopic examination notes typical two major hallmarks for CC CSA, including swollen large chondrocytes with characteristic *vacuolated* cytoplasm and production of metaplastic woven bone within the clear cell cartilaginous stroma. (**g**) Wide resection with reconstruction using an allograft-prosthesis composite was performed. (**h**) Radiograph taken for a severe thigh pain without a history of trauma at 2 years after revision surgery notes a pathologic fracture with comminution and angulation (arrow) in the distal stem area. (**i**) Revision surgery using a tumor prosthesis was performed, and follow-up radiograph at 10 years after second surgery demonstrates a good maintenance with no evidence of local recurrence

sometimes with varying degrees of expansion and internal mineralization with or without a sclerotic margin (Figs. 23.1 and 23.2). They are mostly classified as Grade 1A (thin, sclerotic margin) or 1B (distinct, well-marginated border, but not sclerotic) by the Lodwick classification of lytic bone lesions [10]. The flecks of internal mineralization with a rind of surrounding sclerotic margin mimicking a benign bone tumor were reported in about only 20–30% of cases [8], which can be easily mistaken for CB although CC CSA is often larger and more aggressive-looking (Fig. 23.2). Longstanding lesions may produce expansion of the bone, frequently with cortical thinning. Unlike conventional CSA, cortical breakage with soft tissue mass is not a usual feature, presenting in only fewer than 10% of the cases [1, 8]. However, cortical thinning is observed in about half of the cases [1]. If a blow-out feature is observed, secondary aneurysmal bone cyst needs to be suspected. Periosteal reaction is usually absent to minimal if presents. **Bone scan** usually notes a homogeneous or heterogeneous strong uptake (Figs. 23.3d and 23.4d). **CT scan** is useful to evaluate the extent of the lesion, including the degree of endosteal scalloping and breaches in the cortex, the details of the intralesional calcification, and the status of narrow or wide margin (Fig. 23.4b). **MR images** demonstrate a well-defined intramedullary mass-like lesion with low to intermediate SI on T1-weighted image and heterogeneous high SI on T2-weighted image. The lesion is diffusely or heterogeneously enhanced by contrast medium (Figs. 23.1, 23.2, 23.3, and 23.4). A heterogenous low to intermediate SI on T2-weighted MR images reflects marked mineralization or osseous metaplasia. Perilesional bone marrow edema or periosteal reaction is mostly absent or minimal if presents. Imaging features suggesting CC CSA include a larger lesion, lack of adjacent bone marrow or soft tissue edema, and high signal intensity (SI) on T2-weighted MR images [8]. In contrast, CB is usually smaller and presents with prominent perilesional edema in the adjacent bone marrow and/or surrounding soft tissue, as well as heterogeneous high SI with low to intermediate signal in many cases [10, 11]. Clinical information on the patient's age is also useful. CC CSA usually occurs in young adults with closed growth plate typically 1 to 2 decades older than patients with CB.

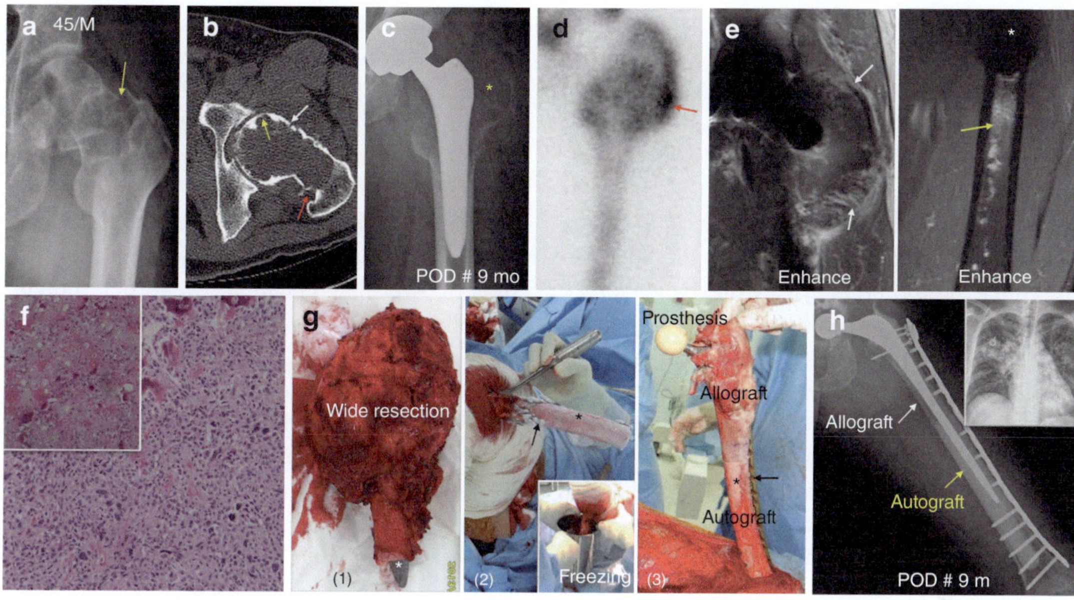

Fig. 23.4 ***Dedifferentiation at local recurrence*.** (**a**) Radiograph taken for right hip pain after slip in a 45-year-old man shows a relatively well-defined, expansile, multilobulated, predominantly osteolytic lesion in the femoral head and neck with a pathologic fracture (arrow). (**b**) CT scan reveals a geographic destruction with focal intralesional densifications with multiple deep cortical scalloping (yellow arrow), cortical breakage (white arrow), and pathologic fracture (red arrow). However, the underlying lesion was not recognized by a primary surgeon, and total hip replacement was performed without a biopsy in a private clinic. (**c**) Follow-up radiograph at 9 months after surgery notes a marked destruction in the greater trochanter (asterisk). He was transferred to our hospital under the impression of a malignant bone tumor. (**d**) Bone scan notes a heterogeneous mild uptake in the trochanteric area with focal strong uptake along the greater trochanter (arrow). (**e**) Enhanced MR image shows a significantly expansile intramedullary lesion with a huge soft tissue mass surrounding the femoral stem, which is heterogeneously enhanced in peripheral and septal pattern (white arrows). Note additional scattered lesions in the distal medullary cavity with good enhancement (yellow arrow), suggesting a seeding of the tumor by insertion procedure of the femoral stem (asterisk). (**f**) Microscopic examination of biopsy specimen shows an area of markedly pleomorphic spindle cells with frequent abnormal mitoses and osteoid to woven bone deposition directly by the tumor cells, indicating a high-grade osteosarcoma. There is another area typically consisting of preexisting CC CSA (inset), allowing a diagnosis of dedifferentiation CC CSA to higher-grade sarcoma. (**g**) Two different surgical procedures were performed for hip and shaft lesions. [1] Firstly, a wide resection including a previously inserted hip prosthesis (asterisks) was performed. [2] Subsequently, the remaining femur distal to the cutting line was treated with extended curettage of the spreading tumor, followed by cryosurgery using liquid nitrogen (inset). Note a whitish freezing bone (asterisk) with iced crystals (arrow). [3] Finally, the large defect was reconstructed by APC fixed to the recycled femur (asterisk) using a long locking plate (arrow). (**h**) Radiograph taken for 9 months after revision surgery shows good maintenance with visible line between the allograft and recycled distal femur junction (red arrow) but no evidence of local recurrence. Unfortunately, however, he died of disseminated pulmonary metastasis and pneumonia 2 weeks later (inset)

23.7 Histologic Findings

Low-power microscopic examination shows a lobular growth pattern of sheets consisting of tumor cells similar to other cartilage tumors, which infiltrate and permeate the host lamellar bone trabeculae as in conventional CSA. The most distinct histologic hallmark is the presence of swollen large chondrocytes with abundant pale to clear cytoplasm, so-called "*clear cell*" chondrocytes, embedded in a loose cartilaginous stroma (Fig. 23.5a). Another major hallmark is the production of woven bone spicules apparently caused by osseous metaplasia of the chondroid matrix. Usually, the woven bone spicules are extensive and arranged in a similar manner to that seen in the osteoblastoma (osteoblastoma-like osseous metaplasia) (Fig. 23.5b). Cortical disruption with soft tissue extension is unusual. Often, multinucleated giant cells are diffusely scattered or clumped (Fig. 23.5c, f). Areas of low-grade CSA lacking cleared cytoplasm are found in about half of the cases [6] (Fig. 23.5d). Foci of coarse calcification are present (Fig. 23.5e), but occasionally large areas can be heavily calcified. Higher-power magnification reveals that individual cells typically show *cleared* or *vacuolated* cytoplasm representing prominent glycogen content within the tumor cells (Fig. 23.5f). The nuclei are round and centrally located with prominent nucleoli. The atypia of the nuclei is usually mild to intermediate and mitoses are rare. Rarely, dedifferentiation to high-grade spindle cell sarcoma may occur (Fig. 23.4f).

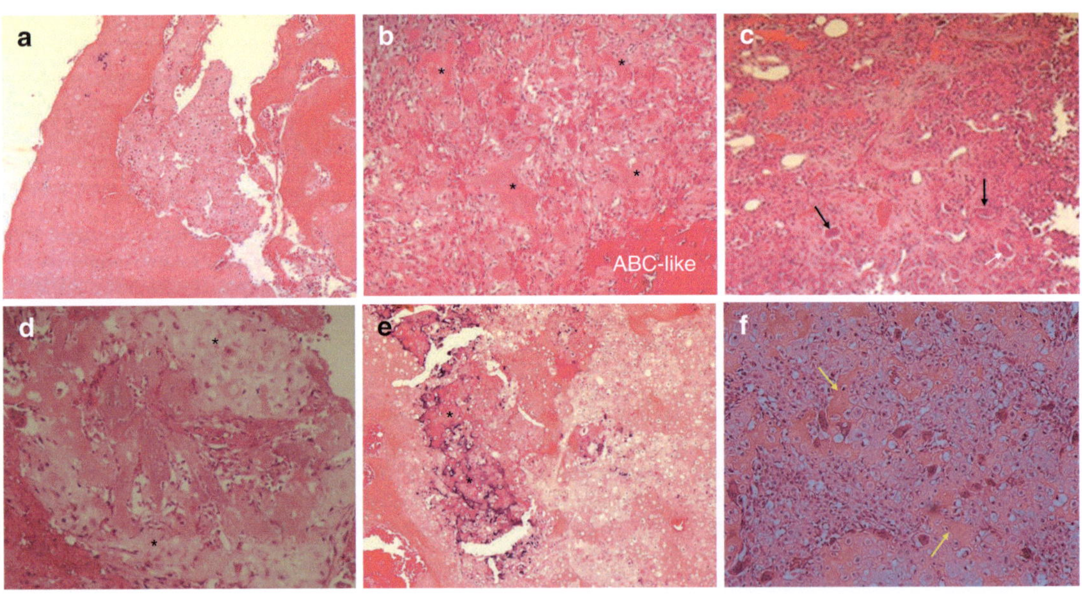

Fig. 23.5 ***Microscopic examination***. (**a**) Low-power magnification shows a lobular architecture of sheets consisting of swollen, large chondrocytes with abundant pale to clear cytoplasm embedded in a loose cartilaginous stroma. (**b**) Extensive production of metaplastic woven bone spicules rimmed by osteoblasts (asterisks) within the clear cell cartilaginous stroma, which simulates osteoblastoma. (**c**) Osteoclast-like multinucleated giant cells are diffusely scattered (arrows) with foci of osteoid deposition. (**d**) Foci of low-grade CSA lacking typical clear cells are seen in this field (asterisks). (**e**) The cartilage is focally calcified in the center of the tumor (asterisks). (**f**) Higher-power magnification demonstrates typical swollen large chondrocytes with round and mildly atypical nuclei, central prominent nucleoli, and typical *cleared or vacuolated* cytoplasm embedded in the chondroid matrix, the most distinct hallmark for a diagnosis of CC CSA. Note another major hallmark of abundant pinkish strands of metaplastic woven bones varying in size and shape apparently formed by osseous metaplasia of the chondroid matrix. There are also numerous scattered and clumped multinucleated giant cells

23.8 Management

En-bloc resection followed by reconstruction is the standard option. Occasionally, inadequate conservative surgical management such as marginal excision or curettage is performed in some cases mistaken for CB due to a relatively indolent clinical course and radiologic overlap, and the cases usually result in recurrence (Fig. 23.2).

23.9 Clinical Course

CC CSA behaves as a low-grade malignancy and carries a much better prognosis than a conventional CSA. En-bloc resection with a negative margin is usually curative. However, inadequate resection leads to a much higher risk of local recurrence and metastatic disease. However, the progression of the disease seems to be slow even after local recurrence. Rarely, dedifferentiation to high-grade spindle cell sarcoma has been reported at initial diagnosis, at recurrence, and at metastasis with a grave prognosis [12] (Fig. 23.4). In a series, 10-year overall survival was reported to be 89%, and disease-free survival was 68% [5]. In another long-term follow-up study, 5 of 7 patients (71%) treated by curettage had local recurrence with a mean interval between surgery and local recurrence of 52.2 months (from 12 to 132), but only 1 of 8 patients (13%) treated by wide or marginal surgical margins had local recurrence [13]. The authors also reported that serum alkaline phosphatase (SAP) level decreased to normal in 7 of 9 patients with high preoperative SAP, and concluded SAP can be used as a good tumor marker in diagnosis and follow-up. More recently, Amer et al. [14] reported 1-year survival rates of 89%, 5-year survival rates of 62%, and a median survival of 79 months in a SEER database analysis of patients with CSA subtypes from 1973 to 2013. Local recurrence may be extremely late, no matter whether treated conservatively by marginal resection or with wide resection [3, 5, 9, 13, 15]. Very late local recurrence was reported at 19 years after surgical resection [16] and even 24 years after initial surgery [13]. The presence of metastasis on presentation was 5.7% of cases among all CSA subtypes [14]. The time to metastasis ranged from 4 to 16 years in the patients who had distant disease [5]. However, very late distant metastasis was reported without local recurrence at 23 years after surgical resection [17] and with local recurrence at 29 years after initial diagnosis [18]. Based on these reports, CC CSAs seemed to have a clear tendency for late local recurrence or metastasis even decades after primary surgery. Therefore, the authors recommended a longer follow-up fordecades or lifelong.

References

1. Mirra JM, Picci P. Clear cell chondrosarcoma. In: Mirra JM, editor. Bone tumors: clinical, radiologic, and pathologic correlations. 2nd ed. Philadelphia: Lea & Febiger; 1989. p. 535–46.
2. Czerniak B. Malignant cartilage lesions. In: Dorfman HD, Czerniak B, editors. Dorfman and Czerniak's bone tumors. 2nd ed (eBook). Elsevier; 2016. p. 474–569.
3. Ayoub KS, Grimer RJ, Carter SR, Mangham DC, Davies A, Tillman RM. Clear cell chondrosarcoma of bone. Sarcoma. 1999;3(2):115–9.
4. Resnick D, Kyriakos M, Greenway GD. Tumors and tumor-like lesions of bone: imaging and pathology of specific lesions. In: Resnick D, editor. Diagnosis of bone and joint disorders. 4th ed. Philadelphia: Saunders; 2002. p. 3897–920.
5. Itälä A, Leerapun T, Inwards C, Collins M, Scully SP. An institutional review of clear cell chondrosarcoma. Clin Orthop Relat Res. 2005;440:209–12.
6. Unni KK, Inwards CY. Clear cell chondrosarcoma. In: Unni KK, Inwards CY, editors. Dahlin's bone tumors: general aspects and data on 10,165 cases. 6th ed. Philadelphia: Lippincott William & Wilkins; 2010. p. 83–91.
7. Rosenthal D, Schiller A, Mankin H. Chondrosarcoma: correlation of radiological and histological grade. Radiology. 1984;150(1):21–6.
8. Murphey MD, Walker EA, Wilson AJ, Kransdorf MJ, Temple HT, Gannon FH. From the archives of the AFIP: imaging of primary chondrosarcoma: radiologic-pathologic correlation. Radiographics. 2003;23(5):1245–78.
9. Bjornsson J, Unni KK, Dahlin DC, Beabout JW, Sim FH. Clear cell chondrosarcoma of bone: observations in 47 cases. Am J Surg Pathol. 1984;8(3):223–30.
10. Kaim AH, Hügli R, Bonél HM, Jundt G. Chondroblastoma and clear cell chondrosarcoma: radiological and MRI characteristics with

histopathological correlation. Skeletal Radiol. 2002;31(2):88–95.
11. Bloem JL, Mulder JD. Chondroblastoma: a clinical and radiological study of 104 cases. Skeletal Radiol. 1985;14(1):1–9.
12. Kalil RK, Inwards CY, Unni KK, Bertoni F, Bacchini P, Wenger DE, et al. Dedifferentiated clear cell chondrosarcoma. Am J Surg Pathol. 2000;24(8):1079–86.
13. Donati D, Yin J-Q, Colangeli M, Colangeli S, Bella CD, Bacchini P, et al. Clear cell chondrosarcoma of bone: long time follow-up of 18 cases. Arch Orthop Trauma Surg. 2008;128:137–42.
14. Amer KM, Munn M, Congiusta D, Abraham JA, Basu Mallick A. Survival and prognosis of chondrosarcoma subtypes: SEER database analysis. J Orthop Res. 2020;38(2):311–9.
15. Unni K, Dahlin D, Beabout J, Sim F. Chondrosarcoma: clear-cell variant. A report of sixteen cases. J Bone Joint Surg Am. 1976;58(5):676–83.
16. Hartwright D, Mangham D, Grimer R. Reactivation of tumor after 19 years? A case of local recurrence in clear cell chondrosarcoma. Int Orthop. 2000;24(2):112–4.
17. Bagley L, Kneeland J, Dalinka MK, Bullough P, Brooks J. Unusual behavior of clear cell chondrosarcoma. Skeletal Radiol. 1993;22(4):279–82.
18. Laitinen M, Nieminen J, Pakarinen T-K. An unusual case of clear cell chondrosarcoma with very late recurrence and lung metastases, 29 years after primary surgery. Case Rep Orthop. 2014;2014:109569.

24 Mesenchymal Chondrosarcoma

24.1 Definition

Mesenchymal chondrosarcoma (MCSA) is a rare, highly malignant variant of CSA, characterized by a bimorphic pattern consisting of undifferentiated mesenchymal cells and islands of cartilaginous differentiation, frequently with multiple vascular spaces, commonly arising in bone and less commonly in meninges and other soft tissues.

24.2 Incidence

MCSA is extremely rare, accounting for less than 5% of all CSAs [1–5], 0.5% of biopsy-analyzed primary bone tumors [6], and 0.7% of all malignant tumors [7]. A more recent analysis of the SEER Database from 1973 to 2011 reported that MCSA accounted for about 4% of the 5110 patients with CSA being similar to previously reported incidence [8].

24.3 Age

Although MCSA can occur in a wide range of age, from the first and eighth decades of life, it mostly affects teenagers or young adults between the second and fourth decades of life, accounting for about 70–80% of the patients [6, 7, 9, 10], which is younger than the typical age of central CSA.

24.4 Location

MCSA involves the long bones or limb less often than other primary bone tumors, representing only about 30–40% of cases. Craniofacial bones or trunk bones are more frequently affected, compring 60–70% of cases [4, 6, 10]. In the Mayo Clinic series, 65% of cases were in bone, 34% in nonskeletal tissues, and the rest in both bone and soft tissue [9]. When bone is affected, it most commonly arises in the axial skeletons such as craniofacial skeleton, especially jaw bones, vertebrae, ribs, chest wall, and pelvic bone. The cranial and spinal central nervous system is also typically involved. In long bones, a diaphysis of femur, humerus, and tibia/fibula is most commonly affected. While conventional CSAs arise from the soft tissues in less than 1% of cases, a high proportion of the MCSA (approximately 30–40% of all cases) occurs in soft tissues (extraskeletal MCSA), including muscle and fat, mainly of the lower extremities, meninges, nasopharynx, and orbital soft tissue [4, 5, 9–11]. Most MCSAs occur as a solitary bony lesion (Fig. 24.1), but multiple lesions of soft tissue and/or multifocal osseous origin were rarely reported [12–14] (Fig. 24.2). In a large series, 72 of 111 MCSAs (65%) occurred in bone, and 5 of 72 MCSA arose in bone (7%) involved multiple skeletal sites [9].

W.-J. Bahk, *Diagnosis and Management of Primary Bone Tumors*,
https://doi.org/10.1007/978-981-96-3484-2_24

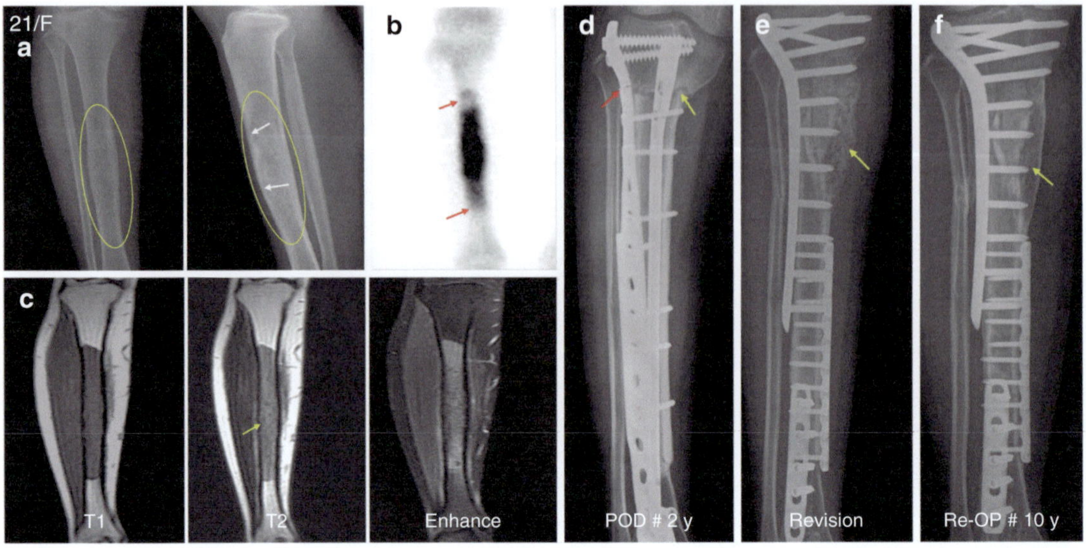

Fig. 24.1 *Osseous MCSA*. (**a**) Radiograph taken for right leg pain of 6 months' duration in a 21-year-old young lady shows a poorly defined, fusiform, medullary radiolucent lesion with mild expansion (red circles), thickening of the cortex, and deep and long endosteal scalloping (arrows) in the tibial shaft. There are typical intralesional *rings and arcs* or *popcorn-like* densities of chondroid material. (**b**) Bone scan reveals a strong uptake with a weak uptake at the periphery of the lesion (arrows). (**c**) MR images demonstrate a well-defined, intramedullary lesion with intermediate signal intensity (SI) on T1-weighted image and intermediate to high SI on T2-weighted image. There are stippled internal dark signals of calcification on both sequences. Note the multiple serpentine vascular structures with low to dark SI within the lesion on T2-weighted image (arrow). The lesion is diffusely enhanced by contrast medium. Incision biopsy confirmed a diagnosis of MCSA based on a bi-morphic histologic pattern including solid mesenchymal areas consisting of undifferentiated small round blue cells and cartilage islands within the solid area, with multiple vascular channels in a "staghorn" pattern reminiscent of hemangiopericytoma. (**d**) Follow-up radiograph at 2 years after wide resection followed by reconstruction using an allograft fixed by intramedullary nail and locking plates shows nonunion at the junction between the proximal host bone and the allograft (yellow arrow) and breakage of the proximal plate (red arrow). (**e**) Removal of the intramedullary nail and broken plate followed by strong fixation using new plates and exuberant autograft and allograft (yellow arrow) was performed. (**f**) Follow-up radiograph at 10 years after revision surgery shows solid union at the host bone-allograft junction (yellow arrow), with no evidence of local recurrence

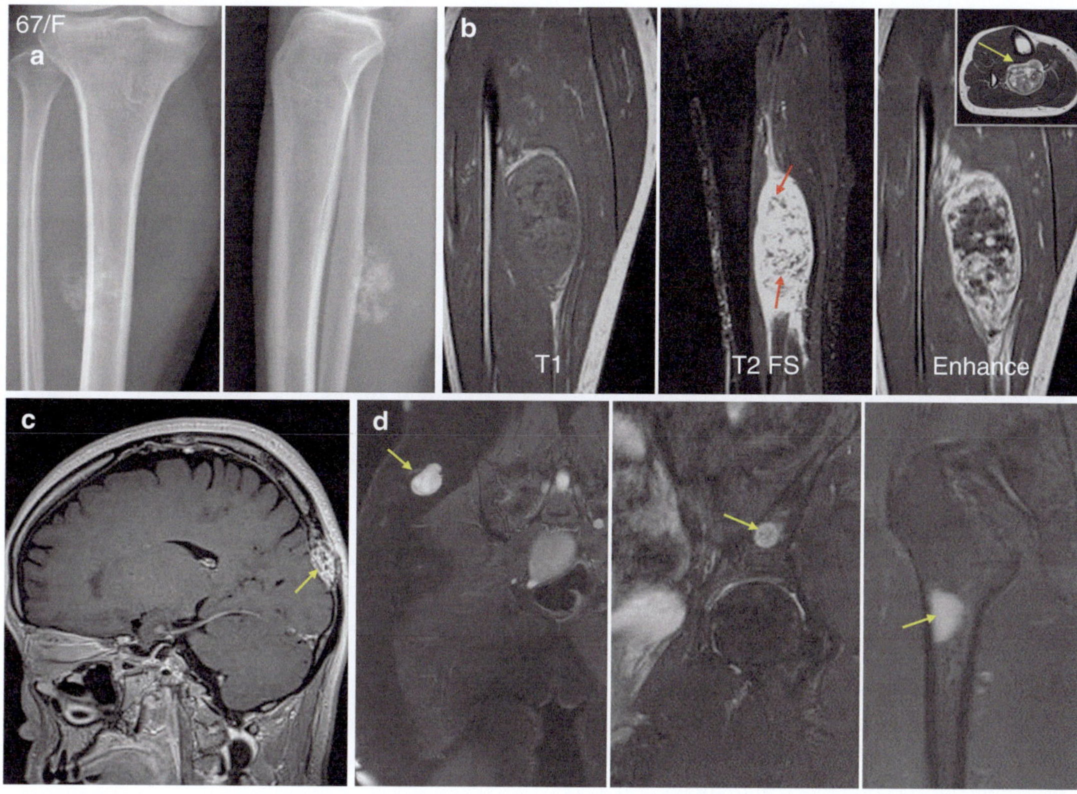

Fig. 24.2 ***Multifocal soft tissue and osseous MCSA***. (**a**) Radiograph taken for right calf mass of 6 months' duration in a 67-year-old woman shows a relatively well-circumscribed radiolucent soft tissue mass with areas of *rings-and-arcs* or *granular* calcification in her right calf. (**b**) MR images reveal a well-defined soft tissue mass adjacent to the tibia with intermediate SI on T1-weighted image and high SI on fat-saturated T2-weighted image. There are characteristic multiple serpentine vascular structures with low to dark SI on fat-saturated T2-weighted image (red arrows), representing hemangiopericytoma-like areas, which are not a feature in other CSAs. The lesion is heterogeneously enhanced in a typical *nodular and peripheral* pattern. The mass is definitely not attached to the tibia or fibula on axial view, indicating a frank soft tissue mass rather than a juxta-cortical lesion (inset). (**c**) A small nodular mass with similar SI is found in the meninges (yellow arrow). (**d**) Additional similar lesions with high SI are also seen in right buttock, left acetabulum, and right proximal femur on T2-weighted image (arrows), suggesting a probable multifocal soft tissue and osseous MCSA

24.5 Clinical Features

Symptoms are often vague and nonspecific, depending upon the location and progression of the tumor. Painful swelling is the most most common presenting complains and may persist for several years. The duration varied from a few days to years, and was for more than 2 years in 16 of 89 patients (18%) with available data regarding symptoms. The tumor may also be incidentally detected on radiographs [9]. Often, MCSA can present as a soft tissue mass. Rarely, limitation of the range of motion in the involved joint can be presented. Tumor compressing the spinal cord can cause paralysis, , and orbital involvement can lead to pain, swelling, visual disturbance, or even protrusion of the eyeball (exophthalmos). Intracranial tumor may manifest with headache.

24.6 Radiologic Finding

Plain radiograph In long bones, the lesion is usually located in the diaphysis and shows a poorly defined, expanding, geographic destruction often with varying degrees of stippled calcifications, simulating conventional CSA (Fig. 24.1). Stippled calcification may coalesce into larger, discrete opacities or heavily calcified mass. Moth-eaten to permeative destruction with ill-defined periosteal reaction is also frequently associated. The degree of expansion of bone with cortical thinning or thickening varies according to tumor duration. Cortical destruction and soft tissue mass formation with stippled calcification are common, strongly suggesting a malignant tumor, particularly when associated with moth-eaten or permeative destruction and poorly defined margin. Prominent extension into soft tissue is seen in about half of cases [5]. Such radiographic appearance is not characteristic, and MCSA is often misdiagnosed as conventional CSA beacuse of its rarity. Surprisingly, the lesion can be occasionally demarcated by a rim of sclerosis as in benign bone tumors despite the high-grade malignant nature [5]. In extra-skeletal location, the lesion is well demarcated and frequently affects the soft tissue adjacent to long bones, often with prominent punctate calcifications (Fig. 24.2). **Bone scan** and **PET/CT scan** generally shows strong uptake of radioisotope (Fig. 24.1b) and FDG in the lesion, respectively. They are also useful to detect multifocal involvement or metastases. **CT scan** more clearly demonstrates aggressive bone destruction, areas of matrix mineralization, and naked soft-tissue mass with intralesional mottled or heavy calcifications. There can be foci of central low attenuation representing tumor necrosis. **MR images** reveal an intramedullary lobular lesion with low to intermediate SI on T1-weighted image and intermediate to high SI on T2-weighted image, with stippled tiny dark signal of calcification or ossification on both sequences. Enhancement by contrast medium vary from nonspecific diffuse patterns (Fig. 24.1c) to characteristic *septal and peripheral* pattern (Fig. 24.2b). Often, MCSA presents a prominent serpentine vascular structure of low to dark SI on fat-saturated T2-weighted and contrast-enhanced images, representing hemangiopericytoma-like structure that is not a feature seen in other CSAs [15] (Fig. 24.2b).

24.7 Histologic Findings

MCSA is characterized by a bimorphic histologic pattern (Fig. 24.3a, b). The first finding is solid primitive mesenchymal areas consisting of undifferentiated small round blue cells, similar to those observed in Ewing's sarcoma. The second finding is multifocal differentiation of the primitive mesenchymal cells into nodules or islands of well-differentiated hyaline cartilage in a lobular pattern. The primitive mesenchymal component can present multiple endothelial-lined vascular spaces often in *staghorn or deer antler* pattern, or pericytoid arrangement which is reminiscent of hemangiopericytoma (Fig. 24.3c). Most lesions present at least small foci with a superficial resemblance to such pattern [6]. Occasionally. the cartilage may undergo some degree of endochondral ossification or calcification (Fig. 24.3c), but osteoid or woven bone is never produced directly by the tumor cells unlike osteosarcoma. The individual mesenchymal cells are round to oval and evenly uniform in size, with hyperchro-

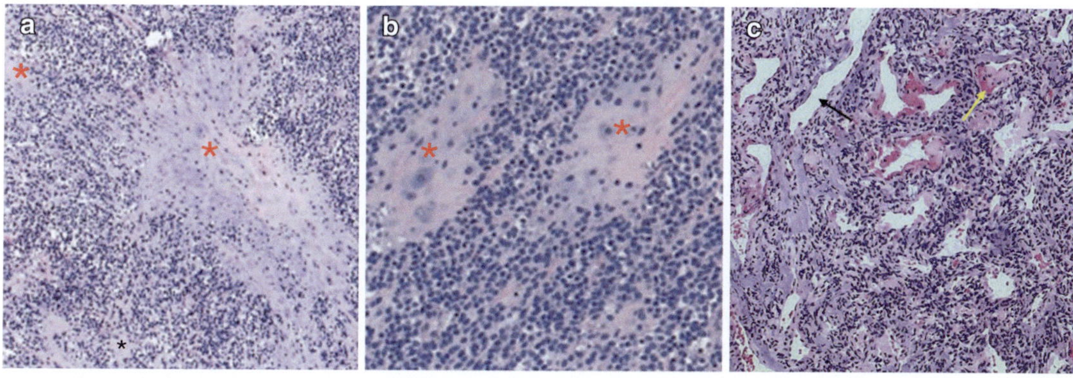

Fig. 24.3 ***Microscopic examination***. (**a**) Low-power magnification shows sheets of small, blue to purple, round to oval, undifferentiated mesenchymal cells similar to Ewing sarcoma in association with several hyaline cartilage nodules of mild to moderate cellularity (asterisks). The differentiating cartilage elements are stained *blue to purple*, unlike typical pink staining of chondroid in chondroblastoma or chondromyxoid fibroma. Thus, they are easier to recognize as cartilage. (**b**) Middle-power magnification reveals poorly differentiated mesenchymal cells with high N/C ratio and hyperchromatic nuclei. The nodules of low cellularity with extracellular eosinophilic matrix are well demarcated or imperceptibly merge into adjacent areas of small round cell component (asterisks). (**c**) A solid tumor area of undifferentiated mesenchymal cells exhibits rich vascular channels in a characteristic *staghorn* pattern or *pericytoid* arrangement of multiple vascular channels (arrow), imparting a hemangiopericytoma. The tiny cartilage nodules undergo a varying degree of endochondral ossification (yellow arrow). However, osteoid or woven bone directly produced by the tumor cells, unlike, is never seen

matic nuclei and high nucleus and cytoplasm (N/C) ratio. The differentiating cartilage elements are usually stained *blue to purple*, unlike the typical pink staining of chondroid in chondroblastoma or chondromyxoid fibroma. Thus, it is easier to recognize them as a cartilage (Fig. 24.3a). The proportion of cartilage and undifferentiated solid area varies among tumors and even in different areas of the same tumor. However, the cartilage element is rarely predominant, typically occupying less than 50% of the surface area. Any amount of malignant cartilage nodules should be observed for a histologic diagnosis, no matter how meager, even as low as 1% [6]. Frequently, cartilage islands can undergo calcification and even ossification. Cases with a predominating noncartilaginous mesenchymal component or the absence of cartilage due to inadequate biopsy sampling may lead to a misdiagnosis of other small, round, blue-cell tumors such as Ewing sarcoma, lymphoma, neuroblastoma, and small cell osteosarcoma. Thus, an adequate and suffient sample is required by incision biopsy, and thus needle or trocar biopsy is not recommended. Necrosis and massive hemorrhage are also occasionally seen. The cartilaginous foci contain cells with strong S-100 protein reactivity, but the undifferentiated mesenchymal cells are negative for this marker [5].

24.8 Management

Wide resection with an adequate margin followed by reconstruction with or without chemotherapy is the standard option. Huvos et al. [16] subdivided MCSA into two distinct groups, the better differentiated hemangiopericytoma-like and the less differentiated small cell variants. They suggested that the variant with less differentiated "Ewing-like" small cells is much more sensitive to the same chemotherapeutic agents in combination with radiation as given for small cell sarcoma than the variant with better differentiated hemangiopericytoma-like areas. However, the effectiveness of chemotherapy is still debatable, but it is often administered concomitantly before and/or after surgery. Radiation therapy after surgery may be considered for a larger tumor with an inadequate surgical margin.

24.9 Clinical Course

A study regarding the prognosis of MCSA is inadequate because of the rarity and variable nature of the disease. However, MCSA is considered as an aggressive malignant tumor with a less favorable prognosis than conventional CSA. Earlier when chemotherapy or radiotherapy was used as the only adjunctive treatment after surgery and its value was difficult to assess, the 5-year survival rate was 54.6% and the 10-year survival rate was only about 27% in the Mayo Clinic series [9]. More recently, chemotherapy has been, however, reported to be related to a significant reduction in the risk of recurrence and death. In a study of 26 patients treated in the Rizzoli institute, the 10-year disease-free survival in the patients who achieved complete surgical remission was 76% with chemotherapy but only 17% without chemotherapy with statistical significance, suggesting that the additional chemotherapy offered a benefit result [11]. The outcome was also similarly favorable in those who received chemotherapy in another series [17]. Among prognostic factors, the presence of metastasis at initial presentation is considered to have the most profound negtive impact, followed to a lesser extent by tumor size and location. In a large series of 113 patients conducted by the European Musculoskeletal Oncology Society, about 15% of the patients had metastases at presentation. The absence of metastases at diagnosis was associated with a significantly better outcome [10]. The authors reported that the 5-year and 10-year overall survival were 84% and 80% in the chemotherapy group and 73% and 46% in the surveillance group. They suggested that chemotherapy can reduce risk of recurrence and death, and concluded that complete resection and adjuvant chemotherapy should be considered as a standard of care for a localized disease. Despite local recurrence being more common in the first 2 years after diagnosis (55% in the present series), late recurrences are also not unusual [9, 16]. Late local recurrence of 27% at 5 years or later and 13% after 10 years were reported in the same series [10]. The distant metastasis rate was very high, up to about 61% in a large series [9]. Metastases sites include lung, bone, and regional and distant lymph nodes. The lung is the most common single site of metastasis, occuring up to half of the cases [9]. Distant metastasis was reported to occur after 10 years in 13% of the patients [10], and in even after a delay of 20 years [9, 10]. Thus, a longer follow-up for decades or life-long follow-up is necessary as in clear cell chondrosarcoma. More recently, Amer et al. [18] reported the presence of metastasis at presentation in 10.6% of patients across all CSA subtypes, with 1-year and 5-year overall survival rate of 76.1% and 37.6%, respectively, in a SEER database analysis of patients encompassing cases from 1973 to 2013.

References

1. Bertoni F, Picci P, Bacchini P, Capanna R, Innao V, Bacci G, et al. Mesenchymal chondrosarcoma of bone and soft tissues. Cancer. 1983;52(3):533–41.
2. Gitelis S, Bertoni F, Picci P, Campanacci M. Chondrosarcoma of bone. The experience at the Istituto Ortopedico Rizzoli. J Bone Joint Surg Am. 1981;63(8):1248–57.
3. Resnick D, Kyriakos M, Greenway GD. Tumors and tumor-like lesions of bone: imaging and pathology of specific lesions. In: Resnick D, editor. Diagnosis of bone and joint disorders. 4th ed. Philadelphia: Saunders; 2002. p. 3897–920.
4. Salvador AH, Beabout JW, Dahlin DC. Mesenchymal chondrosarcoma-observations on 30 new cases. Cancer. 1971;28(3):605–15.
5. Czerniak B. Malignant cartilage lesions. In: Dorfman HD, Czerniak B, editors. Dorfman and Czerniak's bone tumors. 2nd ed (eBook). Elsevier; 2016. p. 474–569.
6. Mirra JM. Mesenchymal chondrosarcoma. In: Mirra JM, editor. Bone tumors: clinical, radiologic, and pathologic correlations. 2nd ed. Philadelphia: Lea & Febiger; 1989. p. 577–89.
7. Unni KK, Inwards CY. Mesenchymal chondrosarcoma. In: Unni KK, Inwards CY, editors. Dahlin's bone tumors: general aspects and data on 10,165 cases. 6th ed. Philadelphia: Lippincott William & Wilkins; 2010. p. 92–7.
8. Schneiderman BA, Kliethermes SA, Nystrom LM. Survival in mesenchymal chondrosarcoma varies based on age and tumor location: a survival analysis of the SEER database. Clin Orthop Relat Res. 2017;475:799–805.
9. Nakashima Y, Unni KK, Shives TC, Swee RG, Dahlin DC. Mesenchymal chondrosarcoma of bone

and soft tissue. A review of 111 cases. Cancer. 1986;57(12):2444–53.
10. Frezza AM, Cesari M, Baumhoer D, Biau D, Bielack S, Campanacci DA, et al. Mesenchymal chondrosarcoma: prognostic factors and outcome in 113 patients. A European Musculoskeletal Oncology Society study. Eur J Cancer. 2015;51(3):374–81.
11. Cesari M, Bertoni F, Bacchini P, Mercuri M, Palmerini E, Ferrari S. Mesenchymal chondrosarcoma. An analysis of patients treated at a single institution. Tumori. 2007;93(5):423–7.
12. Dahlin DC, Henderson ED. Mesenchymal chondrosarcoma. Further observations on a new entity. Cancer. 1962;15(2):410–7.
13. Enzinger FM, Weiss SW. Cartilaginous and osseous soft tissue tumors. In: Enzinger FM, Weiss SW, editors. Enzinger & Weiss's soft tissue tumors. 7th ed. Philadelphia: Elsevier; 2020. p. 1052–84.
14. Schajowicz F. Cartilage-forming tumor. In: Schajowicz F, editor. Tumors and tumor-like lesion of the bone. Berlin: Springer-Verlag; 1994. p. 141–256.
15. Murphey MD, Walker EA, Wilson AJ, Kransdorf MJ, Temple HT, Gannon FH. From the archives of the AFIP: imaging of primary chondrosarcoma: radiologic-pathologic correlation. Radiographics. 2003;23(5):1245–78.
16. Huvos AG, Rosen G, Dabska M, Marcove RC. Mesenchymal chondrosarcoma a clinicopathologic analysis of 35 patients with emphasis on treatment. Cancer. 1983;51(7):1230–7.
17. Dantonello TM, Int-Veen C, Leuschner I, Schuck A, Furtwaengler R, Claviez A, et al. Mesenchymal chondrosarcoma of soft tissues and bone in children, adolescents, and young adults: experiences of the CWS and COSS study groups. Cancer. 2008;112(11):2424–31.
18. Amer KM, Munn M, Congiusta D, Abraham JA, Basu Mallick A. Survival and prognosis of chondrosarcoma subtypes: SEER database analysis. J Orthop Res. 2020;38(2):311–9.

25 Dedifferentiated Chondrosarcoma

25.1 Definition

Dedifferentiation refers to transforamtion of a lower-grade (Grade 1 or 2) malignant tumor, or even a benign tumor into a higher-grade (Grade 3 or 4) malignancy during its clinical course. Dedifferentiated chondrosarcoma (DCSA) is a rare, higher-grade malignant variant transformed from conventional CSA or even benign cartilage tumor such as enchondroma and osteochondroma, with an abrupt transition to higher-grade noncartilaginous malignant tumor.

25.2 Incidence

It accounts for about 1–2% of biopsy-analyzed primary bone tumors [1, 2] and approximately 10–15% of all CSAs in major series [2–6]. However, the SEER data analysis, based on 2757 cases CSA, reported only 5.3% of these tumors fell into the category of DCSA [7].

25.3 Age

Most patients are usually diagnosed between the sixth and eighth decades, which is 1–2 decades older than that of conventional CSA because of the slow indolent process of dedifferentiation. The average age was reported to be about 60 years in major series [2, 3, 7, 8]. Older age may increases the likelihood of distant metstasis at diagnosis.

25.4 Location

The anatomic distribution is identical to that of conventional CSA. The most common sites are the femur, pelvis, and humerus, which are common sites for preexisting conventional CSA (Figs. 25.1, 25.2, and 25.3), accounting for almost 95% of cases [9]. The scapula, ribs, and tibia are less commonly affected. The femur is the most frequently involved bone, occupying 30% of all cases, followed by the pelvis (20%), humerus (16%), ribs (7%), and scapula (7%) [7].

W.-J. Bahk, *Diagnosis and Management of Primary Bone Tumors*,
https://doi.org/10.1007/978-981-96-3484-2_25

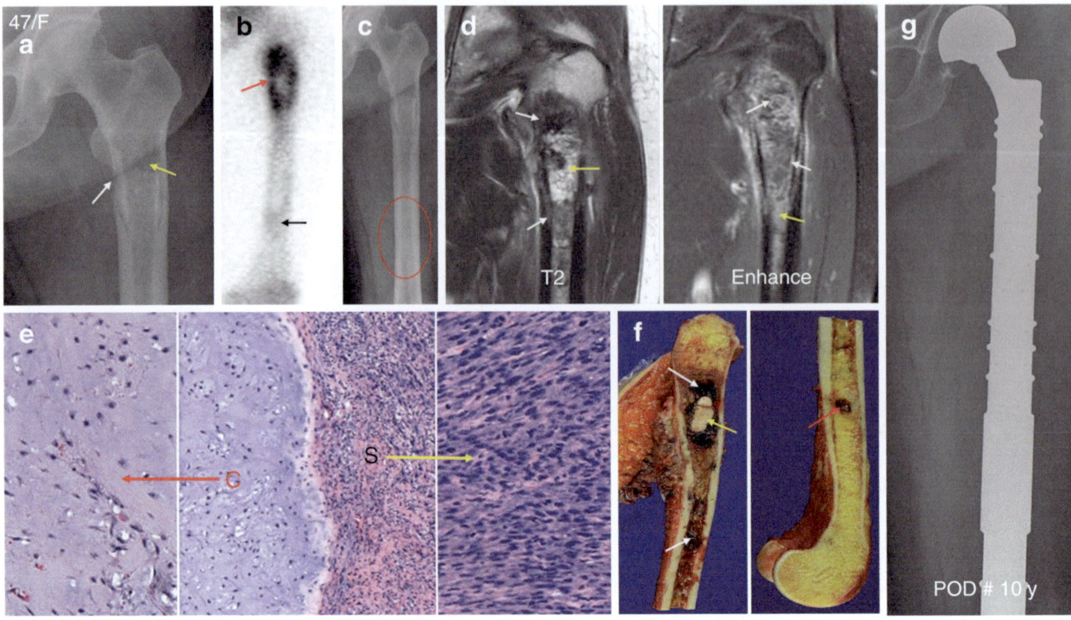

Fig. 25.1 Dedifferentiated to fibrosarcoma. (**a**) Radiograph taken for left proximal thigh pain of 2 months' duration in a 47-year-old woman shows a typical *bimorphic* pattern of a poorly-defined, peripheral radiolucent lesion with cortical thinning and possible disruption, suggesting a more aggressive lesion (white arrow) and central area with internal popcorn-like densities, indicating a less aggressive cartilaginous lesion (yellow arrow) in the proximal femur. (**b**) Bone scan reveals strong uptake with internal void area proximally (red arrow) and mild uptake distally, suggesting a possible skip lesion (black arrow). (**c**) However, there is no discernible skip lesion in the distal femur on plain radiograph (circle). (**d**) T2-weighted MR image demonstrates a characteristic *bimorphic* pattern of a relatively well-defined central lesion of high SI with scattered dark signals centrally indicating a low-grade cartilaginous lesion (yellow arrow), and ill-defined peripheral lesion of cortical destruction and soft tissue extension showing heterogeneous low and intermediate SI, suggesting a more aggressive spindle cell lesion (white arrows). The low-grade cartilaginous lesion is enhanced typically in a *nodular and peripheral* pattern as in other cartilage tumors (white arrows), while the spindle cell lesion is rather diffusely enhanced (yellow arrows). In addition, MRI of distal femur reveals a small lesion with similar signals, suggesting a skip lesion (not shown here). (**e**) Microscopic examination: (Middle) Low-power magnification demonstrates a typical *bimorphic* histology of a cartilaginous component (C) and another spindle cell component (S), separated by an abrupt and sharp demarcation without any transition features between the two tissue types. (Left) The cartilage component shows mild to moderate cellularity and atypia, indicating low-grade CSA. (Right) However, the spindle cell component reveals a markedly high number of pleomorphic spindle cells arranged in a *herringbone* pattern in the absence osteoid production, indicating higher-grade fibrosarcoma. (**f**) Gross specimen reveals a central small area of low-grade CSA (yellow arrow) and peripheral extensive areas of fibrosarcoma (white arrows). Note skip lesion in the distal femur (red arrow), reflecting a distal mild uptake on bone scan. (**g**) Radiograph at 10 years after wide resection and reconstruction using a total femur prosthesis notes good maintenance with no evidence of local recurrence

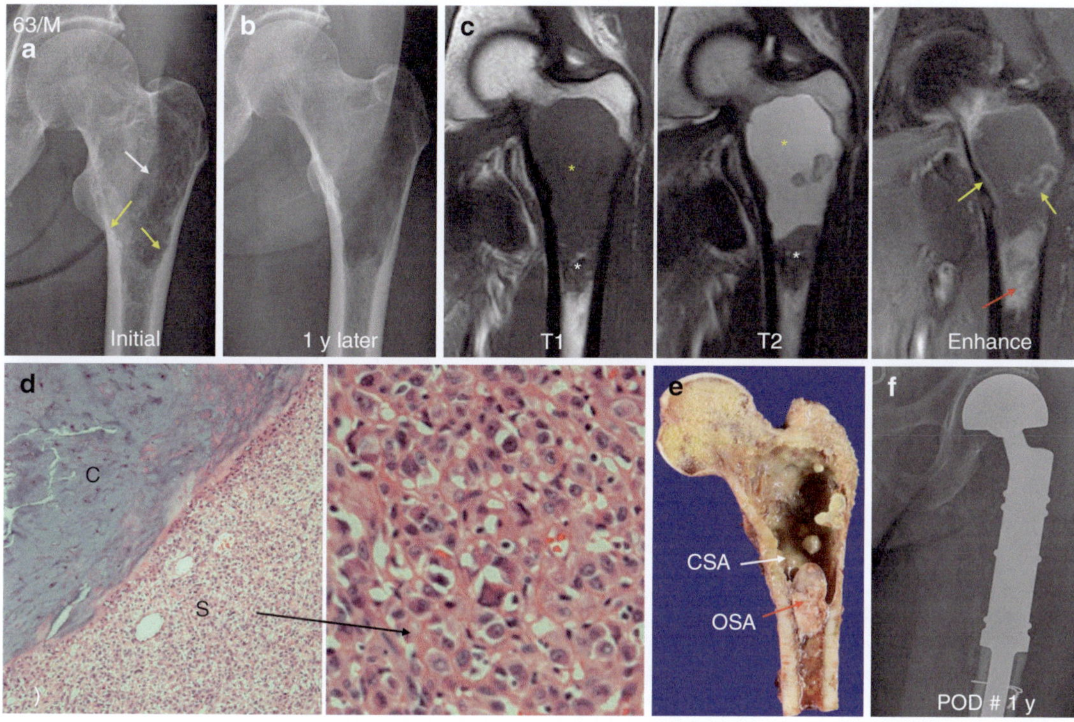

Fig. 25.2 Dedifferentiated to osteosarcoma (OSA). (**a**) Radiograph taken for left hip pain of 3 weeks' duration in a 63-year-old man shows a *bimorphic* pattern of an ill-defined, multilobulated central lesion with *rings and arcs* calcifications (red arrow), suggesting a preexisting low-grade cartilage tumor and more aggressive-looking peripheral radiolucent destructive lesion with cortical scalloping (yellow arrows). He refused further evaluation and treatment for a private reason. (**b**) Radiograph taken for severe aggravation of pain 1 year later reveals that the lesion has become more radiolucent with disappearance of lobulation and calcification, suggesting a progression of the more aggressive lesion with a diminution of the low-grade cartilaginous area. (**c**) MR images demonstrate a proximally located, well-defined, huge, intramedullary mass-like lesion with low SI on T1-weighted image and high SI on T2-weighted image, suggesting a high-water content of nonmineralized hyaline cartilage lesion (yellow asterisks) and distally located, ill-defined, smaller area of low SI on both sequences, indicating a more aggressive spindle cell lesion (white asterisks). The cartilaginous lesion is enhanced in a typical *peripheral and septal* pattern (yellow arrows), while the noncartilaginous spindly lesion is diffusely enhanced (red arrow). (**d**) Microscopic examination: (Left) Lower-power magnification presents a typical *bimorphic* histology of low-grade cartilaginous component (C) and high-grade spindle cell component (S). Note an abrupt and sharp demarcation zone without any transition features between low-grade CSA and spindle sarcoma component. (Right) Higher magnification of the spindle cell area shows marked pleomorphic and bizarre spindle cells directly producing pink osteoid, indicating high-grade OSA. (**e**) Gross specimen reveals low-grade CSA (white arrow) and high-grade OSA (red arrow). (**f**) Radiograph at 1 year after wide resection and reconstruction using a tumor prosthesis notes good maintenance with no evidence of local recurrence

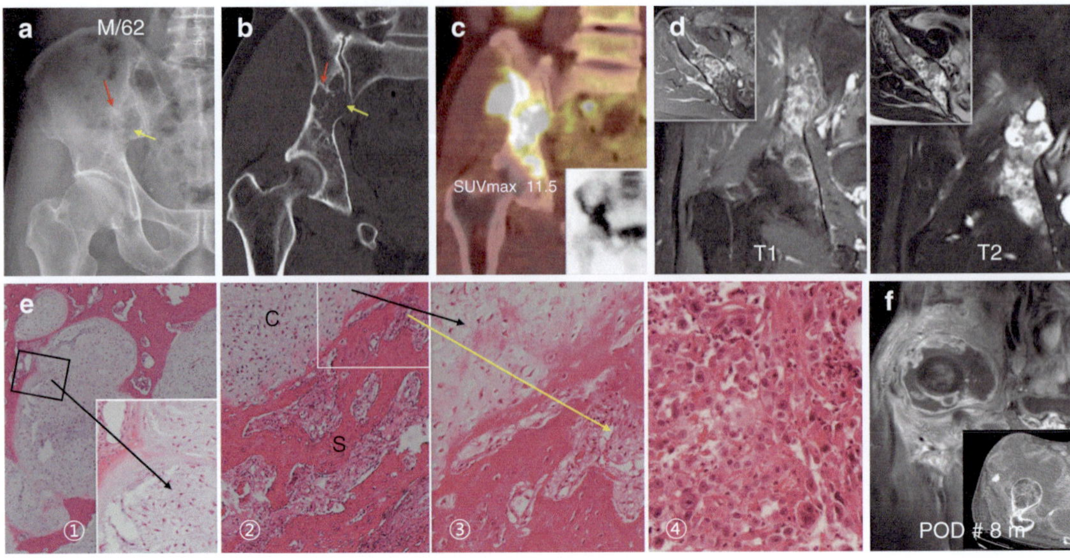

Fig. 25.3 Dedifferentiated to OSA. (**a**) Radiograph taken for right inguinal pain of 1 month's duration in a 62-year-old man shows an ill-defined central sclerotic lesion with stippled calcification (red arrow) and more aggressive-looking peripheral radiolucent lesion (yellow arrow), so-called *bimorphic* pattern, in the ilium adjacent to the sacroiliac joint. (**b**) CT scan reveals more clearly geographic destruction surrounded by a thin sclerotic rim with some internal calcification, suggesting a preexisting low-grade cartilaginous tumor (red arrow) and purely radiolucent lesion with a cortical breakage, suggesting a more aggressive noncartilage lesion (yellow arrow). (**c**) PET/CT scan notes a large destructive lesion in right iliac bone extending to surrounding soft tissue with significantly increased FDG uptake (SUVmax 11.5). Bone scan also shows diffuse strong uptake in the same area (inset). (**d**) MR images demonstrate an ill-defined multilobulated medullary lesion with cortical destruction and soft tissue extension showing heterogeneous intermediate and high to bright SI on both sequences. (**e**) Microscopic examination: (1) Lower-power magnification presents a *CSA permeation* pattern of host bone spicules by cartilage nodules with mild atypia, suggesting a low-grade CSA (2). Another field reveals two different histologic areas of cartilage component (C) and noncartilaginous spindle cell component (S) with a sharp demarcation zone between them (3). Medium-power magnification shows a cartilage component with low to medium degree of cellularity and mild atypia at upper part and another spindle cell component with severe atypia at lower part of the lesion (4). Higher-power magnification of noncartilaginous component reveals pleomorphic and bizarre spindle cells with mitoses producing osteoid to woven bones, indicating conventional high-grade OSA. (**f**) Follow-up CT scan (inset) and MR image taken for severe right inguinal pain at 8 months after internal hemipelvectomy show severe destruction with a huge soft tissue mass indicating a local recurrence. He died of disease progression and distant metastases immediately after hindquarter amputation

25.5 Clinical Features

Pain is the most common symptom. The duration is usually short, but long duration of mild pain may be present in some patients because the lower-grade CSA component slowly transforms into the higher-grade malignancy. A prolonged localized discomfort or mild pain may be associated with the recent development of a rapidly growing mass. A pathologic fracture is associated in about 9–10% of cases [2, 10], and significant aggravation of pain may herald a pathologic fracture. A local recurrence may occasionally be the first sign of the increasing malignancy from lower-grade CSA [6].

25.6 Radiologic Findings

Plain radiographs Radiographs typically reflect the *bimorphic* histologic features of a low-grade area with rings and arcs, punctate, or popcorn-like calcifications, suggesting a lower-grade cartilaginous tumors in the more central area of the lesion, juxtaposed to high-grade area with more aggressive, ill-defined osteolytic area often with moth-eaten to permeative destruction, cortical perforation, and soft tissue mass formation in the more peripheral region (Figs. 25.1, 25.2, and 25.3). The area of lower-grade cartilaginous tumor is prominent, and the high-grade area is relatively minor in early stage. As the differentiation progresses, the high-grade area tend to dominate the lesion and the cartilaginous component area becomes minor or small. Calcification of the bony lesion, and soft tissue mass formation are observed in about half of the cases [6]. Radiographically, DCSA is subclassified into three types by Mercuri et al. [11], which are historically proved. *Type 1* lesion is the most common and reveals features identical to those of a conventional central CSA with additional areas of very aggressive features. *Type 2* lesion resembles the underlying benign enchondroma with destructive changes and/or a large soft tissue mass. *Type 3* lesion, the rarest type, is not distinctive and presents simply as a very high-grade destructive lesion of bone. **CT scan** more clearly shows two distinct areas of different intrinsic characteristics showing a low attenuation with a variably calcified area of low-grade CSA, and another soft-tissue attenuation (iso-attenuation to muscle) of high-grade dedifferentiated component, showing more significant destruction with cortical destruction and naked soft tissue mass. **MR images** demonstrate a characteristic *bimorphic* pattern of a well-defined central lesion of low SI on T1-weighted image and high SI with scattered dark signals on T2-weighted image, indicating low-grade CSA, and more peripherally located another ill-defined lesion with heterogeneous low and high SI on T2-weighted image, suggesting higher-grade dedifferentiated component. The low-grade CSA is enhanced in a characteristic *peripheral and nodular* pattern, but higher-grade component is more strongly and diffusely enhanced in classic cases. These findings are useful to differentiate the two components more clearly. Thus, MRI is also useful in guiding biopsy toward the high-grade area [12]. **Bone scan** presents heterogeneously strong uptake, and is useful to detect a skip lesion or metastasis (Figs. 25.1b, and 25.3c). **PET/CT scan** demonstrates a heterogeneously increased FDG uptake (Fig. 25.3c). It is also useful to detect skip lesions or metastases in the setting of dedifferentiated and other high-grade lesions at high risk of distant metastasis.

25.7 Histologic Findings

The lesion is characterized by the coexistence of two distinct histologic findings of a preexisting lower-grade cartilaginous lesion and another high-grade noncartilaginous spindle cell sarcoma, so-called *bimorphic* pattern. There is a characteristic abrupt and sharp demarcation zone, without any transition features between the two tissue types (Figs. 25.1, 25.2, and 25.3). The cartilaginous component has features of conventional CSA of any grade but usually low-grade, and rarely may show focal high-grade or even enchondroma. Noncartilaginous high-grade components are most often fibrosarcoma, osteosarcoma, or undifferentiated pleomorphic sarcoma [2, 6] (Figs. 25.1, 25.2, and 25.3). Less frequently, they can be rhabdomyoblastic or angioblastic differentiation. Area with high-grade sarcoma can be rich in giant cells, simulating a giant cell tumor of bone [2, 7, 9].

25.8 Management

Wide resection with adequate margin followed by reconstruction is the standard option for the tumors in the long bones. Those involving the pelvis or spine are particularly difficult to manage due to its large size, deep location, and proximity to important adjacent structures such as the bladder or spinal cord. Earlier, DCSA was generally thought to be resistant to chemotherapy [1, 11], and many patients are older with poor medical conditions limiting tolerance to toxicities of chemotherapy. Only very few patients survived for longer than 5 years. Thus, chemotherapy has not been generally included in a standard option for management due to the lack of convincing evidence of the benefit. However, an analysis of large patient collection by Frassica et al. [4] reported adjuvant chemotherapy resulted in an improved 5-year survival rate of up to 22%. A more recent analysis of 72 patients treated at a single institution reported that chemotherapy with doxorubicin and cisplatin seems to improve progression-free survival but not overall survival [13]. Considering the retrospective nature of the study, long time, and heterogeneity in practice of treatment due to the rarity of DDCS, the efficacy of the chemotherapy or radiotherapy is still debatable. Future research, potentially in multicenter prognostic studies, is necessary to evaluate the effectiveness of chemotherapy, including both classical anticancer drugs and novel targeted therapies.

25.9 Clinical Course

DCSA is one of the most highly lethal malignant tumors despite adequate aggressive initial wide surgical resection or even amputation due to frequent early metastasis. On multivariate analysis in a large series, pathological fracture, larger size of the tumor, lymph node involvement, metastasis at diagnosis, extraosseous extension, and undifferentiated pleomorphic sarcoma component were reported to be correlated with worse overall survival, whereas adequate surgical margin and chemotherapy were associated with improved survival [13]. In another large series, 71 patients (21%) had metastases at the time of diagnosis, and the median survival was 5 months with a 10% chance of survival at 2 years [10]. Five-year survival was reported to be only about 10–15%, and patients died most often within 2 years after diagnosis [4, 11]. Other studies reported overall 5-year survival rate of 7–24% [1, 4, 10, 14, 15]. In an analysis of 159 cases from the SEER database (2001–2011), the overall prognosis was also poor with a 5-year overall survival of only 18% [16]. They concluded tumors larger than 8 cm, presence of metastases at diagnosis, and treatment without surgical resection were significant predictors of mortality, whereas adequate surgical resection resulted in improved survival. Despite advances in diagnostic modalities, preoperative imaging, surgical technique, and adjuvant chemotherapy over the past two decades, the survival rate has not drastically improved compared to previous reports. Thus, early recognition of dedifferentiation and resection with a wide margin or amputation for local control with adjuvant chemotherapy for control of distant disease remain the best options for better outcomes up to now.

25.10 Prognosis of Subtypes of Nonconventional CSA

In a recent analysis of survival and prognosis of subtypes of nonconventional CSA based on the SEER database from 1973 to 2013 [17], the only prognostic variable shown to have a significant impact on the survival of each nonconventional CSA subtype was the presence of metastatic disease at diagnosis. The tumor characteristics demonstrated marked differences in the incidence of metastasis at diagnosis among the subtypes, in increasing order: periosteal (2%), clear cell (6%), myxoid (8%), mesenchymal (11%), and dedifferentiated CSA (20%). The median survival depended on the incidence of metastasis; it was highest for the periosteal subtype (97 months), followed by clear cell (79 months), myxoid (60 months), mesenchymal (33.5 months), and lowest for the dedifferentiated subtype (11 months). They also reported 5-year survival rates of about 68%, 62%, 50%, 38%, and 11% for periosteal, clear cell, myxoid, mesenchymal, and dedifferentiated subtypes, respectively.

References

1. Bruns J, Fiedler W, Werner M, Delling G. Dedifferentiated chondrosarcoma—fatal disease. J Cancer Res Clin Oncol. 2005;131(6):333–9.
2. Mirra JM. Dedifferentiated chondrosarcoma. In: Mirra JM, editor. Bone tumors: clinical, radiologic, and pathologic correlations. 2nd ed. Philadelphia, PA: Lea & Febiger; 1989. p. 546–77.
3. Dahlin DC, Beabout JW. Dedifferentiation of low-grade chondrosarcomas. Cancer. 1971;28(2):461–6.
4. Frassica FJ, Unni K, Beabout J, Sim F. Dedifferentiated chondrosarcoma. A report of the clinicopathological

features and treatment of seventy-eight cases. J Bone Joint Surg. 1986;68(8):1197–205.
5. Mitchell A, Ayoub K, Mangham D, Grimer R, Carter S, Tillman R. Experience in the treatment of dedifferentiated chondrosarcoma. J Bone Joint Surg Br. 2000;82(1):55–61.
6. Unni KK, Inwards CY. Chondrosarcoma (primary, secondary, dedifferentiated, and clear cell). In: Unni KK, Inwards CY, editors. Dahlin's bone tumors: general aspects and data on 10,165 cases. 6th ed. Philadelphia: Lippincott William & Wilkins; 2010. p. 60–91.
7. Czerniak B. Malignant cartilage lesions. In: Dorfman HD, Czerniak B, editors. Dorfman and Czerniak's bone tumors. 2nd ed. eBook: Elsevier; 2016. p. 474–569.
8. Johnson S, Tětu B, Ayala AG, Chawla SP. Chondrosarcoma with additional mesenchymal component (dedifferentiated chondrosarcoma): I. A clinicopathologic study of 26 cases. Cancer. 1986;58(2):278–86.
9. Campanacci M. Dedifferentiated central chondrosarcoma. In: Campanacci M, editor. Bone and soft tissue tumors. Wien New York: Springer-Verlag; 1999. p. 319–33.
10. Grimer RJ, Gosheger G, Taminiau A, Biau D, Matejovsky Z, Kollender Y, et al. Dedifferentiated chondrosarcoma: prognostic factors and outcome from a European group. Eur J Cancer. 2007;43(14):2060–5.
11. Mercuri M, Campanacci L. Dedifferentiated chondrosarcoma. Skeletal Radiol. 1995;24(6):409–16.
12. Murphey MD, Walker EA, Wilson AJ, Kransdorf MJ, Temple HT, Gannon FH. From the archives of the AFIP: imaging of primary chondrosarcoma: radiologic-pathologic correlation. Radiographics. 2003;23(5):1245–78.
13. Miao R, Choy E, Raskin KA, Schwab JH, Nielsen GP, Deshpande V, et al. Prognostic factors in dedifferentiated chondrosarcoma: a retrospective analysis of a large series treated at a single institution. Sarcoma. 2019;2019:9069272. https://doi.org/10.1155/2019/9069272. PMID: 31915413; PMCID: PMC6930709
14. Dickey ID, Rose PS, Fuchs B, Wold LE, Okuno SH, Sim FH, et al. Dedifferentiated chondrosarcoma: the role of chemotherapy with updated outcomes. J Bone Joint Surg. 2004;86(11):2412–8.
15. Staals EL, Bacchini P, Bertoni F. Dedifferentiated central chondrosarcoma. Cancer. 2006;106(12):2682–91.
16. Strotman PK, Reif TJ, Kliethermes SA, Sandhu JK, Nystrom LM. Dedifferentiated chondrosarcoma: a survival analysis of 159 cases from the SEER database (2001–2011). J Surg Oncol. 2017;116(2):252–7.
17. Amer KM, Munn M, Congiusta D, Abraham JA, Basu Mallick A. Survival and prognosis of chondrosarcoma subtypes: SEER database analysis. J Orthop Res. 2020;38(2):311–9.

Part IV

Fibro-osseous Tumors and Lesions

Fibrous Dysplasia

26

(***fibrous*** "containing fibers" + ***dys-*** "bad," ***-plasia*** "development")

26.1 Definition

Fibrous dysplasia (FD) is a benign bone neoplasm typified by abnormal fibrous-osseous tissue formed through the fibro-osseous metaplasia, replacing the normal bone marrow. Mostly, the lesion affects a single bone (*monostotic form*) (Figs. 26.1, 26.2, 26.3, 26.4, 26.5, 26.6, 26.7, 26.8, 26.9, 26.10 and 26.11), and rarely multiple bones of a single extremity and/or homolateral scapula or pelvis (*monomelic polyostotic form*) (Fig. 26.2e, 26.4a, 26.9e, 26.11e), or may be distributed in several or many bones throughout the body (*polymelic polyostotic form*) (Figs. 26.12 and 26.13) [1, 2]. A small subset of less than 3% of the cases with the polyostotic form are associated with *McCune-Albright syndrome* [3, 4]. Approximately 1–2% of patients with FD, typically in the polyostotic form, are associated with soft tissue myxomas, so-called *Mazabraud's syndrome* [3, 5].

W.-J. Bahk, *Diagnosis and Management of Primary Bone Tumors*,
https://doi.org/10.1007/978-981-96-3484-2_26

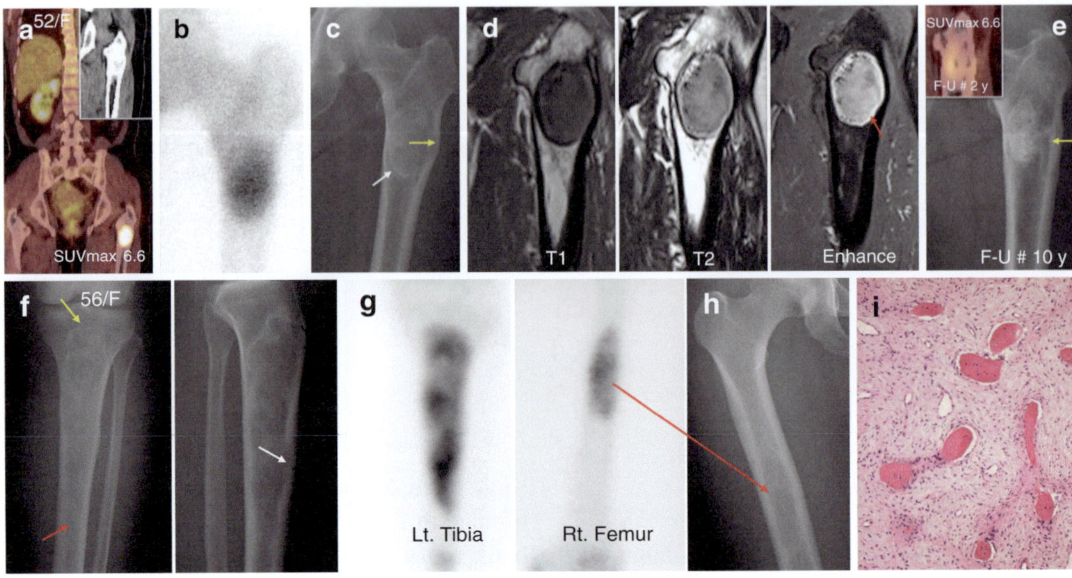

Fig. 26.1 ***Incidentally found lesions***. (**a**) PET/CT scan taken for staging of a known thyroid carcinoma in a 52-year-old lady incidentally shows a high FDG uptake (SUVmax 6.6) in the left proximal femur, which suggests a probable malignant bone tumor or single bone metastasis from thyroid carcinoma. CT scan reveals a well-defined dense mass-like lesion in the same area (inset). (**b**) Pinhole bone scan reveals a moderately increased uptake only in the femoral lesion, indicating an avid monostotic lesion. (**c**) Radiograph reveals a well-defined radiolucent geographic lesion with focal expansion and internal *ground-glass* to focal sclerotic density surrounded by a thin rind of sclerosis (white arrow). The underlying bone is mildly expanded with cortical thinning and superficial endosteal scalloping (yellow arrow). (**d**) MR images demonstrate a well-defined mass-like lesion with low SI on T1-weighted image and intermediate to high SI on T2-weighted image, with: several signal drops of punctate calcification and a thin rim of dark signal. The lesion is peripherally enhanced (red arrow) with internal focal enhancement. Incision biopsy to exclude malignancy of high FDG uptake (SUVmax 6.6) on PET scan confirms a diagnosis of conventional FD. (**e**) Follow-up PET/CT scan at 2 years after biopsy shows markedly decreased FDG uptake (SUVmax 2.7) without any treatment (inset). Follow-up radiograph at 10 years after biopsy notes remodeling of the lesion with opacification and thickening of the cortex (arrow). (**f**) Radiographs taken for left knee pain in a 56-year-old woman incidentally show a large mildly expansile osteolytic lesion with internal *ground-glass* density surrounded by a thin rim of sclerosis proximally (yellow arrow) but no discernible rim distally (red arrow), possibly suggesting an old regressing lesion. There is cortical thinning with deep erosion and endosteal scalloping on the lateral view (white arrow). (**g**) Bone scan reveals a heterogeneous mild to strong uptake in the tibia and mid-shaft of the ipsilateral femur. (**h**) Radiograph of the right femur also notes an ill-defined hazy radiolucent lesion with a mild expansion in the mid-shaft. (**i**) Microscopic examination of the biopsy specimen from the proximal tibia shows irregular short trabeculae of woven bone without osteoblastic rimming and intervening bland-looking fibrous stroma, indicating indicating FD

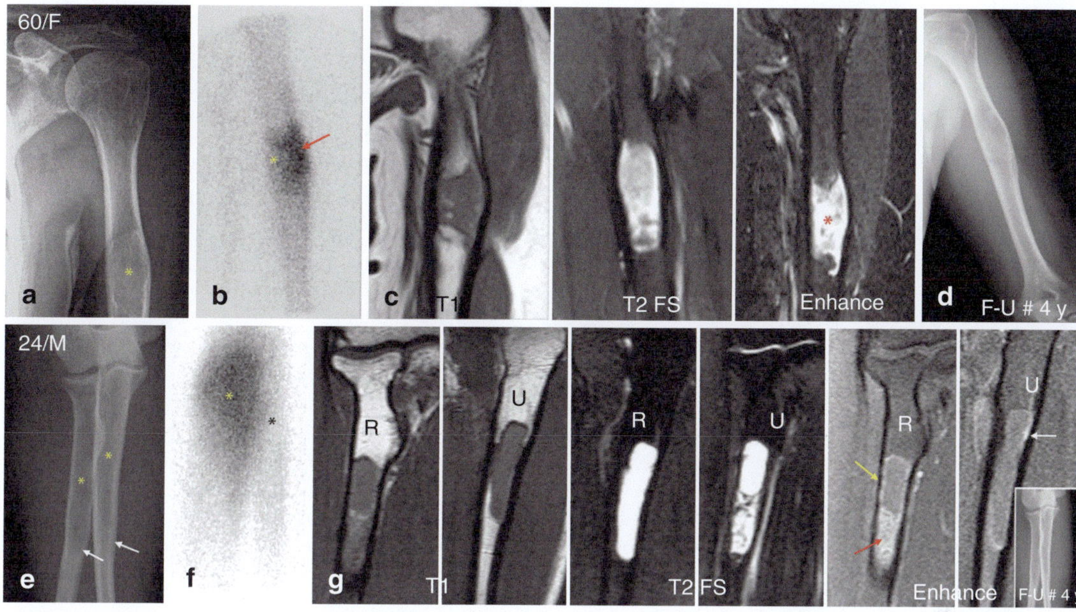

Fig. 26.2 ***Incidentally found lesions***. (**a**) Radiograph taken for left shoulder pain in a 60-year-old woman incidentally shows a mildly expansile, fusiform radiolucent lesion with an internal *ground-glass* density and cortical erosion and thinning (asterisk), typical of FD in the shaft of the humerus. (**b**) Pinhole bone scan reveals eccentrically increased uptake at the lateral aspect of the lesion (arrow) with iso-active to mildly increased uptake at the medial aspect (asterisk). (**c**) MR images note a well-defined medullary lesion with low SI on T1-weighted image and heterogeneous high SI on T2-weighted image. The lesion is diffusely well enhanced by contrast medium (asterisk). (**d**) Follow-up radiograph 4 years later without biopsy shows no definite interval change in the lesion. (**e**) Radiograph taken for right forearm pain after bicycle rider's accident in a 24-year-old young man incidentally shows relatively well-defined lesions of *ground-glass* density (asterisks) with a mild expansion (arrows) affecting both proximal forearm bones. (**f**) Pinhole bone scan notes a heterogenous segmental uptake in the proximal radius (yellow asterisk) but not in the ulna (black asterisk). (**g**) MR images reveal a well-defined mass-like lesion with iso SI on T1-weighted image and bright SI on T2-weighted image in both proximal radius (R) and ulna (U). The radius lesion is heterogeneously enhanced (red arrow) with a peripheral thin enhancement at the proximal lesion (yellow arrow). The entire ulna lesion is almost only peripherally enhanced (white arrow), suggesting a probable extensive cystic change. Follow-up radiograph at 4 years after the initial visit without biopsy shows no definite interval change of the lesion (inset). He is free of right forearm pain

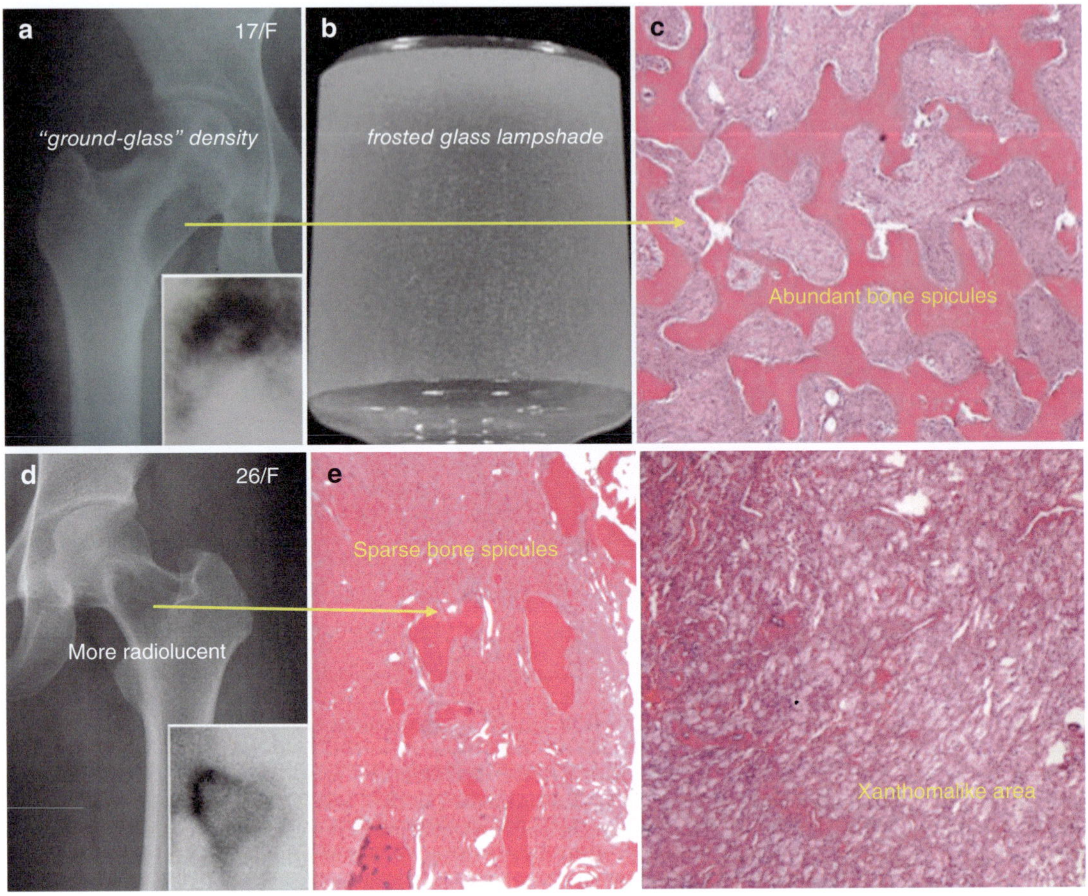

Fig. 26.3 ***The degree of opacity depending on the osseous tissue proportion***. (**a**) Radiograph taken for right hip pain in a 17-year-old girl shows a typical well-marginated osteolytic lesion with a *ground-glass* density surrounded by a thick rim of sclerosis (arrow) in the medial half of the femoral neck. Bone scan reveals a heterogenous strong uptake (inset). (**b**) The lesion's density resembles the *ground-glass* density of a glass bottle. (**c**) Microscopic examination demonstrates abundant woven bone spicules with variable alphabet characters embedded in a bland spindle cell stroma. (**d**) In contrast, another radiograph taken for left hip pain in a 26-year-old lady reveals a well-marginated almost purely radiolucent lesion with a thick rim of sclerosis in the entire femoral neck. Pinhole bone scan reveals a hot uptake along the upper margin of the lesion and milder uptake along the lower margin with a central photon defect (inset). (**e**) Microscopic examination reveals an area of sparse woven bone spicules with more prominent fibrous stromal tissue (Left) and another field of numerous foam cells mimicking xanthoma, which occupies extensive areas of the lesion (Right)

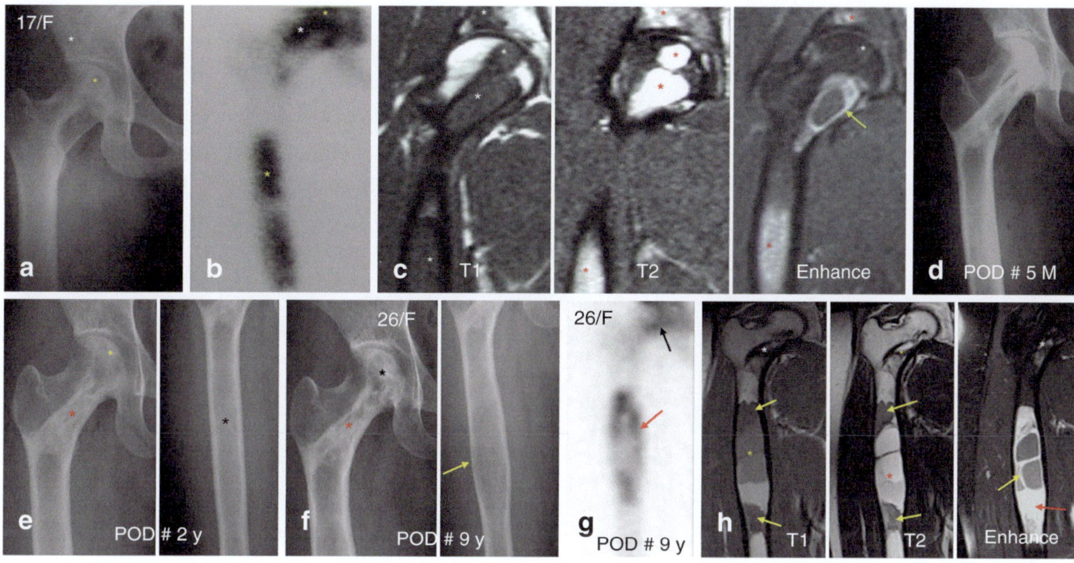

Fig. 26.4 ***Allo-cortical strut bone graft*.** (**a**) The same radiograph of Fig. 26.3a shows additional well-defined small lesion surrounded by a thin sclerotic rim in the femoral neck (yellow asterisk) and ill-defined hazy lesion in the acetabulum (white asterisk). (**b**) Bone scan reveals a strong uptake in the femoral head and neck (white asterisk) and another strong uptake in the acetabulum and femoral diaphysis (yellow asterisks), indicating the monomelic polyostotic lesions. (**c**) MR images demonstrate multiple well-demarcated mass-like lesions (asterisks) with low SI on T1-weighted and high SI on T2-weighted image in the femoral neck and head, proximal shaft and a part of the acetabulum. The main lesion in the neck is peripherally well enhanced (arrow). Those in the acetabulum and proximal shaft are also homogeneously enhanced (red asterisks), but the small lesion in the femoral head is weakly enhanced (white asterisk). (**d**) Follow-up radiograph at 5 months after allo-fibular strut graft without curettage for the main in the femoral neck notes consolidation of the lesion. (**e**) Follow-up radiograph at 2 years after surgery shows a consolidation of the neck lesion (red asterisk), but progression of the head lesion (yellow asterisk). Diaphysis is mildly expanded (black asterisk). (**f**) Follow-up radiograph at 9 years after surgery reveals complete consolidation of the neck lesion (red asterisk) and no further progression of the head lesion (yellow asterisk). However, radiograph taken for right thigh pain of several months' duration shows more degree of expansion with cortical thinning and scalloping (arrow). (**g**) Follow-up bone scan shows a peripheral mild uptake with internal photon defect in the diaphysis (red arrow). The uptake at femoral neck and head area is also significantly decreased (black arrow) when compared to initial bone scan, indicating stabilization or regression of the lesion activity. (**h**) Follow-up MR images demonstrate a well-defined moderately expansile lesion (arrows) with low to intermediate SI on T1-weighted image and slightly higher SI on T2-weighted image, suggesting solid component of FD. There is expanding multiseptated area (asterisks) with iso to low SI on T1-weighted image and high and bright SI on T2-weighted image, indicating nonspecific cystic or secondary ABC change. The solid component is homogeneously enhanced (red arrows) and the cystic component is only peripherally enhanced (yellow arrow). However, the neck lesion is completely consolidated with no local recurrence (asterisks). The patient declined further surgical management for the cystic thigh lesion and lost to follow-up thereafter

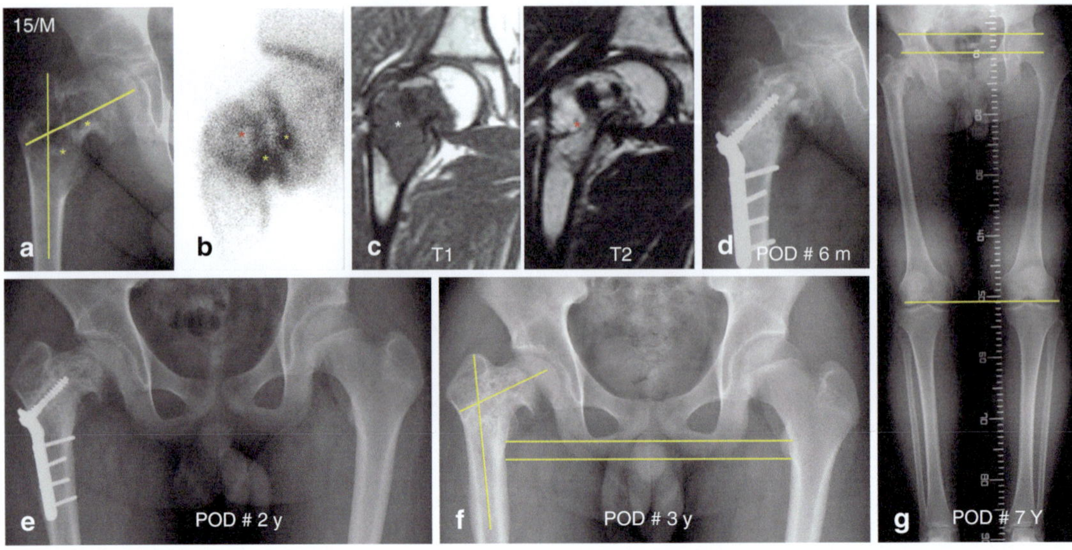

Fig. 26.5 ***Allo-cortical strut bone graft for coxa vara deformity***. (**a**) Radiograph taken for left hip pain with limping gait that had become gradually severe in a 15-year-old boy shows a relatively ill-defined, moderately expansile lesion with *ground-glass* density and multiple sclerotic foci in the intertrochanter and neck areas of the femur. Note a varus deformity (intersecting lines) and bone-forming foci with internal trabeculae, suggesting repeated microfracture and healing callus (asterisks). (**b**) Pinhole bone scan reveals a heterogeneous mild uptake with internal photon defect (red asterisk), suggesting a stabilizing lesion, and strong uptakes (yellow asterisks) reflecting bone-forming foci by repeated microfracture seen on radiograph and MRI. (**c**) MR images demonstrate a well-defined mass-like lesion (asterisks) with low SI on T1-weighted image and high SI on T2-weighted image, with dark signal foci corresponding to callus formation on both sequences. (**d**) Radiograph at 6 months after curettage and allo-cortical strut bone grafting followed by Coventry hip screw fixation notes good maintenance with some consolidation. (**e**) Radiograph at 2 years after surgery shows consolidation of the lesion without further progression of varus deformity. (**f**) Follow-up radiograph at 3 years after surgery reveals a complete consolidation of the lesion with residual varus deformity and mild shortening (between yellow lines). (**g**) Scanogram at 7 years after surgery shows shortening of right thigh length by 3 cm. However, the patient walks tolerably with shoe correction

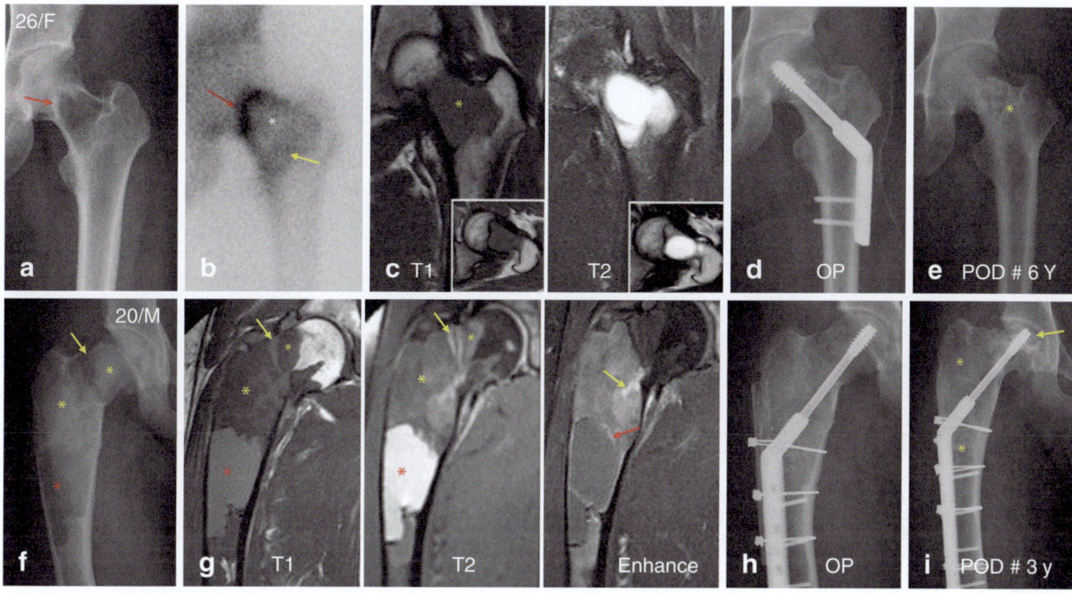

Fig. 26.6 ***Allo-chip bone graft***. (**a**) Radiograph taken for left hip pain of 4 months' duration in a 26-year-old lady shows a well-defined, almost purely radiolucent lesion without discernible trabecular pattern, which is surrounded by a rim of sclerosis in the entire femoral neck (arrow). (**b**) Pinhole bone scan reveals a hot uptake along the upper margin of the lesion (red arrow) and mild uptake along the lower margin (yellow arrow) with a central photon defect area (asterisk), indicating a static or stabilized lesion surrounded by reactive bone. (**c**) MR images reveal a well-defined mass-like lesion with low SI on T1-weighted and high SI on T2-weighted image, simulating cystic lesion. However, microscopic examination confirmed a diagnosis of FD with sparse woven bone production and extensive areas of fibro-histiocytic reaction mimicking xanthoma of bone (Fig. 26.3e). There are no areas of cystic change on histologic examination. (**d**) Curettage and allo-chip bone graft with compression hip screw fixation was performed because the patient was a grown-up adult and the lesion was considered to be stable based on the bone scan and histologic findings. (**e**) Follow-up radiograph at 6 years after surgery shows consolidation of the lesion with no evidence of local recurrence (asterisk). (**f**) Radiograph taken for a sudden severe pain of right hip after jump during military drill in a 20-year-old soldier shows an ill-defined expansile dense lesion with focal *ground-glass* density proximally (yellow asterisks) and a relatively well-defined more radiolucent lesion distally (red asterisk). A pathologic fracture of femoral neck with some gap is associated (arrow). (**g**) MR images reveal two different signal areas of solid component of FD (yellow asterisks) and cystic component (red asterisks) with a pathologic fracture (arrows). There are focal enhancement of solid FD component (yellow arrow) and peripheral thin enhancement of the cystic component (red arrow). Microscopic examination confirmed a FD with a prominent nonspecific cyst, so-called cystic FD. (**h**) Curettage of the lesion and allo-chip bone grafting followed by onlay fibula strut grafting due to poor bone stalk and compression hip screw fixation for a neck fracture was done. (**i**) Follow-up radiograph at 3 years after surgery shows consolidation of the lesions (asterisks) and healing of the fracture. However, avascular necrosis of the femoral head developed (red arrow), and was managed by total hip replacement

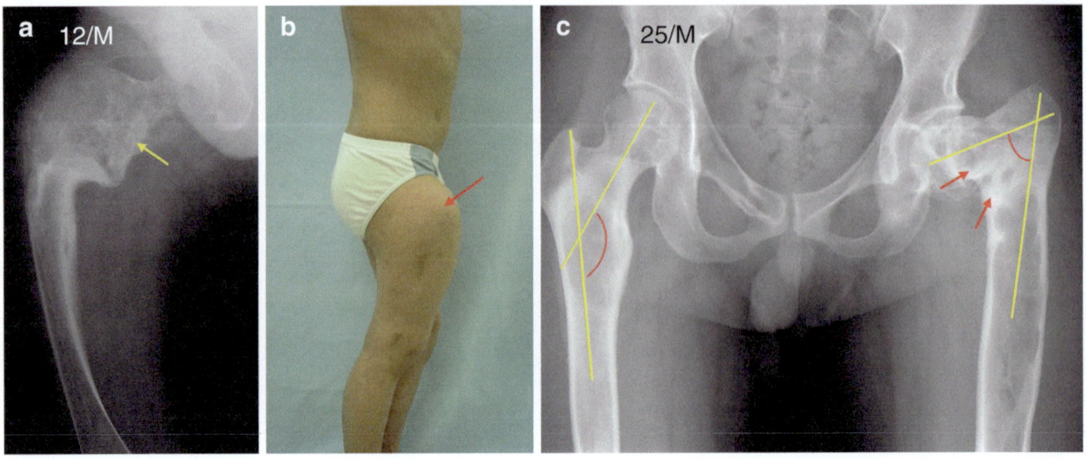

Fig. 26.7 ***Shepherd's crook deformity***. (**a**) Radiograph taken for right hip deformity with limping gait in a 12-year-old boy demonstrates a markedly expansile lesion with *ground-glass* density and a focal area of new bone formation (arrow), suggesting repeated microfracture and healing. Note shepherd's crook deformity with shortening and significant varus deformity of the proximal femur. (**b**) Clinically, the patient presents a deformity simulating the shape of shepherd's crook and shortening of the right thigh (red arrow). (**c**) Radiograph taken for left thigh shortening and limping gait with left hip deformity in a 25-year-old man reveals polyostotic FD of both hips. Right hip shows a valgus deformity and left hip presents a significant varus deformity (intersecting lines) and shortening of left femur with shepherd's crook deformity. There are also dense areas of new bone formation (red arrows), likely reflecting repeated of microfracture and healing

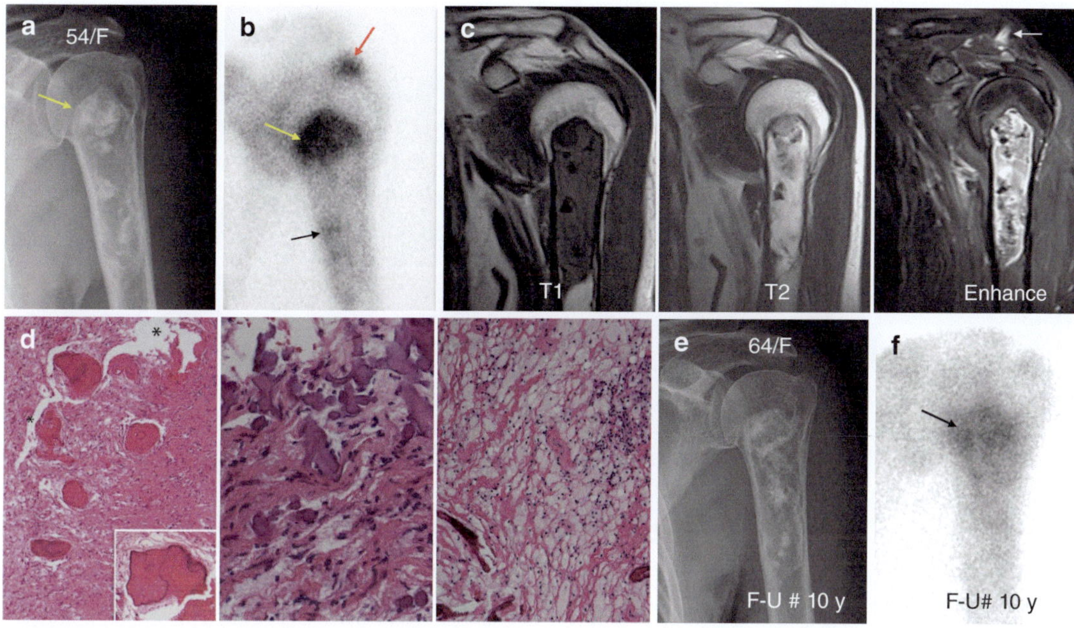

Fig. 26.8 ***Heavy internal calcification***. (**a**) Radiograph taken for left shoulder pain of 5 months' duration in a 54-year-old woman shows a well-defined lesion of *ground-glass* density surrounded by a rim of sclerosis (arrow) and multiple foci of internal punctate or flocculent calcification in the proximal humerus, suggesting an old benign lesion. (**b**) Pinhole bone scan reveals strong uptake in the densely calcifying proximal lesion (yellow arrow) and focal mild uptake in the distal portion of the lesion (black arrow). Note a focal uptake at the AC joint, suggesting a degenerative change (red arrow). (**c**) MR images demonstrate a well-defined mass-like lesion with low SI on T1-weighted image and heterogeneous high SI on T2-weighted image with internal focal dark signals of calcifications on both sequences. The lesion demonstrates internal patchy enhancement with a peripheral enhancing rim. There is another enhancing lesion at the AC joint, suggesting a generative change, which is thought to be the cause of the shoulder pain (white arrow). (**d**) Microscopic examination notes several woven bone spicules devoid of osteoblastic rimming embedded within bland-looking prominent fibrous stroma. There are multiple microscopic cystic foci (asterisks). The bone spicules have irregular cement lines resembling a focal mosaic pattern (Left). Foci of calcification are noted (Middle). A fibro-histiocytic reaction with foam cells and inflammatory cells as well as myxoid stromal change is seen in another field (Right). (**e**) Radiograph at 10 years' follow-up shows stabilization of the lesion with more calcification. (**f**) Follow-up pinhole scan also reveals reduced uptake limited to the previously calcified proximal lesion (arrow), suggesting regression of the lesion

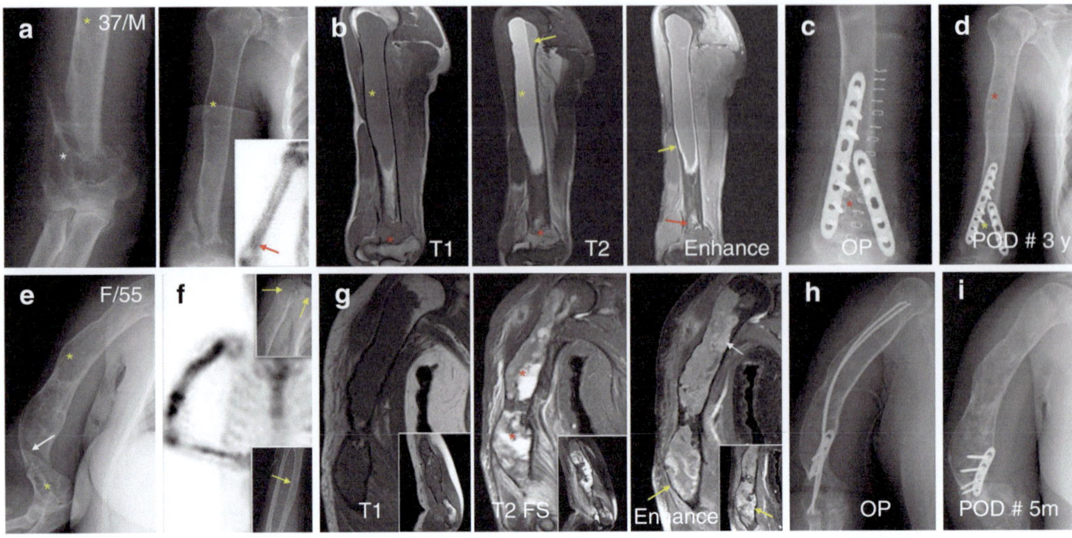

Fig. 26.9 ***Pathologic fracture in monostotic form***. (**a**) Radiograph taken for acute severe pain of right elbow after a slip in a 37-year-old man shows an oblique fracture with a preexisting well-defined osteolytic lesion surrounded by a thin rim of sclerosis in the supracondylar area (white asterisk) and a similar large lesion in the humerus shaft (yellow asterisks). Bone scan notes a localized mild uptake only in the lesion site of the distal humerus (inset). (**b**) MR images reveal a well-defined, large, elongated proximal lesion along the entire shaft and neck of the humerus (yellow asterisks). The SI is low on T1-weighted image and high SI with fluid-fluid level, suggesting a simple cyst with hemorrhage or secondary ABC on T2-weighted image (arrow). There is another smaller lesion with the same SI with mildly displaced fracture in the distal humerus (red asterisks). The large lesion in the shaft and neck is peripherally enhanced, indicating a cystic lesion (yellow arrow), and another small lesion is partially enhanced, suggesting a solid lesion (red arrow). (**c**) Open reduction and internal fixation with allogenic chip bone graft were performed (asterisk). Microscopic examination of the lesion with pathologic fracture confirmed a diagnosis of typical FD with focal areas of cystic change. (**d**) Follow-up radiograph at 3 years after surgery notes healing of the fracture and consolidation of the lesion (yellow asterisk). In addition, the large lesion appears stabilized (red asterisk). *Pathologic fracture in "polyostotic form"*: (**e**) Radiograph taken for right elbow pain after a fall from a ladder shows a short oblique fracture with minimal displacement (red arrow) and a preexisting ill-defined, huge, expansile lesion with *ground-glass* density and diffuse cortical thinning in the entire humerus (asterisks). (**f**) Bone scan reveals intense uptake in the right humeral shaft and head. In addition, there are milder uptake in the scapular, elbow, and shaft of radius, indicating *monomelic, polyostotic form* of the lesion. Note other bone lesions with "ground-glass" density in the additional uptake sites (inset). (**g**) MR images demonstrate a huge mass-like lesion along the deformed entire humeral shaft with low SI on T1-weighted image and heterogeneous intermediate SI with multiple areas of bright signal on fat-saturated T2-weighted image (asterisks), suggesting a cystic change. The lesion exhibits irregular expansion and marked cortical thinning. Pathologic fracture with diffuse surrounding soft tissue edema is associated in the distal humerus. The distal lesion is heterogeneously enhanced (yellow arrows), but the proximal lesion is only focally and weakly enhanced by contrast medium (white arrow). (**h**) Open reduction followed by flexible intramedullary Khai nail insertion with small plate fixation was performed. Microscopic examination confirmed a diagnosis of FD with nonspecific cystic change. The nails were removed a month after surgery because of pus discharge from the insert site. (**i**) Radiograph at 5 months after surgery notes good maintenance of the plate. Unfortunately, however, the patient died of COVID 2019

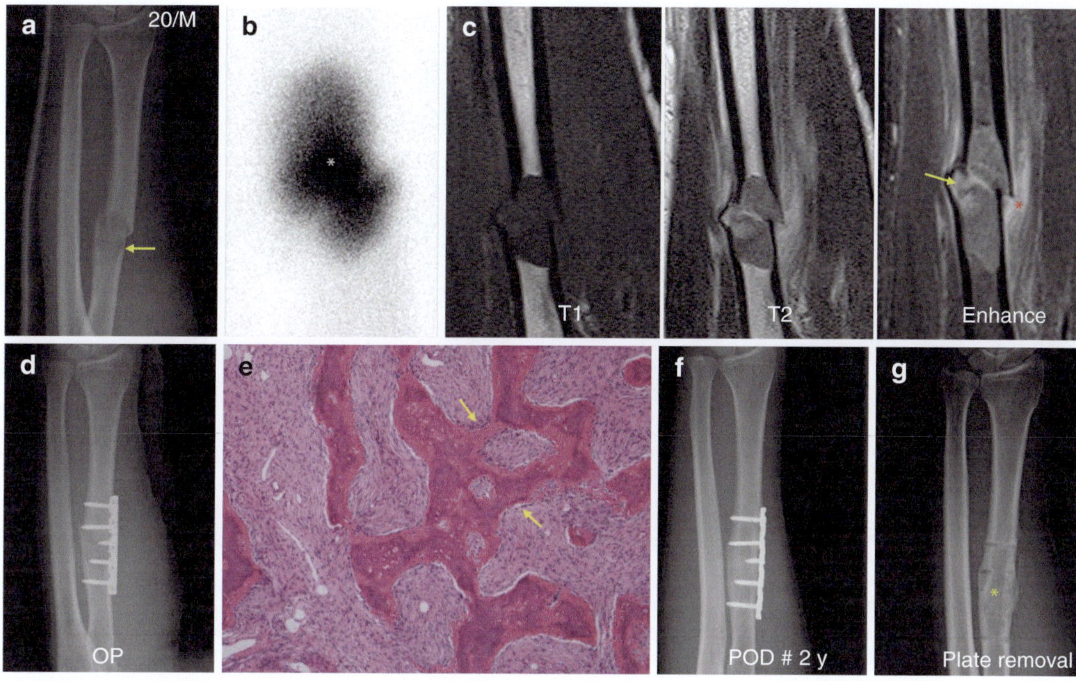

Fig. 26.10 ***A prominent osteoblastic rimming simulating OFD***. (**a**) Radiograph taken for left forearm pain after a slip during skiing in a 20-year-old young man shows a minimally displaced fracture with an underlying hazy radiolucent lesion with *ground-glass* density and cortical thinning (arrow) in the midshaft of radius. (**b**) Pinhole bone scan reveals a homogeneous strong uptake in the lesion with the highest uptake intensity at the mid-level of the lesion (asterisk), suggesting an active bone lesion with recently complicated fracture through the lesion. (**c**) MR images demonstrate a well-defined concentric intramedullary lesion with low SI on T1-weighted image and intermediate SI with focal high signal on T2-weighted image. There is a diffuse adjacent muscle and soft tissue hemorrhage due to pathologic fracture. The preexisting lesion is heterogeneously enhanced (arrow) and the soft tissue hemorrhage or edema is diffusely enhanced (asterisk). (**d**) Open reduction with plate fixation followed by curettage and frozen biopsy was performed. (**e**) Microscopic examination notes branching and anastomosing irregular trabeculae of woven bone embedded within bland spindle stroma. Note a prominent osteoblastic rimming as noted in OFD. However, a final diagnosis of FD is easily made based on the findings of a medullary location rather than eccentric cortical lesion and complete closure of the growth plate on radiograph. (**f**) Follow-up radiograph at 2 years after surgery shows complete union of fracture with no evidence of recurrence. (**g**) Radiograph after plate removal also reveals complete union of fracture with no evidence of recurrence (asterisk)

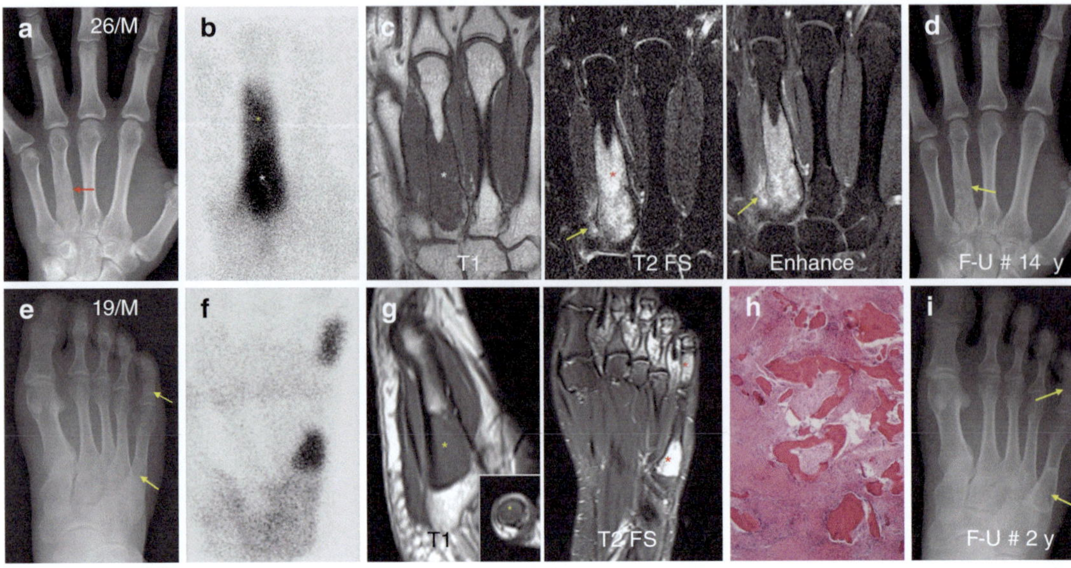

Fig. 26.11 ***Rare location of hand***. (**a**) Radiograph taken for right-hand pain of 2 months' duration in a 26-year-old man shows a mildly expansile lesion with *ground-glass* opacity and marked cortical thinning in the proximal shaft and base of the fourth metacarpal bone (arrow). (**b**) Pinhole bone scan reveals intense uptake in the proximal part of the lesion (white asterisk) with moderate uptake distally (yellow asterisk). (**c**) MR images demonstrate a well-defined, intrmaedullary lesion (asterisks) with SI iso to adjacent muscle on T1-weighted image and intermediate and high SI on T2-weighted image in the proximal 2/3 of the shaft and base of the metacarpal bone. There is diffuse cortical thinning and focal cortical breakage in the base area with focal soft tissue extension, simulating a locally aggressive tumor (arrows). The bone lesion as well as that extending into the adjacent soft tissue is heterogeneously enhanced (arrow). Incision biopsy confirmed a diagnosis of conventional FD. (**d**) Follow-up radiograph at 14 years after incision biopsy without curettage shows a stabilized lesion, and the patient is free of pain. **Rare location of foot:** (**e**) Radiograph taken for right foot pain in a 19-year-old adolescent shows hazy lesions with *ground-glass* density in the proximal half of the fifth metatarsal bone and proximal phalanx of the fifth toe with moderate expansion (arrows). (**f**) Pinhole bone scan notes a moderately increased uptake in both lesions. (**g**) MR image clearly demonstrates a well-defined intramedullary lesion (asterisks) with intermediate SI on T1-weighted image and high SI on fat-saturated T2-weighted image. (**h**) Microscopic examination shows abundant bone spicules embedded within bland fibrous stroma indicative of typical FD. (**i**) Follow-up radiograph at 2 years after initial visit reveals more stabilized lesions (arrows)

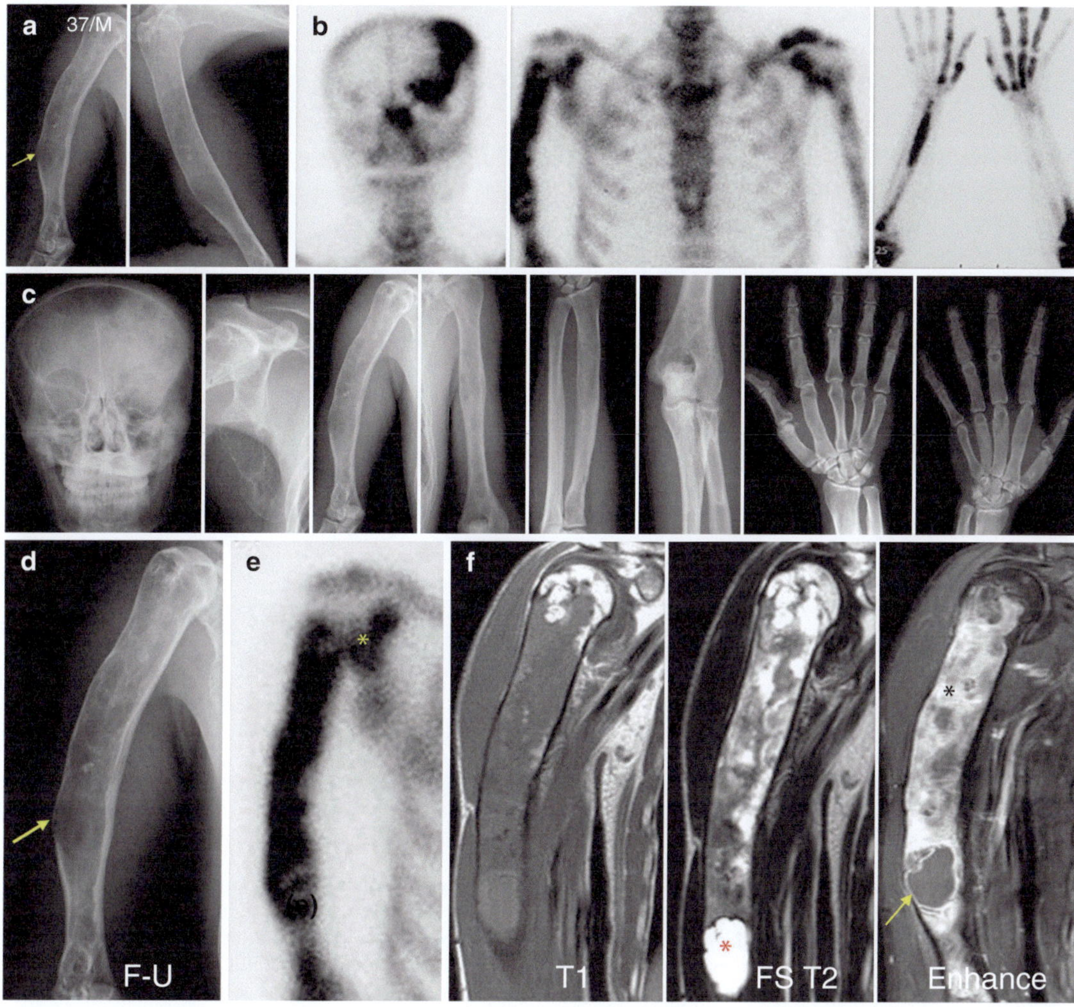

Fig. 26.12 ***Polymelic polyostotic form*.** (**a**) Radiograph taken for intermittent right upper arm pain since childhood that has been aggravated recently in a 37-year-old man shows a large, expansile osteolytic lesion with diffuse *ground-glass* density and irregular cortical thinning and scalloping affecting the entire humerus. The lateral cortex is particularly thinned with a focus of possible impending fracture (arrow). (**b**) Bone scan reveals multiple strong uptakes in the skull bones including the frontal, parietal, and occipital bones, entire right humeris, both elbows, right radius, both scapulae, and short tubular bones of both hands, indicating multifocal bone lesions. (**c**) Radiographs corresponding to hot uptake areas note hazy radiolucent lesions with *ground-glass* opacities, indicative of *polymelic and polyostotic* FD. (**d**) Follow-up radiograph taken for further aggravation of the right upper arm pain by trivial injury notes no definite interval change of the lesion with no evidence of a pathologic fracture (arrow). (**e**) Follow-up pinhole bone scan reveals a homogenous strong uptake along right entire humerus and a part of scapular (asterisk), suggesting still active lesions. (**f**) MR images demonstrate a huge expansile medullary space occupying lesion, exhibiting intermediate SI on T1-weighted and heterogeneous intermediate and high SI with a small distal bright signal, consistent with cystic change (asterisk) on fat-saturated T2-weighted image. The solid lesion is heterogeneously well enhanced (asterisk), and smaller cystic area is only peripherally enhanced by contrast medium (arrow). (**g**) After curettage and frozen biopsy with a confirmation of FD, fibular allogenic strut graft was inserted in the weakest portion and fixed with only two screws. Fracture was developed following a slip at 3 months after surgery. Open reduction with secure fixation by large locking plate and screws was performed, and some of the screws engaged previously inserted fibular graft and far cortex, providing a secure fixtion. Follow-up radiograph at 1 year after re-operation notes consolidation of the lesion with union of the fracture. Last follow-up radiograph at 12 years after re-operation shows incorporation of the fibular graft with consolidation of the lesion and reshaping of the host bone

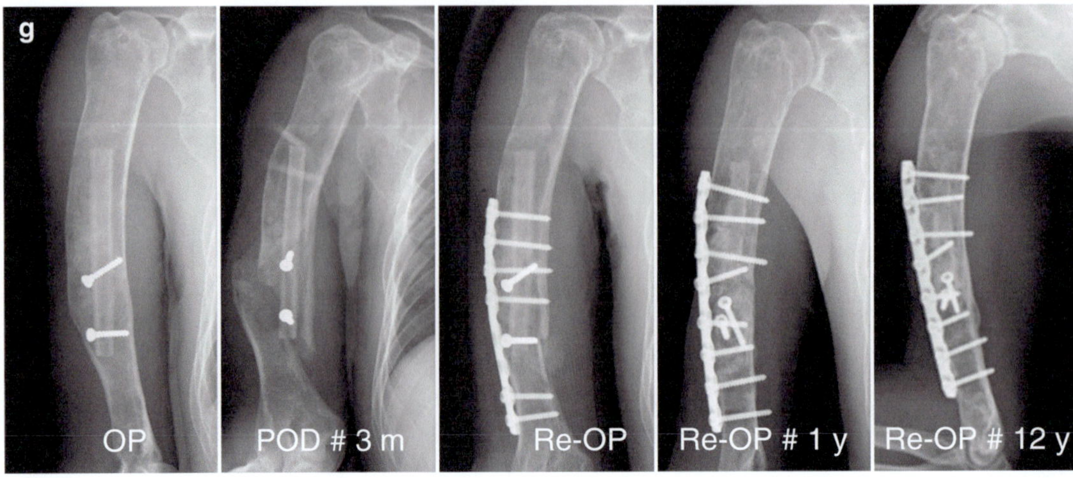

Fig. 26.12 (continued)

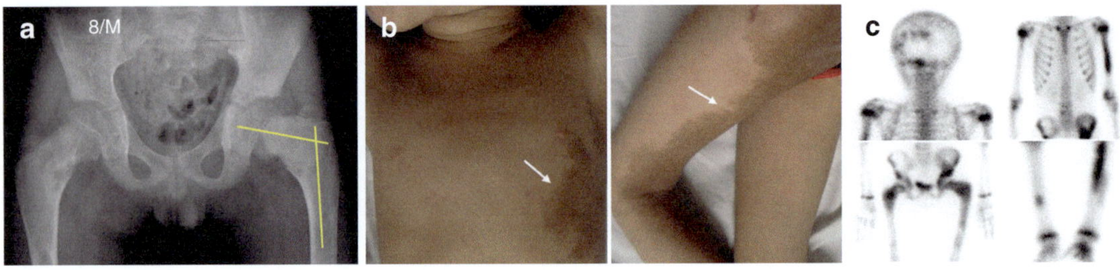

Fig. 26.13 ***McCune-Albright syndrome***. (**a**) Radiograph taken for a painful limping gait in an 8-year-old boy shows an ill-defined ground-glass density to sclerotic lesion with focal radiolucent areas in both proximal femurs with a significantly decreased neck-shaft angle (coxa vara deformity) of the left femur. (**b**) The patient presents prominent multiple *Café-au-lait* skin pigmentations with irregular borders resembling "the coast of Maine" (arrows). However, he has no endocrine abnormalities. (**c**) Bone scan demonstrates multiple areas of increased uptake throughout the body, suggesting multifocal bone lesions. (**d**) Radiographs corresponding to the increased uptake areas on bone scan demonstrate midly expansile, intramedullary lesions with characteristic "*ground-glass*" opacities, consistent with "*polymelic and polyostotic*" FD. (**e**) Corrective valgus osteotomy (red arrow) followed by strut allograft insertion (yellow arrow) and internal fixation using a Coventry hip screw was performed for the left hip FD with coxa vara deformity. (**f**) Corrective valgus osteotomy (red arrow) and internal fixation with a Coventry hip screw were performed on the right hip at 1 year after left hip surgery. The prior left osteotomy site is completely united with normal neck-shaft angle (yellow arrow). (**g, h**) However, both hip pain with limping gait recurred due to varus deformity at 5 and 6 years after initial surgery, respectively. (**i**) After removal of the Coventry hip screw, valgarization with derotation osteotomy fixed by a Richard compression hip screw and plate for both hips was consecutively performed forboth hips. Last follow-up radiograph taken at 10 years after revision surgery shows consolidation of the lesions without varus deformity. (**j**) Radiograph taken for upper arm pain following a trivial blunt injury at 2 years after initial visit shows a transverse to short oblique fracture with underlying medullary lesion with *ground-glass* density in the mid-shaft of the humerus. (**k**) Open reduction with plate fixation was performed. (**l**) Follow-up radiograph at 15 years after surgery shows complete union of the fracture with consolidation of the lesion with a mild bending deformity. (**m**) Follow-up radiographs at 17 years after initial presentation note mild progression of anterior bowing of the tibia with cortical thickening (arrow). The lesions of the short tubular bones of both feet are stabilized with remodeling of the cortices

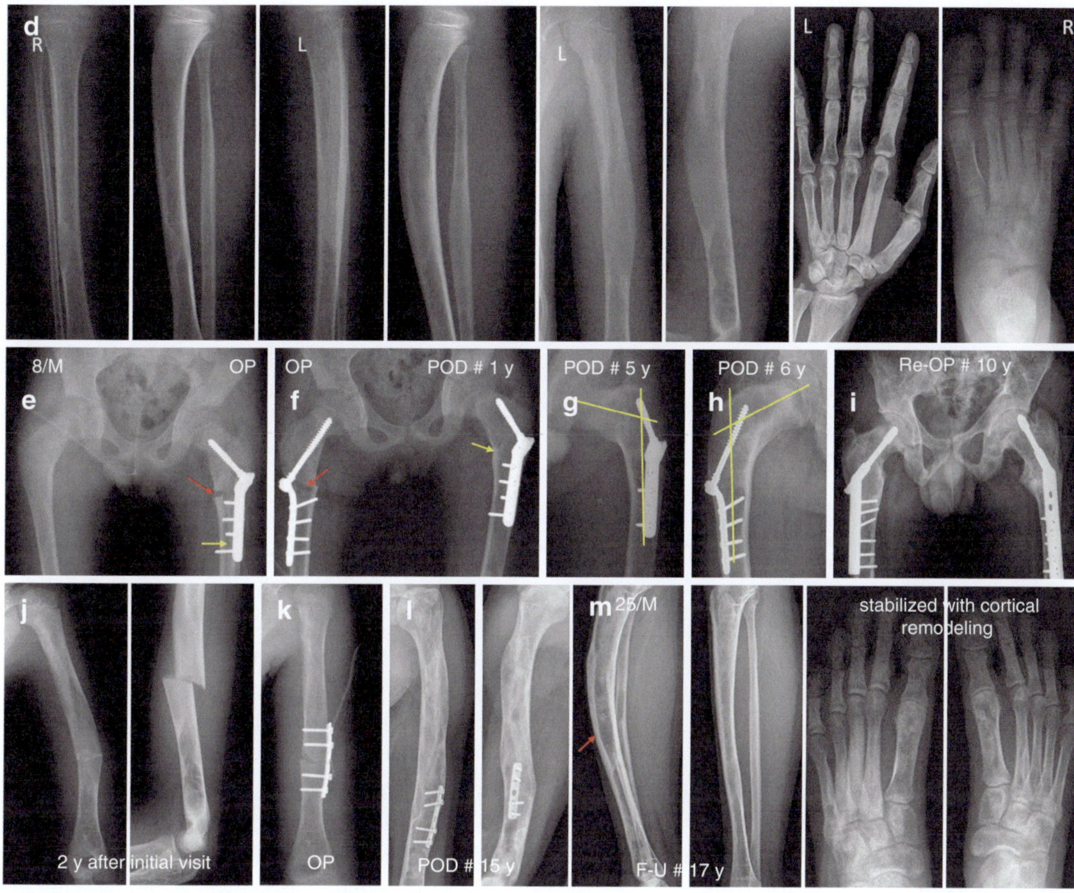

Fig. 26.13 (continued)

26.2 Possible Pathogenesis

A sporadic gene mutation during early gestation may cause a failure of bone-forming cells to normally mature, leading to abnormal fibrous tissue in certain bones. Mutations in the α-subunit of the Gs stimulatory protein (GNAS) lead to an inappropriate overproduction of cyclic adenosine monophosphate (cAMP). The increased serum concentration of cAMP results in abnormally high melanin production in the skin, incomplete differentiation of marrow stromal cells with abnormal maturation of bone matrix arrest at woven bone stage, and hyperfunction of endocrine organs [4, 6]. FD and osteofibrous dysplasia (OFD) have similar histologic features as well as a predilection for childhood or young adolescence. Their histologic relationship and exact nature have remained controversial for many decades. The mutations in the α-subunit of the Gsα stimulatory protein at the Arg201 codon have a role in the development of FD but not in OFD [7, 8]. The data suggest that their pathogenesis is different, and the detection of Gs α mutation at the Arg^{201} codon is quite useful for distinguishing between these lesions. However, the process is not required in clinical practice because a simple clinical-radiologic-pathologic correlation (diagnostic triangle) is enough for a correct diagnosis.

26.3 Incidence

The true incidence is unknown due to being asymptomatic in many cases, but it is estimated to account for almost 1% of biopsy-analyzed primary bone tumors [9] and 5% of all benign bone tumors [10]. The monostotic form is 6–10 times as common as the polyostotic form [1, 9]. In a more recent review, the monostotic form accounts for about 75–80% of cases [3, 4].

26.4 Age

FD usually develops during childhood before puberty and mostly discovered in children and young adults before the age of 30 years. Only 10% of patients are diagnosed in adults older than 40 years of age [9].

26.5 Location

FD lesion can occur in any bones, but particularly in long bones, craniofacial bones, and ribs. Craniofacial bones are the most common location. In the long bones, the femur (particularly proximal part) is the most frequent location, followed by the tibia and humerus (Figs. 26.1, 26.2, 26.3, 26.4, 26.5, 26.6, 26.7, 26.8 and 26.9). The same locations are affected in the polyostotic form [11] (Figs. 26.12 and 26.13). The metaphysis or diaphysis is mostly affected if involving the long bone (Figs. 26.1, 26.2, 26.3, 26.4, 26.5, 26.6, 26.7, 26.8, 26.9, 26.10, 26.11, 26.12 and 26.13). Short tubular bones of the hands and feet are also rarely affected (Fig. 26.11).

26.6 Clinical Features

Monostotic FD is usually asymptomatic and is frequently found incidentally on imaging performed for other reasons (Figs. 26.1 and 26.2). However, the abnormal fibro-osseous tissue weakens the bone over time, which can lead to pathologic fracture (Figs. 26.5, 26.9 and 26.10), pain by fatigue or insufficiency fracture, or varus deformity by repeated microfracture in the weight-bearing area such as medial cortex of the femoral neck (Fig. 26.6). Interestingly, there is no association between the extent of disease and the severity or likelihood of pain. Patients with a mild extent of FD may have debilitating pain while those with extensive disease can be pain-free. Swelling or bone expansion is occasionally observed in superficial bones such as the tibia, fibula, rib, or skull bones. The craniofacial FD is typically seen as a gradual, painless enlargement of the craniofacial region, often leading to facial asymmetry. While many cases of monostotic FD are asymptomatic and discovered incidentally in older children and young adults, the polyostotic form is usually diagnosed during the first decade of life because polyostotic FDs are more commonly symptomatic. However, some patients do not seek medical attention until pain becomes severe, and are diagnosed late in older age (Fig. 26.12). *Polyostotic FD* initially presents with pain with limp, or pathologic fracture in 70% of patients and two-thirds of the patients had such symptoms before the age of 10 years, although it may first manifest as abnormal vaginal bleeding, as reported in an earlier large series of Massachusetts General Hospital [12]. Later study also reported that about 60% of patients with the polyostotic form were symptomatic and diagnosed within the first decade of life [3]. The initial symptoms included pain, limp, spontaneous fracture, bowing, or leg-length discrepancies of varying degrees. Spontaneous fracture occurs most frequently between the ages of 6 and 10 years, declining thereafter [4, 13]. However, misaligned or deformed bone can also lead to a pathologic fracture in adult patients with either the monostotic or polyostotic form (Fig. 26.9). The fracture rate increases with a higher disease burden and fibroblast growth factor 23 levels. Patients with severe polyostotic involvement are prone to disfigurement due to bone expansion, malalignment, and crippling deformities subsequent to repeated process of fracture and healing [9]. Occasionally, the lesion can be a part of complex disease involving not only bones but also extra-skeletal anomalies [4]. An overproduction of melanin on the skin produces *café au lait* pigmentations that have irregular borders resembling the "coast of Maine," which are the most common extra-skeletal abnormalities accompanied by the polyostotic form. When they are associated with endocrinopathy such as precocious puberty in females, diabetes mellitus, goiter, or breast fibroadenomatosis, it is called *McCune-Albright syndrome*. The classic symptom triad includes multiple bone lesions of FD, precocious puberty, and cutaneous pigmentation [14]. However, patients may have only two features of the triad, sometimes lacking the café-au-lait spots or endocrine symptoms [3] (Fig. 26.13). By H. Jaffe [15], manifestation of the full triad is very rare, representing about 1 in 30–40 patients with polyostotic FD. Less frequently, endocrine dysfunction may include Cushing's syndrome, hyperparathyroidism, hyperthyroidism, and acromegaly [1]. Extraordinarily rare patients may have solitary or multiple intramuscular myxoma lesions, typically located in the vicinity of the bone lesions, known as *Mazabraud's syndrome* (Fig. 26.20).

26.7 Radiologic Findings

Plain radiograph Although radiologic features vary widely, they are sufficiently characteristic although not pathognomonic for diagnosis of FD. The spectrum of bone lesions can be classified into one of radiolucent or cystic, sclerotic, and mixed patterns [4]. The normal architecture of bone is altered and remodeled by the FD lesion. The most classic finding is a nonaggressive, intramedullary radiolucent geographic lesion typically with a varying degree of internal *ground-glass* to sclerotic density (Figs. 26.1, 26.2 and 26.3), similar to that of cancellous bone but usually no discernible trabecular pattern although delicate fine trabeculae can be seen within some FD lesions. The density of the lesion is variable depending on the amount of woven bone formation and its degree of mineralization (Fig. 26.3). If the woven woven bone is more prominent, the lesion is closer to ground-glass density (Fig. 26.4), but if sparser, the lesion appears more radiolucent (Fig. 26.5). The lesion in the long bone is usually well-defined with a rind of sclerosis and endosteal scalloping and thinning of the cortex. Finally, the affected bones may undergo mildly to moderately expansile remodeling secondary to the enlarging mass of fibro-osseous tissue [4]. The periosteal reaction is not usually observed except in cases of fracture. Craniofacial FD typically exhibits a rather denser and sclerotic appearance. The lesion may be rapidly enlarged or expanded with prominent radiolucency secondary to cystic change or aneurysmal bone cyst (ABC), often masquerading as malignant transformation [16–19]. Cartilage differentiation is often presented as dense punctate or flocculent spots within the FD lesion when they are mineralized [20]. If cartilage differentiation is extensive enough, the lesion appears similar to a cartilage tumor, so-called "fibro-cartilaginous dysplasia" (FCD) [1]. The lesion is presented as an FD with the addition of ring-like or scattered punctate to flocculent calcifications (Fig. 26.21). The density can also be significantly altered by lesion age and secondary changes, including repeated microfracture and healing (Fig. 26.6), nonspecific cyst or aneurysmal bone cyst (Figs. 26.15, 26.16, 26.17, 26.18 and 26.19), heavy calcification (Fig. 26.8), and even malignant transformation (Fig. 26.24). With time, the classic *ground-glass* appearance changes to a denser and sclerotic pattern with extensive rim of sclerosis or faintly lucent with irregular rind of sclerosis, suggesting regressed or ancient FD [4] (Fig. 26.22). Pathologic fracture or varus deformity due to repeated microfracture might occur less frequently in the monostotic form than in the more severe polyostotic form. The polyostotic FD exhibits the radiographic findings identical to those of the monostatic FD, but the lesions are larger and more often associated with pathological fracture or deformation as a rule [10]. Polyostotic form more often causes repeated microfractures, resulting in bowing of the tibia, leg length discrepancy, coxa vara, acetabular protrusion, crippling deformities such as shepherd's crook deformity as well as occipital prominence, facial asymmetry, or even displacement of one orbit [12]. Therefore, the polyostotic form is usually diagnosed earlier during the first decade of life. Pathological fracture through the thinned cortex is frequent, but the dense fibrous stroma may prevent excessive displacement [2]. In an extensive lesion affecting a weight-bearing proximal femur, curvature of the femur can occur, typically with severe varus bowing deformity (Fig. 26.7). **Bone scan** is very useful to demonstrate the extent and activity of the disease as well as to detect other lesions in monomelic or polymelic polyostotic form (Figs. 26.1, 26.2, 26.3, 26.4, 26.5, 26.6, 26.8, 26.9, 26.10, 26.11, 26.12 and 26.13). It typically shows avid radiotracer uptake in the metabolically active lesion particularly early childhood and periods of skeletal growth (Fig. 26.4b). Increased activity may persist even in old adult throughout the life with a variable intensity. Generally, the intensity of uptake becomes much less active in the stabilized or regressed lesion (Fig. 26.4g). **PET/CT scan** reveals mild to severe hypermetabolic bone lesion(s) which can be mistaken for malignant bone tumor, malignant transformation of preexisting benign bone tumor, or bone metastasis (Fig. 26.1a). Follow-up PET scan may show an increased hypermetabolic activity if combined with a more aggressive secondary change such as ABC or malignant transformation (Fig. 26.19a, e). **CT scan** is the best tool to demonstrate the extent of the lesion, cortical thickness, degree of endosteal scalloping, and mineralization as well as new bone reaction. It is considered the modality of choice particularly in the evaluation of FD in the setting of craniofacial lesions. **MR images** are not particularly useful in distinguishing FD from other entities because the findings are non-specific. The lesion may present marked variabilities in appearance, ranging from definitely benign appearance to locally more aggressive-appearing, with marked cortical thinning, or focal perforation with soft tissue extension particularly if involving a short tubular bone (Fig. 26.11c). The signal intensity (SI) is determined by the amount of fibrous tissue, cellularity, bone matrix production, mineralization, hemorrhage, or edema. In general, the lesion is well-defined with low to intermediate SI on T1-weighted images and heterogeneous intermediate and high SI on T2-weighted images (Figs. 26.1, 26.2, 26.4, 26.5, 26.6, 26.8, 26.10, 26.11 and 26.12). FD lesions may also contain focal to extensive areas of higher to bright SI on T2-weighted image, suggesting non-specific cyst or ABC change. The solid FD lesion is heterogeneously enhanced and the cystic lesion is peripherally enhanced (Figs. 26.4, 26.15, 26.16, 26.17, 26.18 and 26.19).

26.8 Histologic Findings

The lesion consists of branching and anastomosing irregular trabeculae of woven bone and intervening fibrous stroma containing bland spindle cells without prominent cytologic atypia. The woven bone spicules are variably thinned, irregular, curvilinear, or curled typically with alphabet characters including "C, I, L, or Y" shape, so-called "*alphabetic soap*" pattern (Fig. 26.14a). The woven bone spicules are derived directly from the stromal fibrous cells, referred as "*fibro-osseous metaplasia*", and thus the osteoblastic rimming is usually minimal to absent in contrast to OFD, osteoid osteoma, and fracture callus. However, osteoblastic rimming can be prominent, simulating OFD in rare cases (Fig. 26.14b). In such cases, a simple clinical-radiologic-pathologic correlation make it easy to differentiate FD from OFD. A *fibro-osseous metaplasia* is characteristic of FD, but is by no means pathognomonic because a similar pattern can be seen in parosteal and well-differentiated intramedullary OSA [9] (Refer to Fig. 8.1e in Chap. 8 and Fig. 10.5a, b in Chap. 10). In rare cases, the bony spicules may include lamellar bone in a focal mosaic pattern with irregular cement lines resembling a jigsaw puzzle, so-called "*Pagetoid*" appearance (Fig. 26.14b, f). Clear artifact spaces are frequently made between bone spicules and spindle cells of stroma during tissue preparation for H&E stain (Fig. 26.14c). In some cases, the amount of woven bone spicules is sparse, often with numerous foam cells mimicking xanthoma, which corresponds to more radiolucent lesion on radiographs (Fig. 26.14d). The varying proportion of fibrous and osseous tissue is reflected in the degree of ground-glass density and radiolucency on radiographs, or different uptake patterns on bone scan (Fig. 26.3). A peculiar *cementicle* or *cementum-like* material is deposited particularly if involving skull and jaw bones, and multinucleated giant cells can also be scattered in some fields (Fig. 26.14e). Several secondary changes such as fibro-histiocytic reaction with foam cells, giant cell reaction, stromal myxoid change, cystic change, or secondary ABC, and foci of cartilage differentiation may alter the typical histologic findings and make the diagnosis more challenging [1, 3]. Microscopic foci of degenerative cystic change are commonly seen (Fig. 26.14b, d), but macroscopic cystic change reaching many centimeters in diameter is less common [9]. The cystic FD with prominent cystic change is not uncommon in the skull, facial bones, or ribs, but has been reported only sporadically in long bones. However, it is not that rare even in long bones in our experience [18] (Figs. 26.15 and 26.16). Occasionally, secondary ABC with radiographic evidence of an expansile lesion is also associated (Figs. 26.17, 26.18 and 26.19). The cystic or ABC change can be focal or extensive enough to almost completely obliterate the preexisting FD lesion [1]. Cartilaginous foci have been described in at least 10% of cases of FD [21] (Fig. 26.14f). More rarely, the cartilaginous differentiation can be extensive and massive that it can be mistaken for a benign or even malignant cartilage tumor (Fig. 26.21). Foci or even extensive areas of foam cells, myxoid change of the stroma with scanty to few spicules of woven bone are seen in older or ancient lesions (Figs. 26.14g, 26.22d). Exceptionally rarely, significant cytological aberrations but lacking atypical mitoses, so-called *pseudoanaplastic FD*, can be observed in association with classic FD appearing areas (Fig. 26.23).

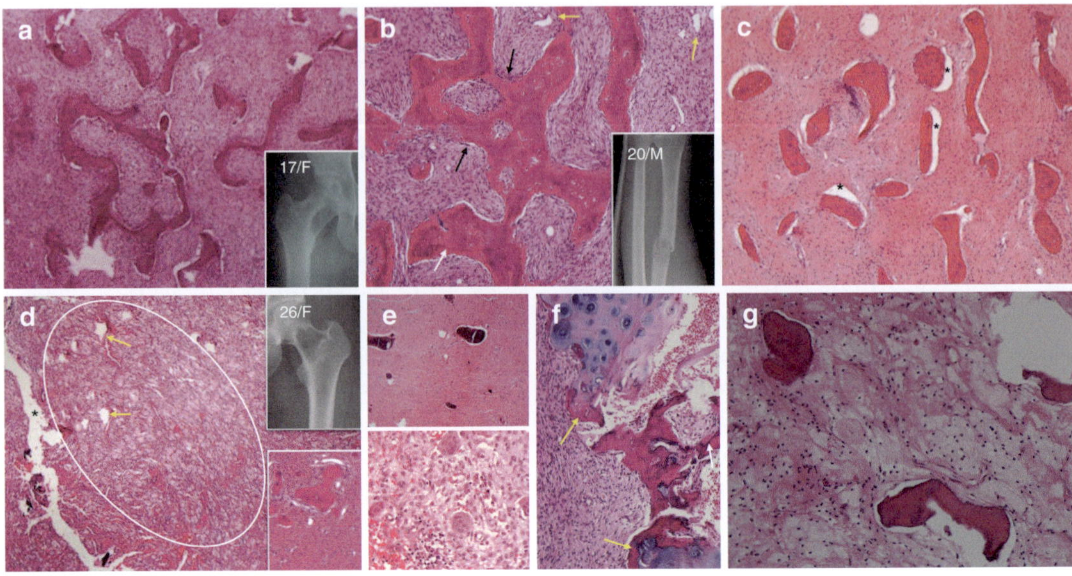

Fig. 26.14 ***Microscopic features***. (**a**) Medium-power magnification typically reveals branching and anastomosing trabeculae of irregular, thin or thick, curled woven bone spicules formed directly from bland spindle cells of the stroma with variable shapes such as "C, I, L, Y," so-called *alphabetic soap* pattern. The abundant woven bone produces a typical *ground-glass* density on radiographs (inset). The woven bone spicules have indistinct edges blending with the fibrous stroma and are usually not rimmed by a prominent single layer of osteoblasts. (**b**) However, osteoblastic rimming is prominent in this case as in OFD (black arrows). In consideration of the concentric medullary location with growth plate closure indicating a grown-up patient on radiographs (inset), a diagnosis of FD is easily rendered rather than OFD. Note bone spicules with irregular cement lines, so-called *Pagetoid* appearance (white arrow). There are multiple microcystic foci as well (yellow arrows). (**c**) Multiple clear artifact spaces are seen between bone spicules and spindle cells of the stroma (black asterisks), which are made during tissue preparation. (**d**) The amount of woven bone spicules is sparse, and there are numerous foam cells mimicking xanthoma (black circle). It can be be misdiagnosis as xanthoma of bone. There are also multiple microfoci of cystic degeneration (arrows). However, another field shows a classic finding of FD with scanty woven bone spicules embedded in bland spindle stroma (lower inset). The sparse amount of woven bone in addition to xanthoma-like areas produces a pure radiolucent lesion on radiographs (upper inset). (**e**) Several small, round to oval, calcified acellular bodies referred to as *cementicles* or *cementum-like* material are deposited particularly if involving the skull and jaw bones (Top). Multinucleated giant cells can also be scattered (Bottom). (**f**) The cartilage islands exhibit prominent endochondral ossification at the periphery resembling the epiphyseal growth plate (yellow arrows), which merge with the adjacent fibro-osseous lesion of typical FD. The dysplastic woven bone shows a focal mosaic pattern with irregular cement lines resembling a jigsaw puzzle, so-called *Pagetoid* appearance (white arrow). (**g**) Focal or even extensive areas with myxoid change of the stroma of foamy histiocytes are seen in this old or ancient FD. The bone spicules are sparse and show a focal mosaic pattern with irregular cement lines

26.9 Management

There is no method of cure for FD. The goals for treatment are pain relief, preventing and managing fractures, and correcting severely misshapen bones. Treatment depends on the extent, location, presence of pain, and severity of the disease including deformities. Only clinical observation with periodic monitoring is necessary without biopsy for asymptomatic patients with typical radiographic findings of *ground-glass* appearance and no risk of pathologic fracture (Fig. 26.2). Antiresorptive therapy with bisphosphonates has been suggested because of the high level of bone resorption in FD tissue. Earlier studies reported promising results of intravenous pamidronate in adults with decreased bone pain, reduced bone turnover markers, and refilling of bone lesions on radiographs in a number of patients [22, 23]. Additional studies with a relatively short follow-up period in a small number of patients reported that intravenous pamidronate therapy also has some beneficial effect with decreased bone pain and bone metabolism markers in pediatrc patients [24–26]. On the contrary, other studies failed to find clear evidence that pamidronate or alendronate has a significant effect on FD-related bone pain [27, 28]. However, the most recent review of 234 articles on the effect of bisphosphonates reported that intravenous therapy significantly decreased bone pain and bone resorption with a proposal for treating persistent and moderate to severe bone pain of FD, but had no effect on the occurence of fracture [29]. Surgical treatment is indicated for weight-bearing bone pain that is not relieved by medical management, correction of deformities interfering with ambulation, or causing functional loss or cosmetic problem, and pathologic fracture as well as cystic or ABC change or malignant transformation [30]. Curettage and bone graft for a painful lesion, preventive or curative fixation for impending or pathologic fracture, and corrective osteotomy for severe deformity would be considered. The grafted bone after curettage in childhood, the lesion is still active, frequently recur because the grafts, even massive, will be resorbed. However, grafting can be successful in older adolescents and adults with static or stabilized lesion [11]. Enneking and Gearen [31] experienced unsatisfactory results after curettage and autogenous cancellous bone grafting in various anatomical sites. Although the cancellous bone grafts were rapidly incorporated, they were subsequently replaced by dysplastic bone resulting in frequent recurrence. Therefore, the authors used an alternative method of cortical bone grafting without curettage. For children or young adolescents with hip pain or varus deformity, strut allo-fibular graft without curettage results in a successful outcome in my practice (Figs. 26.4 and 26.5). Typical orthopedic procedure to remove the lesion and to fill the defect with bone graft is also successful in adult patients with a painful monostotic lesion (Fig. 26.6). In general, open reduction followed by plate fixation is performed for upper extremity fracture with displacement (Figs. 26.9, 26.10, 26.12 and 26.13). Standard closed management is, however, indicated for selected nondisplaced fracture of upper extremity, but residual angulation is not allowed because remodeling and correction of the angulation do not occur as they do in normal bone. Lower extremity fractures will almost always require internal fixation of variable methods, but selected nondisplaced tibia fractures can also be managed by cast immobilization. Internal fixation with intramedullary nails allows stabilization of extensively affected bones (Fig. 26.9h, 26.15c), and is effective for both acute surgery for fractures and elective corrective surgery for major deformities in patients with extensive involvement of the femur or of other long bones [32–34]. Hip screw-plate or proximal femoral nail are usually suitable for proximal femur (Figs. 26.6d, 26.13e–i, 26.17, 26.18 and 26.19), rarely augmented with fibula graft for poor bone stock (Fig. 26.6h). Management of patients with polyostotic FD is very challenging because a majority of these patients are growing children. Significant deformities or limb length discrepancy are more likely to occur in patients with severe disease, requiring multiple corrective procedures. Both fractures and osteotomies can heal in about normal time with periosteal callus [11]. Uncontrollable pain by medication, recurrent fractures, leg length discrepancy, and severe deformity may significantly impair the quality of life (QoL). In a well-characterized cohort study of 255 patients with a full spectrum of FD subtypes including monostotic, polyostotic, McCune-Albright syndrome, and Mazabraud's syndrome, higher skeletal burden scores in the polyostotic form compared the monostotic form reflecting disease severity, were identified as the most consistent predictor of impaired QoL [35]. The authors intended to draw special attention to the clinically unmet need to address QoL in the management of patients with all subtypes of FD, including including its milder forms.

26.10 Clinical Course

FD lesions are not static, and the histological, radiological, and clinical alterations change with the patient's age and the lesion itself. The lesion is metabolically active in early childhood, expands to a varying and unpredictable degree during growth, becomes static in size with decreased metabolic activity after puberty, and finally becomes stabilized or regresses throughout adulthood over time, Kuznetsov et al. [36] evolved the novel concept of *normalization* of FD. Surprisingly, the authors observed a completely normal histology with hematopoietic cells and adipocytes in 4 of 7 specimens from older patients aged 35-51 years, and a nondescript fibrotic change was focally observed in the bone marrow space in the remaining cases. They suggested that activating GNAS mutations disrupt a pathway that is required for skeletal stem cell self-renewal, and their progeny are consumed by apoptosis, whereas residual normal stem cells survive, self-renew, and enable formation of a normal structure with time. The majority of bony lesions become clinically apparent by age 10 years, and new lesions appear no more after the age of 15 [4]. Most individuals with milder forms have an excellent prognosis with normal healthy lives. However, the prognosis may be as variable as the disorder itself based on the bones affected and whether other structures such as nerves are affected, and whether fractures occur. Very rarely, the fibrodysplastic bone may undergo transformation into malignant tumors over time. The prevalence of malignant transformation has been reported to range from 0.4 to 4% [12, 37–40]. In general, the real potential for malignant change is thought to be 1–2% in the monostotic form, but the frequency increases in the polyostotic form. FD lesions treated with irradiation are more likely to develop sarcomatous change. In a Mayo Clinic series, half of the malignancies arising in FD had a history of previous irradiation therapy as a part of the treatment before the sarcoma developed, and the rate of malignant transformation was estimated at about 2% in the monostatic form, but 6.7% in the polyostotic form [38]. With more than 100 reported cases of Mazabraud's Syndrome, 7 cases of sarcoma change of FD have been well reported in this specific setting [41]. The prognosis for patients with sarcomatous change is poor.

26.11 Clinical Spectrum of FD

Radiologic and histologic findings of FD are usually typical enough for a correct diagnosis. However, the classical findings are frequently modified by supervening microfracture with healing, hemorrhage, myxoid degeneration, cartilaginous foci, and degenerative changes such as fibro-histiocytic reaction, nonspecific cystic or secondary ABC, or even malignant transformation. This section deals with such more complicated forms of FD including (1) *cystic FD,* (2) *FD with secondary ABC,* (3) *FD with myxoma (Mazabraud's syndrome),* (4) *FD with enchondroma-like nodules* (fibrocartilaginous dysplasia), (5) *pseudoanaplastic FD,* (6) *ancient FD, and* (7) *malignant transformation.* When the lesion becomes more prominently osteolytic with rapid enlargement or expansion, complications such as cystic change, secondary ABC, and malignant transformation should be suspected. MRI can easily differentiate cystic change from malignant change. However, it is often difficult to distinguish nonspecific cystic change from secondary ABC on MRI when *fluid-fluid* levels are not associated. FD is occasionally associated with cartilage nodules embedded in the fibroblastic stroma, which can be extensive enough simulating a cartilage tumor. With aging, the lesion regresses with scanty bony spicules in the loose myxofibrous tissue with foamy histiocytes, so-called *ancient FD* resembling liposclerosing myxofibrous tumor (LSMFT). Extraordinarily rarely, FD can present significant bizarre-looking, atypical cells with smudged nuclei but no definite abnormal mitosis, so-called *pseudoanaplastic* FD. The lesion may very rarely undergo *malignant transformation*, usually into to osteosarcoma (OSA), fibrosarcoma (FSA), or chondrosarcoma (CSA), in less than 1% of all FD cases. The incidence is increased in the polyostotic form of FD, especially in the setting of McCune-Albright syndrome or Mazabraud's syndrome. Radiologists, pathologists, and orthopedic surgeons should be aware of all presentations of FD in various clinical settings to avoid misdiagnosis and to provide adequate management.

1. **Cystic FD**

Microscopic foci of degenerative cystic change are often seen in FD (Fig. 26.14b, d), but macroscopic cystic change reaching many centimeters in diameter is less common [9]. Furthermore, the phenomenon of large cystic change with accumulation of serous fluid can occur. Occasionally, the cystic change is prominent enough to nearly or totally obliterate the underlying FD [1], and it can be mistaken for a nonspecific cyst or a simple bone cyst if the FD area is not exists or so scant that it is missed by a pathologist in the absence of suspicion of *cystic* FD (Fig. 26.15). Since Jaffe first described a case of rapidly enlarging bone tumor of the caused by hemorrhagic cystic degeneration in a "fibrodysplastic" lesion [16], cystic FD has been reported to be not uncommon in the skull, facial bones, and ribs. The phenomenon has been thought to be rare and reported only sporadically in long bones [17, 42–45]. However, it is not that rare even in the long bones if physicians are aware of this phenomenon [18]. Clinically, it is important to differentiate cystic FD from secondary ABC because simple curettage with allogenic chip-bone graft is sufficient treatment even for extensive cystic FD [18] (Figs. 26.6h and 26.15c) but thorough curettage with or without adjuvant therapy may be necessary for locally more aggressive ABC to reduce the recurrence (Figs. 26.17, 26.18 and 26.19).

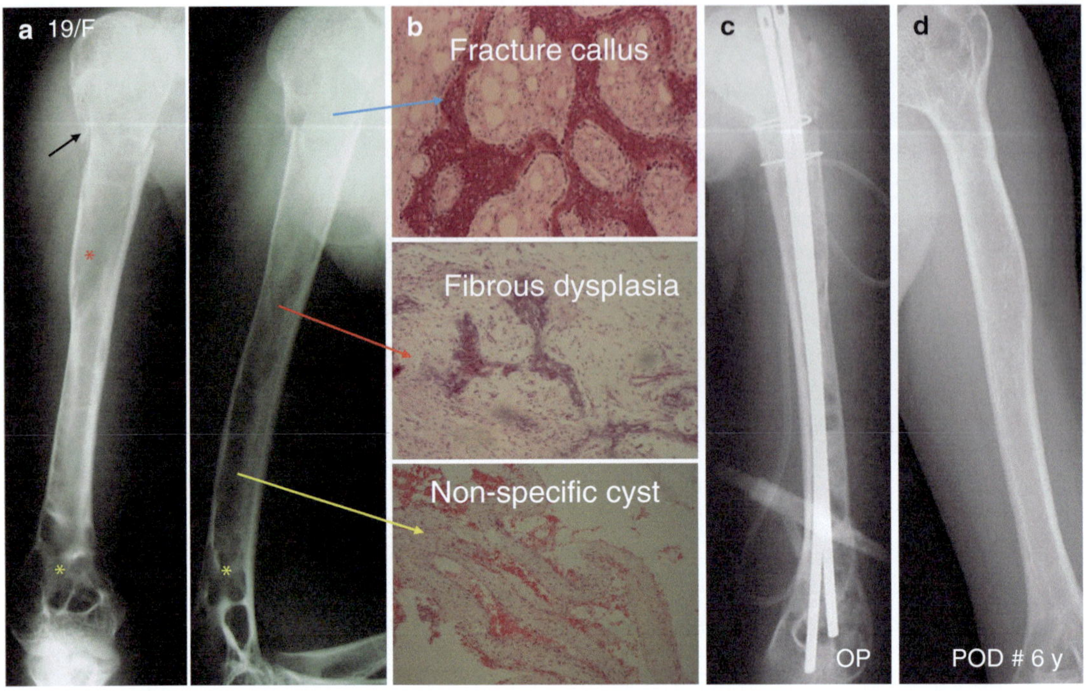

Fig. 26.15 (**a**) Radiographs taken for right shoulder pain after lifting a heavy object in a 19-year-old adolescent show a pathologic fracture of the surgical neck of the humerus (arrow) and an incidental finding of diffusely expanding medullary lesion (red asterisk) with *ground-glass* density and multilobulated sclerotic and lucent area, indicating typical FD as well as more radiolucent bubbly, multilobulated radiolucent areas (yellow asterisks) suggesting cystic change, which involves nearly entire humerus. (**b**) Microscopic examination reveals three different components of fracture callus, classic FD, and a nonspecific cystic component, which correspond to the pathologic fracture, *ground-glass* density, the radiolucent cystic area on on radiographs, respectively. A small field shows a peripheral network of lamellar bone laid down over primitive woven bone spicules with bubbly to vacuolated stroma and primitive fat marrow, suggesting a fracture callus with estimated age of 5–7 weeks (Top). The vast majority of the areas are occupied by a nonspecific cystic structure (Bottom). The initial pathologic report was a nonspecific cyst with fracture callus. However, I requested the pathologist to review the histology slides again to find any preexisting solid lesion because I believed the lesion was a huge cystic FD. A tiny focus of FD was finally found by scrutinized examination (Middle). In this case, the cystic degeneration is prominent enough to nearly obliterate the underlying FD. (**c**) Intramedullary flexible nails were inserted to fix the fracture after medullary rimming from the proximal entry for the nails to achieve a curettage effect. (**d**) Although the humerus is entirely affected, the lesion was completely healed without evidence of local recurrence by a simple surgery of medullary rimming and nailing, shown on the final follow-up radiograph at 6 years after surgery

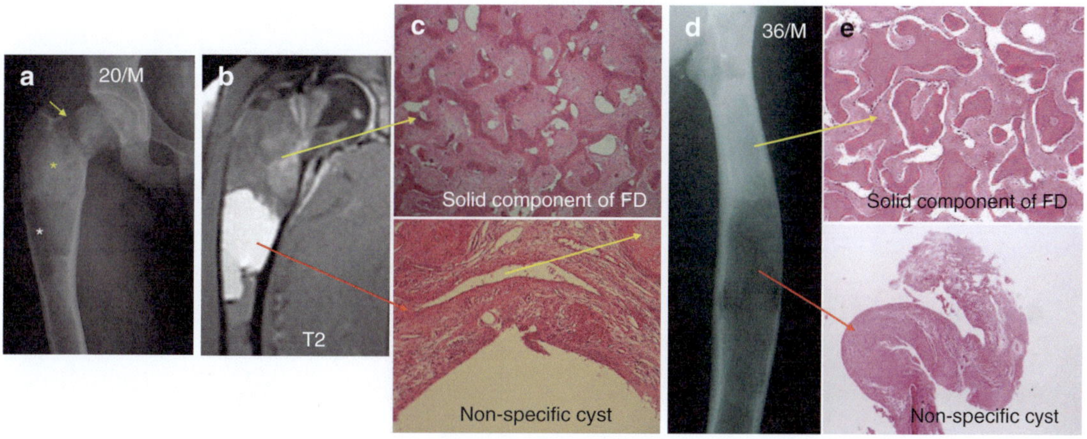

Fig. 26.16 (**a**) Radiograph taken for right hip pain during military drill in a 20-year-old soldier shows an expansile medullary lesion with marked thinning of the cortex in the proximal femur. There are two different densities of a proximal *ground-glass* density to somewhat sclerotic area (yellow asterisk) suggesting FD, and a distal radiolucent area (white asterisk) probably suggesting cystic degeneration, secondary ABC, or even malignant change. There is an associated pathologic fracture of the femoral neck (arrow). (**b**) T2-weighted MR image more clearly shows a solid area of heterogeneous intermediate and high SI proximally and a cystic area of bright SI distally, indicating FD with cystic degeneration or secondary ABC rather than malignant change. (**c**) Microscopic examination notes findings of classic FD and nonspecific cyst, corresponding to the proximal solid and distal cystic areas on MRI, respectively. (**d**) Another radiograph taken for left thigh pain in a 36-year-old man shows a moderately expanding large lesion in the diaphysis of the femur. There are also two different densities of a proximal *ground-glass* density to more sclerosis, and a distal radiolucency with significant expansion, cortical thinning, and endosteal scalloping, suggesting FD with cystic degeneration, secondary ABC, or even possibly malignant change. (**e**) Microscopic examination confirms that the proximal "ground-glass" to a rather sclerotic lesion is classic FD and that another osteolytic area is mostly cystic degeneration with scanty area of FD, respectively

2. **Secondary ABC Change**

Occasionally, secondary ABC can be superimposed on FD and present an aggressive-looking appearance with rapid enlargement and radiolucency (Figs. 26.17, 26.18 and 26.19). Secondary ABC is most frequently associated with giant cell tumor, chondroblastoma, and FD in decreasing order, occupying about 70% of secondary ABC [19]. Secondary ABC can also be extensive enough to almost completely obliterate the preexisting FD lesion as cystic FD does [1]. Standard management for ABC is thorough extended curettage using high-speed burr and bone grafting or cementing for the resultant defect as in primary ABC. Various adjuvant therapies including argon beam cauterization (burning the tumor bed), phenol (a chemical), or cryotherapy (liquid nitrogen) have also been recommanded to reduce local recurrence in contrast to treatment of cystic FD.

3. **Mazabraud's Syndrome (FD with Intramuscular Myxoma)**

Early in 1926, the first case of fibro-osseous lesions associated with myxomas was noted by Henschen [46]. Later in 1967, Mazabraud [47] fully documented the association between fibromyxomas of the soft tissues and FD of the bones, and named it *Mazabraud's syndrome* (MS). The vast majority of cases are accompanied by the

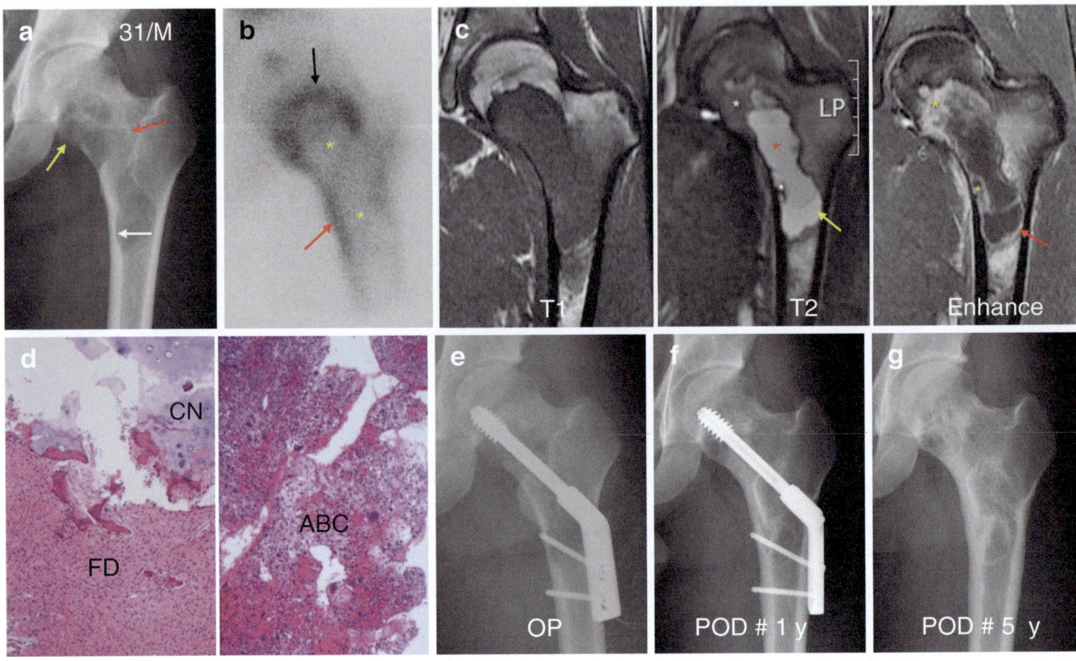

Fig. 26.17 (**a**) Radiograph taken for left hip intermittent pain of 4 months' duration with recent aggravation of the pain in a 31-year-old man shows an ill-defined, moderately expansile, osteolytic and sclerotic lesion with *ground-glass* density surrounded by a thin rim of sclerosis (red arrow), suggesting a possible preexisting FD in the proximal femur. In addition, findings of expansion, cortical thinning with possible cortical breakage (yellow arrow), and deep endosteal scalloping (white arrow) suggest more aggressive secondary change such as nonspecific cystic or ABC change or even malignant transformation. (**b**) Pinhole bone scan reveals moderately increased uptake along the superomedial margin of the lesion (black arrow) and mild uptake along the medial cortex (red arrow) with an internal photon defect (asterisks), which corresponds to the sclerotic reactive bone formation and either type of cystic change, respectively. (**c**) MR images shows a large well-defined lesion with low SI on T1-weighted image and mostly intermediate to high SI (red asterisk) with higher signal of *fluid-fluid* level (yellow arrow) and focal areas of intermediate signals of solid FD (white asterisks) on T2-weighted image, suggesting a focal residual FD with extensive ABC change. The solid lesion is heterogeneously enhanced (yellow asterisks) and the cystic lesion presents peripheral and septal enhancement (red arrow). The perilesional bone marrow and soft tissue edema are diffusely well enhanced. (**d**) Microscopic examination demonstrates two different findings of an area of FD with focal cartilage nodules (CN) and another area of ABC. (**e**) Extended curettage using a high-speed bur followed by allogenic chip bone graft and prophylactic compression hip screw fixation was performed. (**f**) Follow-up radiograph at 1 year after surgery notes consolidation of the lesion. (**g**) Follow-up radiograph at 5 years after surgery shows consolidation of the lesion with no recurrence

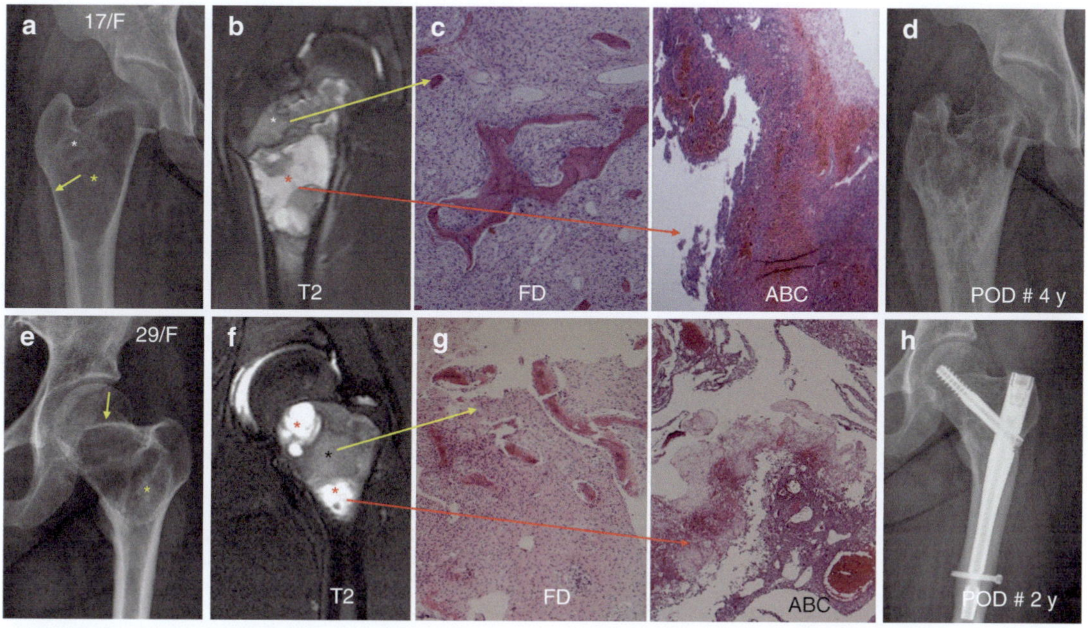

Fig. 26.18 (**a**) Radiograph taken for right hip pain of 2 weeks' duration in a 17-year-old girl shows a well-defined, moderately expansile, predominantly radiolucent lesion (yellow asterisk) with areas of *ground-glass* density (white asterisk) in the trochanteric and neck area of the femur. There is cortical thinning with endosteal scalloping (arrow). (**b**) T2-weighted MR image reveals an expansile multilobulated lesion with two distinct signals of a proximal intermediate SI indicating solid lesion of FD (white asterisk) another distal heterogeneous high SI of nonspecific cystic or ABC change (red asterisk). (**c**) Microscopic examination demonstrates two disticnt aeas of typical FD and secondary ABC, respectively. (**d**) Follow-up radiograph at 4 years after extended curettage and allogenic bone grafting shows consolidation of the lesion with no evidence of local recurrence. (**e**) Radiograph taken for left hip of 3 months' duration in a 29-year-old lady shows a multilobulated expansile radiolucent lesion with hazy internal *ground-glass* density and sclerotic foci (yellow asterisk) surrounded by a complete sclerotic rim (arrow) in the trochanteric and neck area of the femur. (**f**) T2-weighted MR image reveals intermediate SI of the solid lesion (black asterisk) with higher to bright SI of the cyst (red asterisks), indicating FD with either type of cystic change. (**g**) Microscopic examination also demonstrates two distinct components of FD and secondary ABC rather than nonspecific cyst. (**h**) Radiograph at 2 years after extended curettage and allogenic bone grafting without adjuvant therapy followed by internal fixation shows consolidation of the lesion with no evidence of recurrence

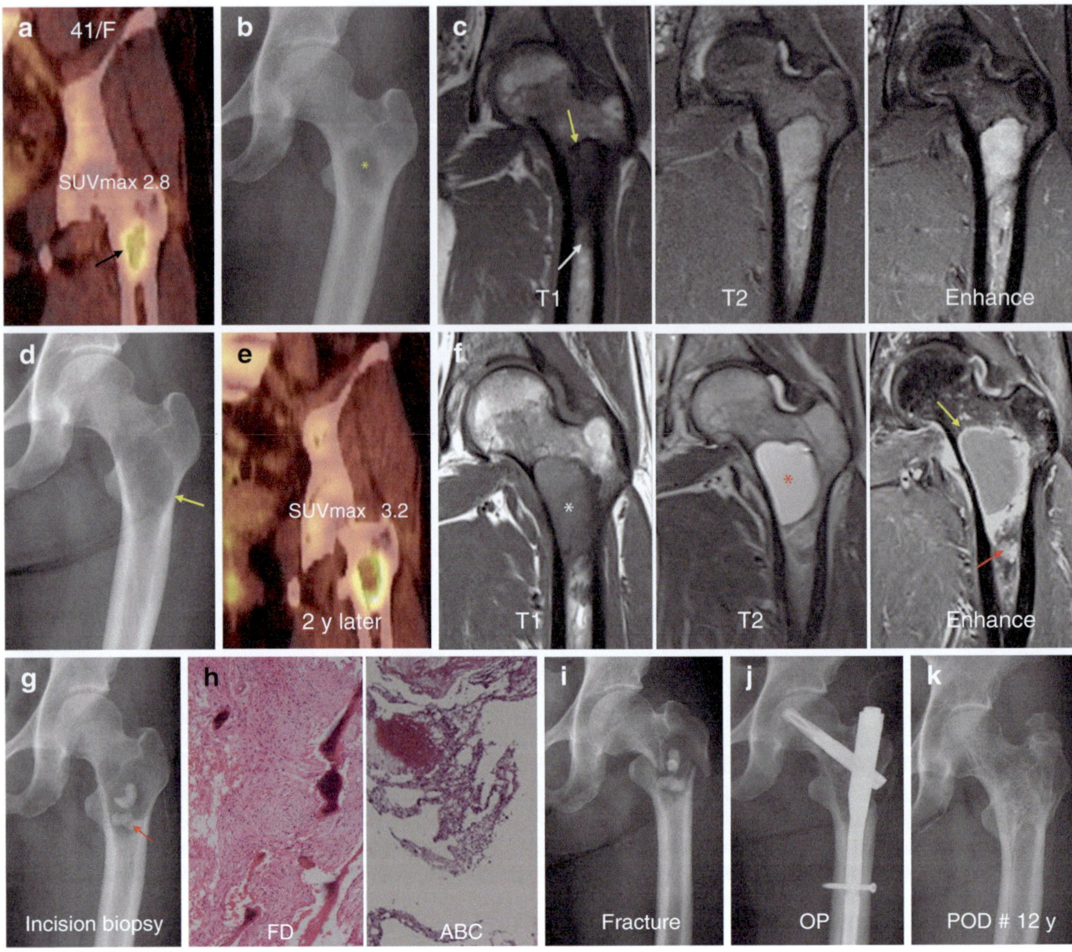

Fig. 26.19 ***ABC change during follow-up***. (**a**) PET/CT scan for staging of known breast cancer in a 41-year-old woman incidentally shows moderately increased FDG uptake (SUVmax 2.8) along the sclerotic shell of the medullary lesion (black arrow) with inner FDG-void region, indicating a less active benign bone lesion in the left proximal femur. (**b**) Radiograph reveals an ill-defined radiolucent lesion with *ground-glass* density (asterisk). (**c**) MR images note a proximally well-defined and distally ill-defined lesion with low to intermediate SI on T1-weighted image and intermediate to high SI on T2-weighted image. The proximal margin of the lesion is surrounded by a thin dark signal of sclerotic rim (yellow arrows), whereas the distal margin is not defined by a sclerotic rim. The lesion is diffusely well enhanced (asterisk). The image studies suggested FD, and surgical management including biopsy was not performed because she was free of pain at this time. (**d**) Two years later, follow-up radiograph taken for newly developed right hip pain of 2 week's duration reveals that the lesion has become larger and more radiolucent with deep endosteal scalloping and cortical thinning (arrow) compared with the initial radiograph, suggesting more aggressive secondary change of FD such as either form of cystic change or even malignant transformation. (**e**) Follow-up PET/CT scan shows slightly increased FDG uptake (SUVmax increased to 3.2). (**f**) MR images reveal an increased size of the lesion (asterisks) with low to intermediate SI on T1-weighted image and high SI on T2-weighted image. The proximal lesion is only peripherally enhanced suggesting either form of cystic change (yellow arrow), whereas the distal lesion is heterogeneously well enhanced indicating a preexisting solid lesion (red arrow). (**g**) Incision biopsy followed by cement plugging to prevent bleeding (arrow) was performed to distinguish a nonspecific cyst from a more aggressive ABC. (**h**) Microscopic examination shows an area of sparse bone spicules embedded in bland fibrous stroma suggesting FD and another area of secondary ABC rather than nonspecific cystic change. (**i**) Pathologic fracture occurred with a slip at 1 week after biopsy. (**j**) Extended curettage and allogenic chip bone graft followed by closed reduction with internal fixation using a proximal femoral nail was performed. (**k**) Follow-up radiograph at 12 years after surgery reveals consolidation of the lesion with no local recurrence

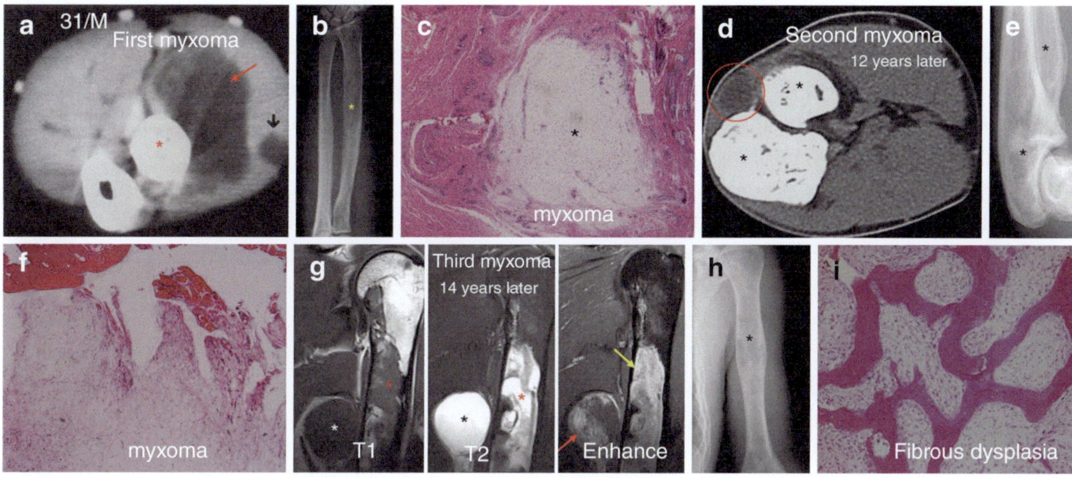

Fig. 26.20 ***Metachronous multiple myxomas. The first myxoma:*** (**a**) CT scan taken for a slowly growing mass of the right forearm during 6 months in a 31-year-old man shows a large intramuscular lucent mass (red arrow) with a satellite small lucent mass (black arrow). The large mass is adjacent to the sclerotic lesion fully obliterating the medullary space of the radius (asterisk). (**b**) Radiograph reveals an ill-defined mildly expanding lesion with *ground-glass* density involving nearly the entire radius, suggesting FD (asterisk). (**c**) Microscopic examination of excised intramuscular soft tissue mass demonstrates a myxoid mass with abundant mucoid material and loose reticulin fibers and an infiltrative indistinct margin, which is consistent with intramuscular myxoma (asterisk). ***The second myxoma:*** (**d**) Twelve years later, CT scan taken for newly developed mass of the right forearm shows a lucent soft tissue mass (red circle) neighboring the sclerotic medullary lesions of both ulna and radius (asterisks). (**e**) Radiograph reveals a mildly expanding lesion with *ground-glass* density and diffuse cortical thinning, indicating FD (asterisks). (**f**) Microscopic examination of excised mass also notes the same findings of previously excised intramuscular myxoma. ***The third myxoma:*** (**g**) Another 2 years later, MR images taken for a newly deveoped third mass of the left upper arm demonstrate a well-defined round to oval soft tissue mass (asterisks) with low SI on T1-weighted image and high SI on T2-weighted image. The mass is also typically located in the vicinity of the mildly expanding humerus lesion (red asterisks) with heterogeneous intermediate SI on T1-weighted image and heterogeneous bright SI on T2-weighted image. The soft tissue mass (red arrow) and bony lesion (yellow arrow) are heterogeneously well enhanced. (**h**) Radiograph notes a mildly expanding lesion with a typical *ground-glass* density (asterisk). (**i**) Microscopic examination shows classic findings of FD of the humerus. The excised mass is also confirmed as a myxoma. Note that all myxomas are located in the vicinity of the long bones affected with FD

polyostotic FD rather than the monostotic form. Most patients have intramuscular myxoma(s) most often located in the vicinity of the bone lesions [48] (Fig. 26.20). The syndrome usually occurs in adults aged 17 to 82 years adults aged a mean age of 46 years in reported cases. Intramuscular myxomas are multiple in the majority of cases, which grow slowly and are usually painless. Recently, the prevalence of MS is reported to be 2.2% (32 patients) in a multicenter study of 1446 patients with FD from the European Musculo-Skeletal Oncology Society (EMSOS) [5]. MS was diagnosed at a mean of 10 years after diagnosis of FD, and myxomas were predominantly localized in the upper leg. The authors identified GNAS mutations in the myxoma tissue in 5 of 6 patients (83%), possibly suggesting a common origin of FD and myxomas. Local recurrence of myxoma occurred in 6 of 20 patients in whom surgical resection was performed (30%) at a median of 8.5 years (range, 1.9–16.0 years). High cellularity of myxoma was associated with recurrence. The authors failed to find malignant change in their review of 32 patients with MS. However, 7 cases of malignant change from FD in the setting of MS have been sporadically reported with more than 100 reported cases to date, and OSA was the most common malignant diagnosis [41]. However, malignant change from myxomas in the setting of MS has never been identified to date.

4. **Fibrocartilaginous Dysplasia (FD with Enchondroma-Like Nodules)**

In earlier 1930, Telford [49] first fully documented the occurrence of cartilaginous differentiation described as masses of cartilage in FD. And in 1942, Lichtenstein and Jaffe [50] described a cartilage component which was thought to be an integral part of the dysplastic process in FD. Decades later in 1980, Pelzmann et al. [51] reported a case of polyostotic FD with an exceptionally large amount of hyaline cartilage, and called it *fibro-chondrodysplasia*. Years later in 1984, Dahlin and colleagues [52] described a new entity of 5 cases previously classified with FD consisting of fibro-osseous and extensive cartilage components and termed it as *fibrocartilaginous mesenchymoma with low-grade malignancy*, because of unusual histologic features with propensity of local recurrence in some cases. However, Bulychova et al. [53] did not find any instances showing malignant behavior or distant spread although it may recur in longer term follow-up study of 12 patients. Thus, the authors favored to call *fibrocartilaginous mesenchymoma* (FCM) of bone. Ishida and Dorfman [54] suggested this phenomenon should be considered as a variant of FD rather than a distinct bone tumor based on their observation of massive chondroid differentiation, and designated the lesion as *fibrocartilaginous dysplasia* (FCD) or *FD with massive cartilaginous differentiation*. It has been well known that hyaline cartilage islands similar to growth plate or enchondroma (EC) are often seen in a fibro-osseous lesion [1, 9, 15, 16, 55–57]. To date, there have been controversies in the literature regarding FCM as a separate neoplasm or one that coincides with FCD [1, 58–60]. Gambarotti and colleagues [61] reported, however, that FCM was genetically related to FCD, based on their molecular investigation finding of no GNAS (guanine nucleotide-binding protein α-stimulating polypeptide) mutation in FCM, which is known to be characteristic of FCD. The authors concluded FCM did not seem to be related genetically to FD, low-grade OSA, and dedifferentiated CSA. More recently in 2020, FCM was listed as an independent tumor entity in the WHO classification of bone tumors [62]. The incidence of FCD is extremely rare. There is a sharp demarcation between the cartilage nodules and fibro-osseous tissue, but it can be frequently detached by curettage during surgery. The amount of cartilage varies from case to case, and the exact ratio of the cartilage and fibro-osseous tissue has not been proposed for the diagnosis. Generally, the cartilage nodules are small less than 1 cm in diameter, but the chondroid differentiation can be massive in amount and large in size reaching several centimeters in diameter on rare occasion [12, 50], which may be mistaken for benign or even malignant cartilage tumor. The cartilage islands, between 0.1 and 3.0 cm in diameter, were present in 14% of patients with polyostotic form and in none of the patients with monostotic form in a large series of FD [12]. However, another series with eight cases of FCD (massive chondroid differentiation in FD) reported that only two cases occurred in polyostotic FD and six cases in the monostotic FD [54]. The average age of the patients was 15.3–17.5 years, ranging from 4 to 26 years, and the lesion usually occurred in the proximal femur as the common site, followed by the fibula, tibia, or humerus. The individual cells in cartilage islands may show mild to moderate atypism with high cellularity, binucleated chondrocytes, and plump chondrocytes in focal areas, which may be misinterpreted as benign or even malignant cartilage tumor particularly if the cartilage differentiation is extensive and a general pathologist is not aware of this phenomenon. The cartilage islands exhibit an enchondral ossification at the periphery resembling a growth plate, which merge with the adjacent fibro-osseous lesion of typical FD (Fig. 26.21). This finding is not usually seen in true cartilage tumor, and the cartilage islands in EN are partially or completely typically encased by various thickness of reactive host lamellar bone at the periphery of cartilaginous lobules, so-called *lamellar bone encasement* pattern. In addition, the individual lobules are also separated by normal bone marrow spaces with hematopoietic

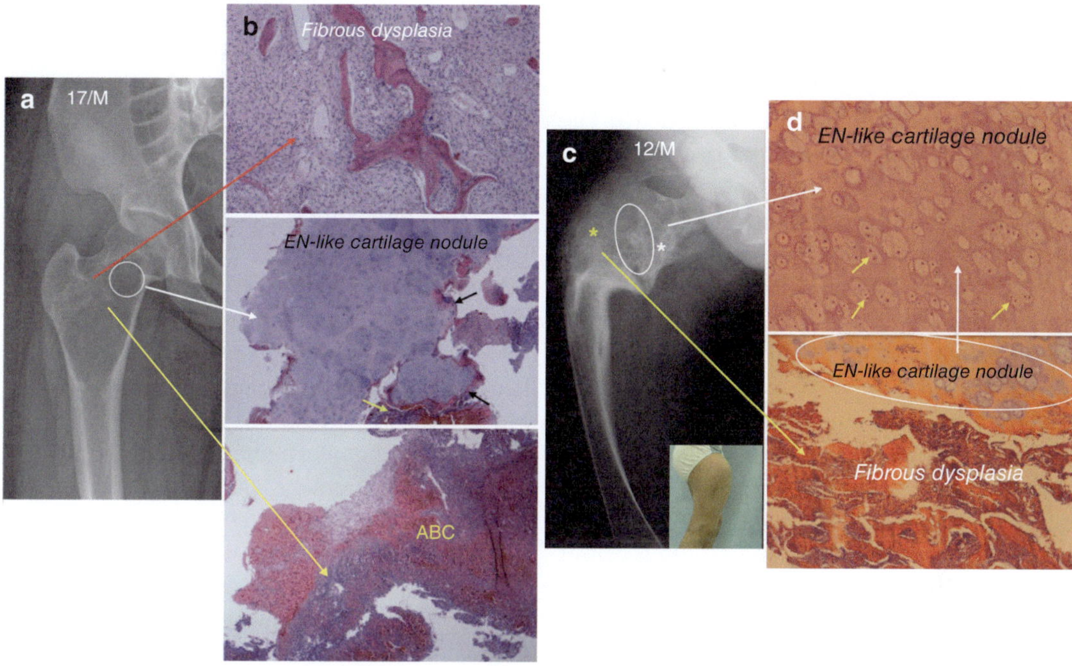

Fig. 26.21 (**a**) Radiograph taken for right hip pain of 2 weeks' duration in a 17 year-old adolescent shows a mostly radiolucent geographic lesion with focal *ground-glass* density to sclerotic area and stippled calcification (circle) abutting the apophyseal plate which is still partially opened. (**b**) Microscopic examination reveals features of typical FD and extensive EC-like cartilage nodules, as well as secondary ABC, corresponding to the *ground-glass* density, stippled calcification, and radiolucent area on radiograph, respectively. While the cartilage islands of EC are typically encased by reactive host lamellar bone of varying degree periphery and separated by normal bone marrow spaces with hematopoietic elements, the nodules of FCD reveal peripheral endochondral ossification (black arrows) adjacent to the fibro-osseous elements of FD (yellow arrow). (**c**) Radiograph taken for right hip deformity with limping gait in a 12-year-old boy demonstrates an expansile lesion with *ground-glass* density to dense sclerosis (asterisk), internal flocculent calcifications, and focal radiolucency (circle). There is also a dense sclerotic area of a healing callus by repeated microfracture (white asterisk). Severe coxa vara with shepherd's crook deformity is also noted. (**d**) Microscopic examination reveals areas of massive cartilage differentiation producing EC-like cartilage nodules adjacent to areas of typical FD, which were detached by curettage during surgery (Bottom). Higher-power view of an individual cartilage nodule shows moderately increased cellularity with mild atypia and frequent binucleated chondrocytes (arrows), which can be mistaken for low-grade CSA if the FD area is absent due to inadequate biopsy or of lack of this phenomenon (Top)

elements. Thus, it is very important to identify the fibro-osseous elements of FD adjacent to the cartilage nodules with peripheral ossification to avoid the misdiagnosis of EC or CSA in cases with a dominant cartilage component. The cartilage nodules may arise from the epiphyseal rests, direct spontaneous metaplasia of the fibrous tissue, or abortive callus formation after trauma or fracture [12]. FD could produce cartilage nodules embedded in the fibroblastic stroma if the lesion abuts the epiphyseal plate in a growing child. To date, the other reported fibrous tumors with similar phenomenon have included desmoplastic fibroma [63] and low-grade FSA of bones [64]. The possible developmental modes of cartilage nodules in parent fibrous tumors including FD, desmoid tumor, and FSA were suggested by Mirra [65]. The hypothesis is as follows: (1) The fibrous lesion abuts the growth plate during the growth phase. (2) The lesion interferes with physiologic endochondral ossification along the metaphyseal side of the physeal plate. (3) The interference with the normal physiologic processes leads to lack of normal calcification of the growth plate cartilage. (4) The abnormal calcification process results in the deposition of poorly calcified nodules within the metaphysis analogous to those seen in EC. (5) The cartilage nodules derived from the physis are embedded in the parent fibrous tumor that abuts the plate. (6) The nodules grow within the fibrous stroma and become variably calcified. (7) After years, the growth of calcified cartilage nodules stops spontaneously. However, malignant change to CSA should be suspected if growth continues.

5. **Regressed or Ancient FD**

With time, mesenchymal cells that carry GNAS mutations undergo apoptosis and GNAS-mutated skeletal stem cells diminish, leading to regression of FD. The classic *ground-glass* appearance on radiograph changes into a denser and sclerotic pattern with extensive rim of sclerosis or faintly lucent with irregular rind of sclerosis [4]. The enlarged fibro-osseous masses usually cause cortical thinning and scalloping as well as expansile remodeling. The rind of reactive sclerosis varies from thin to extensive and may be interrupted or incomplete. Histologically, most areas have significantly diminished stromal cells and dysplastic bone spicules with prominent foamy histiocytes, but the typical area of FD remains only in small foci, suggesting, regression of the lesion (Fig. 26.22). Kuznetsov et al. [36] proposed the novel concept of *normalization* of FD. Interestingly, the authors observed a completely normal histology with hematopoietic cells and adipocytes in 4 out of 7 specimens, and nondescript fibrotic change along with normal bone trabeculae in the rest, whereas bone scintigraphy and radiographic images still show mild activity and a hazy appearance of FD in older patients (35–52 years of age). As a lesion ages, the mutated stem cells fail to self-renew, and their progeny are consumed by apoptosis but residual normal stem cells survive, self-renew, and form a normal structure.

6. **Pseudoanaplastic FD**

Anaplasia includes the histologic characteristics that typify cancer, and consists of sufficient nuclear, cytoplasmic, and mitotic pleomorphism to enable a trained pathologist to recognize the lesion as malignant. Extremely rarely, similar cytological aberrations lacking atypical mitoses can be seen in a number of benign bone lesions such as giant cell tumor [66], osteoblastoma [65–68], chondromyxoid fibroma [65, 69], and fibrous cortical defect [65, 66] as well as FD [66]. The terms *pseudoanaplastic* or *pseudomalignant* have been used to describe those pleomorphic but benign tumors which typically lack atypical mitoses and follow a benign clinical course, for which only conservative surgical management is necessary. A diagnostic guideline for *pseudoanaplastic* tumors of bone was suggested as follows [66]. Firstly, mitotic figures should not present, or should be extremely scarce and typical if they exists. Rare cases may contain a few typical mitoses, but far fewer than would be expected for bizarre, highly anaplastic-looking true malignant tumors. Careful attention should be paid to distinguish true abnormal mitoses and karyorrhectic pseudomitoses. Special immunohistochemical stains for cellular proliferation, such as Ki-67, can be useful. Because the majority of lesions with significant cytological aberrations are true sarcomas, another adequate biopsy should be recommended if the first biopsy sample is inadequate, particularly when obtained using core or trocar biopsy. Secondly, the clinical and radiographic features should be within the range of the benign lesion being considered *pseudoanaplastic*. Such lesions are generally small to moderate in size with a complete surrounding rim of sclerosis, growth is absent to imperceptible, or it may be found incidentally during evaluation for another process. Finally, the clinical behavior of the lesion should be benign without any evidence of aggressive local recurrence in bone and/or adjacent soft tissue, regional or distant metastases. Out of over 4000 cases of bone tumors retrieved from the personal database of Mirra, only 15 cases (0.35%) met these criteria [66].

7. **Malignant Transformation**

In general, the potential for malignant transformation has been estimated to be 1% in the monostotic form, but the frequency increases with the polyostotic form. In the Mayo Clinic series, 13 of 28 (46%) cases of malignancies in FD had

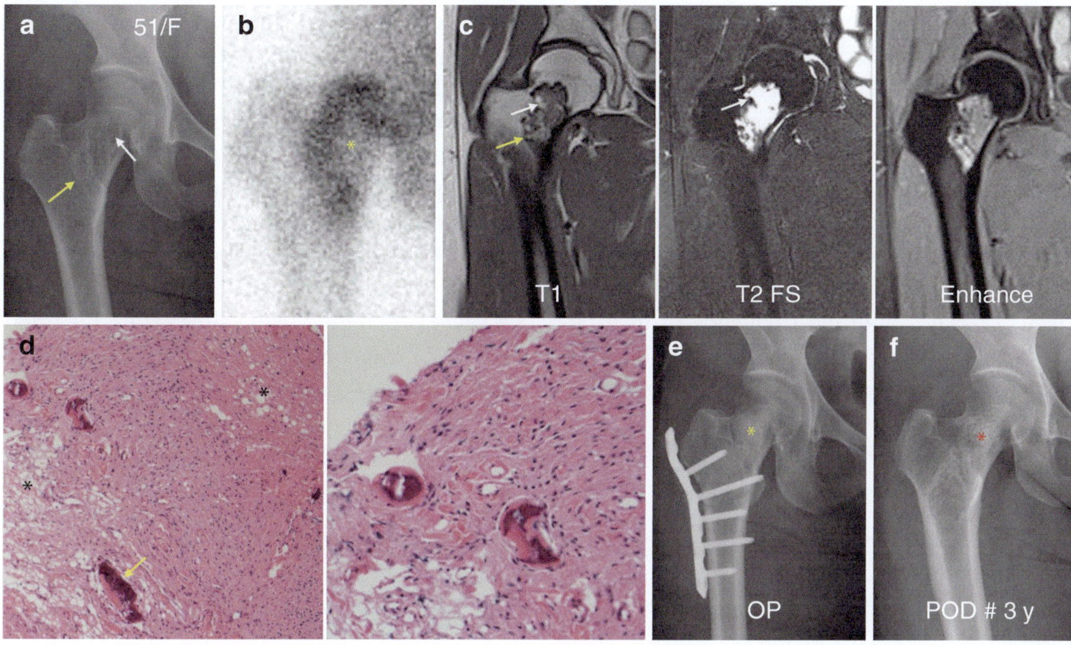

Fig. 26.22 (**a**) Radiograph taken for right hip pain of 4 months' duration in a 51-year-old woman shows a relatively well-defiend, faintly lucent lesion absent of typical *ground-glass* density but with an abnormal trabecular pattern (white arrow) surrounded by an irregular rim of sclerosis (yellow arrow) in the femoral head and neck. (**b**) Pinhole scan view reveals marginally increased uptake photon defect in the center (yellow asterisk). (**c**) MR images demonstrate a relatively well-defined medullary mass-like lesion with low SI on T1-weighted image and bright SI on fat-saturated T2-weighted image. There is a focal high signal on T1-weighted image which appears as a focal low signal on T2 FS image (white arrows), possibly indicating a small amount of fat tissue. The lesion is surrounded by a dark signal of thin rim of sclerosis which is partially destructed and incomplete (yellow arrow), suggesting a long-standing benign lesion with regression. The lesion is heterogeneously enhanced by contrast medium. (**d**) Microscopic examination: (Left) Lower-power magnification notes bland spindle cell stroma with small and sparse woven bone spicules (yellow arrow) and focal areas of fat cell aggregation (black asterisks). (Right) Higher magnification reveals a paucity of small spicules of partly calcified woven bone with a Pagetoid appearance devoid of osteoblastic rimming embedded in more or less cellar stroma with some blood vessels, suggesting regression of the lesion. (**e**) Curettage with allogenic chip bone graft and plate fixation for prevention of perioperative fracture was performed because of moderate but bothersome hip pain. (**f**) Follow-up radiograph at 3 years after surgery shows consolidation of the lesion and she is free of hip pain

received irradiation before the sarcoma developed, and thus these can be considered post-irradiation sarcoma. The rate of malignant change was 1.9% in the monostatic form but 6.7% in the polyostotic form [38]. The malignant tumor associated with FD usually develops in the third or fourth decade of life. The most frequent anatomic sites were the craniofacial bones and the proximal femur followed by the tibia and the humerus, which correlates with the frequency of distribution of bones involved in FD. The interval between irradiation and the occurrence of sarcoma ranged from 3 to 52 years with a mean of 19 years. OSA is the most common type of tumor followed by FSA and CSA [38, 40]. Patients with Mazabraud syndrome also have a high risk of malignant transformation up to 6–7% [41]. The outcomes are disappointing, with a lower overall survival rate compared with that of primary OSA. Pulmonary metastasis develops in most patients, and the mean survival is reported to be only 3.4 years [1]. In the Mayo Clinic series, the prognosis of malignancy in FD was also poor with a mortality rate of 53.6% [38].

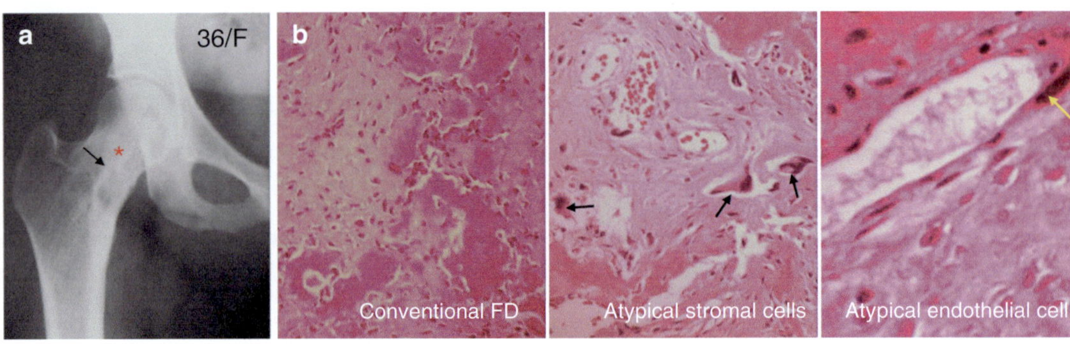

Fig. 26.23 (**a**) Radiograph taken for right hip pain in a 36-year-old woman shows a relatively well-defined radiolucent lesion with typical *ground-glass* density (asterisk) surrounded by a complete rim of sclerosis (arrow) in the medial aspect of the femoral neck, suggestive of a long-standing benign lesion, most consistent with FD. (**b**) Microscopic examination: (Left) This field reveals an area of conventional FD with variable bone spicules embedded in bland fibrous stroma. (Middle) another field shows several bizarre-looking, atypical cells with smudged nuclei (arrows). (Right) Higher-power magnification shows an atypical endothelial cell of the blood vessel (arrow). However, not a single mitosis was seen on all pathologic slides despite scrutinized observation. Both osteoblastic stromal cells and endothelial cells exhibit bizarre morphology with marked atypia, even though they are from different cell lineages, which possibly attributes to ischemia. The radiographic finding of benignancy with a complete rind of sclerosis, in correlation with the pathologic finding of bizarre-looking, atypical cells but no definite abnormal motoses, supports a diagnosis of *pseudoanaplastic FD*. The patient was treated with simple curettage and bone grafting, and the patient remains free of local recurrence or metastasis at 5 years after surgery (Courtesy by Dr. Mirra)

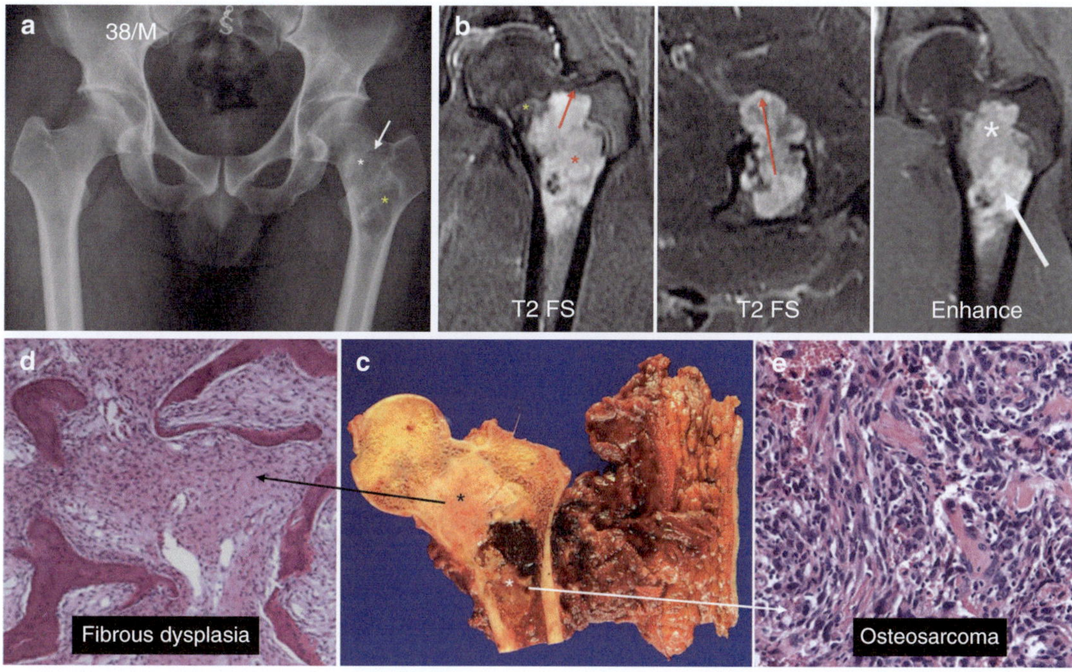

Fig. 26.24 (**a**) Radiograph taken for left hip pain of 3 months' duration in a 38-year-old man shows a focal area of *ground-glass* to sclerotic density (white asterisk) with an ill-defined, mildly expanding, osteolytic lesion (yellow asterisk), suggesting FD possibly with cystic or malignant change. In addition, a more aggressive-looking appearance with an incomplete surrounding rim of sclerosis and partial destruction (arrow) heralds more likely a malignant change. The patient denied a history of irradiation before the lesion developed. (**b**) Fat-saturated T2-weighted coronal image reveals an iill-defined, intramedullary lesion with intermediate to high SI and focal dark signal (red asterisk), which infiltrates into the adjacent marrow through the partially destructed surrounding rim of sclerosis (arrow). Note destruction of the cortex with naked soft tissue formation on axial view (red arrow). The proximal lesion is mildly enhanced (asterisk) and the distal lesion is more strongly enhanced (arrow). (**c**) Gross specimen from wide resection clearly demonstrates a proximal area of white to yellowish color (black asterisk) and a distal area of orange to red color (white asterisk) with dark clots of hemorrhage. Microscopic examination shows an area of typical FD (**d**) and another area of bizarre pleomorphic spindle cells, producing abundant osteoid to primitive woven bones with abnormal mitoses, indicating OSA (**e**). The preexisting FD is typically transformed to OSA without prior irradiation therapy

References

1. Czerniak B. Fibrous dysplasia and related lesions. In: Dorfman HD, Czerniak B, editors. Dorfman and Czerniak's bone tumors. 2nd ed. Elsevier; 2016. p. 570–616.
2. Stewart MJ, Gilmer WS, Edmonson AS. Fibrous dysplasia of bone. J Bone Joint Surg Br. 1962;44(2):302–18.
3. Riddle ND, Bui MM. Fibrous dysplasia. Arch Pathol Lab Med. 2013;137(1):134–8.
4. Kushchayeva YS, Kushchayev SV, Glushko TY, Tella SH, Teytelboym OM, Collins MT, et al. Fibrous dysplasia for radiologists: beyond ground glass bone matrix. Insights Imaging. 2018;9(6):1035–56.
5. Majoor BC, van de Sande MA, Appelman-Dijkstra NM, Leithner A, Jutte PC, Vélez R, et al. Prevalence and clinical features of Mazabraud syndrome: a multicenter European study. J Bone Joint Surg. 2019;101(2):160–8.
6. Weinstein LS, Shenker A, Gejman PV, Merino MJ, Friedman E, Spiegel AM. Activating mutations of the stimulatory G protein in the McCune–Albright syndrome. N Engl J Med. 1991;325(24):1688–95.
7. Alman BA, Greel DA, Wolfe HJ. Activating mutations of Gs protein in monostotic fibrous lesions of bone. J Orthop Res. 1996;14(2):311–5.
8. Sakamoto A, Oda Y, Iwamoto Y, Tsuneyoshi M. A comparative study of fibrous dysplasia and Osteofibrous dysplasia with regard to GSα mutation at the Arg201 Codon: polymerase chain reaction-restriction fragment length polymorphism analysis of paraffin-embedded tissues. J Mol Diagn. 2000;2(2):67–72.

9. Mirra JM, Gold RH. Fibrous dysplasia. In: Mirra JM, editor. Bone tumors: clinical, radiologic, and pathologic correlations. 2nd ed. Philadelphia: Lea & Febiger; 1989. p. 191–266.
10. DiCaprio MR, Enneking WF. Fibrous dysplasia: pathophysiology, evaluation, and treatment. J Bone Joint Surg. 2005;87(8):1848–64.
11. Campanacci M. Fibrous dysplasia. In: Camapanacci M, editor. Bone and soft tissue tumors. Wien/New York: Springer-Verlag; 1999. p. 435–61.
12. Harris W, Dudley HR, Barry R. The natural history of fibrous dysplasia: an orthopaedic, pathological, and roentgenographic study. J Bone Joint Surg. 1962;44(2):207–33.
13. Leet AI, Chebli C, Kushner H, Chen CC, Kelly MH, Brillante BA, et al. Fracture incidence in polyostotic fibrous dysplasia and the McCune-Albright syndrome. J Bone Miner Res. 2004;19(4):571–7.
14. Albright F, Butler AM, Hampton AO, Smith P. Syndrome characterized by osteitis fibrosa disseminata, areas of pigmentation and endocrine dysfunction, with precocious puberty in females: report of five cases. N Engl J Med. 1937;216(17):727–46.
15. Jaffe HL. Fibrous dysplasia. In: Jaffe HL, editor. Tumors and tumorous conditions of the bones and joints. Phildelphia: Lea & Febiger; 1958. p. 117–42.
16. Jaffe H. Fibrous dysplasia of bone. Bull N Y Acad Med. 1946;22(11):588–604.
17. Schlesinger PT, Keats S, Ruoff AC III. Fibrous dysplasia: report of a case. J Bone Joint Surg. 1949;31(1):187–91.
18. Bahk WJ, Kang YK, Rhee SK, Chung YG, Lee AH, Bahk YW. Cystic fibrous dysplasia in the long bone. Orthopedics. 2007;30(10):871–3.
19. Bahk WJ, Mirra JM. Differential diagnostic value of "blue reticulated chondroid-like material" in aneurysmal bone cysts: a classic histopathologic analysis of 215 cases. Am J Clin Pathol. 2015;143(6):823–9.
20. Sanerkin N, Watt I. Enchondromata with annular calcification in association with fibrous dysplasia. Br J Radiol. 1981;54(648):1027–33.
21. Van Horn P Jr, Dahlin D, Bickel W, editors. Fibrous dysplasia: a clinical pathologic study of orthopedic surgical cases. Proc Staff Meet Mayo Clin. 1963:38, 175–189.
22. Chapurlat RD, Delmas PD, Liens D, Meunier PJ. Long-term effects of intravenous pamidronate in fibrous dysplasia of bone. J Bone Miner Res. 1997;12(10):1746–52.
23. Liens D, Delmas PD, Meunier P. Long-term effects of intravenous pamidronate in fibrous dysplasia of bone. Lancet. 1994;343(8903):953–4.
24. Lala R, Matarazzo P, Bertelloni S, Buzi F, Rigon F, De Sanctis C. Pamidronate treatment of bone fibrous dysplasia in nine children with McCune-Albright syndrome. Acta Paediatr. 2000;89(2):188–93.
25. Pfeilschifter J, Ziegler R. Effect of pamidronate on clinical symptoms and bone metabolism in fibrous dysplasia and McCune-Albright syndrome. Med Klin. 1998;93(6):352–9.
26. Zacharin M, O'Sullivan M. Intravenous pamidronate treatment of polyostotic fibrous dysplasia associated with the McCune Albright syndrome. J Pediatr. 2000;137(3):403–9.
27. Plotkin H, Rauch F, Zeitlin L, Munns C, Travers R, Glorieux FH. Effect of pamidronate treatment in children with polyostotic fibrous dysplasia of bone. J Clin Endocrinol Metab. 2003;88(10):4569–75.
28. Boyce AM, Kelly MH, Brillante BA, Kushner H, Wientroub S, Riminucci M, et al. A randomized, double blind, placebo-controlled trial of alendronate treatment for fibrous dysplasia of bone. J Clin Endocrinol Metab. 2014;99(11):4133–40.
29. Chapurlat R, Legrand MA. Bisphosphonates for the treatment of fibrous dysplasia of bone. Bone. 2021;143:115784.
30. Stanton RP. Surgery for fibrous dysplasia. J Bone Miner Res. 2006;21(S2):P105–P9.
31. Enneking WF, Gearen P. Fibrous dysplasia of the femoral neck. Treatment by cortical bone-grafting. J Bone Joint Surg Am. 1986;68(9):1415–22.
32. Feuillan P. McCune-Albright syndrome. Curr Ther Endocrinol Metab. 1997;6:235–9.
33. Ippolito E, Bray EW, Corsi A, De Maio F, Exner UG, Robey PG, et al. Natural history and treatment of fibrous dysplasia of bone: a multicenter clinicopathologic study promoted by the European Pediatric Orthopaedic Society. J Pediatr Orthop B. 2003;12(3):155–77.
34. Stanton RP, Diamond L. Surgical management of fibrous dysplasia in McCune-Albright syndrome. Pediatr Endocrinol Rev. 2007;4:446–52.
35. Majoor BC, Andela CD, Bruggemann J, van de Sande MA, Kaptein AA, Hamdy NA, et al. Determinants of impaired quality of life in patients with fibrous dysplasia. Orphanet J Rare Dis. 2017;12(1):1–8.
36. Kuznetsov SA, Cherman N, Riminucci M, Collins MT, Robey PG, Bianco P. Age-dependent demise of GNAS-mutated skeletal stem cells and "normalization" of fibrous dysplasia of bone. J Bone Miner Res. 2008;23(11):1731–40.
37. Huvos A, Higinbotham N, Miller T. Bone sarcomas arising in fibrous dysplasia. J Bone Joint Surg. 1972;54(5):1047–56.
38. Ruggieri P, Sim FH, Bond JR, Krishnan Unni K. Malignancies in fibrous dysplasia. Cancer. 1994;73(5):1411–24.
39. Schwartz D. The malignant transformation of fibrous dysplasia. Am J Med Sci. 1942;247:1–20.
40. Yabut SM, Kenan S, Sissons HA, Lewis MM. Malignant transformation of fibrous dysplasia. A case report and review of the literature. Clin Orthop Relat Res. 1988;228:281–9.
41. Multani I, Popovic S, Parasu N, Ghert M. Osteosarcomatous transformation in the setting of

Mazabraud's syndrome: a case report and review of the literature. Case Rep Orthop. 2019;2019:2638478.
42. De Iure F, Campanacci L. Clinical and radiographic progression of fibrous dysplasia: cystic change or sarcoma? Description of a clinical case and review of the literature. La Chirurgia degli organi di movimento. 1995;80(1):85–9.
43. Fisher AJ, Totty WG, Kyriakos M. MR appearance of cystic fibrous dysplasia. J Comput Assist Tomogr. 1994;18(2):315–8.
44. Okada K, Yoshida S, Okane K, Sageshima M. Cystic fibrous dysplasia mimicking giant cell tumor: MRI appearance. Skeletal Radiol. 2000;29(1):45–8.
45. Simpson A, Creasy T, Williamson D, Wilson D, Spivey J. Cystic degeneration of fibrous dysplasia masquerading as sarcoma. J Bone Joint Surg Br. 1989;71(3):434–6.
46. Henschen F. Fall von ostitis fibrosa mit multiplen tumoren in der umgebenden muskulatur. Verh Dtsch Ges Pathol. 1926;21(2):93–7.
47. Mazabraud A, Semat P, Roze R. Apropos of the association of fibromyxomas of the soft tissues with fibrous dysplasia of the bones. La Presse medicale. 1967;75(44):2223–8.
48. Sundaram M, McDonald DJ, Merenda G. Intramuscular myxoma: a rare but important association with fibrous dysplasia of bone. Am J Roentgenol. 1989;153(1):107–8.
49. Telford E. A case of osteitis fibrosa (with formation of hyaline cartilage). Br J Surg. 1931;18(71):409–14.
50. Lichtenstein L. A condition affecting one, several or many bones, the Graver cases of which may present abnormal pigmentation of skin, premature sexualdevelopment, hyperthyuroidism or still other extra-skeital abnormalities. Arch Pathol. 1942;33:777–816.
51. Pelzmann K, Nagel D, Salyer W. Polyostotic fibrous dysplasia and fibro chondrodysplasia-case report 114. Skeletal Radiol. 1980;5(2):116–8.
52. Dahlin DC, Bertoni F, Beabout JW, Campanacci M. Fibrocartilaginous mesenchymoma with low-grade malignancy. Skeletal Radiol. 1984;12(4):263–9.
53. Bulychova IV, Unni KK, Bertoni F, Beabout JW. Fibrocartilagenous mesenchymoma of bone. Am J Surg Pathol. 1993;17(8):830–6.
54. Ishida T, Dorfman HD. Massive chondroid differentiation in fibrous dysplasia of bone (fibrocartilaginous dysplasia). Am J Surg Pathol. 1993;17(9):924–30.
55. Schajowicz F. Fibrous dysplasia. In: Schajowicz F, editor. Tumors and tumorlike lesions of bone and joints. New York: Springer-Verlag; 1981. p. 478–90.
56. Lichtenstein L. Polyostotic fibrous dysplasia. Arch Surg. 1938;36(5):874–98.
57. Schajowicz F. Tumors and tumor-like lesions of bone and joints. New York: Springer; 1981. p. 47–64.
58. Bhaduri A, Deshpande RB. Fibrocartilagenous mesenchymoma versus fibrocartilagenous dysplasia: are these a single entity? Am J Surg Pathol. 1995;19(12):1447–8.
59. Kyriakos M, McDonald DJ, Sundaram M. Fibrous dysplasia with cartilaginous differentiation ("fibrocartilaginous dysplasia"): a review, with an illustrative case followed for 18 years. Skeletal Radiol. 2004;33:51–62.
60. Lin J, Shulman SC, Steelman CK, Oskouei SV, Reith JD, Simoneaux SF, et al. Fibrocartilaginous mesenchymoma, a unique osseous lesion: case report with review of the literature. Skeletal Radiol. 2011;40:1495–9.
61. Gambarotti M, Righi A, Vanel D, et al. Fibrocartilaginous mesenchymoma of bone: a single-institution experience with molecular investigations and a review of the literature. Histopathology. 2017;71:134–42.
62. Gambarotti M, Inwards CY. Fibrocartilaginous mesenchymoma. In: WHO Classification of Tumours Editorial Board, editor. Soft tissue and bone tumours. 5th ed. Lyon: International Agency for Research on Cancer; 2020. p. 470–1.
63. Bahk WJ, Kang YK, Lee AH, Mirra JM. Desmoid tumor of bone with enchondromatous nodules, mistaken for chondrosarcoma. Skeletal Radiol. 2003;32:223–6.
64. Mirra JM. Fibrous tumors with enchondroma-like nodules. In: Mirra JM, editor. Bone tumors: clinical, radiologic, and pathologic correlations. 2nd ed. Philadelphia: Lea & Febiger; 1989. p. 674–90.
65. Mirra JM, Kendrick RA, Kendrick RE. Pseudomalignant osteoblastoma versus arrested osteosarcoma. A case report. Cancer. 1976;37(4):2005–14.
66. Bahk WJ, Mirra JM. Pseudoanaplastic tumors of bone. Skeletal Radiol. 2004;33(11):641–8.
67. Cheung F, Wu W, Lam C, Fu Y. Diagnostic criteria for pseudomalignant osteoblastoma. Histopathology. 1997;31(2):196–200.
68. Mitchell ML, Ackerman LV. Metastatic and pseudomalignant osteoblastoma: a report of two unusual cases. Skeletal Radiol. 1986;15:213–8.
69. Bahk WJ, Mirra JM, Sohn KR, Shin DS. Pseudoanaplastic chondromyxoid fibroma. Ann Diagn Pathol. 1998;2(4):241–6.

27 Liposclerosing Myxofibrous Tumor (LSMFT)

27.1 Definition

Liposclerosing myxofibrous tumor (LSMFT) is a benign bone lesion with distinct radiographic features and a complex mixture of diverse histologic paterns, showing a significant predilection for the intertrochanteric region of the femur.

27.2 Synonym

Polymorphic fibro-osseous lesion/polymorphic fibrous dysplasia (FD)/polymorphic fibrocystic disease.

27.3 Possible Pathogenesis

LSMFT may arise from involutional and ischemic changes in the altered fat of a lipogenic bone lesion with superimposed proliferative changes [1]. The lesion can be the end result of repeated reactions to stresses on the bone altered by a fibro-osseous proliferation such as FD [2]. It may occur by gene mutations of the α-subunit of the Gs protein (GNAS mutations) as in FD [3, 4].

27.4 Incidence

LSMFT is not described as a distinct entity in the WHO classification of soft tissue and bone tumors or major textbooks on orthopedic pathology. It is reported as rare, but the true incidence is likely higher than reported due to asymptomatic and incidentally found nature in many cases.

27.5 Age

The patients ranged widely from 15 to 80 years of age with a mean age of 42–46 years in major series dealing with LSMFT [1, 5].

27.6 Location

LSMFT has a striking predilection for the intertrochanteric region of the femur, occupying over 85% of cases [1, 5] (Figs. 27.1, 27.3, 27.4 and 27.5). Rarely, non-hip locations have also been eported in the femoral shaft, tibia, humerus, rib, pelvic bone, and cranial vault [1, 6–8] (Fig. 27.2).

W.-J. Bahk, *Diagnosis and Management of Primary Bone Tumors*,
https://doi.org/10.1007/978-981-96-3484-2_27

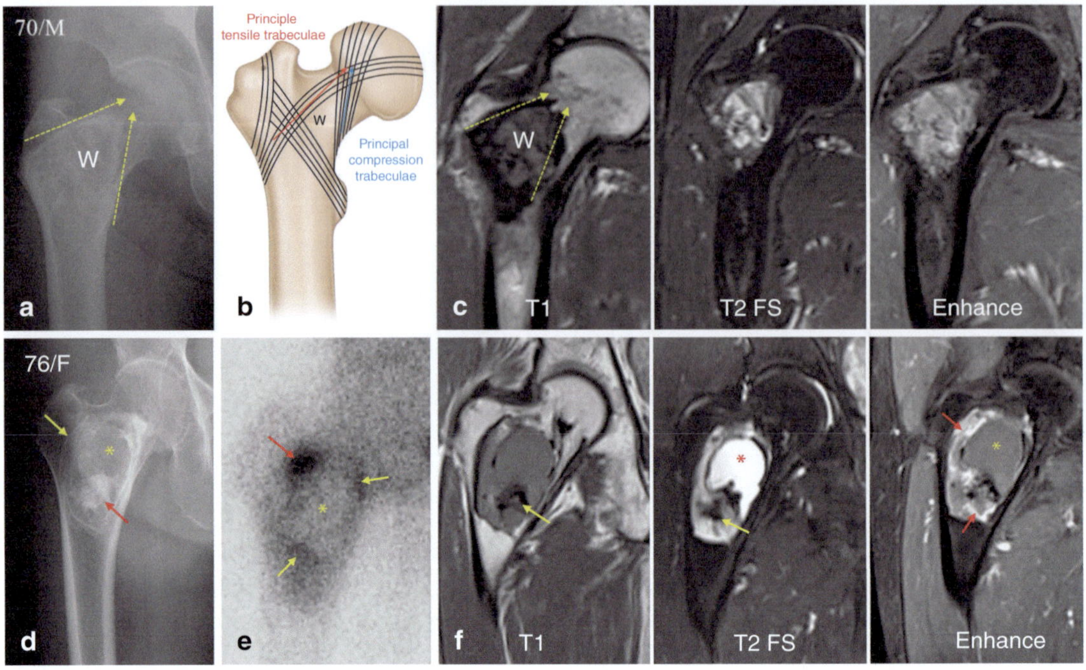

Fig. 27.1 ***Incidentally found on radiograph***. (**a**) Pelvis radiograph obtained as a part of routine radiographs for lower back pain with right sciatica in a 70-year-old man incidentally shows a well-defined, triangular-shaped lesion of *ground-glass* to sclerotic density with radiolucent foci in the femoral neck and trochanteric region. The full-size lesion exhibits prominent patchy-like central density and peripheral thick sclerosis with a tendency for the proximal border to forms a pointed cornical shape, producing the characteristic shape of ship's bow (dotted arrows) in Ward's triangle (W). (**b**) A schematic figure shows the lateral margin of the lesion running parallel to the principal tensile trabeculae (red arrow) and the medial margin paralleling the principal compression trabeculae (blue arrow). (**c**) MR images demonstrate a well-defined multilobulated lesion with low and intermediate SI on T1-weighted image and heterogeneous high SI on fat-saturated T2-weighted image. The lesion also presents the characteristic shape of the ship's bow (dotted arrows) in Ward's triangle (W). The lesion is heterogeneously enhanced by contrast medium. (**d**) Another pelvis radiograph obtained as a part of routine radiographs for lower back in a 76-year-old man also shows the incidental finding of a well-defined, radiolucent lesion with *ground-glass* density (asterisk) and internal dense opacification (red arrow), surrounded by a thin rim of peripheral sclerosis (yellow arrow) in the femoral neck and trochanteric region. (**e**) Pinhole bone scan reveals a focal hot uptake (red arrow) with mild uptake (yellow arrows) at the periphery of the lesion. However, most of the internal area shows a photon defect (asterisk). (**f**) MR images demonstrate a large, intramedullary mass-like lesion with intermediate SI on T1-weighted image and high SI with area of bright signal on fat-saturated T2-weighted image, suggesting cystic or myxoid change (red asterisk). There are internal dark signals of calcification on both images (yellow arrows). The lesion is focally enhanced (red arrows). The area with bright signal on T2-weighted image is not enhanced at all, even peripherally (yellow asterisk), suggesting a more likely myxoid rather than cystic change. (**g**) Microscopic examination notes (**a**) *myxofibrous* area with low cellularity and significant myxoid change occupying a large portion of the lesion, which reflects the bright signal on fat-saturated T2-weighted image and non-enhanced areas on contrast-enhanced image, (**b**) other small areas of fat cells with early fibrous change and focal osseous metaplasia, (**c**) combination of lamellar bones and pagetoid mosaic woven bones with fat cells, so-called *Liposclerosing* area, (**d**) abundant foamy macrophages, (**e**) scanty woven bone spicules reminiscent of FD, and (**f**) dystrophic calcification

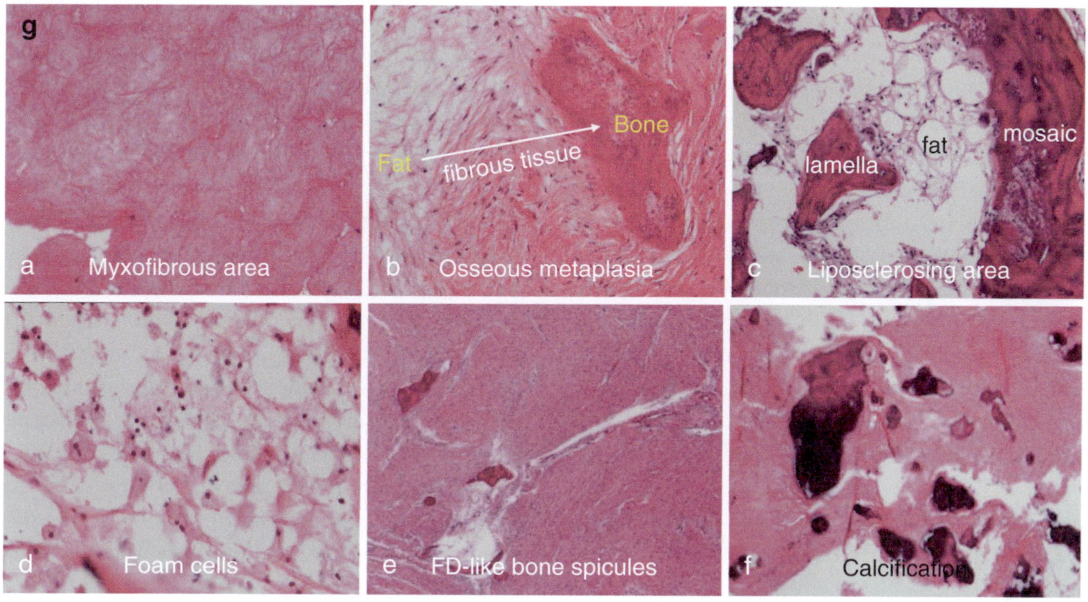

Fig. 27.1 (continued)

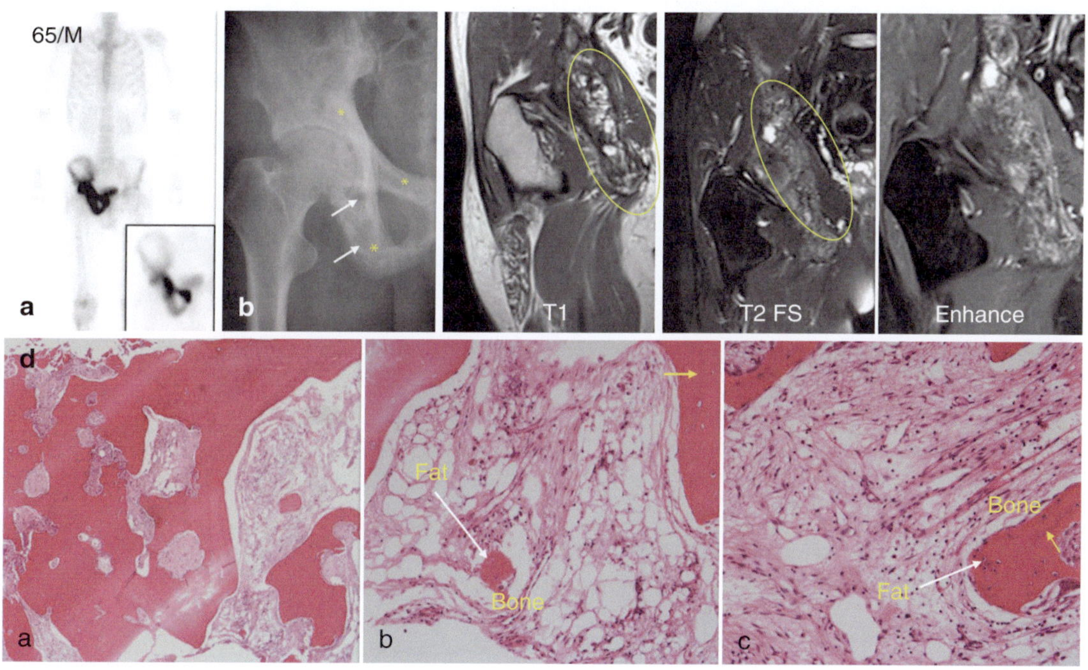

Fig. 27.2 ***Incidentally found on bone scan***. (**a**) Bone scan taken for evaluation of increased serum alkaline phosphatase on routine serum chemistry in a 65-year-old man shows an extensive area of strongly increased uptake in the right pelvic bones. (**b**) Radiograph reveals a mildly expansile sclerotic lesion (asterisks) in the right acetabulum, ischium, and pubic rami with focal radiolucent areas (arrows). (**c**) MR images demonstrate an ill-defined, mildly to moderately expansile, mass-like lesion with mixed low and high SI on both T1- and T2-weighted images (circles). The lesion is heterogeneously and focally enhanced. (**d**) Microscopic examination: (a) Low-power magnification shows heavy woven to lamellar bone formation with fibrous spindle cells and fat tissue, as well as focal myxofibrous areas. Higher-power magnification reveals abundant fat cells (b) and foamy macrophages (c). Some fat cells reveal early fibrous change and focal osseous metaplasia (white arrows). The lamellar bone spicules exhibit a mosaic pattern with hazy cement lines (yellow arrows)

27.7 Clinical Features

Although many lesions are incidentally found on imaging studies including plain radiograph (Figs. 27.1 and 27.5), bone scan (Figs. 27.2 and 27.5), or abdomen CT scan for other reasons, pain is the most frequent presenting symptom probably because of mechanical weakening of the bone secondary to abnormal osseous replacement (Fig. 27.3). An earlier series reported that approximately 40% of patients were incidentally found, pain was the most common presenting symptom in 48% of the patients, and pathologic fracture was associated in 10% of patients [1].

27.8 Radiologic findings

Plain radiogrpah are usually quite characteristic with a striking predilection for intertrochanteric and neck regions of the femur. Typically, radiograph reveals a well-defined radiolucent lesion of geographic destruction surrounded by a sclerotic rim with normal to mildly expanded bone contour, indicating an indolent growth pattern of benign bone tumor (Figs. 27.1, 27.2, 27.3, 27.4 and 27.5). The degree of sclerotic rim thickness, internal ground-glass density, or mineralized matrix is variable (Fig. 27.4). The degree of sclerosis is mild in 10% of cases, but the majority of lesions show considerable sclerosis, moderate in 60% and extensive in 30%, suggesting an old benign lesion [1]. The lesion in the intertrochanteric region and neck of the femur has a tendency to show a proximal border with a pointed cone-shape resembling a shape of ship's bow (Fig. 27.1a). The conical configuration is the consequence of reinforcement of normal trajectorial array proximal to the lesion in the Ward's triangle. The lateral margin of the lesion runs parallel to the principal tensile trabeculae and the medial margin parallels the principal compression trabeculae (Fig. 27.1b). This distinctive configuration can conclusively distinguish an LSMFT from other lesions if presents [9]. LSMFT may present a variety of patterns individually reminiscent of FD, fibroxanthoma, myxofibroma, lipoma, cyst, bone infarct, or Paget's disease. **Bone scan** shows heterogeneous mild to strong uptake of radioisotope within the lesion depending on the avidity of

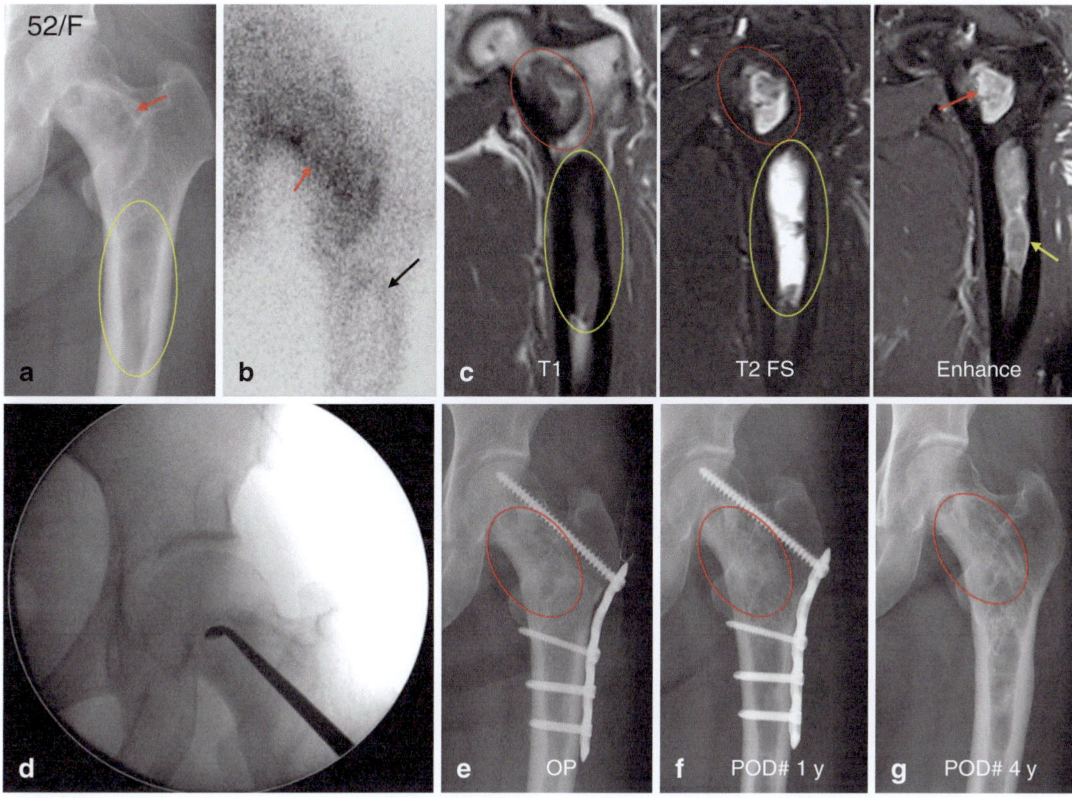

Fig. 27.3 ***Painful lesion***. (**a**) Radiograph taken for left hip pain of 3 months' duration in a 52-year-old woman shows two separated-looking radiolucent lesions with internal *ground-glass* density. The proximal lesion in the femoral neck area is well-defined by a thin complete rim of sclerosis (red arrow), but the distal lesion in the proximal shaft is ill-defined, lacking a discernible rim of sclerosis (yellow circle). (**b**) Pinhole bone scan reveals a focal moderate uptake in the proximal lesion, suggesting a focally active lesion (red arrow), and a faint peripheral uptake in the distal lesion, indicating a minimally active or stable lesion (black arrow). (**c**) MR images demonstrate a smaller proximal lesion (red circles) with low to intermediate SI on T1-weighted image and heterogeneous high SI with focal low signals on fat-saturated T2-weighted image. The larger distal lesion (yellow circle) shows intermediate SI on T1-weighted image and bright SI on T2-weighted image, suggesting cystic or myxoid change. The proximal lesion is heterogeneously enhanced (red arrow) suggesting a solid tumor, but distal lesion notes a thin peripheral enhancement, indicating possible cystic change. (**d**) Curettage followed by allo-chip bone grafting was performed under the guidance of a C-arm image intensifier in the proximal active lesion that was believed to be a cause of the hip pain. (**e**) Additional plate fixation was performed to prevent postoperative fracture. (**f**) Follow-up radiograph at 1 year after surgery shows a partial consolidation of the lesion. (**g**) Follow-up radiograph at 4 years after surgery shows a complete consolidation of the lesion with residual focal radiolucency. (**h**) Microscopic examination: (**a**) Low-power magnification shows a constellation of various tissue patterns including myxofibrous tissue with low cellularity, ischemic-bone with calcification, mosaic bone, fat cells, foamy macrophages with sclerotic change, and scanty woven bone spicules embedded in the fibrous background reminiscent of FD. Higher-power magnification reveals (**b**) early fibrous change from hypertrophic fat cells (black arrow) and focal metaplasia to woven bone spicules (white arrows), (**c**) the Pagetoid or mosaic bone of ischemic type with irregular mosaic lines (white arrow), (**d**) foamy macrophages, (**e**) area of fibrous tissue with sclerotic change and collagen production adjacent to the foamy cell-rich area (circle), and (**f**) area of bland fibrous tissue with scanty metaplastic woven bone (yellow arrows) reminiscent of FD that may not be found in many cases

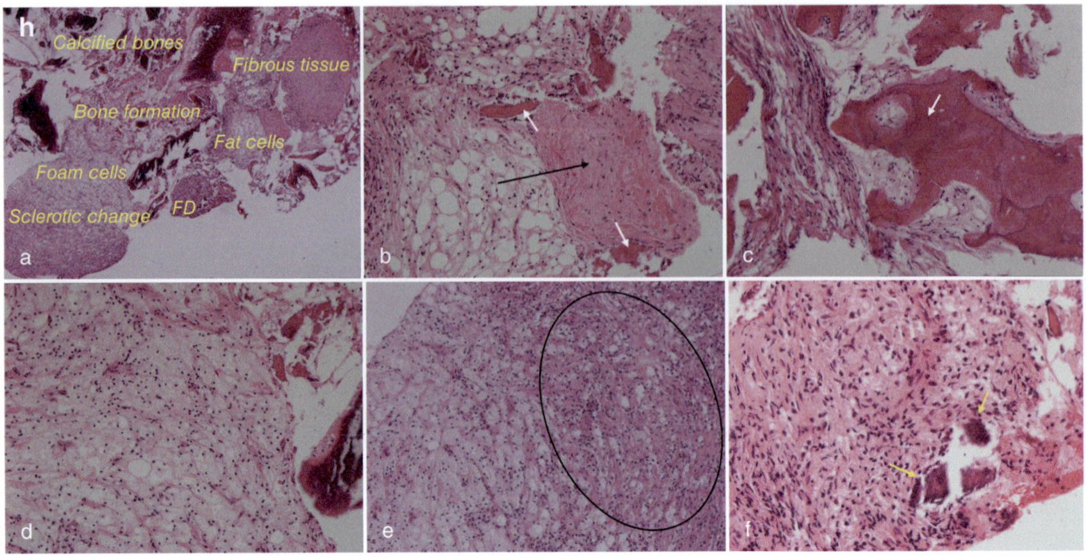

Fig. 27.3 (continued)

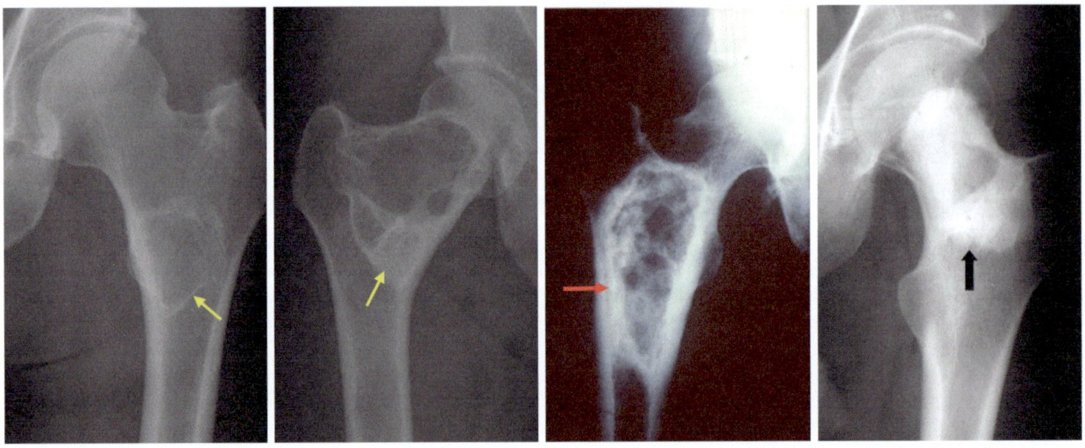

Fig. 27.4 ***Varying amounts of reactive sclerotic rim***. Plain radiographs show a geographic lesion of variable size and shape with a varying degree of *ground-glass* density, mineralized matrix as well as a thin (yellow arrows), moderately thick (red arrow), and significantly thick (black arrow) reactive rim of surrounding sclerosis

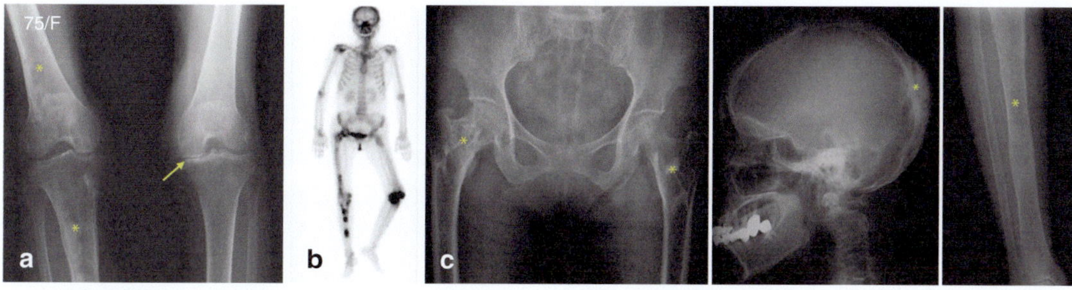

Fig. 27.5 ***Malignant change to FSA***. (**a**) Radiograph taken for left knee pain of 5 months' duration in a 75-year-old woman shows a severe narrowing of medial joint space with subchondral sclerosis (yellow arrow), indicating advanced osteoarthritis of the knee. Note the incidentally found lobular radiolucent lesions with an irregular *ground-glass* density in the contralateral right distal femur and proximal tibia (asterisks). (**b**) Bone scan reveals intense uptake at the left arthritic knee and other multiple areas of focal hot uptake at the right proximal and distal femur, proximal tibia, left seventh rib, and calvarium, suggesting a polyostotic lesion. (**c**) The corresponding radiographs of both proximal femurs, right tibia, and occipital bone show similar multiple lesions with *ground-glass* density and radiolucent foci, suggesting a polyostotic FD (asterisks). (**d**) Total knee replacement was performed for the left knee osteoarthritis, and other asymptomatic lesions were left to follow-up without biopsy. (**e**) MR images of the right hip demonstrate a huge irregular intramedullary lesion with heterogeneous low and intermediate SI on T1-weighted image and intermediate and high SI on T2-weighted image in the femoral neck, intertrochanteric area, and proximal diaphysis. There is no local aggressiveness such as discernible cortical breakage at that time. The lesion is peripherally and focally enhanced. (**f**) Follow-up radiograph at 18 months after the initial visit shows no definite interval change. However, radiograph taken for newly developed right hip pain at 30 months after the initial visit shows a more significant radiolucency proximally (circles) and a newly developed small lucent lesion distally (yellow arrow). In addition, there is significant cortical thinning and a possible breakage (white arrow). (**g**) Follow-up MR images at 30 months after the initial visit reveal diffuse spreading of the lesion with mild bony expansion, cortical thinning, and cortical breakage (white arrows). The lesion is more strongly enhanced than before with cortical breakage and enhanced soft tissue masses (yellow arrows). (**h**) Post-biopsy radiograph shows a pathologic fracture through the medial cortical breakage site (yellow arrow). Cement plug (asterisk) is visible in the biopsy site. (**i**) PET/CT scan reveals inhomogeneous high FDG activity (SUVmax 6.9) along the periphery of the lesion with a central FDG-void area, suggesting a probable malignant change of the benign preexisting lesion. In addition, multifocal low activities are noted in the right proximal tibia, left proximal femur and iliac bone, sternal manubrium, and T11 vertebra, suggesting a preexisting polyostotic benign lesion. (**j**) Limited surgery including resection of the fracture fragment with curettage followed by cementing, hemi-arthroplasty, and plate fixation was performed because the patient did not want more radical surgery. (**k**) Follow-up radiograph at 6 months after surgery shows multiple periprosthetic radiolucent areas, suggesting local recurrence (arrows). She died of disease progression with multiple pulmonary metastases. (**l**) Microscopic emanation demonstrates a complex mixture of various tissue patterns including: (**a**) Prominent fat and areas of fibrous sclerotic change with focal osseous metaplasia (inset). (**b**) Atypical bone formation with ischemic ossification (white asterisk) and myxofibrous stroma (black asterisk). There are curvilinear and circular metaplastic bone spicules typically reminiscent of FD (inset). (**c**) Woven bone spicules with irregular mosaic lines of calcification (Pagetoid bone), and xanthomatous change with foam cells and fat cells (inset). The abovementioned findings are indicative of LSMFT or ancient regressing FD. (**d**) In another area, a transitional area is clearly observed between the benign myxofibrous component and the pleomorphic malignant cell component. (**e**) Higher-power magnification reveals a hypercellular area with pleomorphic spindle cells arranged in a storiform pattern with abundant collagen production but no bone formation, indicating malignant transformation to FSA. This case of malignant change from LSMFT affecting the proximal femur in the setting of the polyostotic form suggests that LSMFT is likely an ancient regressing or a variant of FD rather than a distinct bone tumor, because there are areas with curvilinear and circular metaplastic bone spicules, typically reminiscent of FD and the polyostotic form of LSMFT has not been reported to date

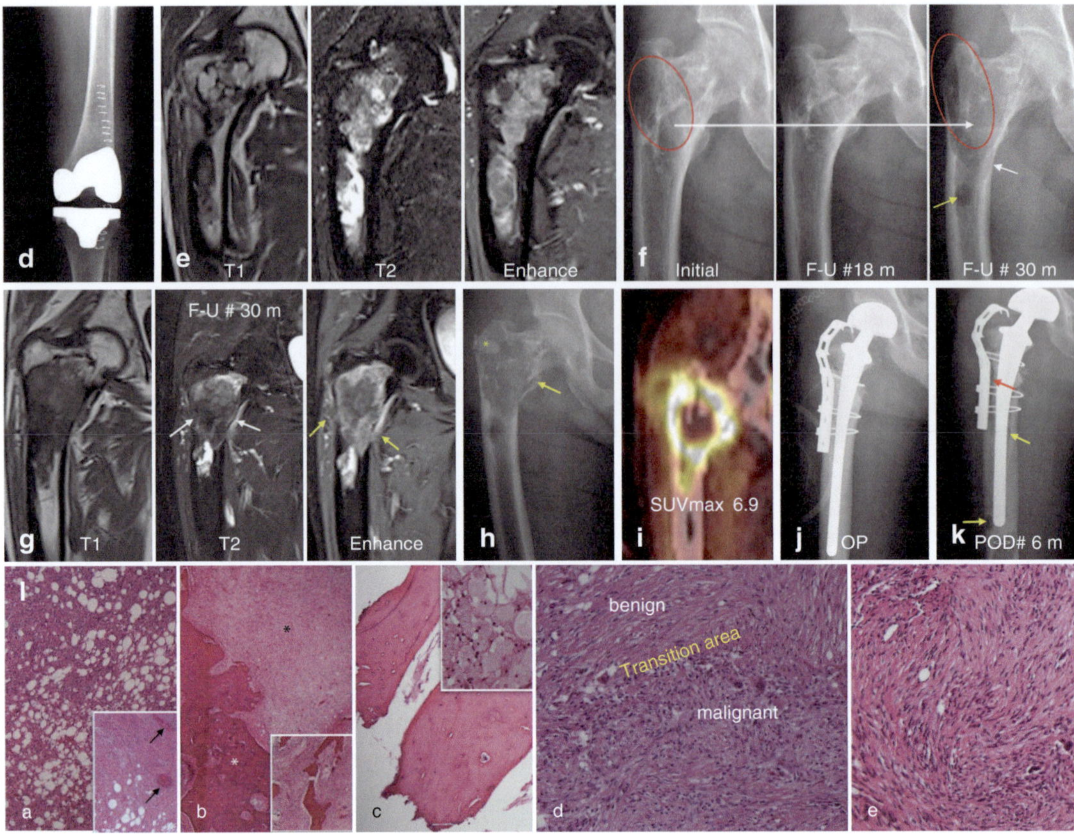

Fig. 27.5 (continued)

the lesion (Figs. 27.1, 27.2, 27.3 and 27.5). **MR findings** Despite the name including *Lipo*, distinct fatty components are usually not seen on MR images, probably because the lipomatous component is usually too small and mixed with other more prominent myxofibrous or fibro-osseous tissue [1]. The signal intensity (SI) is highly variable, depending on the amount of myxofibrous tissue, fat cells, various types and amount of bone spicules, calcification, and cystic change. However, in general, the SI is relatively homogeneous iso-intense to skeletal muscle on T1-weighted image and heterogeneous high due to prominent myxoid component on T2-weighted image with variable thickness of dark signal of peripheral sclerotic rim on both sequences. The lesion is heterogeneously or focally enhanced (Figs. 27.1, 27.2, 27.3 and 27.5).

27.9 Histologic Findings

A complex mixture of various tissue patterns, including fat, myxofibrous tissue, ischemic-bone with calcification, curvilinear trabeculae of woven bone in the fibrous background reminiscent of FD as well as woven bone spicules with irregular mosaic lines of calcification (Pagtoid bone), is observed. The area reminiscent of FD with curvilinear bone trabeculae embedded within the fibrous stroma may be absent in some cases. Other components such as fat necrosis, foamy macrophage (xanthoma cells), rounded cementum-like ossicles, cystic change, and rarely cartilage may also be seen [1, 2, 9–11]. The term "*LipoSclerosing*" refers to lesional bone within altered fat, consisting of lamellar, Pagetoid (mosaic), woven, and/or ischemic type, which is independent of reactive sclerotic bone (Figs. 27.1, 27.2 and 27.3). The term "*MyxoFibrous*" refers to myxoid areas of mucopolysaccharide-rich ground substance and fibrous areas of collagen, which may also have characteristic curvilinear and circular ossicles reminiscent of FD, and/or dystrophic calcification in the necrotic fat [1].

27.10 Clinical Relevance

In 1986, Ragsdale and Sweet [9] first described atypical ossifying fibrocystic lesions of almost site-specific proximal femoral variant under the term of *polymorphic FD* at that time. Years later, they used the more descriptive term "LSMFT" to cover the variety of tissue types that exceeds the usual FD [12]. Subsequently, Kransdorf et al. [1] accepted the lesion as a distinct bone tumor and described it in more details in 39 patients with LSMFT. However, Heim-Hall and Williams [2] suggested that LSMFT is a traumatized variant of FD. A wide variety of tissue patterns may represent reactive fibro-osseous proliferation caused by repeated stresses on bone, particularly in the proximal femur where weight-bearing stress is considerably higher than other bones. Furthermore, point mutation in the G-protein subunit or somatic mutation of the GNAS gene, which characterizes both monostotic and polyostotic FD, has also been observed in several cases of LSMFT [3, 4]. More recently, it is suggested that LSMFT may not be a distinct entity because the lesions almost always share histologic features of either FD or interosseous lipoma. Dattilo et al. [5] reported 12 patients with degenerative FD and 3 patients with degenerative intraosseous lipoma in their series. Thus, they suggested LSMFT may not be a distinct lesion and use of the term would be discontinued. Such studies support that LSMFT may be a variant or ancient regression of FD. However, other current reports indicate that the lesion would be considered as a separate lesion [13–16]. Whether LSMFT is a distinct entity remains controversial. To the best of my knowledge, polyostotic LSMFT has not been documented in the literature to date. However, my colleagues and I experienced a case with histologic features equivalent to LSMFT in the proximal fermus, which transformed to fibrosarcoma, in the setting of in the setting of polyostotic form on imaging studies (Fig. 27.5). Therefore, I would like to carefully suggest that LSMFT may be a variant of FD rather than a distinct entity in itself.

27.11 Management

Asymptomatic lesions do not require any surgical treatment, but biopsy and periodic follow-up are necessary due to higher incidence of malignant change. Simple curettage with bone graft or cement filling is indicated for painful lesions. Patients presenting with pathologic fracture usually require curettage and bone graft followed by open reduction with internal fixation or joint arthroplasty when the femoral neck is fractured.

27.12 Clinical Course

Typically, a favorable prognosis is expected after complete removal of the tumor in painful patients. However, a higher incidence of malignant change (10–16%) has been reported in patients with LSMFT when compared to that in patients with FD [1, 9, 10, 17], although the exact incidence is unknown and probably overestimated in a consultative series. The increased incidence of malignant change in LSMFT is likely attributed to its extensive involution and ischemic change [9]. The malignant change is thought to occur secondary to its involutional and ischemic damage or through increasing atypism of fibroxanthomatous components [1, 9]. Secondary sarcoma generally occurs in the reactive border of the ischemic bone marrow with transition area (Fig. 27.5l), as in infarction-associated sarcoma (Chap. 9). Reported secondary sarcomas from

LSMFT include conventional OSA, telangiectatic OSA, FSA, and MFH [1, 9, 10, 17, 18].

References

1. Kransdorf MJ, Murphey MD, Sweet DE. Liposclerosing myxofibrous tumor: a radiologic-pathologic-distinct fibro-osseous lesion of bone with a marked predilection for the intertrochanteric region of the femur. Radiology. 1999;212(3):693–8.
2. Heim-Hall JM, Williams R. Liposclerosing myxofibrous tumour: a traumatized variant of fibrous dysplasia? Report of four cases and review of the literature. Histopathology. 2004;45(4):369–76.
3. Matsuba A, Ogose A, Tokunaga K, Kawashima H, Hotta T, Urakawa S, et al. Activating Gs α mutation at the arg201 codon in liposclerosing myxofibrous tumor. Hum Pathol. 2003;34(11):1204–9.
4. Corsi A, De Maio F, Ippolito E, Cherman N, Robey PG, Riminucci M, et al. Clinical vignette: monostotic fibrous dysplasia of the proximal femur and liposclerosing myxofibrous tumor: which one is which? J Bone Miner Res. 2006;21(12):1955–8.
5. Dattilo J, McCarthy EF. Liposclerosing myxofibrous tumor (LSMFT), a study of 33 patients: should it be a distinct entity? Iowa Orthop J. 2012;32:35–9.
6. Choi JW, Kim CH, Choi JS, Lee YS, Kim HK, Yeom BW, et al. Liposclerosing Myxofibrous tumor in tibia-a case report and review of the literature. Korean J Pathol. 2005;39(3):207–10.
7. Ploof J, Shaikh H, Melli J, Jour G, Turtz A. Liposclerosing myxofibrous tumor of the cranial vault: a case report. Neurosurgery. 2019;84(3): E207–E10.
8. Regado ER, Garcia PBL, Caruso AC, de Almeida ALB, Aymoré IL, Meohas W, et al. Liposclerosing myxofibrous tumor: a series of 9 cases and review of the literature. J Orthop. 2016;13(3):136–9.
9. Ragsdale BD, Sweet DE. Bone. In: Henson E, Albores-Saavedra J, editors. The pathology of incipient neoplasia. Philadelphia: WB Saunders; 1986. p. 381–423.
10. Ragsdale BD. Polymorphic fibro-osseous lesions of bone: an almost site-specific diagnostic problem of the proximal femur. Hum Pathol. 1993;24(5):505–12.
11. Deel C, Hassell L. Liposclerosing Myxofibrous tumor: a review. Arch Pathol Lab Med. 2016;140(5):473–6.
12. Ragsdale BD, Sweet DE, Vinh TN. Radiology as gross pathology in evaluating chondroid lesions. Hum Pathol. 1989;20(10):930–51.
13. Abraham JA. Cystic and radiolucent bone lesion. In: Biermann JS, editor. Orthopaedic knowledge update musculoskeletal tumors 3. Rosemont: American Academy of Orthopaedic Surgeons; 2014. p. 92.
14. Saupe NM. Extra-articular conditions. In: Kim Y, Mamisch TC, editors. Hip magnetic resonans imaging. Berlin: Springer; 2014. p. 188–9.
15. Wei S, Siegal GP. Fibroosseous lesions. In: Wei S, Siegal GP, editors. Atlas of bone pathology. New York: Springer; 2013. p. 203–5.
16. Manaster BJ, David AM, David GD. Fibrous tumors and Tumorlike conditions. In: Manaster BJ, David AM, David GD, editors. Musculoskeletal imaging: the requisites. 4th ed. Philadelphia: Elsevier Saunders; 2013. p. 404.
17. Campbell K, Wodajo F. Case report: two-step malignant transformation of a liposclerosing myxofibrous tumor of bone. Clin Orthop Relat Res. 2008;466(11):2873–7.
18. Illac C, Delisle M-B, Bonnevialle P, Chiavassa-Gandois H, de Pinieux G, Gomez-Brouchet A, editors. Telangiectatic osteosarcoma secondary to a liposclerosing myxofibrous tumor: a case report. Ann Pathol. 2012;32(4):259–62.

28 Osteofibrous Dysplasia

(***osteo*** "bone" + ***fibrous*** "containing fibers" + ***dys-*** "bad," ***-plasia(plasis)*** "development")

28.1 Definition

Osteofibrous dysplasia (OFD) is a benign fibro-osseous lesion almost exclusively arising from the cortex of the mid-diaphysis of the tibia or fibula in children.

28.2 Synonyms

Ossifying fibroma/juvenile adamantinoma/intra-cortical fibrous dysplasia/Kempson-Campanacci lesion.

28.3 Possible Pathogenesis

Fibrous dysplasia (FD) and OFD sometimes share quite similar histologic findings and predilection for age of occurrence during childhood or adolescence. However, their exact nature has remained controversial for many decades. Mutations of the α-subunit of the Gsα stimulatory protein at the Arg201 codon have a role in the development of FD but not in OFD [1, 2]. The data suggest their pathogenesis is different, and detection of the Gs α mutation at the Arg201 codon is quite useful for distinguishing between these lesions. However, this test is not clinically required because a simple diagnostic triangle (clinical-radiologic-pathologic correlation) is sufficient to make an accurate diagnosis.

28.4 Incidence

OFD is rare, accounting for less than 1% of all bone tumors [3] and only about 0.2% of primary biopsy-proven bone tumors [4].

28.5 Age

The lesion is characterized by very early onset either at birth or in the first 2 decades of life [3–6], although ages have been reported to range from 3 weeks to 35 years in the Mayo Clinic series [7].

28.6 Location

OFD is almost exclusively localized to the anterior cortex of the tibia and/or fibula. Occasionally, the ipsilateral tibia and fibula can be simultaneously affected in up to 12% of cases, but isolated involvement of the fibula alone is very rare, representing only 3–7% [4, 7]. In extremely rare cases, both tibias are affected in 3% of OFD [4] (Fig. 28.3a). The ulna, radius, clavicle, and humerus have also been reported as extremely rare locations [8–13] (Fig. 28.6).

W.-J. Bahk, *Diagnosis and Management of Primary Bone Tumors*,
https://doi.org/10.1007/978-981-96-3484-2_28

28.7 Clinical Presentations

OFD is usually painless, and the most common presentation is localized swelling or protrusion of the anterior shin due to moderate expansion of the affected tibia often with anterior bowing of the leg. Stress or pathologic fracture is not infrequent [4–6]. Localized pain is the most common complaint in 25%, localized swelling is present in only 9%, and 12.5% of patients have sustained a pathologic fracture in a large series of 80 patients [7]. OFD can be incidentally found on radiograph obtained for unrelated reasons such as pain after a traffic accident, slip, or trivial injury (Figs. 28.4, 28.5, 28.6 and 28.7).

28.8 Radiologic Findings

Plain radiograph Typically, OFD shows a well-defined, eccentrical, cortical-based, osteolytic lesion extending into the medullary space occasionally with a *ground-glass* density surrounded by a sclerotic rim as seen fibrous dysplasia (FD). However, OFD exclusively arises from the anterior cortex of the diaphysis of the tibia and/or fibula, and often typically presents with with anterior bowing as well as cortical thinning and thickening (Figs. 28.1, 28.2, 28.3, 28.4 and 28.5). The varying degree of anterior bowing is usually present at the time of diagnosis, which may become more severe with sclerotic changes as the disease progresses after biopsy or simple curettage (Figs. 28.4 and 28.5). Generally, most lesions are oriented longitudinally parallel to the long axis of the bone (Figs. 28.1, 28.2, 28.3, 28.4, 28.5, 28.6 and 28.7). Initially, it may present as a single or multiple small lesion(s) confined to cortex (Fig. 28.1) or occasionally with focal medullary extension (Fig. 28.2). The multiple lesions become confluent to produce saw-toothed or bubbly multilobulated expansile osteolytic lesions (Figs. 28.3, 28.4, 28.5 and 28.6). At the time of diagnosis, many lesions can appear as large multilobulated shape with osteolytic foci spreading along the long axis of the anterior cortex and extensively extending into the medullary cavity. In more advanced cases, the radiographic appearance is typical, with an enlarged underlying bone, thinning or disappearance of the external cortex, sclerotic reaction on the medullary aspect, and medullary extension of the lesion producing a narrow medullary canal (Figs. 28.5, 28.6 and 28.7). An aggressive periosteal reaction is not seen in the absence of fracture. Stress or pathologic fracture is frequently associated (Figs. 28.4, 28.5 and 28.6). **Bone scan** and **SPECT scan** show a varying degree of increased uptake (Figs. 28.1, 28.2, 28.3, 28.4, 28.5, 28.6 and 28.7). **MR findings** are not specific but useful for assessing the extent of intramedullary involvement ranging from the lesion confined to the cortex to the more aggressive lesion with varying degrees of medullary extension or perilesional marrow and soft tissue edema. A mutilobulated appearance caused by internal low-signal bands with or without tiny dark foci is seen in the larger lesions (Figs. 28.3c and 28.6c). The cortical lesion can expand to the medullary cavity without aggressive cortical destruction and adjacent soft tissue extension if pathologic fracture is not associated. The signal intensity (SI) is intermediate on T1-weighted images and heterogeneous intermediate and high on T2-weighted images. All lesions present diffuse and heterogeneous moderate to strong enhancement by contrast medium (Figs. 28.1, 28.2, 28.3, 28.4, 28.5, 28.6 and 28.7).

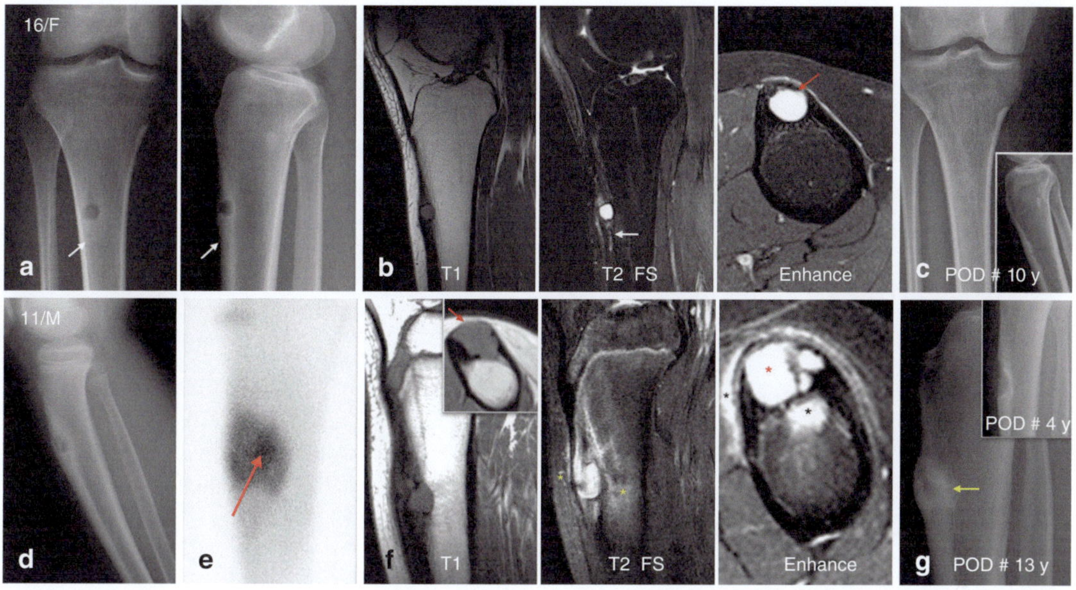

Fig. 28.1 ***Small lesion confined to the cortex with pain***. (**a**) Radiographs taken for the right leg swelling of 1 year's duration with newly developed pain in a 16-year-old girl show a small, well-defined, round to oval, radiolucent lesion surrounded by a thin rim of sclerosis with multiple tiny satellite lesions confined to the thickened cortex (arrows). (**b**) MR images reveal a well-defined, small, intracortical, round, main lesion with intermediate SI on T1-weighted image and bright SI on fat-saturated T2-weighted image, with a thin dark signal of sclerotic rim on both sequences. Several tiny satellite lesions are also seen (white arrow). Simple curettage was done for severe pain and frozen biopsy confirmed a diagnosis of OFD. (**c**) Follow-up at 10 years after simple curettage shows a complete healing of the lesion with remodeling of the anterior cortex. (**d**) Radiograph taken for painful swelling of the left proximal shin in a 11-year-old boy shows a multilobulated radiolucent lesion with a *ground-glass* density confined to the thickened anterior cortex of the proximal tibia. (**e**) Pinhole bone scan reveals a heterogeneous uptake in the lesion, suggesting an active lesion. (**f**) MR images demonstrate a well-defined, lobulated lesion confined to the thickened cortex with intermediate SI on T1-weighted image and bright SI on fat-saturated T2-weighted image. The anterior outer cortex is significantly thinning and almost disappeared on the axial image (inset). There are severe perilesional bone marrow and soft tissue edema (yellow arrows). Post-contrast image demonstrates strong enhancement of the intracortical lesion (red asterisk) as well as adjacent soft tissue and bone marrow edema (black asterisks). Intracortical abscess or OO was initially suspected over OFD because of uptake pattern on pinhole bone scan and marked perilesional and soft tissue inflammation with edema. However, frozen biopsy during curettage confirmed a diagnosis of OFD. (**g**) Radiograph at 4 years after curettage reveals a radiolucent lesion with internal haziness and sclerotic rim (inset). Last follow-up radiograph at 13 years after surgery shows a small residual radiolucent lesion with internal *ground density* surrounded by a significantly thickened sclerosis (arrow), suggesting a static lesion. And the patient is free of pain

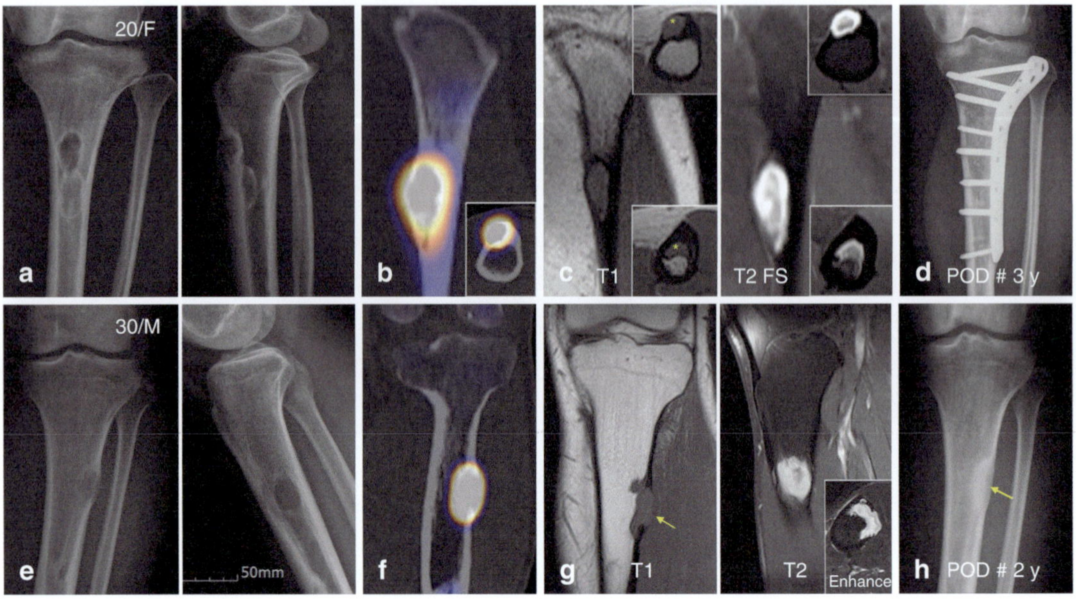

Fig. 28.2 ***A focal extension into the medullary cavity***. (**a**) Radiographs taken for painful swelling of the left proximal shin of 3 years' duration in a 20-year-old young woman show a multilobulated oval radiolucent lesion with *ground-glass* density surrounded by a thin sclerotic rim confined to the cortex proximally and another lesion affecting the medullary cavity distally in the proximal tibia. (**b**) Bone SPECT scan reveals a hot uptake along the periphery of the lesion. (**c**) MR images demonstrate a well-defined, oval, cortical-based lesion extending into the medullary cavity with intermediate SI on T1-weighted image and heterogeneous high and bright SI on fat-saturated T2-weighted image, with a thin dark signal of sclerosis on both sequences. Axial images clearly exhibit an intracortical lesion (upper inset) and focal medullary extension (lower inset) with the same signal. There is a marked cortical thinning but no breakage and soft tissue extension. (**d**) Follow-up radiograph at 3 years after thorough curettage and allograft followed by plate fixation shows consolidation of the lesion without evidence of recurrence. (**e**) Radiographs taken for the left proximal leg pain of 6 months' duration in a 30-year-old man show a cortex-based round to oval radiolucent lesion extending into the medullary cavity with a *ground-glass* density, which is surrounded by a hazy incomplete thin sclerotic rim in the proximal tibia. (**f**) Bone SPECT scan reveals a focally increased uptake in the periphery of the lesion. (**g**) MR images demonstrate a well-defined intracortical lesion focally extending into the medulla with intermediate SI on T1-weighted image and high SI on fat-saturated T2-weighted image. Note cortical ballooning and thinning with focal disappearance of the outer cortex but no discernible soft tissue extension (arrow). The lesion is well enhanced by contrast medium (inset). (**h**) Follow-up radiograph at 2 years after curettage reveals consolidation of the lesion with sclerotic change (arrow)

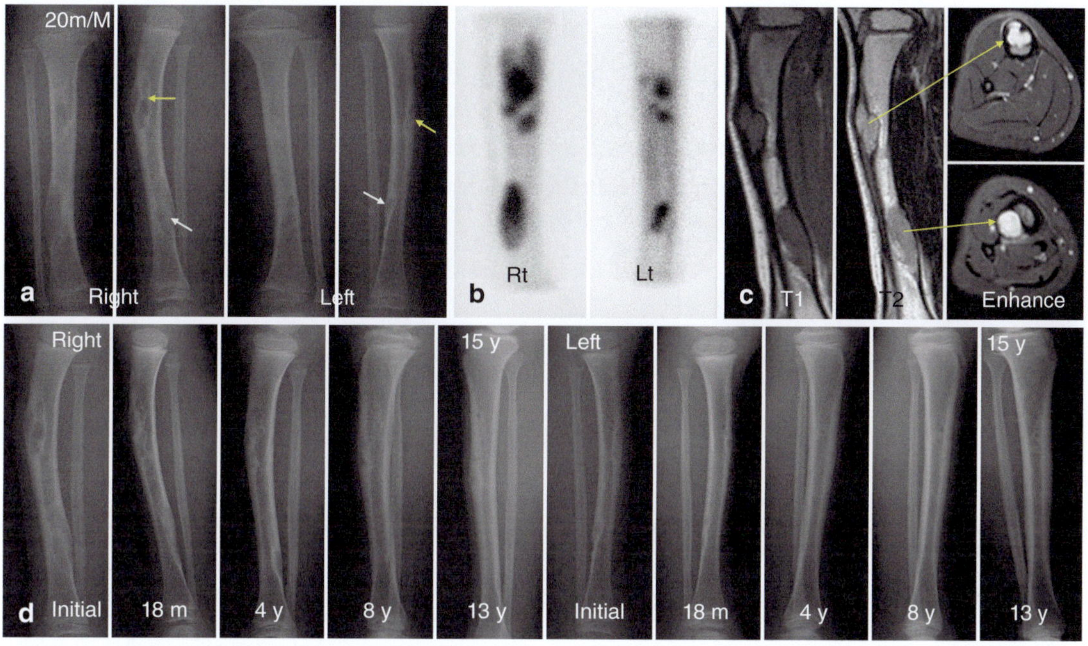

Fig. 28.3 ***Bilateral tibia involvement with spontaneous healing***. (**a**) Radiographs taken for swelling of both legs in a 20-month-old infant boy show an eccentric, cortical-based, multilobulated, two separate proximal and distal multilobulated osteolytic lesions with internal *ground-glass* density and marked cortical thinning, which are surrounded by rinds of sclerosis in the shaft of both tibias. Extraordinarily, the lesions are located simultaneously at the anterior and posterior cortices of both tibias (arrows). Note moderate anterior bowing in the right tibia and mild bowing in the left tibia. (**b**) Bone scan reveals heterogeneous strong uptakes in the separate lesions of both tibias, suggesting active lesions. (**c**) MR images demonstrate well-defined two separate lobulated intracortical lesions extending into the medullary cavity with intermediate SI on T1-weighted image and intermediate to high SI on T2-weighted image. Both anterior and posterior lesions are well enhanced by contrast medium. (**d**) Follow-up serial lateral radiographs show gradual and chronological regression of the lesions. Follow-up radiographs at 13 years after the initial visit demonstrate nearly complete healing of the lesion with spontaneous correction of anterior bowing and a remodeling of the cortices of both tibias

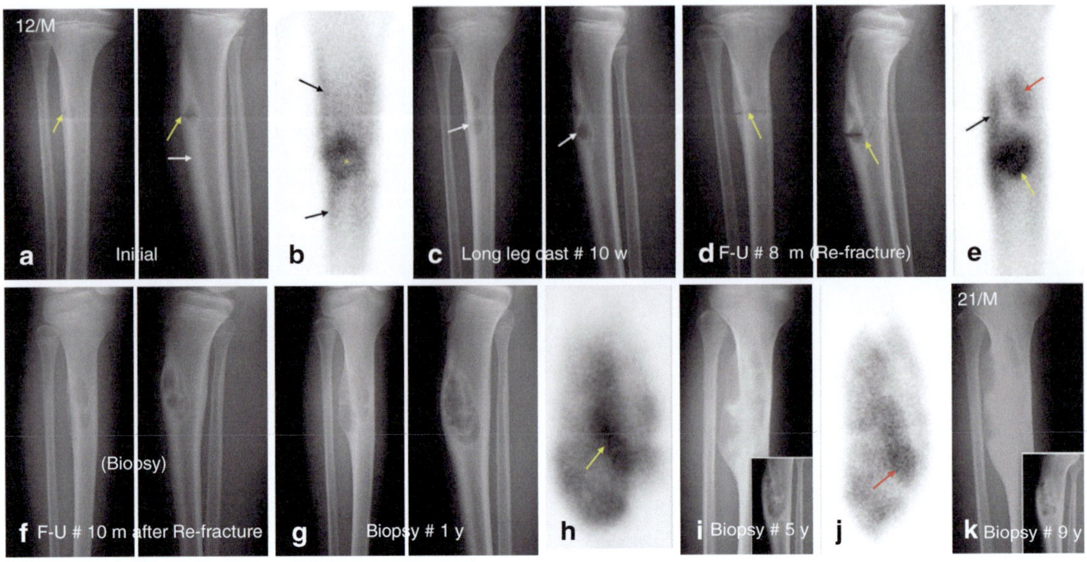

Fig. 28.4 ***Linear pathologic fracture***. (**a**) Radiographs taken for right leg pain developed during skipping rope in a 12-year-old boy show a single, small radiolucent lesion confined to the anterior cortex of the proximal tibia. The lesion has *ground-glass* density, and the anterior cortex is markedly thickened (red arrow). A very thin linear line indicating a patholgic fracture is seen through the lesion (yellow arrow). (**b**) Pinhole bone scan reveals moderately increased uptake with an internal photon defect in the lesion (asterisk). A long segmental, diffuse mild uptake along the anterior cortex suggests reactive bone change (black arrows). The exact activity of the cortical lesion is undetermined due to the pathologic fracture. (**c**) The associated fracture is healed well with cast immobilization, but the lesion enlarge with a newly developed small satellite lesion on follow-up radiograph at 10 weeks after long leg cast immobilization (arrows). (**d**) Radiographs taken for a recurrent painful swelling of the right leg during running at 8 months after the first fracture show a stable-looking lesion with more clearly visible re-fracture line (arrows). (**e**) Follow-up pinhole scan demonstrates more intense uptake within the main lesion (yellow arrow) and newly developed smaller, weaker uptake (red arrow). The reactive segmental uptake along the lateral cortex is also seen (black arrow). (**f**) Follow-up radiograph at 10 months after re-fracture shows the lesion enlarged with a complete healing of the fracture. Incision biopsy was done because of parents' concern about the possiblity of progression to adamantinoma. Microscopic examination confirmed a typical OFD without areas of epithelial nest. (**g**) Follow-up radiographs at 1 year after biopsy show further progression of the disease. (**h**) Follow-up pinhole scan reveals a much greater increase in extent and intensity of the uptake, suggesting progression of the lesion (yellow arrow). (**i**) Follow-up radiographs at 5 years after biopsy demonstrate an increase in size of the lesion but appearing stabilized. (**j**) Follow-up pinhole scan shows a decreased intensity of uptake, suggesting a stabilized lesion (arrow). (**k**) Follow-up radiographs at 9 years after biopsy show no further increase in size with diffuse sclerotic change of the lesion. He is doing well with mild protrusion of the proximal shin but no pain

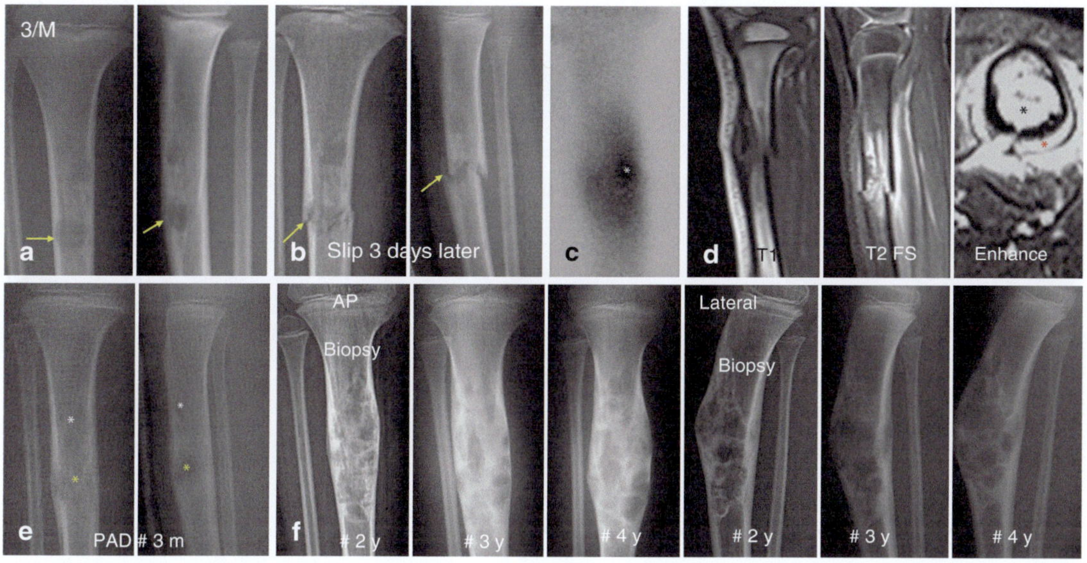

Fig. 28.5 ***Mildly displaced pathologic fracture***. (**a**) Radiograph taken for right leg pain after slip in a 3-year-old boy incidentally shows an ill-defined multilobulated cortex-based radiolucent lesion extending into the medullary cavity in the proximal tibia. There is significant cortical thinning and scalloping but no bowing or fracture line at that time (arrows). (**b**) However, pathologic fracture occurs after a second slip 3 days later while waiting for MRI evaluation (red arrow). (**c**) Pinhole bone scan reveals mildly increased uptake with a focal stronger uptake at upper lesion (asterisk), suggesting a single active lesion. Minimal increased uptake is noted along the fracture line. (**d**) MR images demonstrate a lobulated intracortical lesion invading the medullary cavity with low and intermediate SI on T1-weighted image and heterogeneous high SI on fat suppression T2-weighted image. Extensive hemorrhage and edma related to fracture is noted in the bone marrow and adjacent soft tissue. Post-contrast image shows a strong enhancement of the main lesion with hemorrhage and edema (black asterisk). In addition, subperiosteal and soft tissue hemorrhage are also strongly enhanced (red asterisk). (**e**) Follow-up radiographs at 3 months after cast immobilization note a complete healing of the fracture with near resolution of the upper lesion (white asterisk) and a hazy, larger, lower portion of the lesion (yellow asterisk). Incision biopsy was performed because of the parents' concern about the possibility of progression to adamantinoma. Histologic diagnosis was typical OFD in the absence of epithlial clusters indicative of adamantinoma. (**f**) After incision biopsy, serial radiographs reveal a gradual progression of the lesion. Note significant expansion and anterior bowing of proximal tibia on lateral view. (**g**) Follow-up radiographs at 5 years after biopsy show further expansion expansion and anterior bowing of the proximal tibia. (**h**) En-bloc resection of diseased tibia shaft (OFD) was performed and the defect was reconstructed by vascularized fibular graft (VFG). (**i**) Immediate postoperative radiograph shows good position of VFG from the ipsilateral side (red arrow) fixed with dual plates. (**j**) Follow-up radiograph at 2 years after surgery reveals good incorporation of VFG with some hypertrophy. (**k**) However, radiograph taken for right leg pain after a fall at 8 months after removal of plates notes a fracture of the grafted bone (red arrow). (**l**) Follow-up radiograph at 1 year after surgical management of the graft fracture and (**m**) immediate radiograph after removal of the plates demonstrate complete union of fracture with hypertrophy of the grafted fibula. (**n**) Follow-up radiograph at 4 years after VFG demonstrates an overgrowth resulting in lengthening of the tibia by 4.5 cm. (**o**) Shortening osteotomy was performed at the hypertrophied VFG (red arrow) to equalize the legs. (**p**) Radiograph at 12 years after initial visit when the patient became a 15-year-old adolescent shows a healing of the lesion with hypertrophied grafted fibula and no leg length discrepancy on scanogram

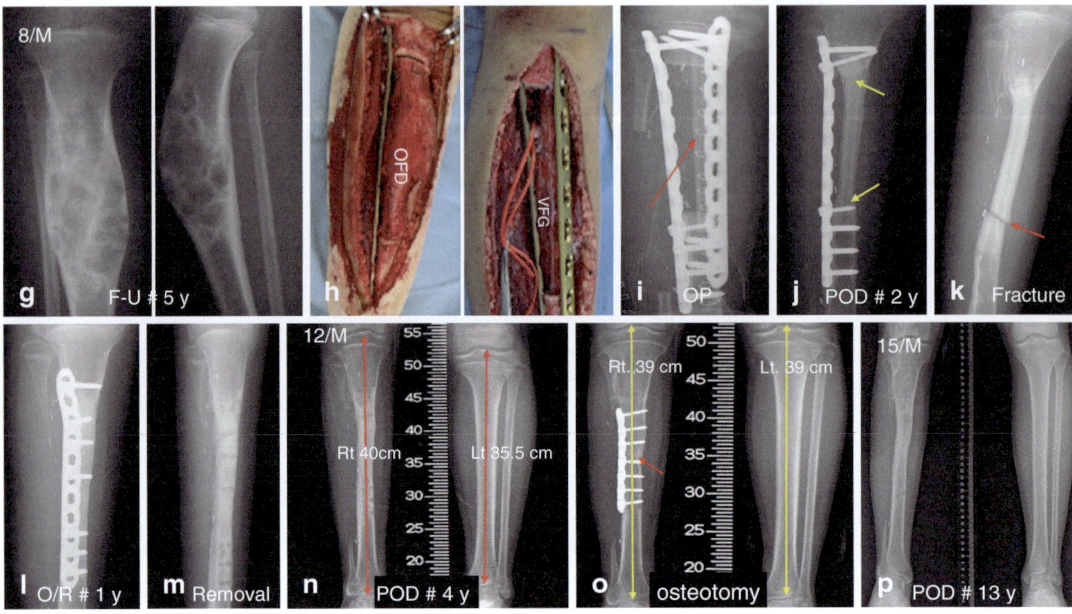

Fig. 28.5 (continued)

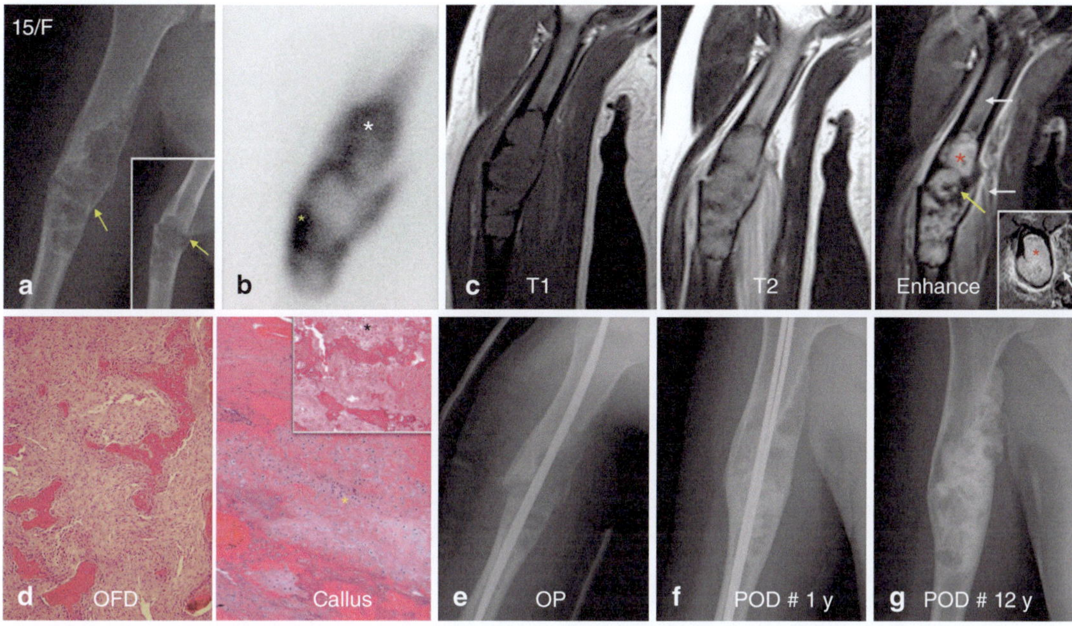

Fig. 28.6 ***Rare location of humerus***. (**a**) Radiograph taken for acutely developed pain in the right upper arm during exercise on a horizontal bar in a 15-year-old girl shows a well-defined, multilobulated, bubbly, eccentric osteolytic lesion which is surrounded by an irregular thin rim of sclerosis with *ground-glass* density in the mid-shaft of the humerus. The underlying bone is moderately expanded with markedly thinned cortex and pathologic fracture (arrows). (**b**) Pinhole bone scan reveals moderate and strong uptake in the peripheral areas of the lesion (asterisks) with a central photon *"defect, reffered to as doughnut sign"*. (**c**) MR images demonstrate a well-demarcated multilobulated mass-like lesion occupying the cortex and medullary cavity with intermediate SI on T1-weighted image and heterogeneous intermediate to high SI T2-weighted images. The lesion is surrounded by a thin dark signal of reactive sclerosis with internal multiple tiny foci of dark signal on both sequences. Contrast-enhanced image shows diffuse intense enhancement of the lesion (red asterisks) with a focal irregular nonenhancing area of calcification (yellow arrow). There is also diffuse enhancement of adjacent bone marrow and soft tissue hemorrhage (white arrows). (**d**) Microscopic examination reveals irregular, curvilinear trabeculae of woven bone with prominent osteoblastic rimming embedded in a bland fibrous stroma, indicative of OFD (Left). Note another area with emanation of messes with chondroid to primitive cartilage from a bland stroma simulating chondrosarcoma, as well as primitive osteoid converting to primitive woven bone with *regularly ominous* plump stromal cells (asterisks), indicating fracture callus with estimated age between the first and second week. Practically, the patient suffered a pathologic fracture 10 days before the biopsy. (**e**) A flexible intramedullary nailing was performed for a pathologic fracture, but curettage with bone graft was not done. (**f**) Follow-up radiograph at 1 year after surgery reveals complete healing of fracture with consolidation of the lesion. (**g**) Follow-up radiograph at 12 years after surgery notes a stabilization of the lesion with sclerotic change. The patient is doing very well without any pain by simple surgery

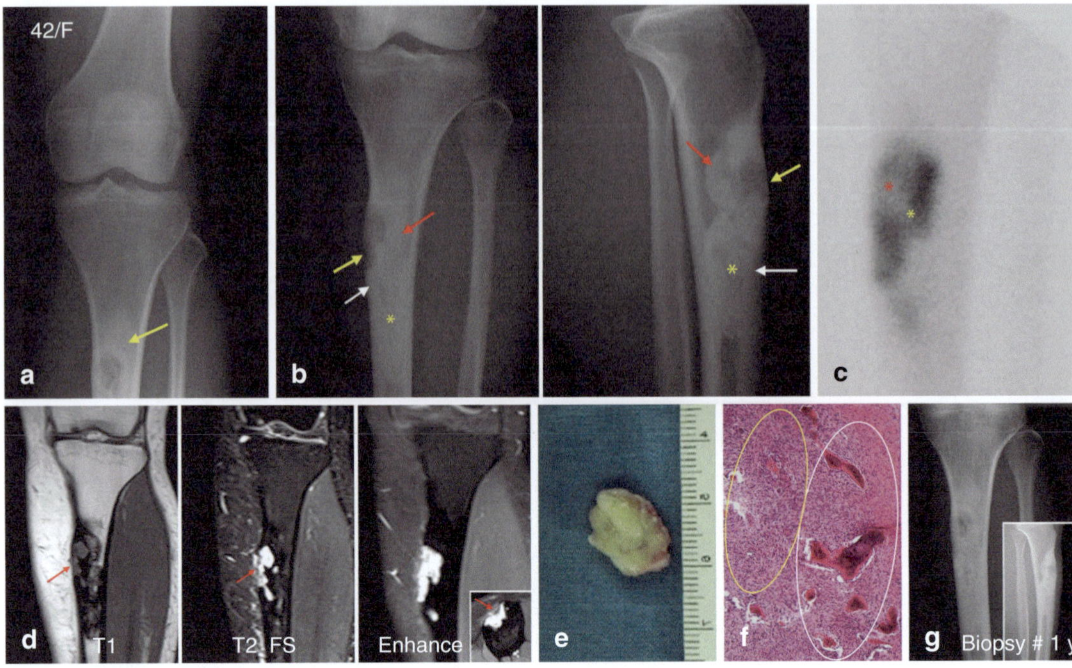

Fig. 28.7 ***Incidentally found regressing OFD***. (**a**) Radiograph taken for left knee pain in a 42-year-old lady shows no definite abnormal finding of the knee joint. However, there is an incidentally found radiolucent lesion with hazy internal densities surrounded by thick sclerosis in the diaphysis of the proximal tibia (arrow). (**b**) Additional radiographs of tibia reveal a hazy, eccentric, cortex-based, multilobulated radiolucent lesion with focal thinning of the overlying cortex (yellow arrow) and diffuse thickening of the adjacent cortex (white arrow). A surrounding sclerotic reaction is prominent (red arrows) and even produces a complete obstruction of the medullary canal (asterisks). (**c**) Pinhole bone scan notes eccentrically moderate and strong uptake in the periphery of the lesion (yellow asterisk) with a central photon defect (red asterisk), indicating an inactive regressed old lesion surrounded by prominent surrounding reactive sclerotic bone. (**d**) MR images demonstrate a multilobulated, cortex-based, eccentric, mass-like lesion extending into the medullary cavity with intermediate SI on T1-weighted image and bright SI on fat suppression T2-weighted image, which is surrounded by a thick dark signal of sclerosis with focal loss of anteromedial cortex on both sequences. However, there is no discernible soft tissue extension (arrows). The lesion is homogeneously well enhanced by contrast medium. (**e**) Gross specimen of the excised lesion notes a whitish to yellowish, soft to robbery, fibrous mass. The surface of the mass is gritty by a deposition of bone spicules. (**f**) Microscopic examination shows a prominent bland spindle cell stroma with scanty, tiny to small primitive woven bone spicules in the central area (yellow circle) and more abundant, larger, matured, mineralized woven to lamellar bone in the periphery (white circle), referred to as *zonal architecture*. The central paucity of bone spicules reflects a photon defect of minimum uptake on bone scan (red asterisk on bone scan) and the peripheral abundancy with moderate to strong uptake in the periphery of the lesion on pinhole bone yellow asterisk. (**g**) Follow-up radiographs at 1 year after biopsy shows no interval change of the lesion

28.9 Histologic Findings

Irregular, curvilinear trabeculae of woven bone with prominent osteoblastic rimming (Fig. 28.8a, b) unlike classic FD which usually shows only minimal to absent osteoblastic rimming. However, rare cases of FD may also present prominent osteoblastic rimming as in OFD (Refer Fig. 26.14b in Chap. 26). In such rare cases, radiologic-pathologic correlation is crucial for differentiation of both entities. Intervening stroma consists of bland fibroblast-like spindle cells arranged in a storiform pattern with varying degrees of myxoid and fibrous tissue. The stromal cells produce an abundant collagenous matrix usually with delicate collagen fibers. A *zonal architecture* can be observed in appropriately sampled cases [3–6]. It is characterized by a

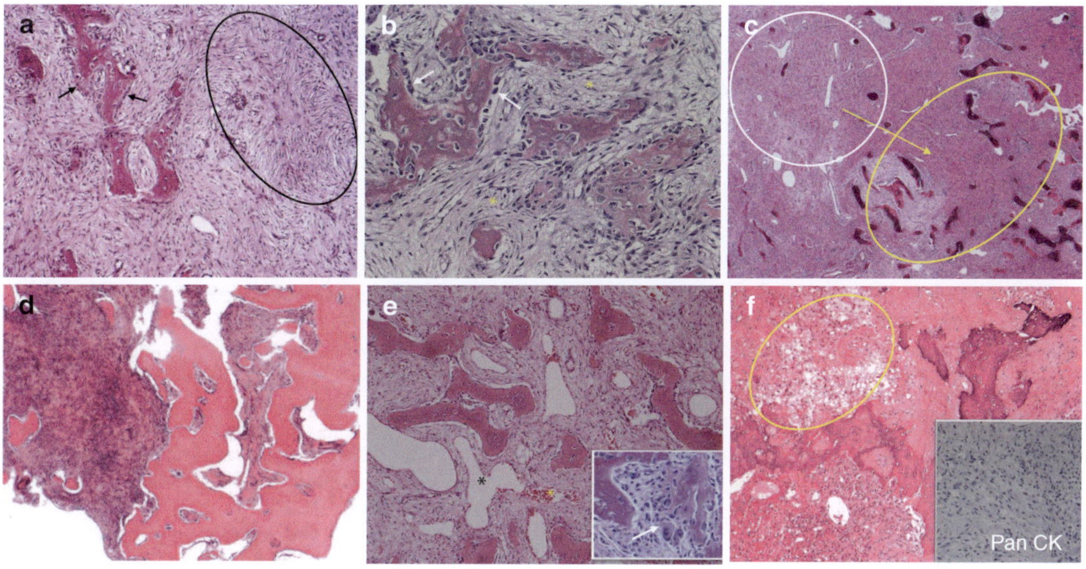

Fig. 28.8 *Microscopic features*. (**a**) The lesion is typified by irregular, curvilinear trabeculae of woven bone with prominent osteoblastic rimming (arrows) embedded within bland fibrous stroma producing a collagen matrix. The stroma tissue arranged in a whirling or storiform pattern is noted in this field (black circle). (**b**) Higher magnification reveals a single row of prominent cubic osteoblasts rimming the woven bone spicules (arrows). The spindle stroma cells are bland-looking with delicate to coarse fibers in the fibro-myxoid background (asterisks). (**c**) An adequately obtained sample can demonstrate that the bone trabeculae are scanty, tiny to small, and woven, and even predominantly fibrous in the center (white circle) and gradually more abundant, larger, more mature toward the periphery (yellow circle), a characteristic *zonal architecture*. (**d**) In the periphery, the bone trabeculae become coarse, anastomosing, and lamellar, and blend with the overlying host cortex. (**e**) Myxomatous or cystic changes (black asterisk) and dilated vessels with red blood cells (yellow asterisk) are observed, and some scattered multinucleated giant cells (inset) are also seen, which may alter the typical findings. (**f**) A focal area of xanthomatous change with foamy histiocytic infiltration is observed in this older lesion (yellow circle). IHC for keratin reveals scattered keratin-positive stromal cells, but clusters of keratin-positive cells are usually not seen (inset). Positive for cytokeratin is quite useful to differentiate OFD from FD in which the stain is always negative

central prominent fibrous area with sparse and thin woven bone and a middle zone of fibro-osseous tisue with pure woven bone rimmed by osteoblasts with a gradual transition showing an increased number of mature and mineralized bone trabeculae toward the periphery (Fig. 28.8c). Finally, the bone trabeculae and fibrous tissue anastomose and blend into the surrounding host bone (Fig. 28.8d). The central zone may exhibit myxomatous or cystic change in older lesions [3]. Myxomatous and cystic changes as well as dilated vessels with red blood cells are often seen (Fig. 28.8e). There can also be a small collection of multinucleated giant cells. In addition, foci of foam cells can be seen in older lesions (Fig. 28.8f), which may alter the typical findings and make the diagnosis more confusing. **Immunohistochemical stain** (IHC) with cytokeratin is quite useful to differentiate FD and OFD. IHC for keratin reveals scattered keratin-positive stromal cells, but clusters of keratin-positive cells are not seen (Fig. 28.8f). In an IHC study of 30 cases of OFD, isolated cytokeratin-positive cells were seen in the stroma of 28 cases (93%), but not found in any of the 47 FD cases. However, hyperchromatic epithelial clusters indicative of adamantinoma were never observed in any of the 30 cases of OFD [14].

28.10 Management

Conservative care is favored in general and surgery, even a biopsy, is usually not indicated [6]. However, surgical treatment is considered for growing or extensive lesions, pathologic fracture, significant bowing or pain, or rare case of pseudarthrosis. Pathologic fracture could be managed well by cast immobilization (Figs. 28.4 and 28.5). Progression of the lesion may be followed after simple curettage or even incision biopsy (Figs. 28.4g and 28.5f). Surgical management should be delayed as long as possible, preferably after puberty, if curettage is planned because intralesional curettage before complete stabilization of the lesion is often followed by a local recurrence. En-bloc resection may be necessary if surgical management is planned before puberty (Fig. 28.5h). When necessary, the correction of residual bowing can be performed safely after the age of 10–12 years when the lesion slowly and partially repairs through peripheral bone thickness.

28.11 Clinical Course

The clinical course is slow and usually self-limiting. However, it can occasionally be unpredictable ranging from a nonprogressive static lesion (Fig. 28.7) to a locally aggressive with a progressive enlargement and severe bowing (Figs. 28.4 and 28.5). OFD may considerably progress during the first decade of life, thereafter remain static or stabilized, and slowly and gradually heals with cortical thickening after 10–12 years of age [6] (Fig. 28.3). The lesions rarely continue to grow after the age of 15 years [4]. The younger the patient, the more likely recurrence occurs especially if only intralesional curettage is performed. The relationship between OFD and adamantinoma is still controversial. Mirra [4] and Campanacci [6] suggested a small minority of OFD may progress into adamantinoma. However, other studies reported OFD did not show a progression to adamantinoma [7, 15]. In an IHC study where cytokeratin-positive cell clusters indicative of adamantinoma were never observed in OFD, the authors also failed to demonstrate a progression of OFD to adamantinoma [14].

References

1. Alman BA, Greel DA, Wolfe HJ. Activating mutations of Gs protein in monostotic fibrous lesions of bone. J Orthop Res. 1996;14(2):311–5.
2. Sakamoto A, Oda Y, Iwamoto Y, Tsuneyoshi M. A comparative study of fibrous dysplasia and Osteofibrous dysplasia with regard to GSα mutation at the Arg201 codon: polymerase chain reaction-restriction fragment length polymorphism analysis of paraffin-embedded tissues. J Mol Diagn. 2000;2(2):67–72.
3. Czerniak B. Adamantinoma of long bone. In: Dorfman HD, Czerniak B, editors. Dorfman and Czerniak's bone tumors. 2nd ed. Elsevier; 2016. p. 1142–73.
4. Mirra JM, Picci P. Osteofibrous dysplasia. In: Mirra JM, editor. Bone tumors: clinical, radiologic, and pathologic correlations. 2nd ed. Philadelphia: Lea & Febiger; 1989. p. 1217–31.
5. Campanacci M. Osteofibrous dysplasia of long bones a new clinical entity. Ital J Orthop Traumatol. 1976;2(2):221–37.
6. Campanacci M. Osteofibrous dysplasia. In: Campanacci M, editor. Bone and soft tissue tumors. Wien/New York: Springer-Verlag; 1999. p. 714–20.
7. Park YK, Unni KK, McLeod RA, Pritchard DJ. Osteofibrous dysplasia: clinicopathologic study of 80 cases. Hum Pathol. 1993;24(12):1339–47.
8. Gopinathan NR, Prakash M, Saibaba B, Das A. Osteofibrous dysplasia of clavicle clinically mimicking chronic osteomyelitis. Indian J Radiol Imaging. 2016;26(02):290–3.
9. Kamineni S, Briggs T, Saifuddin A, Sandison A. Osteofibrous dysplasia of the ulna. J Bone Joint Surg Br. 2001;83(8):1178–80.
10. Ozaki T, Hamada M, Sugihara S, Kunisada T, Mitani S, Inoue H. Treatment outcome of osteofibrous dysplasia. J Pediatr Orthop B. 1998;7(3):199–202.
11. Sissons HA, Kancherla PL, Lehman W. Ossifying fibroma of bone. Report of two cases. Bull Hosp Jt Dis. 1983;43(1):1–14.
12. Wang JW, Shih CH, Chen WJ. Osteofibrous dysplasia (ossifying fibroma of long bones): a report of four cases and review of the literature. Clin Orthop Relat Res. 1992;278:235–43.
13. Yoshida S, Watanuki M, Hayashi K, Hosaka M, Hagiwara Y, Itoi E, et al. Osteofibrous dysplasia arising in the humerus: a case report. Rare Tumors. 2018;10:2036361318808852.
14. Sweet DE, Vinh TN, Devaney K. Cortical osteofibrous dysplasia of long bone and its relationship to adamantinoma: a clinicopathologic study of 30 cases. Am J Surg Pathol. 1992;16(3):282–90.
15. Unni KK, Inwards CY. Osteofibrous dysplasia. In: Unni KK, Inwards CY, editors. Dahlin's bone tumors: general aspects and data on nnnn165 cases. 6th ed. Philadelphia: Lippincott William & Wilkins; 2010. p. 327–30.

Part V

Fibrous (Fibrogenic) and Fibro-histiocytic Tumors and Lesions

29 Fibrous Cortical Defect/ Non-ossifying Fibroma

29.1 Definition

Fibrous cortical defect (FCD) is an ephemeral small benign lesion of fibroblastic proliferation which is limited to the cortex in younger children. FCD is mostly less than 3 cm in maximum dimension [1]. Nonossifying fibroma (NOF) is a larger-sized, common nonneoplastic benign fibrogenic lesion eccentrically involving the medullary cavity in older children or adolescents. NOF is considered as a larger version (>3–5 cm) of FCD. These lesions are histologically identical and thought to be non-neoplastic but a group of developmental abnormalities related to dysfunctional ossification. Most NOF is single, but multifocal NOFs may be occasionally present, and rarely found in the setting of the Jaffe-Campanacci syndrome (multiple NOFs of considerable size, café au-lait spots, mental retardation, hypogonadism, cryptorchidism, ocular/cardiovascular anomalies, or skin alterations) [2–4].

29.2 Synonym

Metaphyseal fibrous defect/cortical desmoid / fibrous cortical defect/non-osteogenic fibroma/ fibroxanthoma.

29.3 Incidence

The actual incidence is unknown because most lesions are asymptomatic and found incidentally. It has been estimated that approximately 30–40% of all normal children and adolescents with open growth plates may have one or more undetected FCDs [4–7]. NOF accounts for about 2% of biopsy-analyzed primary bone tumors [1]. It has been almost twice as often in boys as in girls, and a greater number of patients are also boys in our collection probably because boys more commonly seek medical attention, probably due to more frequent pain from hyperactivity with a trivial injury or even pathologic fracture during activity.

29.4 Possible Pathogenesis

The etiology is not clear. Repeated pulling of muscle or ligament at the bone insertion can produce focal subperiosteal hemorrhage and fibroblastic metaplasia during childhood when the periosteum is loosely attached to the bone. This may explain the predominant incidence in boys generally with more hyperactivity than girls. Thereafter, there is no more subperiosteal hemor-

W.-J. Bahk, *Diagnosis and Management of Primary Bone Tumors*,
https://doi.org/10.1007/978-981-96-3484-2_29

rhage because the periosteum is is firmly attached to the underlying bone, and the lesion gets regressed with abundant collagen production and profuse foamy macrophages acting as scavengers when patients become older (personal communication to Dr. Mirra). Ritschl et al. [8] supported this theory by noting that FCD always arose from the bone where tendons, joint capsule, and ligaments insert onto the metaphysis adjacent to the growth plate, but never was observed in areas including medial aspect of the distal tibia and femoral neck. A boy predominance in incidence may also support the possible pathogenesis of repeated minor injury.

29.5 Age

The lesions are mostly found during the first and second decades of life before the age of 20 years in more than 80% of patients [1]. FCD is usually found before the age of 10 years and NOF between ages age of 10 and 15 years. They are rarely seen beyond the age of 30 years because they spontaneously heal before this age. The oldest patient in our series is 25 years of age (Fig. 29.11).

29.6 Location

The lesion most commonly affects the metaphysis near the physis of the long bone, particularly around the knee (distal femur and proximal tibia) and ankle (distal tibia and fibula). NOF is rarely seen in the proximal femur and upper extremity, where it may be found more often in the proximal humerus [4] (Fig. 29.8). The vast majority of lesions are single (Figs. 29.1, 29.2, 29.3, 29.4, 29.5, 29.6, 29.7, 29.8, 29.9, 29.10 and 29.11), but may be multifocal (Figs. 29.12 and 29.13). In a large series, 72 out of 900 biopsy-proven cases (8%) had more than one lesion [9].

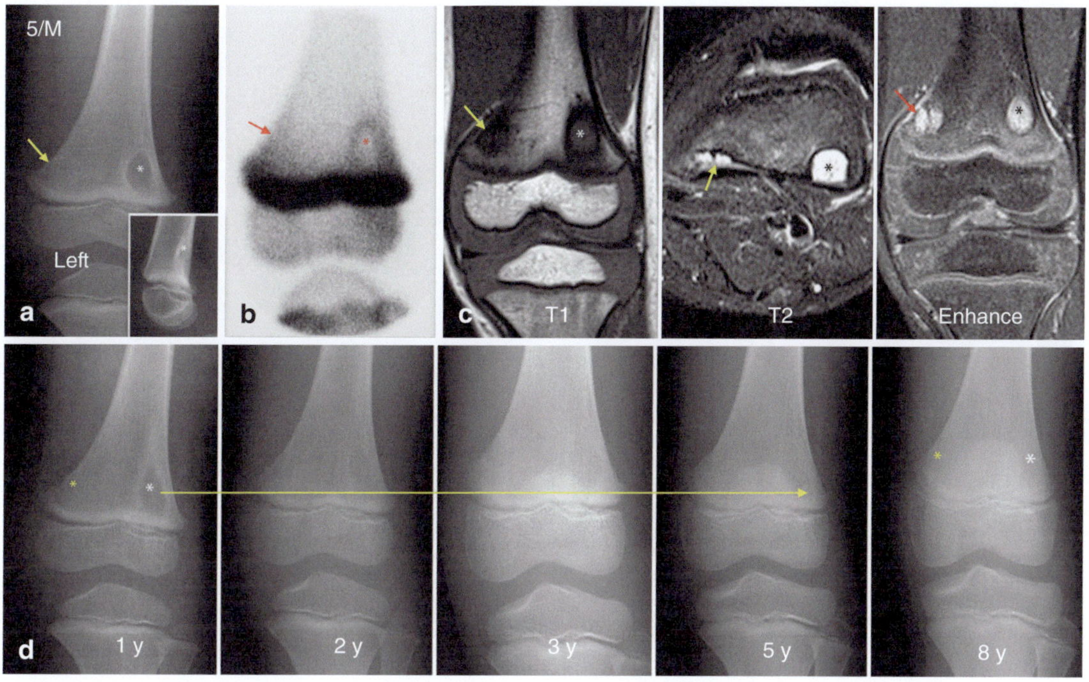

Fig. 29.1 ***Multifocal FCD***. (**a**) Radiograph taken for right knee pain in a 5-year-old boy incidentally shows a well-defined, eccentric, round to oval, cortical-based radiolucent lesion surrounded by a thin rim of sclerosis at the lateral condyle of the contralateral left distal femur (asterisk) and another smaller very hazy lesion in the medial condyle (arrow). (**b**) Pinhole bone scan reveals a moderately increased peripheral uptake with a central photon defect, so-called *doughnut sign*, in the lateral condyle, suggesting a still active lesion (asterisk). However, the medial lesion presents very subtle uptake, suggesting another regressing lesion (arrow). (**c**) MR images demonstrate a well-defined, small, eccentric, cortex-based, round to oval lesion in the posterolateral aspect of the right femoral condyle (asterisks) with low SI on T1-weighted image and high SI on T2-weighted image, exhibiting a thin dark signal of surrounding sclerosis on both sequences. The lesion is measures about 1.8 cm in maximum diameter, indicating FCD. The lesion is heterogeneously well enhanced (asterisk). Another smaller lesion with the same nature is seen at the posteromedial aspect with good enhancement, suggesting smaller FCD (arrows). (**d**) Follow-up radiographs note chronologic regression of the both lesions. Radiograph at 5 years' follow-up shows a complete resolution of the lesions. The last follow-up radiographs at 8 years show normal appearance of the bones

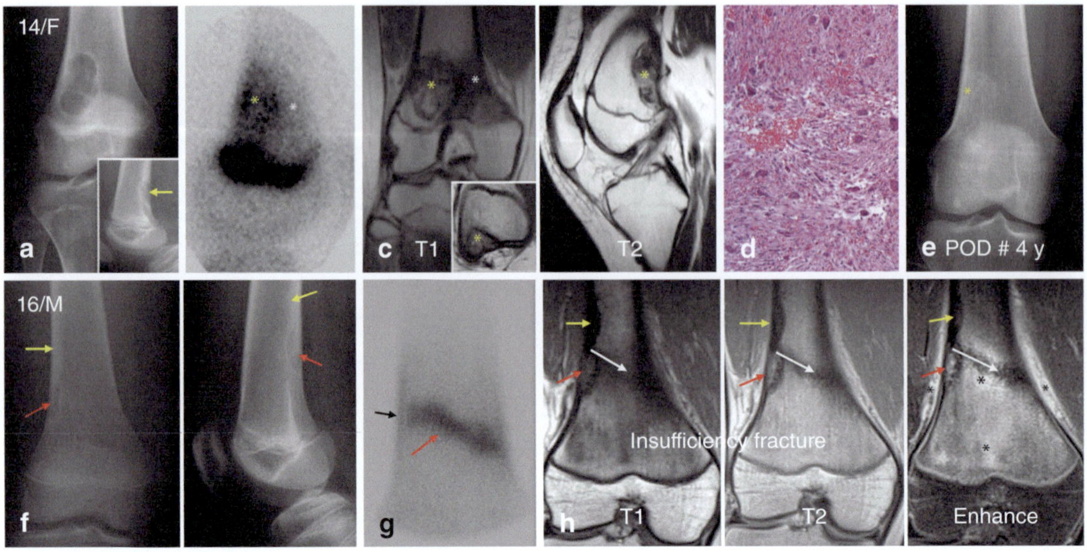

Fig. 29.2 ***The distal femur***. (**a**) Radiograph taken for right knee pain of 3 month's duration in 14-years-old girl shows a multilobulated, eccentric, radiolucent lesion surrounded by a thin rim of sclerosis in the meta-diaphysis of the distal femur. The lesion is mainly confined to the cortex with focal mild expansion into the medullary cavity on lateral view (inset). (**b**) Pinhole bone scan presents a heterogeneous moderate and strong uptake, suggesting an active lesion (yellow asterisk), and peripheral mild uptake, corresponding to low signal on T1-weighted image (white asterisk). (**c**) MR images demonstrate a multilobulated, eccentric, cortex-based lesion extending into the medullary cavity (yellow asterisks). The SI is heterogeneous low and intermediate on both T1- and T2-weighted images, suggesting a solid fibrous lesion. Another area with low SI on T1-weighted image (white asterisk) may suggest bone marrow edema, which shows no increased uptake on bone scan. (**d**) Microscopic examination notes a fibro-histiocytic proliferation arranged in a *storiform pattern* with extensive hemorrhagic foci. Numerous multinucleated giant cells are diffusely sprinkled throughout the spindly stroma, simulating GCT at first glance. However, a diagnosis of NOF can be easily rendered if her age of 14 years before closure of growth plate and the location in the meta-diaphysis rather than the epiphysis are considered. (**e**) Radiograph at 4 years after curettage and allogenic chip-bone graft shows a complete healing of the lesion (asterisk). **Stress fracture:** (**f**) Radiograph taken for right distal thigh pain of 1 week's duration in a 16-year-old boy shows a hazy, eccentric, small, cortical-based, radiolucent lesion (red arrows) with more proximal sclerotic to dense lesion (yellow arrows) in the meta-diaphysis of the distal femur. (**g**) Pinhole bone scan reveals an oblique band-like hot uptake (red arrow) from the area of weak uptake along the cortex of the distal femur (black arrow). A stress fracture is suspected to arise from the lesion as a stress riser for the fracture origin, which is not visible on the standard radiographs. (**h**) MR images demonstrate two separate well-defined, cortical-based, small, oval lesions with different signals. The proximal lesion shows low SI on both sequences (yellow arrows) and the distal lesion reveals intermediate SI on T1-weighted image and intermediate to high SI on T2-weighted image (red arrows). Both lesions are surrounded by a peripheral low signal sclerotic rim. There is a thick oblique band of low SI in the distal femur starting from the junction between both lesions, suggesting a linear stress fracture to arise from the junction as a stress riser (white arrows). The proximal lesion is not enhanced (yellow arrow), but the distal lesion is well enhanced by contrast medium (red arrow). The edema and hemorrhage of distal bone marrow and adjacent soft tissue are also diffusely enhanced (asterisks)

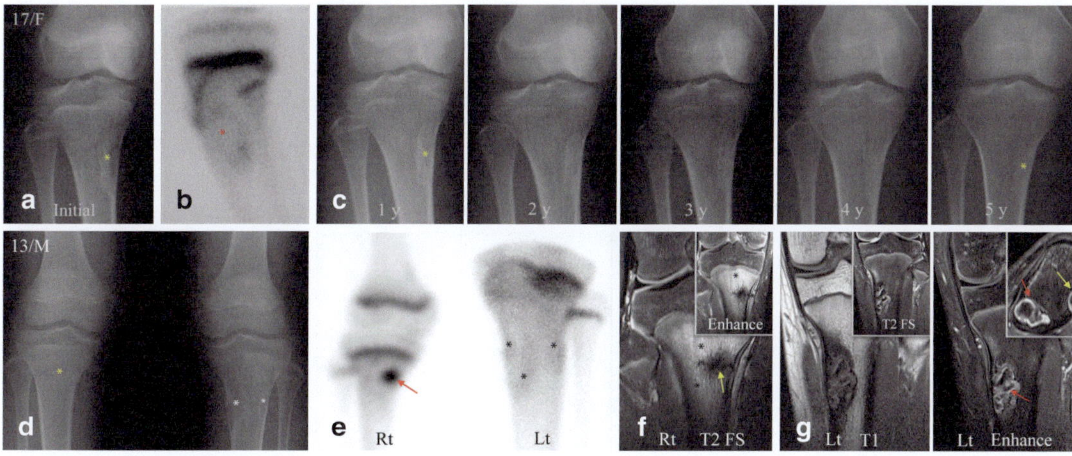

Fig. 29.3 ***Proximal tibia***. (**a**) Radiograph taken for right knee pain by blunt trauma in a 17-year-old girl incidentally shows a well-defined, eccentric, multilobulated radiolucent lesion with internal sclerotic area (asterisk) and surrounding sclerotic rim in the medial aspect of the right proximal tibia. (**b**) Pinhole bone scan reveals very mild uptake along the periphery of the lesion with central photon defect (asterisk), suggesting a stabilized lesion. (**c**) Serial follow-up radiographs demonstrate chronological slow regression of the lesion as the patient grows. The lesion is completely healed with sclerotic change (asterisk) at 5 years' follow-up at the age of 22 years. (**d**) Radiograph taken for right knee pain of 10 days' duration with no memorable history of injury in a 13-year-old boy shows no abnormal finding in the symptomatic right proximal tibia (yellow asterisk), but incidentally notes an eccentric, larger, multilobulated radiolucent, medial lesion and another smaller lateral lesion with rim of sclerosis in the contralateral asymptomatic left proximal tibia (white asterisks). (**e**) Pinhole bone scan reveals a small focal hot uptake in the medial portion of the metaphysis of the right proximal tibia (arrow), indicating a probable concealed insufficiency or stress fracture not seen on radiograph. Incidentally, heterogeneous subtle multiple uptakes are seen in the contralateral left proximal tibia, suggesting inactive lesions (asterisks). (**f**) Fat-suppressed T2-weighted image of the painful right knee demonstrates a linear dark signal (arrow) and high signal of hemorrhage in the perilesional bone marrow (black asterisks). There are enhanced bone marrow edema/hemorrhage and periosteal reaction (asterisks) but no enhanced main lesion, suggesting an insufficiency or stress fracture with no preexisting lesion (inset). (**g**) However, MR images of the asymptomatic contralateral left knee demonstrate a well-defined, eccentric, cortex-based, multi-lobulated lesion with heterogeneous low and intermediate SI on T1-weighted image and intermediate and peripherally high SI on T2-weighted image (inset) with multiple foci of signal void on both sequences, suggesting incidentally found old OFs. The lesions are heterogeneously and peripherally enahnced (arrows)

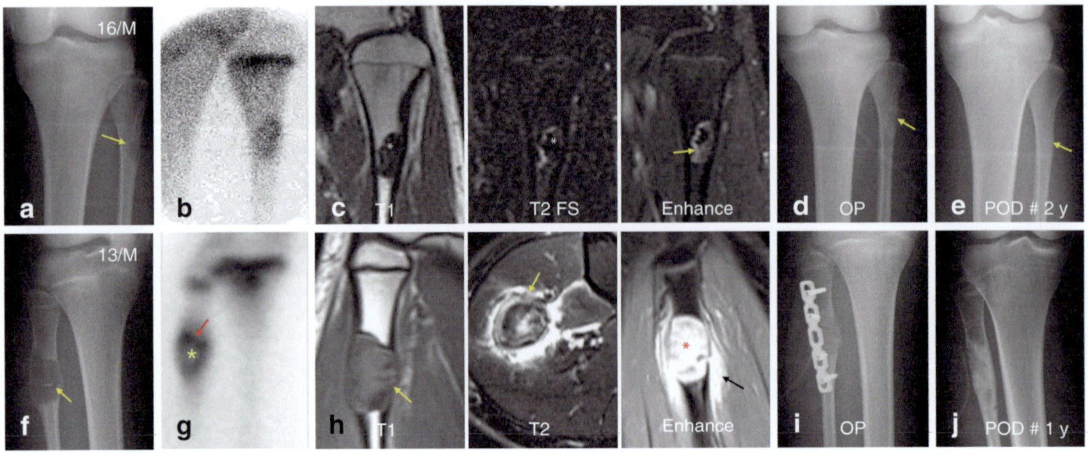

Fig. 29.4 ***Proximal fibula***. (**a**) Radiograph taken for right knee pain of 3 month's duration in 16-years-old adolescent shows a well-defined, eccentric, small round to oval, radiolucent lesion with a thin sclerotic rim in the left proximal fibula. (**b**) Pinhole bone scan reveals a moderately increased uptake in the lesion. (**c**) MR images demonstrate a well-defined lobulated oval lesion (asterisks) with low SI on T1-weighted image and internal low to dark SI with peripheral high signal on fat-saturated T2-weighted image, suggesting maturation of the lesion with profuse collagen deposition and ossification. The lesion is irregularly and peripherally enhanced (arrow). (**d**) Curettage and allogenic chip-bone graft were performed because of continuous bothering pain with moderate uptake on the bone scan. Microscopic examination of curetted specimen confirmed a diagnosis of NOF. (**e**) Follow-up radiograph at 2 years after surgery shows a complete healing of the lesion (arrow). (**f**) Radiograph taken for right proximal leg pain of several 4–5 months duration with a recent aggravation in a 13-year-old boy shows a well-defined geographic destruction with moderate expansion and cortical thinning as well as bone fragment in it, suggesting a possible pathologic fracture without a history of trauma in the proximal fibula (arrow). (**g**) Pinhole bone scan reveals a peripheral hot uptake along the shell of the radiolucent bone lesion (arrow) with central photon defect (asterisk), referred to as *doughnut sign*. (**h**) MR images demonstrate a well-defined, lobular, expansile mass-like lesion with intermediate SI on T1-weighted image and heterogeneous high SI on T2-weighted image. Cortical thinning with breakage and surrounding hemorrhage/edema are associated (yellow arrows). The lesion (asterisk) and soft tissue hemorrhage (arrow) are strongly enhanced. (**i**) Curettage and allogenic chip-bone graft with plate fixation to avoid long-term use of cast brace were performed. (**j**) Follow-up radiograph at 1 year after surgery notes consolidation of the lesion

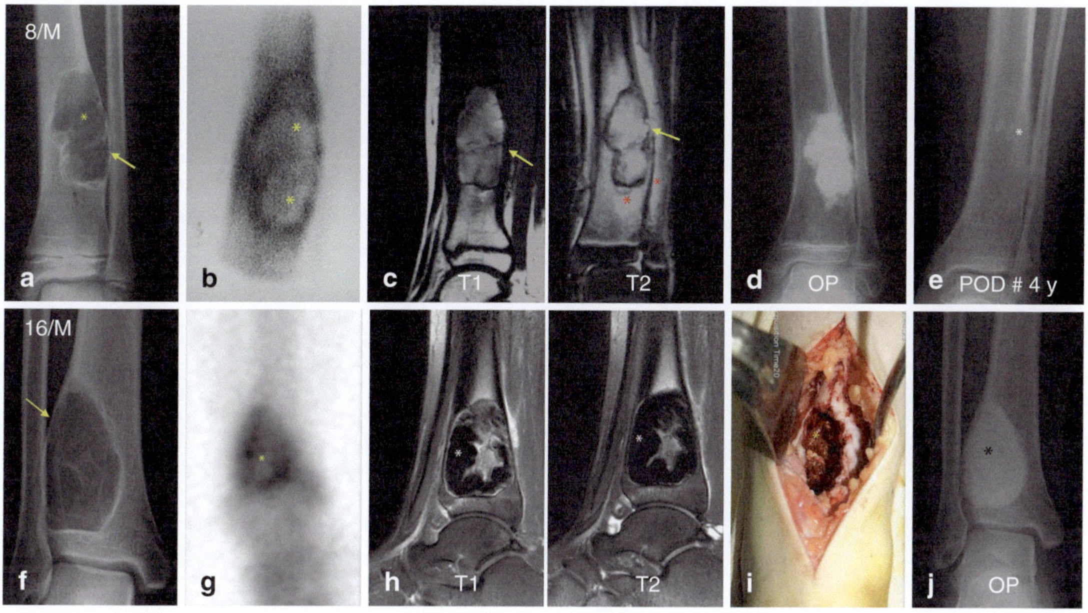

Fig. 29.5 ***Distal tibia***. (**a**) Radiograph taken for left ankle pain of 3 weeks' duration in an 8-year-old boy shows a well-defined, eccentric, bubbly radiolucent lesion (asterisk) surrounded by a thin rind of sclerosis in the diaphysis of the distal tibia. The lesion is mildly expanded with significant cortical thinning (arrow). (**b**) Pinhole bone scan reveals increased peripheral uptake with internal photon defect (asterisks). (**c**) MR images present a well-defined, multilobulated large lesion with heterogeneous intermediate and high SI on T1-weighted image and high to bright SI on T2-weighted image, surrounded by a thin rim of dark signal on both sequences. The lesion is mildly expansile with significant cortical thinning and breaches (arrows). There are prominent perilesional bone marrow and adjacent soft tissue hemorrhage or edema (red asterisks). (**d**) Curettage and allogenic chip-bone graft was performed. (**e**) Follow-up radiograph at 4 years after surgery notes a complete healing of the lesion with consolidation (asterisk). (**f**) Radiograph taken for right ankle of 4 months' duration in a 16-year-old adolescent shows an eccentric, well-defined, ballooning lesion with internal multiple septations, which is surrounded by a thin rind of sclerosis affecting the metadiaphysis of the distal tibia. The lateral cortex is markedly thinned but no discernible destruction or fracture (arrow). (**g**) Bone scan reveals diffusely increased uptake with a focal internal photon defect (asterisk). (**h**) MR images demonstrate a well-defined, large lesion with heterogeneous SI with marked internal dark signal (asterisks) on both T1- and T2-weighted images. There is no periosteal reaction or correactive edema. (**i**) Note the glistening, brownish-tanned component reflecting the tumor itself with hemorrhage and hemosiderin pigmentation (asterisk). (**j**) Immediate postoperative radiograph shows a good filling of the defect with allograft chips

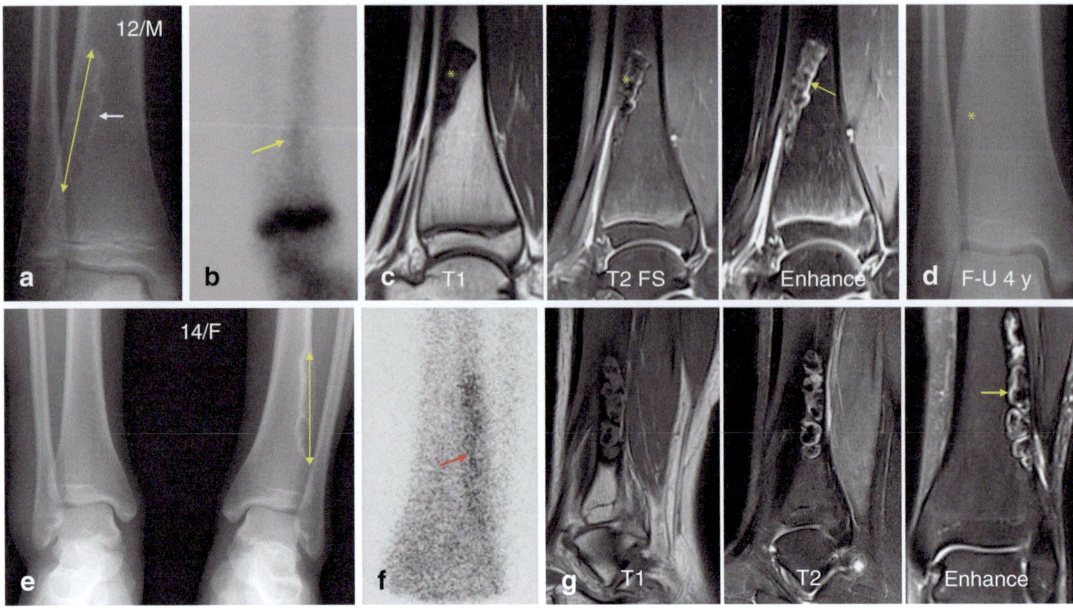

Fig. 29.6 ***Typical longitudinal orientation***. (**a**) Radiograph taken for intermittent swelling of right distal leg of 3 years' duration in a 12-year-old boy shows an eccentric, longitudinally oriented (double head arrow), *bubbly* lesion surrounded by a thin sclerotic rim in the meta-diaphysis of the distal tibia. (**b**) Bone scan reveals minimal uptake along the lesion (arrow), suggesting a stable benign lesion. (**c**) MR images note a well-defined, eccentric, multilobulated, longitudinally oriented lesion (asterisks) with low SI on T1-weighted image and heterogeneous low and high SI on T2-weighted image. Post-contrast image shows peripheral and septal enhancement (arrow). (**d**) Follow-up radiograph at 4 years after the initial visit presents complete disappearance of the lesion without any treatment (asterisk). (**e**) Both ankle radiograph taken for right ankle pain after a sprain in a 14-year-old girl shows no abnormal finding in the right ankle but incidentally notes a well-defined, eccentric, intracortical, multilobulated lesion in the contralateral left tibia, which is typically oriented along the growth axis of the tibia (double head arrows). (**f**) Pinhole bone scan reveals moderately increased activity along the lesion. (**g**) MR images demonstrate a longitudinal, intracortical lesion with heterogeneous intermediate SI on T1-weighted image and high SI on T2-weighted image, with internal dark signals on both sequences. Post-contrast image shows peripheral and septal enhancement (arrow)

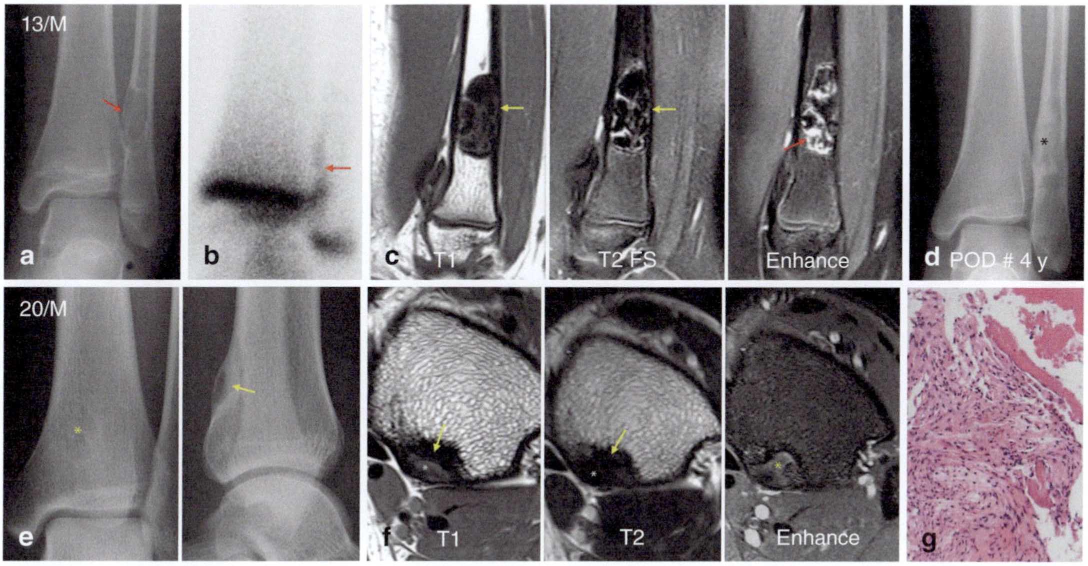

Fig. 29.7 ***Distal fibula*.** (**a**) Radiograph taken for left ankle pain of 2 weeks' duration in a 13-year-old boy shows an eccentric, well-defined, bubbly lesion surrounded by a thin rind of sclerosis in the diaphysis of the distal fibula. The lesion is medially expanded with marked cortical thinning (arrow). (**b**) Pinhole bone scan reveals eccentrical mild uptake along the medial cortex of the bone lesion (arrow). (**c**) MR images demonstrate a well-defined, multilobulated mass-like lesion with thinned but intact cortex (yellow arrows) with low SI on T1-weighted image and focal high SI on T2-weighted images, with prominent internal dark signals on both sequences. Contrast enhancement is noted at the margin and internal septa of the lesion (red arrow). (**d**) Follow-up radiograph at 4 years after curettage and allogenic chip bone graft notes healing of the lesion with consolidation and some remodeling of the fibula. **Longstanding regressing lesion:** (**e**) Radiograph taken for left ankle pain of 6 months' duration in a 20-year-old young man shows a subtle hazy lesion on anteroposterior view (asterisk). However, it is a clearly visible intracortical radiolucent lesion surrounded by a thick rim of sclerotic bone involving anterior cortex of the distal tibia on lateral view (arrow). (**f**) MR images reveal a well-defined, intracortical, small, oval lesion (asterisks) with low and intermediate SI on T1-weighted image and low SI on T2-weighted images, which is surrounded by a thick dark signal of reactive sclerosis (arrows). The lesion is heterogeneously enhanced (asterisk). (**g**) Microscopic examination notes moderate fibro-histiocytic cell proliferation arranged in *storiform* pattern with abundant collagen deposition and a focus of foam cells, suggesting an old regressing NOF

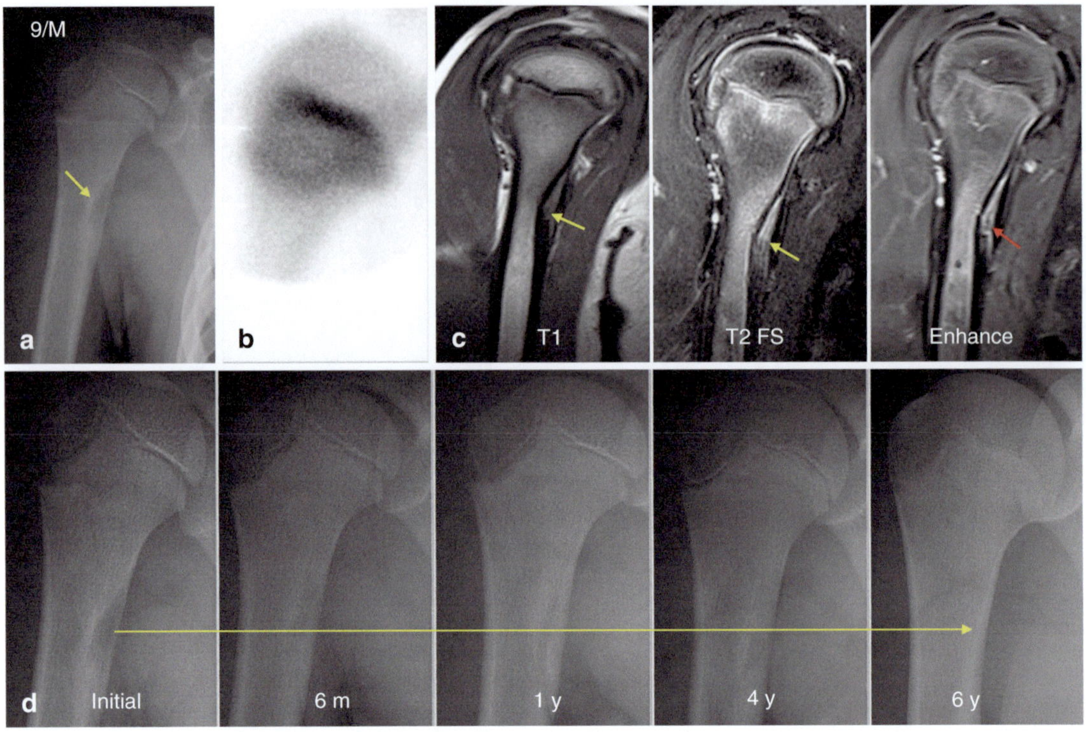

Fig. 29.8 ***Proximal humerus*** (**a**) Radiograph taken for intermittent shoulder pain of several months' duration in a 9-year-old boy incidentally shows a well-defined, eccentric, radiolucent radiolucent lesion with internal *ground-glass* density surrounded by a thin rim of sclerosis (arrow) in the proximal humerus. (**b**) Pinhole bone scan reveals no uptake in the lesion, suggesting an inactive benign lesion. (**c**) MR images demonstrate a well-defined, elongated lesion confined to the cortex (yellow arrows) with intermediate SI on T1-weighted image and heterogenous high SI on fat-saturated T2-weighted image. The lesion is heterogeneously well enhanced (red arrow). (**d**) Follow-up radiographs gradual, chronogical, spontaneous regression of the lesion. Radiograph at 6 years' follow-up shows complete healing of the lesion with a normalized cortical thickness

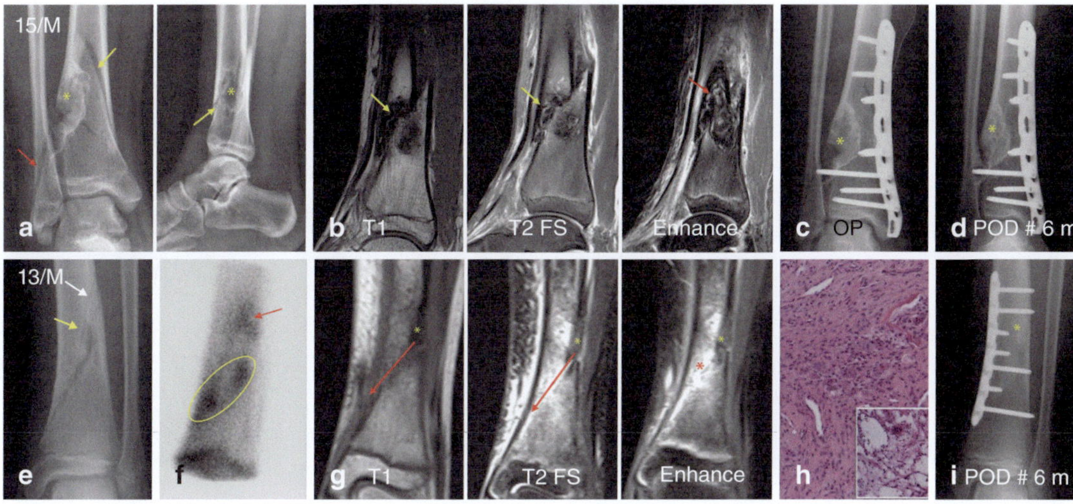

Fig. 29.9 ***Mildly displaced fracture***. (**a**) Radiograph taken for right ankle pain by a slip during snowboarding in a 15-year-old boy shows a mildly displaced spiral fracture of the distal tibia (yellow arrows) with a large, well-defined, eccentric, bubbly, cortex-based, sclerotic, and lucent lesion (asterisk) surrounded by a thin rind of sclerosis, indicating underlying NOF. A distal fibular fracture is also associated but without a preexisting underlying lesion (red arrow). (**b**) MR images reveal a moderately displaced oblique fracture with a preexisting lesion with low SI on T1-weighted image and heterogeneous low and intermediate SI with focal high signals on T2-weighted image. The lesion is focally and peripherally enhanced by contrast medium (red arrow). (**c**) Immediate postoperative radiograph after open reduction with internal fixation using plate and curettage with allogenic-chip bone graft for the preexisting NOF demonstrates good reduction and filling of the lesion with aoolgenic-bone chips (asterisk). (**d**) Follow-up radiograph at 6 months after surgery shows a consolidation of the lesion (asterisk) with radiologic union of the fracture. (**e**) Radiograph taken for left ankle pain after a slip on the stairs in a 13-year-old boy shows a minimally displaced oblique fracture (yellow arrow) with a small, ill-defined, dense lesion surrounded by a thin sclerotic rim (white arrow) in the distal tibia, suggesting a preexisting lesion with pathologic fracture. (**f**) Pinhole bone scan reveals heterogeneous hot uptake along the fracture line (circle) and milder uptake in the preexisting lesion (arrow). (**g**) MR images demonstrate a small intracortical lesion (asterisks) with low SI on T1-weighted image and intermediate to high SI on T2-weighted image, which seems to act as a stress riser for the oblique fracture. The lesion is weakly enhanced (yellow arrows), but bone marrow hemorrhage/edema by the fracture is diffusely well enhanced (red asterisk). It is clinically important that even a regressing small NOF with mild uptake on bone scan can act as a stress riser to trigger a pathologic fracture as in this case. (**h**) Microscopic examination exhibits a fibroblastic cell proliferation with scattered multinucleated giant cells and scar-like tissue. Another field shows prominent foam cells (inset), indicating a regressing NOF. (**i**) Follow-up radiograph at 6 months after internal fixation using plate shows complete consolidation of the underlying NOF with union of the fracture (asterisk)

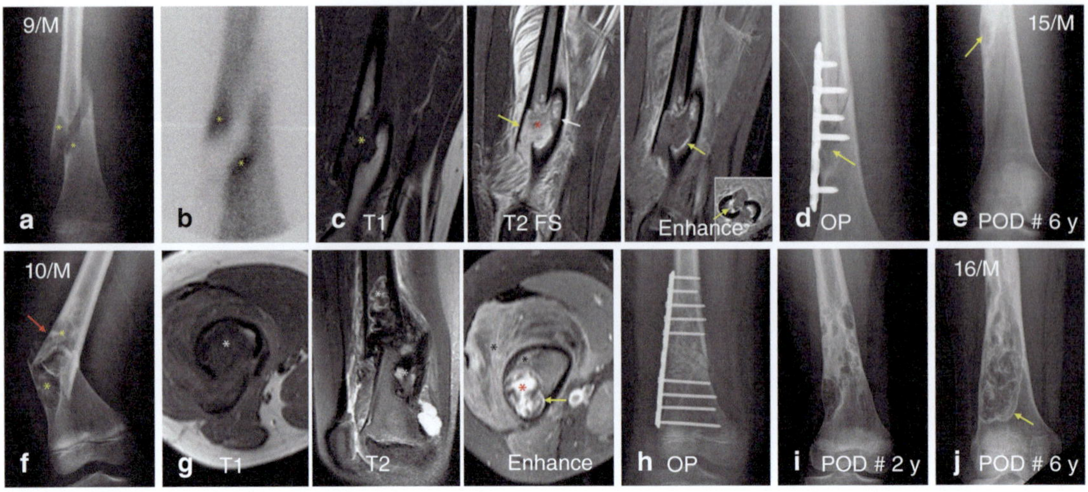

Fig. 29.10 ***Moderately to severely displaced fracture***. (**a**) Radiograph taken for left distal thigh pain immediately following blunt trauma during playing in a 9-year-old boy shows a more moderately displaced spiral fracture of the shaft of the distal femur and a preexisting small radiolucent lesion with cortical thinning surrounded by a thin sclerotic rim (asterisks). (**b**) Pinhole bone scan reveals focal areas of strong uptake in the corresponding regions of the preexisting radiolucent lesion on radiograph, suggesting still active lesion (asterisks). (**c**) MR images demonstrate a well-defined, medulla-occupying, mass-like lesion with thinning of the anterior cortex (yellow arrow) but normal thickness of the posterior cortex (white cortex), suggesting eccentric, anterior cortex-based lesion. SI is low on T1-weighted image and heterogeneous high SI on fat-saturated T2-weighted image. The displaced fracture is associated with significant surrounding bone marrow, muscle, and soft tissue hemorrhage with inflammation. The lesion is focally and peripherally enhanced (arrows). (**d**) Open reduction and plate fixation followed by curettage and allogenic bone graft (arrow) was performed. Frozen biopsy during surgery confirmed a diagnosis of NOF. (**e**) Follow-up radiograph at 6 years after surgery when the patient was 15 years old shows consolidation of the lesion still with hazy focal radiolucency (arrow). The patient is free of pain (asterisk). (**f**) Radiograph taken for left distal thigh pain with pseudomotion immediately after a slip while running in a 10-year-old boy shows a fracture with severe angulation of the distal femur and a large, poorly defined, multilobulated underlying lesion (yellow asterisks) with marked cortical thinning (red arrow). (**g**) MR images reveal an eccentric, cortex-based, multi-lobulated, medulla-occupying mass-like lesion with low SI on T1-weighted and heterogeneous low and high on T2-weighted image with dark signal areas on both sequences, suggesting mature bone formation with increasing mineralization. Significantly angulated and displaced fracture is associated with prominent adjacent bone marrow and surrounding soft tissue hemorrhage. Post-contrast image shows intense internal (asterisk) and peripheral enhancement (arrow). The soft tissue and bone marrow hemorrhage/edema with inflammation are diffusely enhanced (black asterisks). (**h**) Open reduction and plate fixation followed by curettage and allogenic bone graft were performed. (**i**) Follow-up radiograph at 2 years after surgery notes some consolidation area with multiple radiolucent small areas. (**j**) Follow-up radiograph at 6 years after surgery shows further consolidation of the lesion with multiple hazy radiolucent areas, surrounded by a thin rim of reactive sclerosis (arrow). The patient completely pain-free.

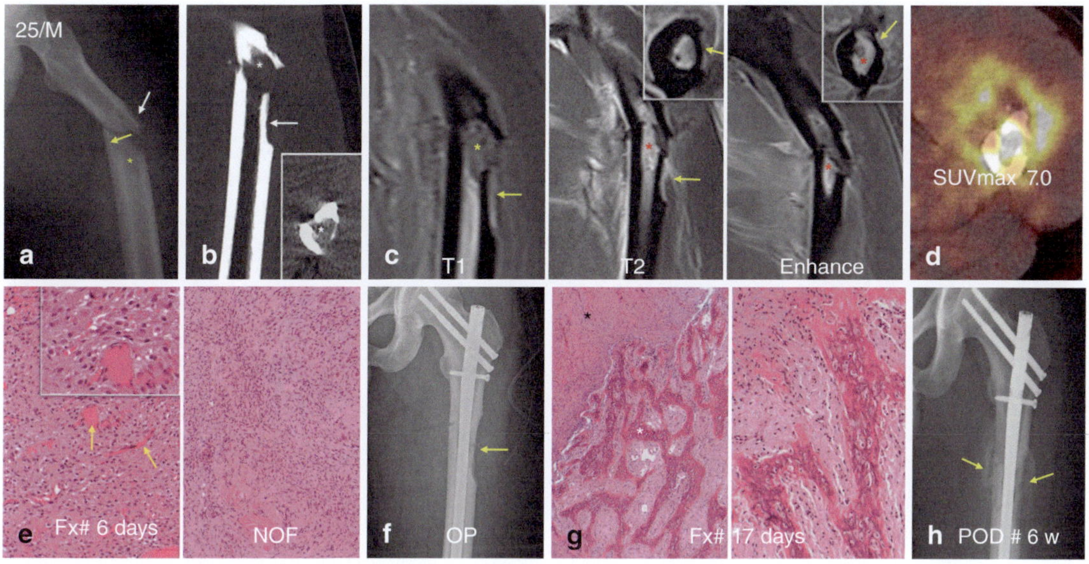

Fig. 29.11 ***Severely angulated fracture in regressing NOF***. (**a**) Radiograph taken for left thigh pain with pseudomotion following a collision during playing basketball in a 25-year-old soldier shows a fracture of the femoral midshaft with severe angulation. A subtle preexisting radiolucent lesion in the medullary cavity (asterisk) with endosteal scalloping (yellow arrow) is observed upon careful scrutiny. There is cortical erosion by extrinsic pressure (white arrow). (**b**) CT scan reveals a comminuted fracture with a suspicious intramedullary mass lesion (asterisk) with an eroded outer surface of the cortex by extrinsic pressure (arrow). (**c**) MR images demonstrate an ill-defined, small cortex-based mass-like lesion extending into the medullary cavity (asterisks) with low SI on T1-weighted image and high SI with focal bright signal on T2-weighted image. The anterolateral cortex is compressed and eroded by external soft tissue mass with similar signal (red arrows). However, there is no definite periosteal reaction. The medullary lesion (asterisks) and external soft tissue mass compressing the outer surface of the cortex (yellow arrow) are weakly enhanced. (**d**) PET/CT scan notes hypermetabolic activity (SUVmax 7.0) at fracture site and adjacent soft tissue or hematoma due to fracture. However, there is no definite mass-like uptake. (**e**) Microscopic examination: (Left) Most areas show explosive growth of tightly packed mesenchymal cells and a few wisps of primitive osteoid (arrows), suggesting early callus estimated age of the end of 1 week. Practically, biopsy was performed at 6 days after the fracure. Higher-power magnification (inset) reveals that the individual cells appear high nuclear to cytoplasmic ratio, larger nucleoli, and typical mitoses. (Right) In addition, a focal area of fibro-histiocytic cells in *storiform* pattern with abundant collagen deposition and sparse multinucleated giant cells, indicaive of NOF, is also identified upon close examination, suggesting a possible preexisting tumor. (**f**) Delayed surgery of open reduction and intramedullary nailing followed by curettage was performed at 17 days after the fracture due to a delayed confirmatory diagnosis of underlying NOF. The erosion by an external compression is clearly visible after reduction (arrow), but an exact histologic diagnosis of the external mass was not rendered. (**g**) Microscopic examination of biopsy specimens obtained during medullary rimming for nail insertion: (Left) Lower-power magnification reveals an area of fibro-histiocytic cells with abundant collagen deposition, suggesting NOF (black asterisk) and another area of osteoid to woven bone trabeculae prominently rimmed by a single layer of osteoblasts osteoblasts. connected together, to form to form variable-sized circles with less cellular marrow, indicating a callus estimated age of 2–3 weeks. Practically, the surgery was performed exactly 17 days after the fracture. (Right) Higher-power magnification notes woven trabeculae beginning with mineralization and less cellular *regularly ominous* marrow, which can be interpreted as osteosarcoma without histologic knowledge of fracture callus. (**h**) Radiograph at 6 weeks after surgery shows good maintenance of fixation with moderate external callus (arrows)

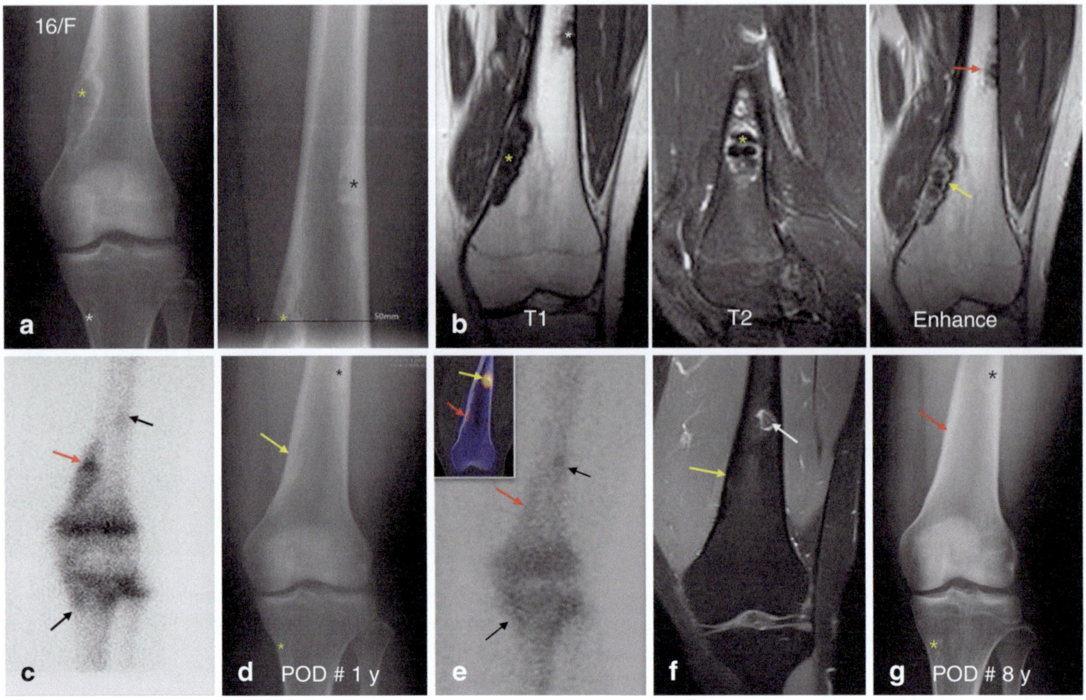

Fig. 29.12 ***Synchronous multiple NOFs*.** (**a**) Radiographs taken for recently developed right distal thigh pain in a 16-year-old girl show a well-defined, eccentric, multilobulated, intracortical lesion in the medial aspect of distal femur (yellow asterisks). The lesion is typically oriented along the growth axis of the involved femur. There are incidentally found smaller lesions in the lateral aspect of the femoral mid-shaft (black asterisk) and medial aspect of the proximal tibia (white asterisk), indicating a polyostotic lesion. (**b**) MR images reveal an eccentric, intracortical, multilobulated main lesion (yellow asterisks) with low SI on T1-weighted image and heterogeneous high SI on T2-weighted image, with internal dark signals on both sequences. There is a more proximally located smaller lesion of the same nature (white asterisk). The lesions are heterogeneously and peripherally enhanced (arrows). (**c**) Bone scan demonstrates mild peripheral and intense central uptake in the main lesion of the medial distal femur, suggesting still-active lesion (red arrow). However, the uptake is very subtle in other inactive lesions (black arrows). Simple curettage with bone graft of the main lesion was performed due to focal strong uptake and newly developed pain. (**d**) Follow-up radiograph at 1 year after surgery notes healing of the lesion (arrow). Other lesions are also decreased in size with consolidation (asterisks). (**e**) Follow-up bone scan shows no definite uptake in the surgically treated main lesion (red arrow). However, subtle uptake remains in other lesions (black arrows). Bone SPECT scan shows very tiny uptake in the curetted lesion (red arrow), but focal increased uptake persists in the femoral shaft lesion that received no treatment (yellow arrow). (**f**) Follow-up MR image demonstrates complete disappearance of the lesion treated by curettage (yellow arrow). However, the untreated lesion affecting the femoral shaft is still visible (white arrow). (**g**) Follow-up radiograph at 8 years after surgery notes complete healing with no recurrence of the curetted lesion (red arrow). Untreated lesions are also healed with sclerotic change (asterisks). Surgical management of curettage and bone graft shortens the healing process compared to spontaneous healing

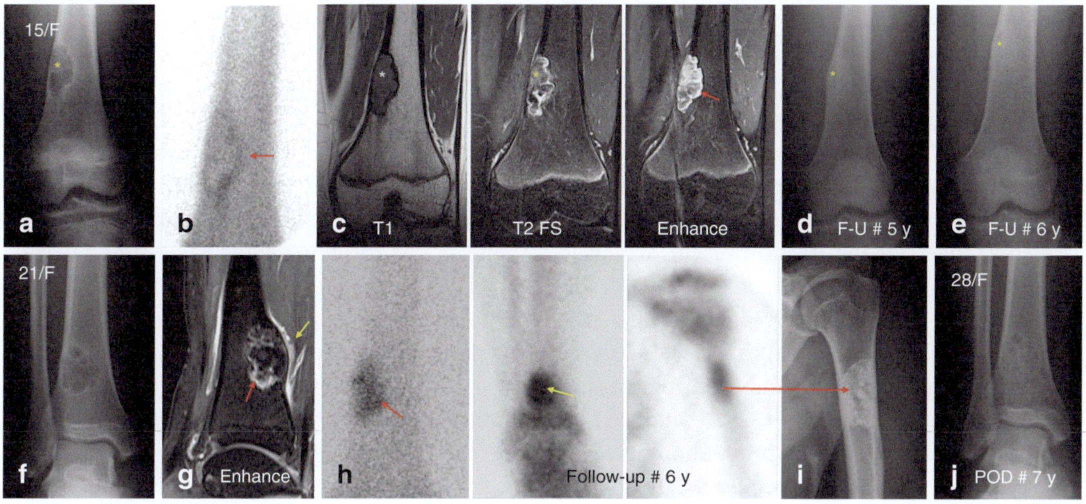

Fig. 29.13 ***Metachronous multiple NOFs*** (**a**) Radiographs taken for right knee pain after a traffic accident in a 15-year-old girl incidentally shows a well-defined, eccentric, lobulated, radiolucent lesion surrounded by a thin rind of sclerosis in the diaphysis of the distal femur (asterisk). (**b**) Pinhole bone scan reveals mild to moderate uptake along the margin of the lesion (red arrow), but whole-body scan notes no definite uptake in areas, suggesting a monostotic lesion. (**c**) MR images demonstrate a well-defined, multilobulated, cortex-based, eccentric lesion (asterisks) with intermediate SI on T1-weighted and heterogeneous intermediate and high SI on fat-saturated T2-weighted image, with internal focal dark dots and surrounded by a thin dark signal on both sequences. Post-contrast image shows peripheral and septal enhancement (red arrow). (**d**) Follow-up radiograph at 5 years the initial visit notes hazy consolidation of the lesion (asterisk). (**e**) One year later, radiograph notes nearly complete regression of the lesion with some remodeling of the cortex (asterisk). (**f**) Radiograph taken for newly developed right ankle at the patients' age of 21 reveals a well-defined, eccentric, bubbly, osteolytic lesion surrounded by a thin rim of sclerosis in the meta-diaphysis of the distal tibia, indicating newly developed NOF. (**g**) Post-contrast image shows a well-defined, eccentric lesion with posterior bulging with heterogeneous peripheral and septal enhancement (red arrow) with a marked periosteal reaction (yellow arrow). (**h**) Follow-up bone scan reveals newly developed strong uptake in the right distal tibia (yellow arrow) and mild uptake in the left proximal humerus (black arrow), both of which were not seen on the initial bone scan. The uptake in the distal femur lesion becomes more more intesne (red arow) compared with that on the initial pinhole scan. (**i**) Radiograph for the area of increased uptake on bone scan shows a well-defined lesion with a complete homogeneous sclerosis in left proximal humerus (stage D). (**j**) Radiograph at 7 years after curettage and allogenic chip bone graft, at her age of 28, reveals a consolidation of the lesion with no ankle pain

29.7 Clinical Features

These lesions are usually asymptomatic and found incidentally. However, larger lesions can produce pain and/or swelling, and potentially weaken the bone enough to predispose to microfracture, fatigue, or stress fracture with the lesion as a stress riser for the fracture origin, which is usually not visible on standard radiograph (Fig. 29.2f). A pathologic fracture is also frequently associated with varying lesion sizes, following a slip or or blunt trauma during playing and sports activity (Figs. 29.9, 29.10 and 29.11). Even regressing small lesion or junction between the separated lesions can act as a stress riser (Figs. 29.2h and 29.9g).

29.8 Radiologic Findings

Plain radiograph They are usually distinctive and diagnostic on conventional radiographs without biopsy. Characteristically, FCD is a small eccentric purely intracortical, radiolucent lesion in the metaphyseal area, which is mostly less than 3 cm in maximum diameter [1]. NOF is usually larger than 3–5 cm and extends from the cortex into the medullary space (cortical-based) near the physis of long bones. In early to mid-phase, NOF typically exhibits an eccentric, well-defined, multilobulated radiolucent lesion surrounded by a thin sclerotic rim generally involving the metaphysis to meta-diaphysis of long bones. The lesion can be separated by thin septa or lines to produce *bubbly* appearance, and is usually oriented along the growing axis of the involved bone (longer than its width). With age, the distance from the growth plate gradually increase, and the lesion eventually moves to the diaphysis in older adolescence or young adulthood (Fig. 29.10a, g and 29.11a). And, the internal density becomes denser due to increasing mineralization, and may exhibit complete homogeneous sclerosis at the final stage. The cortex may be thinned, and the affected bone can be expanded in some cases. Ritschl et al. [8] described stages in the evloution of NOF. *Stage A lesion* is a small, oval to slightly polycyclic in shape with or without a thin sclerotic rim, which is located eccentrically in the cortex near the growth plate (Fig. 29.1a). *Stage B lesion* moves toward the metaphysis as the bone grows and is located at a variable distance from the epiphysis, depending on growth rate. The shape is clearly demarcated by a thin sclerotic rim. The lesion becomes larger with cortical thinning and more polycyclic, grape-shaped borders, but periosteal reaction is not seen (Fig. 29.2a). *Stage C lesion* shows increasing mineralization which typically tends to start from the diaphyseal side and proceeds toward the growth plate (Fig. 29.2f). *Stage D lesion* is typified by complete homogeneous sclerosis (Fig. 29.13g). Rarely, aneurysmal bone cyst (ABC) can be superimposed resilting in a rapid enlargement and expansion of the underlying bone, and ABC associated with NOF was reported to account for about 3% of secondary ABC in a large series [10]. **Bone scan** A degree of the tracer uptake depends on the evolution stage of the lesion. In general, NOF itself is usually not associated with markedly increased activity. Bone scan is useful to classify active, healing, or inactive lesions based on the intensity of uptake corresponding to the degree of hyperemia and osteoblastic activity and to detect multiple lesions as well (Figs. 29.3, 29.12 and 29.13). Intense uptake suggests a more active process in the early stage (Fig. 29.2b), concealed microfracture or stress fracture which is not seen on plain radiograph (Fig. 29.2g), or even secondary ABC change. Mild to moderate uptake may be observed during the healing phase. Uptake is not present if the lesion is stabilized or has completely healed. The strong uptake in addition to the clinical symptom of pain and large size with marked cortical thinning of the lesion may indicate surgical management. **CT scan** is useful for assessing the exact size of the lesion, subtle changes in lesion size over time, and the presence of cortical integrity. However, CT scan is not appropriate for young patients due to the concern of a significant radiation exposure. **MRI** is not routinely necessary for diagnosis due to characteristic clinical and radiographic features. In the early stage, MR images demonstrate an eccentric, well-defined, multilobulated lesion with a peripheral thin dark signal of sclerotic rim. The signal intensity (SI) varies with amounts of fibrous tissue, hemosiderin, hemorrhage, collagen, foamy histiocytes, and bone trabeculae present in a given lesion [11]. Initially, SI is low on T1-weighted image and heterogeneous intermediate and high on T2-weighted image, with a dark signal peripheral rim. However, the lesion shows heterogenous low to dark signal on all sequences when the lesion matures with profuse collagen deposition, and begins to ossify. Contrast enhancement is also variable.

29.9 Histologic Findings

(1) *Early to middle (active or proliferative) stage:* The essential component of the NOF is a dense network of exuberant fibro-histiocytic cells arranged in *storiform, pinwheel, or whirling* pattern (Fig. 29.15a). The lesion is usually hypercellular, and the individual cells may have plump nuclei even with mild atypia. However, the nuclei are monotonously regular, chromatin is even, and there may be occasional typical mitosis but no frank pleomorphism and abnormal mitosis (Fig. 29.15b). Osteoclast-like multinucleated cells can be evenly scattered throughout the lesion. In general, they are less prominent and smaller than those seen in a conventional giant cell tumor (GCT) of bone. However, they may be prominent throughout the spindly stroma as in a GCT, which necessitate clinical, radiologic, and pathologic correlation to differentiate NOF from GCT in rare cases (Fig. 29.2d). GCT occurs rarely in patients younger than 20 years with an open growth plate, and almost always affects the epiphysis and often extends to the metastasis but does not purely involve but not purely involves the metaphysis. A number of sprinkled inflammatory cells, mainly lymphocytes and hemorrhagic foci, are often seen around the prominent multinucleated giant cells (Fig. 29.15c) (2). *Advanced middle to late (inactive or reparative) stage:* With aging, the cellularity of the stromal cells decreases gradually and the collagen deposition is accelerated particularly in hemorrhagic areas or degenerative foci. The collagen fibers are usually delicate and scarce. Woven to lamellar bone can be found, which is not produced by the lesional tissue itself but is reactive. The reactive bone spicules usually begin to be deposited at the periphery and spread to the center in the late healing or regressing stage. The *Storiform* or *whirling* pattern is more prominent in this stage than the earlier stage, and focal myxoid change with well-oriented reactive bone trabeculae lined by a single layer of osteoblasts, which may simulate a fracture callus of 2–3 weeks' age (Fig. 29.15d). Lipid laden foamy macrophages are increased in number being directly proportional to the lesion's maturation. Hemosiderin pigmentation can be seen in all phases and is often observed predominantly, and even cluters of cholesterol crystal clefts may also be seen (Fig. 29.15e). Cystic changes and necrotic areas can be seen particularly when pathological fracture is associated. The number of multinucleated giant cells, diminishes, becoming sparse or even absent. Ghost multinucleated giant cells can be observed in necrosis areas, and typical mitotic figures are occasionally seen, which are not worrisome features for malignancy (Fig. 29.15f). However, atypical mitoses are never seen. Rarely, secondary ABC change can be focally or extensively associated (Fig. 29.15f), producing a rapid enlargement by "blowout" expansion on radiograph if it is extensive [12]. Some individual cells in exceptionally rare case may exhibit significantly bizarre-looking pleomorphic nuclei mimicking a malignant tumor, a condition referred to as *pseudonanplastic* FCD [10] (Fig. 29.14).

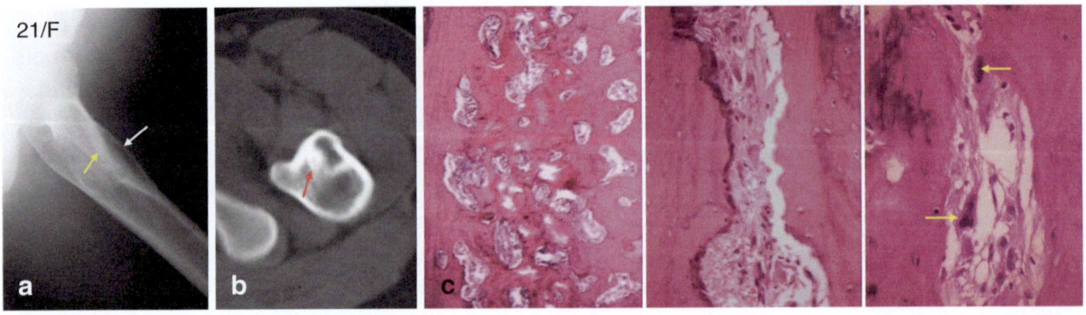

Fig. 29.14 ***Pseudoanaplastic FCD***. (**a**) Lateral radiograph reveals a well-defined radiolucent lesion confined to the cortex of the proximal femur. The lesion is oriented along the growing axis of the involved femur (longer than its width). It is surrounded by a significantly thickened sclerotic rim (yellow arrow) and the outer cortex is mildly bulged out and markedly thinned (white arrow), indicating a long-standing benign process. (**b**) CT scan shows a well-defined intracortical lucent lesion surrounded by abundant reactive bone (arrow). (**c**) Microscopic examination: (Left) Low-power examination notes a thickened lamellar bone with numerous cement lines. There are tiny nests with mild cellularity within the sclerotic bone. (Middle) Medium-power magnification reveals a small number of fibro-histiocytic cells, some of which have bizarre-looking nuclei embedded within loose fibrous stroma, which produce delicate collagen fibers. (Right) Higher-power magnification shows markedly atypical spindle cells with large, bizarre-looking nuclei resembling fibrosarcoma. However, not a single mitotic figure is found. In correlation with radiographic findings of a long-standing benign process, a diagnosis of *pseudoanaplastic FCD* was rendered by Dr. Mirra JM. No local recurrence or metastasis was observed at 4 years after simple curettage, which clinically supports a benign nature of the lesion

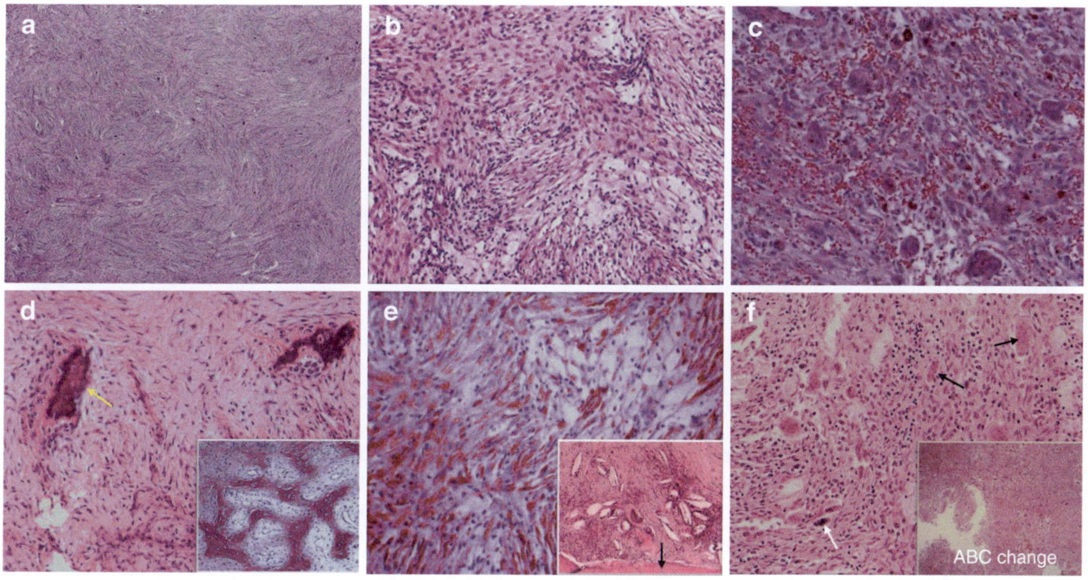

Fig. 29.15 *Microscopic features*. **(1) Early to middle active or proliferative phases:** (**a**) Low-power magnification shows a prominent spindle cell proliferation characteristically arranged in intersecting fascicles forming a *storiform or whirling* pattern. (**b**) Medium-power magnification reveals a large number of fibro-histiocytic stromal cells with plump but monotonously regular nuclei. (**c**) Numerous multinucleated giant cells are diffusely scattered throughout this filed, mimicking conventional GCT. Diffuse fresh hemorrhage is also seen around the giant cells. **(2) Advanced middle to late inactive or healing phases:** (**d**) With the age of the lesion, collagen production is accelerated with reactive osteoid to woven bone spicules which are not produced by lesional tissue itself but reactive on nature. The reactive bone spicules are rimmed by plump osteoblasts and partially ossified or calcified (arrow). The bone formation usually begins at the periphery and spreads to the center. Note focal myxoid change with well-oriented prominent reactive bone trabeculae lined by a single layer of osteoblasts (inset), which simulates fracture callus of 2–3 weeks' age in Fig. 29.11g. (**e**) Hemosiderin pigmentation may manifest in all phases. Xanthomatous reaction with foamy macrophages having rich lipid is observed in direct proportion to the degree of maturation of the lesion. In this late phase, the foamy cells are abundantly found in the form of sheets with scar tissue, but osteoclast-like giant cells are absent. Cholesterol clefts are also focally seen and there is a sharp border between the tumor and the underlying cortex (arrow in inset). (**f**) Cystic changes and necrotic areas are observed in association with sprinkled inflammatory cells. Ghost multinucleated giant cells are observed in the necrotic area (black arrows), and a typical mitotic figure is also seen (white arrow), neither of which is a worrisome feature for malignancy. Of course, there is not a single discernible atypical mitosis. Secondary ABC change with areas of massive hemorrhage is also observed (inset)

29.10 Management

FCD and small, asymptomatic NOF are considered "do not touch" lesions which need only serial radiographic follow-up without biopsy until growth or regression is confirmed. (Fig. 29.1). Simple curettage with or without bone graft is necessary when the lesion is symptomatic, large large, and expansile, or shows increased uptake on bone scan. Surgical management of curettage and bone graft can drastically shorten the healing period compared to spontaneous healing. Pthlogic fracutres with mild displacement are treated with cast immobilization, resulting callus formation is expected to strengthen the diseased bone. However, open reduction and internal fixation with biopsy may be necessary for a displaced fracture with expanded lesion or unclear diagnosis (Figs. 29.9, 29.10 and 29.11). Prophylactic curettage with bone graft may be considered for large lesions, particularly if there is significant chance of impending fracture (Fig. 29.5).

29.11 Clinical Course

Basically, FCD and NOF are self-limiting lesions. Most FCDs gradually disappear and eventually become resolve as the host bone grows in length. It has been described to take about 5 years in NOF and 10 years in NOF for spontaneous resolution [1]. However, it is difficult to predict the exact time required for complete disappearance, as the lesion's age at the time of first radiographic detection is unknown. Regression usually begins at the end of adolescence, and almost or completely disappears by about 25 years of age [1] (Fig. 29.3c). The prognosis after simple curettage and bone graft is excellent. However, the lesion recurred in 6.7% of nonsyndromic NOFs without the café-au-lait spot and 60% of syndromic NOFs with the spots after curettage and bone grafting in a series of 35 multiple NOFs. Therefore, the authors recommended a more strict curette of the multiple NOF lesions, particularly in the setting of syndromic NOFs with other extra-skeletal anomalies [13]. In a review of 23 cases of pathologic fractures through NOFs, all fractures except one (96%) were located in the lower extremity, mostly in the tibia and fibula (78%). The fractured bones showed more than 50% lesion involvement by the lesion on both radiologic planes, and, and the vertical length of the lesion exceeded about 3 cm in all non-fibular lesions. The authors suggested that lesions of that size should be monitored closely, or prophylactic curettage and bone grafting need to be considered to prevent fracture [14]. Other studies suggested that *stage B* lesions were at an increased risk of fracture, whereas no fractures were observed in the other 3 stages. Therefore, periodic follow-up is necessary for the case of larger *stage B* lesions until they reach *stage C* [15]. However, another study reported that about 60% of large lesions exceeding these measurements had no pathologic fracture at the time of diagnosis. Thus, the authors suggested that the majority of patients with large NOFs can be monitored without intervention [16]. However, our cases with pathologic fracture were *stage C* lesion with migration of the lesion to the diaphysis (Figs. 29.9, 29.10 and 29.11). A stress fracture was not visible on standard radiograph but detected on bone scan and MRI occurs in a case with concomitant *Stages C* and *D* lesions (Fig. 29.2f–h). The stress fracture is believed to arise from the junction between the distal hazy radiolucent lesion (*Stage C*) and the proximal radiodense lesion (*Stage D*). Malignant transformations have been extremely rarely reported [1, 17–21].

References

1. Mirra JM. Fibrocortical defect and nonossifying fibroma. In: Mirra JM, editor. Bone tumors: clinical, radiologic, and pathologic correlations. 2nd ed. Philadelphia: Lea & Febiger; 1989. p. 692–735.
2. Jaffe HL. Non-ossifying fibromata. In: Jaffe HL, editor. Tumors and tumorous conditions of the bones and joints. Phildelphia: Lea & Febiger; 1958. p. 117–41.
3. Cherix S, Bildé Y, Becce F, Letovanec I, Rüdiger HA. Multiple non-ossifying fibromas as a cause of pathological femoral fracture in Jaffe-Campanacci syndrome. BMC Musculoskelet Disord. 2014;15(1):1–6.
4. Campanacci M, Laus M, Boriani S. Multiple non-ossifying fibromata with extraskeletal anomalies: a new syndrome? J Bone Joint Surg Br. 1983;65(5):627–32.
5. Jaffe HL, Lichtenstein L. Non-osteogenic fibroma of bone. Am J Pathol. 1942;18(2):205–21.
6. Nielsen GP, Kyriakos M. Fibrohistiocytic tumours. In: Fletcher CDM, Bridge J, Hogendorn PCW, Mertens F, editors. World Health Organization classification of Tumours. Pathology and genetics of tumours of soft tissue and bone. Lyon: IARC; 2002. p. 301–4.
7. Caffey J. On fibrous defects in cortical walls of growing tubular bones: their radiologic appearance, structure, prevalence, natural course, and diagnostic significance. Adv Pediatr Infect Dis. 1955;7:13–51.
8. Ritschl P, Karnel F, Hajek P. Fibrous metaphyseal defects-determination of their origin and natural history using a radiomorphological study. Skeletal Radiol. 1988;17(1):8–15.
9. Moser R, Sweet D, Haseman D, Madewell J. Multiple skeletal fibroxanthomas: radiologic-pathologic correlation of 72 cases. Skeletal Radiol. 1987;16(5):353–9.
10. Bahk WJ, Mirra JM. Pseudoanaplastic tumors of bone. Skeletal Radiol. 2004;33(11):641–8.
11. Jee WH, Choe BY, Kang HS, Suh KJ, Suh JS, Ryu KN, et al. Nonossifying fibroma: characteristics at MR imaging with pathologic correlation. Radiology. 1998;209(1):197–202.
12. Czerniak B. Fibrous and fibrohistiocytic lesions. In: Dorfman HD, Czerniak B, editors. Dorfman and Czerniak's bone tumors. 2nd ed. Elsevier; 2016. p. 617–91.

13. Jamshidi K, Motaghi P, Bagherifard A, Eigi M, Al-Baseesee HH, Mirzaei A. Comparison of characteristic features and local recurrence in syndromic versus non-syndromic multifocal non-ossifying fibroma. J Orthop Sci. 2021;26(4):655–9.
14. Arata MA, Peterson H, Dahlin D. Pathological fractures through non-ossifying fibromas. Review of the Mayo Clinic experience. J Bone Joint Surg. 1981;63(6):980–8.
15. Herget GW, Mauer D, Krauß T, El Tayeh A, Uhl M, Südkamp NP, et al. Non-ossifying fibroma: natural history with an emphasis on a stage-related growth, fracture risk and the need for follow-up. BMC Musculoskelet Disord. 2016;17(1):1–7.
16. Easley ME, Kneisl JS. Pathologic fractures through nonossifying fibromas: is prophylactic treatment warranted? J Pediatr Orthop. 1997;17(6):808–13.
17. Bhagwandeen S. Malignant transformation of a non-osteogenic fibroma of bone. J Pathol Bacteriol. 1966;92(2):562–4.
18. Biazzo A, Errani C, Gambarotti M, De Paolis M, Donati DM, Giannini S. Spindle cell sarcoma of bone arising from a non-ossifying fibroma: a case report. J Clin Orthop Trauma. 2013;4(2):80–4.
19. Kyriakos M, Murphy WA. Concurrence of metaphyseal fibrous defect and osteosarcoma. Skeletal Radiol. 1981;6(3):179–86.
20. Picci P, Sieberova G, Alberghini M, Balladelli A, Vanel D, Hogendoorn PC, et al. Late sarcoma development after curettage and bone grafting of benign bone tumors. Eur J Radiol. 2011;77(1):19–25.
21. Hastrup J, Jensen TS. Osteogenic sarcoma arising in a non-osteogenic fibroma of bone. Acta Pathol Microbiol Scand A. 1965;63(4):493–9.

30 Benign Fibrous Histiocytoma

30.1 Definition

Benign fibrous histiocytoma is a rare mesenchymal tumor composed of fibroblasts and histiocytes in varying proportions, which is usually found in subcutaneous or deep soft tissue of the extremities of aduls, but rarely in the bones of adults. Benign fibrous histiocytoma of bone (BFHB) is histologically composed of interlacing bundles of bland fibroblasts and histiocytes arranged in a storiform pattern, which is indistinguishable from fibrous cortical defects (FCD) or nonossifying fibroma (NOF) without clinical and radiologic correlation [1, 2]. BFHB can be distinguished from them on the basis of atypical locations including the ilium, rib, sacrum, and vertebra and unusual older patient's age over 20 years [3].

30.2 Synonyms

Xanthoma/xanthofibroma/fibroxanthoma.

30.3 Incidence

BFHB occurs very rarely, accounting for less than 1% of primary bone tumors [1, 3–5].

30.4 Possible Pathogenesis

BFH may be the end product of preexisting lesion such as fibrous dysplasia, giant cell tumor (GCT), and NOF/OFD with fibro-histiocytic repair tissue and prominent foam cells. Mirra [3] described that about 5–10% of conventional GCT are rich in fibro-histiocytic tissue and foam cells, simulating BFHB (Refer Chapter 1 Giant Cell Tumor in Volume 2). Bertoni et al. [1] reported that 10 out of 350 cases (2.9%) of GCT showed histologic features of extensive, distinct fibroblastic cells arranged in a storiform pattern with scattered multinucleated cells, foam cells, and large necrotic areas that were identical to those of BFHB and all cases were located in long bones. Spjut et al. [6] also described BFHB may represent a secondary regressive or degenerative phenomenon in the above-mentioned preexisting lesions which cannot be easily identified. However, there is still controversy about whether BFHB is a distinct benign bone tumor or merely a reactive lesion superimposed on such preexisting conditions.

W.-J. Bahk, *Diagnosis and Management of Primary Bone Tumors*,
https://doi.org/10.1007/978-981-96-3484-2_30

30.5 Age

Most patients are adults over 20 years of age with a wide range from 21 to 68 years [2, 4, 7]. It is about the similar age for GCT except for a few much older patients, while FCD/NOF is mostly found during the first and second decade of life. BFH can often occur in older patients between the sixth and eighth decades (Fig. 30.1), and GCT is also rarely seen in patients older than 60 years. Thus, an age over 60 years would not be considered a diagnostic parameter.

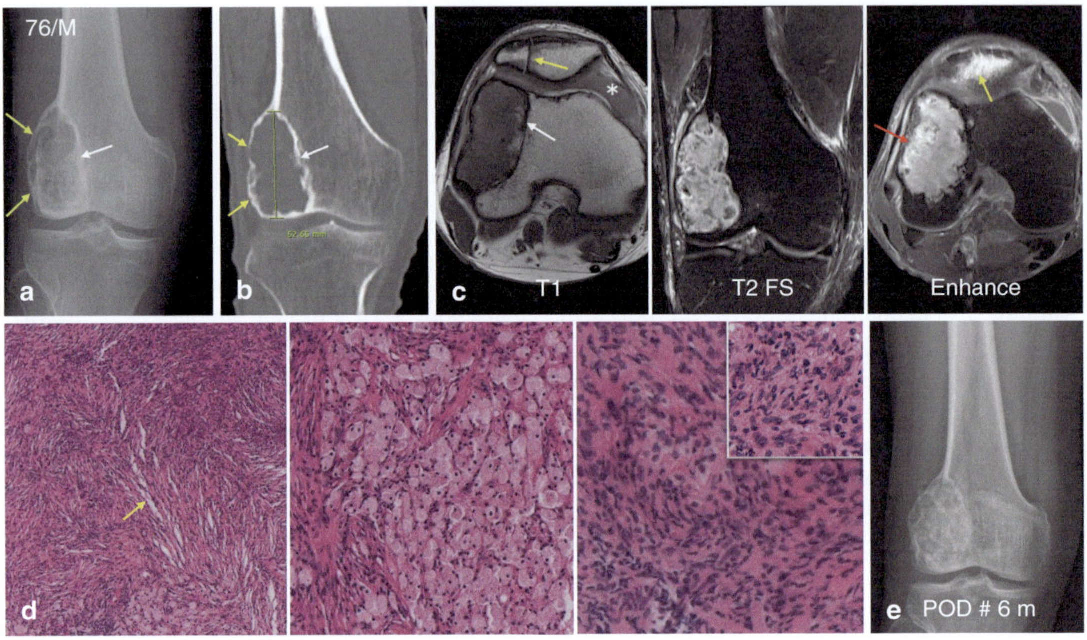

Fig. 30.1 (**a**) Radiograph taken for right knee pain of 6 months' duration which was aggravated following a slip in a 76-year-old man shows a well-defined, eccentric, bubbly, radiolucent lesion surrounded by a thin rim of sclerosis (white arrow) in the epi-metaphysis of the medial femoral condyle. Note irregular thinning of cortex with lucent lines, suggesting repeated insufficiency or stress fractures, which can be a probable cause of chronic pain (yellow arrows). (**b**) CT scan more clearly reveals an eccentric, well-defined, radiolucent lesion with irregular surrounding sclerotic rim (white arrow). There is also significant cortical thinning and irregular thickening with no definite destruction (yellow arrows). There is no internal density or periosteal reaction. (**c**) MR images demonstrate a well-defined eccentric mass-like lesion with low SI on T1-weighted image and high SI with focal low and dark signals on fat-suppressed T2-weighted image in the epi-metaphysis abutting the distal femoral articular surface. The lesion well demarcated by a thi sclerotic rim of dark signal (white arrow). There is cortical erosion and thinning but no discernible cortical destruction. The patella shows vertical dark signal (yellow arrow) with low SI of extensive hemorrhage and edema in the joint space on T1-weighted image (asterisk), indicating a fracture caused by a direct blow during slip, which should be a cause of acute aggravation of the chronic pain. The femoral lesion is heterogeneously enhanced (red arrow) and the fractured patella, assocated with hemorrhage and edema, is strongly enhanced (yellow arrow). (**d**) Microscopic examination: (Left) Low-power magnification presents a large number of spindle cells with interspersed foamy macrophages arranged in a *storiform* pattern. Inflammatory cells are diffusely scattered. There are areas of prominent microscopic cystic change (arrow). However, multinucleated giant cells are completely absent in all slides. (Middle) The foamy macrophages with clear vacuolated cytoplasm due to abundant intracytoplasmic lipid are forming larger solid clusters in this field. (Right) Higher-power magnification shows mildly atypical spindle cells with elongated plump nuclei and small prominent nucleoli, but no abnormal mitosis. (**e**) Follow-up radiograph at 6 months after thorough curettage and allogenic-chip bone graft reveals consolidation of the lesion

30.6 Location

The lesion occurs most commonly in flat bones including the spine, rib, pelvis, and skull which are not a typical place for FCD/NOF. In long bones, the metaphysis of the proximal and distal femur as well as proximal tibia is most commonly affected, and the diagnosis is less commonly involved [2, 4]. The reported cases involving the epiphysis of long tubular bones can be controversial in diagnosis because it is very difficult, or perhaps even impossible, to exclude ancient regressive form of GCT with a prominent fibro-histiocytic component [7].

30.7 Clinical Features

Pain with variable duration of months to several years is the most frequent symptom, although it can be asymptomatic and discovered incidentally. Rarely, it can present with a pathological fracture.

30.8 Radiologic Findings

Plain radiograph The lesion in the long bone appears as an eccentrically located, well-defined, radiolucent lesion surrounded by a reactive sclerotic rim usually affecting the metaphysis, simulating NOF. The lesion may be multilobulated with septa or ridges, producing a *soap-bubble* appearance. The lesion is often fusiform in shape with cortical erosion, thinning or thickening, and mild expansion. Irregular thinning and thickening of cortex may show multiple lucent lines, indicating tiny insufficiency fractures, which may be a possible cause of pain in patients with BFHB [4] (Fig. 30.1a). However, cortical destruction with soft tissue invasion is rare, and periosteal reaction or calcification of the lesion is usually not seen. **CT scan** more clearly reveals a well-defined, osteolytic lesion with a prominent sclerotic margin and a thinned or thickened cortex with or without breakage. There is no internal density or periosteal reaction (Fig. 30.1b). **MR images** show a well-defined, eccentric, mass-like lesion with low to intermediate SI on T1-weighted images and heterogeneous high SI on T2-weighted images. The lesion is sharply demarcated by a dark signal of surrounding sclerotic rim on all sequences. Hemorrhagic or cystic areas can be seen with or without fluid-fluid levels. The lesion is heterogeneously enhanced by contrast medium (Fig. 30.1c).

30.9 Histologic Findings

BFH consists of fibroblast-like spindle cells and variable numbers of interspersed foamy macrophages (xanthoma cells). The individual spindle cells show bland elongated plump nuclei and small prominent nucleoli, which are arranged in short intersecting fascicles that typically present a *storiform or whirling* pattern, at least focally. The foamy macrophages with clear vacuolated cytoplasm due to an abundant intracytoplasmic lipid are interspersed among the spindle cells and occasionally form small or larger solid clusters. Multinucleated giant cells are sparsely distributed among the other components often with inflammatory cells. However, they can be totally absent from most or all fields (Fig. 30.1d). Areas of fresh or old hemorrhage with hemosiderin deposition or cholesterol clefts are commonly seen. Microscopic cystic change can often be observed. Reactive or reparative new bone formation is also occasionally found. A few mitoses can be scattered but atypical mitosis is never found. These histologic findings overlap with those seen in FCD/NOF or even regressive ancient GCT. Therefore, clinical and radiologic correlation is mandatory for a correct diagnosis. However, it is very difficult, or even impossible, to rule out regressive ancient form of GCT presenting a prominent fibro-histiocytic component particularly when multinucleated giant cells are sparse to absent with the location of epi-metaphysis of the distal femur or proximal tibia in patients between 20 and 40 years of age.

30.10 Management

Complete curettage with bone graft is the treatment of choice (Fig. 30.1e). En-bloc resection can be considered for large expansile lesions or for lesions involving resectable bones such as fibula and rib.

30.11 Prognosis

The prognosis is not conclusive due to very small numbers of cases. Healing seems to be expected when the lesion is completely removed by surgical management. Bertoni et al. [1] reported that there was no recurrence regardless of the surgical margin achieved, including curettage, marginal excision, or wide excision. However, a high incidence of local recurrence was reported after incomplete curettage in another series [2]. Grohs et al. [4] added cauterization using phenol after extensive curettage and burring, and they concluded a thorough local treatment was sufficient to prevent local recurrence and fully restore daily activity. Although recurrences can occur after curettage, locally aggressive behavior or particularly distant metastasis indicates that the diagnosis of BFH would be inappropriate. Possibly, these cases can be misdiagnosed examples of GCT or low-grade malignant fibrous histiocytoma of bone [8].

References

1. Bertoni F, Calderoni P, Bacchini P, Sudanese A, Baldini N, Present D, et al. Benign fibrous histiocytoma of bone. J Bone Joint Surg Am. 1986;68(8):1225–30.
2. Clarke BE, Xipell JM, Thomas DP. Benign fibrous histiocytoma of bone. Am J Surg Pathol. 1985;9(11):806–15.
3. Mirra JM. Fibrous histiocytoma. In: Mirra JM, editor. Bone tumors: clinical, radiologic, and pathologic correlations. 2nd ed. Philadelphia, PA: Lea & Febiger; 1989. p. 759–66.
4. Grohs JG, Nicolakis M, Kainberger F, Lang S, Kotz R. Benign fibrous histiocytoma of bone: a report of ten cases and review of literature. Wien Klin Wochenschr. 2002;114(1–2):56–63.
5. Unni KK, Inwards CY. Xanthoma of bone. In: Unni KK, Inwards CY, editors. Dahlin's bone tumors: general aspects and data on 10,165 cases. 6th ed. Philadelphia, PA: Lippincott William & Wilkins; 2010. p. 225–42.
6. Spjut HJ, Dorfman HD, Fechner RE, Ackerman LV. Tumors of bone and cartilage. In: Atlas of tumor pathology. Second series, Fascicle 5. Washington, DC: Armed Forces Institute of Pathology; 1983. p. 16–8.
7. Matsuno T. Benign fibrous histiocytoma involving the ends of long bone. Skeletal Radiol. 1990;19:561–6.
8. Czerniak B. Fibrous and Fibrohistiocytic lesions. In: Dorfman HD, Czerniak B, editors. Dorfman and Czerniak's bone tumors. 2nd ed. eBook: Elsevier; 2016. p. 617–91.

31 Solitary Fibrous Tumor

31.1 Definition

Solitary fibrous tumor of bone (SFTB) is an extremely rare benign or malignant neoplasm consisting of oval to spindle-shaped cells derived from the pericytes of Zimmerman having long processes wrapping around capillaries characterized by strong morphologic heterogeneity with a wide spectrum of biologic features. In early 1871, Wagner [1] first mentioned a spindle cell mesenchymal tumor of poorly understood origin in the pleura. Later in 1931, Klemperer and Rabin described five cases of primary neoplasms in the pleura, and called it *localized fibrous mesothelioma* [2], and subsequently reported in extrapleural sites such as skin, nervous system, soft tissue, liver, lung, kidney, thyroid, and even bone. More later in 1956, Stout [3] first described the primary bone counterpart of this rare tumor.

31.2 Synonym

It was previously termed hemangiopericytoma (HPC) which is, however, no longer accepted in the WHO classification of soft tissue and bone tumors [4, 5]. The histological findings and clinical behavior of SFT and HPC are closely related, although not identical, and thus the unifying term "SFT/HPC" was proposed [6].

31.3 Incidence

SFTB is exceptionally rare. Earlier in 1956, Stout reported only 2 out of 197 cases (1%) of HPCs at various sites were primarily in bone. Since then, SFTB has been reported mainly in single case reports, and described as exceedingly rare even in major series [7–9], occupying only 0.14% (15 from 10,165 cases) of bone tumors in a more recent Mayo Clinic series [10]. In the earlier series on 8452 bone tumors from the same institute, the incidence was 0.08% of primary bone tumors, 0.1% of malignant primary bone tumors, 4.7% of primary vascular bone tumors, and 11% of malignant vascular bone tumors [11].

31.4 Age

It may occur at any age, but usually affects middle-aged adults [2, 5, 12] with a peak incidence in the fourth and fifth decades of life [10, 13].

31.5 Location

Any bone can be involved. However, the axial skeleton including sacroiliac region, lumbosacral spines, skull bones, and other flat bones

W.-J. Bahk, *Diagnosis and Management of Primary Bone Tumors*,
https://doi.org/10.1007/978-981-96-3484-2_31

such as scapula and sternum as well as the long bones such as femur, tibia, fibula, and humerus are most frequently affected [14, 15].

31.6 Clinical Features

Most SFTBs tend to grow slowly and may not cause signs and symptoms until they become very large. Pain or swelling of long duration is the usual presentation. Extraordinarily, SFT can primarily arise from bone [16], and rarely metastasize to bone from various anatomic sites including meninges, peritoneum, head and neck, extremities, and viscera [2, 17–20].

31.7 Radiologic Findings

Plain radiograph SFTB presents a nonspecific, locally aggressive-looking, osteolytic lesion with a geographic or moth-eaten pattern of bone destruction. The lesion often exhibits a cortical destruction with extension into the adjacent soft tissue (Fig. 31.1a). **CT scan** more clearly reveals a well-circumscribed, smooth, and lobulated soft tissue mass that may contain scattered calcifications. Central focal low-attenuation areas can be observed in larger lesions, suggesting cystic or necrotic changes. **MR images** demonstrate a relatively well-defined medullary mass-like lesion with heterogeneous low to intermediate SI on T1-weighted image and variable SI T2-weighted image, with low signal foci on both T1- and T2-weighted images attributable to abundant collagen or fibrous tissue content. However, hemorrhage, nonspecific cystic change or necrotic foci may result in areas of high signals on T2-weighted image. Frequently, internal serpentine black signal or focal dark signal suggesting abundant vasculature can be seen (Fig. 31.1b). A locally aggressive appearance can also be noted with multiple areas of cortical breakage with soft tissue extension mimicking a malignant tumor. The lesion shows heterogeneous strong enhancement by contrast media, with nonenhancing cystic or necrotic areas.

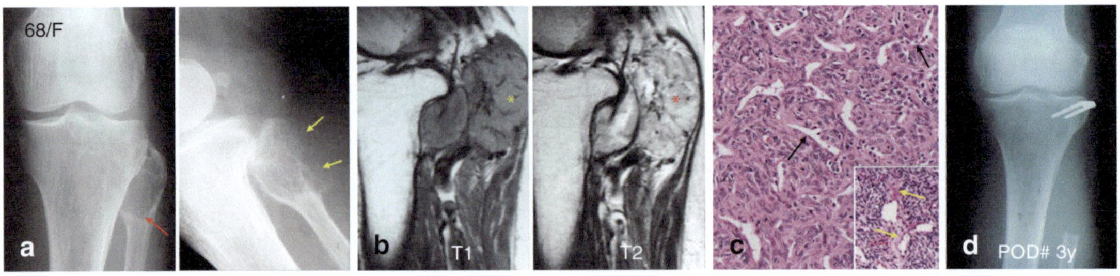

Fig. 31.1 (**a**) Radiograph taken for left knee pain of 1 year's duration in a 68-year-old woman shows a well-defined, multilobulated, mildly expanding, geographic destruction (red arrow) in the fibular head and neck on anteroposterior radiograph. However, there is a significant cortical destruction with soft tissue extension, suggesting a locally aggressive or even malignant bone tumor on lateral view (yellow arrows). (**b**) MR images reveal a multilobulated mass-like lesion showing cortical destruction and huge soft tissue mass with intermediate SI on T1-weighted image and heterogeneous intermediate and high SI on T2-weighted image. Note internal serpentine black signal or focal dark signal particularly in the soft tissue mass, suggesting abundant vasculature (asterisks). The lesion was strongly enhanced by contrast medium, but the image is not available here. (**c**) Microscopic examination notes sheets of haphazardly arranged oval to spindle-shaped fibroblastic cells embedded in prominent collagenous stroma. The cellularity is moderate to high and the individual cells have a small amount of cytoplasm, enlarged nuclei with dense chromatin, atypical nucleoli, and a few mitoses, indicating Grade 2 SFTB. Note characteristically numerous, variable sized and shaped, thin-walled, sharply branched in *staghorn-like* appearance (black arrows). Areas of perivascular hyalinization are clearly seen (arrows in inset). Stains for CD34, CD99, and Bcl-2 were strongly positive, which supported a diagnosis of SFTB. (**d**) Follow-up radiograph at 3 years after wide resection of the proximal fibula reveals no evidence of local recurrence. The patient is doing well without disease at 20 years after surgery, which was confirmed recently by a telephone communication with the patient

31.8 Histologic Findings

The lesion typically presents a varying degree of cellularity, nuclear atypia, and mitotic activity with a wide spectrum of biologic features from benign to intermediate or even malignant behavior. The lesion is composed of round to oval or spindle-shaped fibroblastic cells embedded in collagenous stroma arranged haphazardly (*pattern-less*) or in short fascicles. The cells are usually monotonous lacking frank anaplasia in benign or low-grade tumors. Cellularity is variable from low or medium to high with varying grades of anaplasia including bizarre nuclei and number of mitoses depending on the grade of the disease. Mitotic activity and necrosis are the major criteria for distinguishing benign from malignant SFT. A higher-grade malignant tumor has higher cellularity with severe atypia, necrosis, infiltrative growth pattern, and increased mitotic activity. Characteristically, the tumor cells are arranged around vascular spaces, and the clusters of the tumor cells may alter the vascular shape in a typical "*antler-like*" or "*staghorn-like*" appearance, consisting of multiple, large calibered, thin-walled, sharply branched (Fig. 31.1c). The focal HPC-like pattern of *staghorn-like* vascular channels can be seen in other sarcomas including mesenchymal chondrosarcoma, fibroblastic osteosarcoma, fibrosarcoma, or undifferentiated pleomorphic sarcoma. However, the tumor cells and characteristic vascular spaces are intimately related and spread throughout the lesion only in SFT/HPC. Areas of necrosis, cystic or myxoid change, calcification, hemorrhage as well as perivascular hyalinization (Fig. 31.1c) may also be found. Tang and colleagues suggested a grading system from Grade 1 to 3 for SFTB [13]. Grade 1 is a hypocellular lesion containing cells with small, ovoid nuclei set in fairly abundant cytoplasm, no prominent nucleoli, and with zero to one mitosis. A *staghorn-like* vascular pattern is striking and characteristic. Grade 3 is characterized by more numerous cells with small amounts of cytoplasm and enlarged nuclei containing atypical chromatin patterns, atypical nucleoli, and mitoses more than 4 per 10 high power fields. A *staghorn-like* vascular pattern is much less discernible than in lesions of other grades. Grade 2 is a lesion with findings between Grade 1 and 3.

31.9 Immunohistochemical Stains

CD34, CD99, and Bcl-2 are constantly positive. However, they are less specific, and the absence of CD34 does not rule out SFT [21–24]. CD34 expression is strongly positive in more than 80% of SFTs, but its expression may be lost in most aggressive SFTs [25, 26]. More recently, STAT6 nuclear staining as a surrogate marker of NAB2-STAT6 gene fusion has been reported to be a highly sensitive and specific marker for SFT [14, 25, 27–29]. Bianchi et al. [14] reported expression of CD34 and of STAT6 immunopositivity in 95% and in 100% of cases, respectively. The *staghorn* vascular appearance with the presence of the NAB2-STAT6 gene rearrangement is considered pathognomonic feature for SFT/HPC. Cytokeratin, S-100, and p53 proteins have shown increased expression in malignant SFTs, but are not specific.

31.10 Management

Surgical resection is the gold standard of treatment. Thorough or extended curettage is carefully considered for an absolutely benign lesion. Because even bland-looking SFTB can, however, be locally recurrent and metastatic, initial management by wide resection with an adequate margin is reasonable for both benign and malignant SFTBs [8] (Fig. 31.1d). Radiation therapy (RT) is the treatment of choice for the inoperable cases. Preoperative RT may shrink the tumor and improve local control. In a multicenter study of perioperative RT in 549 patients with primary extra-meningeal SFT, Hass and colleagues suggested that combining RT with surgery significantly improved local control, especially in patients with less favorable resection margins and in those who have tumors with a high mitotic count. However, the authors failed to prove an overall survival benefit [30]. Another recent multicenter study supports the role of postoperative radiation in disease control for intracranial SFT/HPC, irrespective of surgical extent and grade [31]. Chemotherapy has also been used in patient with advanced or metastatic setting of SFT, but antiangiogenic compounds including pazopanib, sunitinib, or axitinib have shown higher efficacy with longer survival than the historical use of chemotherapy [32].

31.11 Clinical Course and Prognosis

Although most SFTs at different sites are relatively benign, about 10% to 20% of cases may display aggressive behavior with local invasion, recurrence, and distant metastasis [29, 33]. However, Wold et al. [8] reported SFTBs were benign in 4 cases (27%), intermediate in 2 (13%), and malignant in 9 (60%) out of 15 cases in their series. More recently, Unni and Inwards [10] suggested most HPCs exhibit at least low-grade malignancy. Due to the unpredictable biological behavior of these tumors and the possibility of recurrence many years after the initial diagnosis the initial diagnosis, long-term follow-up is required. In a review of 41 cases from the literature and 4 additional cases of primary HPC of bone, the 5-year and 10-year survival rates were 75% and 44%, respectively, and late recurrence or metastases tended to develop long afterward as late as 6, 7, 8, 9, 18, and 26 years after their original diagnosis [13]. Thus, the authors believed that adequate surgical removal of the lesion either by en-bloc resection or even amputation is the most appropriate form of therapy. Recent analysis of 24 patients with SFTB in a single institution reported disease-specific survival of 64% at 5 years and 49% at 10 years. No local recurrence occurred in patients considered to have low-grade malignancy. In particular, the authors reported that 10-year recurrence-free survival was 64% for high-grade patients compare to 100% in low-grade patients, although this disdifference was not statistically significant, likely due to the limited number of patients with a bias [14]. The authors concluded that the aggressive behavior of primary SFTB seems to be independent from mitotic count or any other clinicopathological and molecular features.

References

1. Wagner E. Das tuberkelähnliche Lymphadenom: (Der cytogene oder reticulirte Tuberkel.). Von E. Wagner Mit zwei Tafeln: Otto Wigand; 1871.
2. Klemperer P, Rabin CB. Primary neoplasms of the pleura. A report of five cases. Arch Pathol. 1992;22(1):1–31.
3. Stout A. Tumors featuring pericytes; glomus tumor and hemangiopericytoma. Lab Investig. 1956;5(2):217–23.
4. Fletcher C. The evolving classification of soft tissue tumours: an update based on the new WHO classification. Histopathology. 2006;48(1):3–12.
5. Demicco EG, Fritchie KJ, Han A. Solitary fibrous tumor. In: In: WHO Classification of Tumours Editorial Board, editor. WHO classification of tumours of soft tissue and bone, vol. 5. 5th ed. Lyon: IARC Press; 2020. p. 104–8.
6. Unni KK, Mertens F, Fletcher CD, Guillou L, Fletcher JA, Fletcher CDM, Mandahl N. Extrapleural solitary fibrous tumour and haemangiopericytoma. In: Unni KK, Mertens F, Fletcher CD, editors. WHO classification of tumours of soft tissue and bone. Lyon: IARC Press; 2002. p. 86–90.
7. Unni KK, Ivins JC, Beabout JW, Dahlin DC. Hemangioma, hemangiopericytoma, and hemangioendothelioma (angiosarcoma) of bone. Cancer. 1971;27(6):1403–14.
8. Wold LE, Unni KK, Cooper KL, Sim FH, Dahlin DC. Hemangiopericytoma of bone. Am J Surg Pathol. 1982;6(1):53–8.
9. Huvos AG. Hemangiopericytoma of bone. In: Huvos AG, editor. Bone tumors: diagnosis, treatment and prognosis. Philadelphia: WB Saunders; 1979. p. 358–72.
10. Unni KK, Inwards CY. Hemangiopericytoma. In: Unni KK, Inwards CY, editors. Dahlin's bone tumors: general aspects and data on 10,165 cases. 6th ed. Philadelphia, PA: Lippincott William & Wilkins; 2010. p. 282–5.
11. Dahlin DC. Hemangioendothelioma (hemangiosarcoma) and hemangiopericytoma. In: Dahlin DC, editor. Bone tumors: general aspects and data on 8,542 cases. 4th ed. Springfield: Charles C Thomas; 1986. p. 368–70.
12. Picci P, Manfrini M, Donati DM, Gambarotti M, Righi A, Vanel D, Dei Tos AP. Diagnosis of musculoskeletal tumors and tumor-like conditions: clinical,

radiological and histological correlations-the Rizzoli case archive. 2nd ed. Cham: Springer; 2020. p. 3–11.
13. Tang JS, Gold RH, Mirra JM, Eckardt J. Hemangiopericytoma of bone. Cancer. 1988;62(4):848–59.
14. Bianchi G, Lana D, Gambarotti M, Ferrari C, Sbaraglia M, Pedrini E, et al. Clinical, histological, and molecular features of solitary fibrous tumor of bone: a single institution retrospective review. Cancers. 2021;13(10):2470.
15. Mirra JM, Tang JS, Gold R. Hemangiopericytoma. In: Mirra JM, editor. Bone tumors: clinical, radiologic, and pathologic correlation. Philadelphia: Lea & Febiger; 1989. p. 1436–53.
16. Verbeke SL, Fletcher CD, Alberghini M, Daugaard S, Flanagan AM, Parratt T, et al. A reappraisal of hemangiopericytoma of bone; analysis of cases reclassified as synovial sarcoma and solitary fibrous tumor of bone. Am J Surg Pathol. 2010;34(6):777–83.
17. Bikmaz K, Cosar M, Kurtkaya-Yapicier O, Iplikcioglu AC, Gokduman CA. Recurrent solitary fibrous tumour in the cerebellopontine angle. J Clin Neurosci. 2005;12(7):829–32.
18. Chan J. Solitary fibrous tumour-everywhere, and a diagnosis in vogue. Histopathology. 1997;31(6):568–76.
19. Colia V, Provenzano S, Morosi C, Collini P, Renne SL, Dagrada PG, et al. Solitary fibrous tumour presenting with a single bone metastasis: report of six cases and literature review. Clin Sarcoma Res. 2016;6(1):1–6.
20. Hoshi M, Araki N, Naka N, Koizumi M, Hashimoto N, Onishi M, et al. Bone metastasis of intracranial meningeal hemangiopericytoma. Int J Clin Oncol. 2005;10(3):208–13.
21. Chilosi M, Facchetti F, Dei Tos AP, Lestani M, Morassi ML, Martignoni G, et al. Bcl-2 expression in pleural and extrapleural solitary fibrous tumours. J Pathol. 1997;181(4):362–7.
22. Hasegawa T, Matsuno Y, Shimoda T, Hirohashi S, Hirose T, Sano T. Frequent expression of bcl-2 protein in solitary fibrous tumors. Jpn J Clin Oncol. 1998;28(2):86–91.
23. Mosquera JM, Fletcher CD. Expanding the spectrum of malignant progression in solitary fibrous tumors: a study of 8 cases with a discrete anaplastic component-is this dedifferentiated SFT? Am J Surg Pathol. 2009;33(9):1314–21.
24. Kayser K, Trott J, Böhm G, Huber M, Kaltner H, André S, et al. Localized fibrous tumors (LFTs) of the pleura: clinical data, asbestos burden, and syntactic structure analysis applied to newly defined angiogenic/growth-regulatory effectors. Pathol Res Pract. 2005;201(12):791–801.
25. Ouladan S, Trautmann M, Orouji E, Hartmann W, Huss S, Büttner R, et al. Differential diagnosis of solitary fibrous tumors: a study of 454 soft tissue tumors indicating the diagnostic value of nuclear STAT6 relocation and ALDH1 expression combined with in situ proximity ligation assay. Int J Oncol. 2015;46(6):2595–605.
26. Yokoi T, Tsuzuki T, Yatabe Y, Suzuki M, Kurumaya H, Koshikawa T, et al. Solitary fibrous tumour: significance of p53 and CD34 immunoreactivity in its malignant transformation. Histopathology. 1998;32(5):423–32.
27. Doyle LA, Vivero M, Fletcher CD, Mertens F, Hornick JL. Nuclear expression of STAT6 distinguishes solitary fibrous tumor from histologic mimics. Mod Pathol. 2014;27(3):390–5.
28. Yoshida A, Tsuta K, Ohno M, Yoshida M, Narita Y, Kawai A, et al. STAT6 immunohistochemistry is helpful in the diagnosis of solitary fibrous tumors. Am J Surg Pathol. 2014;38(4):552–9.
29. Vogels RJ, Vlenterie M, Versleijen-Jonkers YM, Ruijter E, Bekers EM, et al. Solitary fibrous tumor. Clinicopathologic, immunohistochemical and molecular analysis of 28 cases. Diagn Pathol. 2014;9(1):1–9.
30. Haas RL, Walraven I, Lecointe-Artzner E, van Houdt WJ, Strauss D, Schrage Y, et al. Extrameningeal solitary fibrous tumors-surgery alone or surgery plus perioperative radiotherapy: a retrospective study from the global solitary fibrous tumor initiative in collaboration with the Sarcoma patients EuroNet. Cancer. 2020;126(13):3002–12.
31. Lee JH, Jeon SH, Park CK, Park SH, Yoon HI, Chang JH, Suh CO, et al. The role of postoperative radiotherapy in intracranial solitary fibrous tumor/hemangiopericytoma: a multi-institutional retrospective study (KROG 18-11). Cancer Res Treat. 2022;54(1):65–74.
32. Martin-Broto J, Mondaza-Hernandez JL, Moura DS, Hindi N. A comprehensive review on solitary fibrous tumor: new insights for new horizons. Cancers. 2021;13(12):2913.
33. Keraliya AR, Tirumani SH, Shinagare AB, Zaheer A, Ramaiya NH. Solitary fibrous tumors: 2016 imaging update. Radiol Clin North Am. 2016;54(3):565–79.

32 Desmoplastic Fibroma

32.1 Definition

Desmoplastic fibroma of bone (DFB) is an extremely rare benign, locally aggressive fibroblastic bone tumor composed of thin, wavy fibroblasts set in abundant dense intercellular collagen, which is histologically identical to the desmoid tumor of soft tissue.

32.2 Incidence

DFB is extraordinarily rare, accounting for about 0.2–0.3% of biopsy-analyzed primary bone tumors [1] or less than 0.1% of all bone tumors [2–5].

32.3 Age

The lesion may occur at any age, but the majority of patients are adolescents and young adults during the first three decades of life [3, 4, 6].

32.4 Location

Any bone can be involved. In a large series with 107 cases in the literature and 7 cases from the authors' institution, long bones including the femur, tibia, humerus, and radius, pelvic bones, as well as craniofacial bones are most frequently affected. The mandible was the most common single site of involvement, representing about one-fourth of all cases, followed by the femur, pelvis bone, and humerus in that order [6]. Other series of 27 cases reported approximately 60% occurred in the pelvis and long bones and 33% in skull bone. The mandible was also the single most frequent site of involvement, occupying about 26% of all cases [4]. The lesion usually occurs in the meta-diaphysis often extending into the epiphysis in adults, but rarely in the mid-diaphysis if the long bone is affected [1, 6, 7]. Only about 5% of all cases have been reported to arise in the diaphysis [6].

32.5 Clinical Features

The clinical manifestations are nonspecific and similar to those of other bone tumors. Pain with or without palpable mass or swelling is the most common symptom, although it can be asymptomatic in some patients. The pain is usually mild in the beginning and becomes bothersome to severe. Less than 10% of patients initially complain of swelling alone without pain [1]. Pathologic fracture is occasionally associated, being reported in 10–15% of the patients [4, 6].

W.-J. Bahk, *Diagnosis and Management of Primary Bone Tumors*,
https://doi.org/10.1007/978-981-96-3484-2_32

32.6 Radiologic Findings

Plain Raduiogrph The lesion usually presents as a well-defined or partially well-defined, multilobulated, geographic destruction with a narrow zone of transition containing no internal mineralized matrix. The affected bone is mildly to moderately expanded and the cortex can be thinned and even absent, but it is usually replaced by a thin shell of reactive bone. The margin of lesion can also be surrounded by a reactive sclerotic bone, somtimes significantly thick reactive sclerosis. In long bones, the lesion is usually oval to oblong in shape with its longest dimension parallel to the long axis of the involved bone (Figs. 32.1 and 32.2). It usually occurs in the metaphysis and may extend to the epiphysis and eventually to the subchondral bone in skeletally mature patients. In a radiographic analysis of 114 cases, Crim et al. [6] reported that geographic bone destruction, with a narrow zone of transition and nonsclerotic wide margin (96%) as well as internal pseudotrabeculation (91%) were the most consistent findings. The lesion slowly grows and erodes or even breaches the cortex, but the periosteum is usually preserved without destruction. Thus, the host bone is widened by gradual apposition of periosteal new bone formation and eventually expands in a *globe-like* shape. Typically, the uneven destruction of the medulla and cortex can lead to variably thickened ridges, imparting a *reticulated*, *trabeculated*, or *bubbly* appearance (Fig. 32.3). The cortex can be significantly thinned even with cortical breakage and a focal extension into the soft tissue indicating a locally aggressive lesion in about 30% of cases [6] (Figs. 32.1 and 32.3). A periosteal reaction or periosteal new bone formation is rare except with pathologic fracture. **CT scan** clearly reveals a well-defined purely osteolytic or mixed osteolytic or mildly sclerotic lesion, occasionally with varying degrees of surround sclerosis (Fig. 32.2c). CT scan more clearly shows cortical erosion or disruption possibly with a soft tissue mass extending beyond the original destroyed cortex. **MR images** reveal the extent of the lesion and small cortical perforations with soft tissue extension (Fig. 32.1c) and the zone of transition or thickness of marginal sclerosis with dark signal (Fig. 32.2d). The SI is low to intermediate on T1-weighted image and heterogeneous high background with foci of low intensity on T2-weighted image (Figs. 32.1, 32.2 and 32.3). The low SI on T2-weighted images may reflect the presence of dense fibrous matrix and the low to acellularity of the tumor [8, 9]. The SI of the tumor may vary with the amount of collagen within the tumor. Generally, the lesion is surrounded by a varying degree of dark signal of reactive sclerosis on both sequences. The lesion is heterogeneously enhanced by contrast medium (Figs. 32.1c and 32.2d). **Bone scan** The lesion shows a variable uptakes from subtle or mild to moderate degree (Fig. 32.1b).

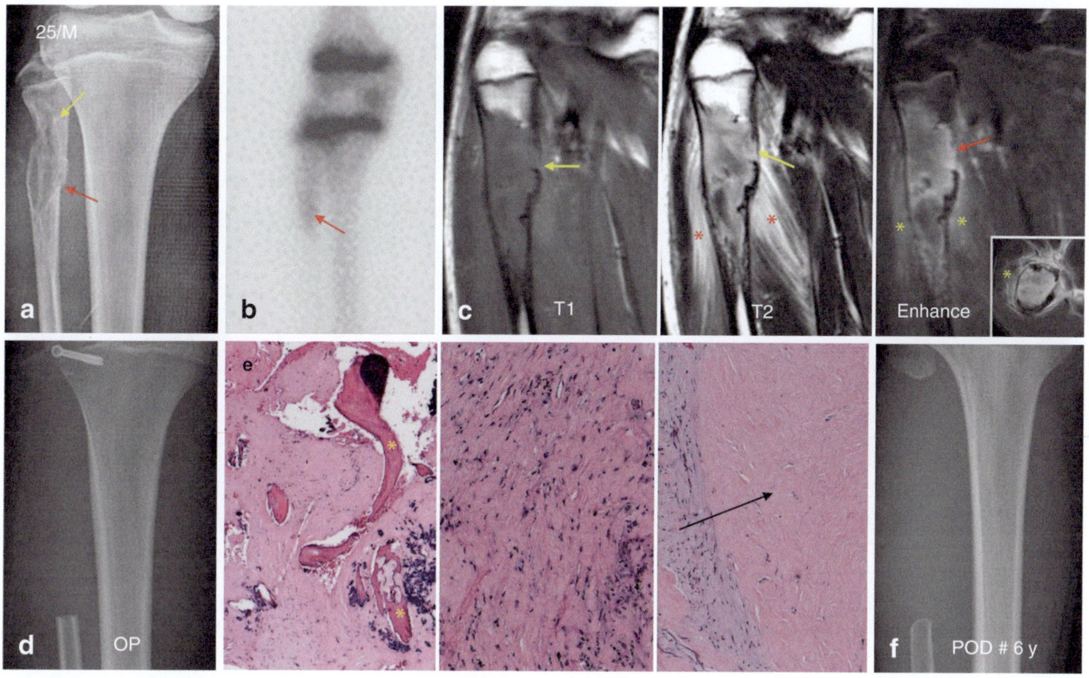

Fig. 32.1 (**a**) Radiograph taken for right knee pain of 2 weeks' duration in a 25-year-old young man shows a relatively well-defined, multilobulated, radiolucent lesion with an irregular rim of surrounding sclerosis (yellow arrow) in the meta-diaphysis of the proximal fibula. The cortex is markedly thinned and cortical breakage or pathologic fracture is suspected (red arrow). The lesion is typically oblong with its longest dimension parallel to the long axis of the fibula. (**b**) Bone scan reveals only a subtle to mild uptake in the lesion (red arrow). (**c**) MR images demonstrate a relatively well-defined, intramedullary mass-like lesion lacking the dark signal of a slcerotic rim, with intermediate SI on T1-weighted image and intermediate and high SI with focal low to dark signal foci on T2-weighted image. Note cortical thinning and breakthrough with mild soft tissue extension (yellow arrows). There are also diffuse high to bright signals in the surrounding soft tissues and muscles on T2-weighted image (red asterisks) with diffuse enhancement on contrast-enhanced image (yellow asterisks), suggesting prominent hemorrhage and inflammation probably due to concealed fracture. The lesion itself is heterogeneously enhanced (red arrow). (**d**) En-bloc resection with adequate margin was done under impression of locally aggressive or malignant bone tumor without biopsy. (**e**) Microscopic examination: (Left) Low-power magnification presents a focal infiltrative growth pattern of scanty spindle-shaped fibroblasts embedded within abundant collagen bundles, with permeation of the host lamella bone at the periphery of the lesion (asterisks), as in FSA. (Middle) Higher-power magnification reveals that the stroma cells are bland and scanty in the central area, but the cellularity is higher with thin-walled, dilated vascular channels in the peripheral area. (Right) The focal higher cellular area with a lesser amount of collagen is gradually merging into the pinkish, dense fibrous area with sparse fibroblasts, simulating scar tissue (long arrow). The wavy collagen is typically laid down in *"broad and parallel"* fashion rather than *"herringbone"* pattern in FSA or *"storiform"* pattern in fibrohistiocytic lesions. (**f**) Follow-up radiograph at 6 years after surgery shows no evidence of local recurrence

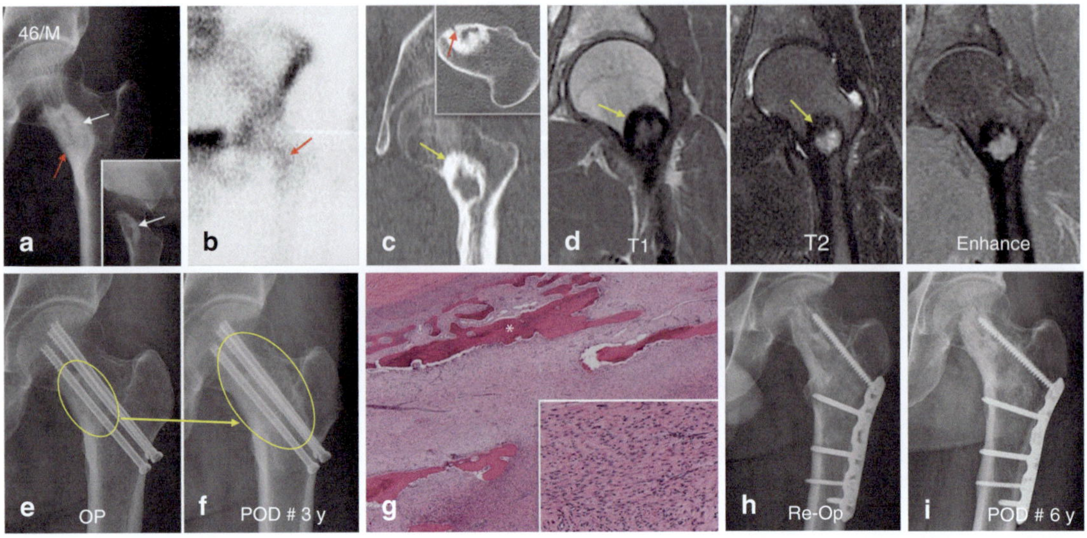

Fig. 32.2 (**a**) Radiograph taken for left hip pain of 5 months' duration, accutely aggravated after running in a 46-year-old man shows a well-defined, eccentric, oval to oblong, radiolucent lesion surrounded by markedly thick sclerotic bone (white arrows) in the medial aspect of left femoral neck. Note its oval shape with the longest dimension aligned with the long axis of the femoral neck and a radiolucent line, suggesting insufficiency or stress fracture induced by running (red arrow). (**b**) Bone scan reveals only peripheral mild uptake (arrow). (**c**) CT scan notes a radiolucent lesion surrounded by a thick sclerotic rim (yellow arrow) with a cortical crack indicating incomplete fracture (inset). (**d**) MR images demonstrate a well-defined mass-like lesion with low to intermediate SI on T1-weighted image and high SI on T2-weighted image, which is surrounded by a thick dark signal of reactive sclerotic bone on both sequences (yellow arrows). However, there is no discernible fracture line, which is seen as a crack on CT scan. The main internal lesion is homogeneously well enhanced. (**e**) In situ fixation with cannulated screws was performed under the radiologic impression of old benign tumor with an incomplete pathologic fracture without biopsy. (**f**) Follow-up radiograph taken for intermittent pain with mild limp at 3 years after surgery shows radiologic union of the linear fracture but progression of the lesion (yellow circle). (**g**) Microscopic examination of biopsy material reveals spindle-shaped fibroblastic cells producing bundles arranged of collagen fibers but no bone or cartilage matrix. The tumor destructs and infiltrates the bone marrow space associated with permeation of the host lamellar bone (asterisks). However, the individual cells are bland-looking with monotonous nuclei in size and shape, and collagen bundles are typically arranged in *parallel* fashion, indicating DFB (inset). (**h**) Extended curettage using high-speed bur followed by bone graft and plate fixation was performed after removal of the cannulated screws. (**i**) Follow-up radiograph at 6 years after second surgery reveals consolidation of the lesion with no evidence of recurence, and the patient is pain-free

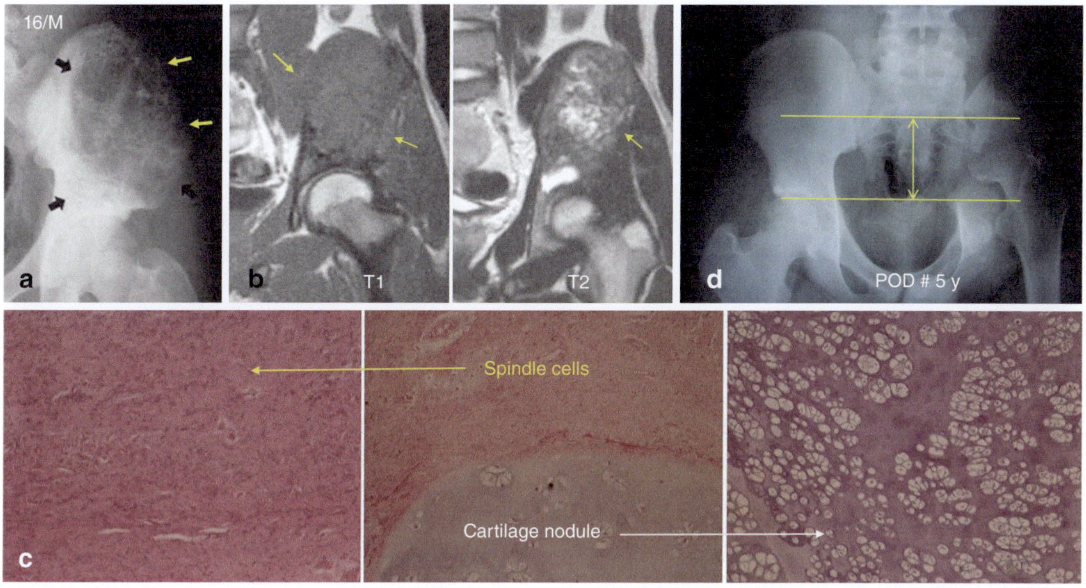

Fig. 32.3 (**a**) Radiograph taken for a large palpable mass of the left pelvic area of 2 years' duration in a 16-year-old adolescent shows a relatively well-defined, huge, multilobulated, geographically destructive lesion with a typical *trabeculated* to *bubbly* appearance in nearly the entire left iliac wing and a part of the acetabulum (black arrows). There is significant thinning of the cortex with possible cortical destruction and soft tissue extension (yellow arrows). (**b**) MR images reveal a large expansive mass-like lesion with intermediate SI on T1-weighted image and heterogeneous intermediate and high SI with focal areas of low signal on T2-weighted image. The cortex is ballooned and irregularly destructed with soft tissue extension (arrows). (**c**) Microscopic examination: (Middle) Lower-power magnification notes that the tumor consists of two different tissue components; an area with bland spindle cells embedded within a wavy collagenous stroma in the upper field and another area of bland hyaline cartilage nodule in the lower field. There is a sharp demarcation between the spindle lesion and the cartilage nodule. (Left) Higher magnification of the upper field shows that the spindled stromal cells are bland-looking with monotonous nuclei and the collagen is fine, wavy, and fibrillar. There is no bone or cartilage matrix production by the spindle cells in this area, suggesting DFB. (Right) Higher magnification of the enchondroma-like nodule in the lower field reveals hypercellularity with occasional bi-nucleated chondrocytes, simulating CSA. (**d**) Internal hemipelvectomy was performed in another hospital with a misdiagnosis of CSA by the general pathologist who was not aware of the phenomenon that DFB abutting the epiphyseal plate in growing children can produce enchondroma-like cartilage nodules with high cellularity, mild atypia, or frequent bi-nucleated chondrocytes. The final diagnosis was revised to DFB with hyaline cartilage nodules after consultation with Dr. Mirra. The patient is disease-free without evidence of local recurrence or distant metastasis 5 years after surgery

32.7 Histologic Findings

DFB is histologically identical to the desmoid type of fibromatosis in soft tissue. The lesion dominantly consists of bland, spindle-shpaed fibroblasts, producing a variable amount of collagen, but no bone or cartilage matrix. The fibrous tissue is rather compact and mature with varying proportions of fibroblasts and collagen fibers. The cellularity is variable from areas to areas and can be focally high but never very cellular, with lesser amount of collagen gradually merging into the pinkish dense eosinophilic areas with sparse fibroblasts, simulating scar tissue (Fig. 32.1e). The individual cells show bland-looking monotonous nuclei in size and shape, which are uniform in size and shape, and are round to ovoid with finely stippled chromatin but minute to absent nucleoli. Mitoses are always typical and the number is scanty. The collagen is laid down typically in a "*broad and parallel*" fashion unlike the "*herringbone*" pattern in fibrosarcoma (FSA) or "*storiform*" pattern in other fibro-histiocytic lesions. The collagen fibers run parallel with variable thickness, which may be straight or wavy depending on the degree of contraction during fixation [1]. Thin-walled, dilated vascular channels may be observed within the stroma as well. The lesion may exhibit a focal infiltrative growth pattern at the periphery of the lesion with permeation of the host bone marrow, simulating FSA or fibroblastic osteosarcoma particularly when it is extensive (Fig. 32.2g). Extraordinarily, DFB present with extensive chondroid metaplasia as in fibrocartilaginous dysplasia [10, 11] (Fig. 32.3c). Fibrous tumors including DFB, fibrous dysplasia, and FSA abutting the epiphyseal plate, prticularly in grwoing children, can produce eposits of the hypercellular nodules of hyaline cartilage within fibroblastic stroma of the parent tumor. The nodules may show varying degrees of cytologic atypia with occasional bi-nucleated chondrocytes, simulating chondrosarcoma (CSA) [12]. Physicians should be aware of this phenomenon for a correct diagnosis to prevent overtreatment with misdiagnosis of CSA (Fig. 32.3).

32.8 Management

En-bloc resection with a marginal or, better, a wide margin is the treatment of choice, especially in DFB with cortical breakage and soft tissue extension [1, 5, 7]. Campanacci described a high incidence of local recurrence up to about half of cases after curettage with or without local adjuvants [7]. Radiotherapy is another therapeutic option when the surgical margin is not enough or surgery is not feasible [13–15].

32.9 Prognosis and Clinical Course

Due to its rarity, the prognosis is difficult to predict. However, DFB is considered a slow-growing progressive tumor with locally aggressive behavior but no capacity to metastasize. An analysis of 191 patients in the literature reported a recurrence rate of 55–72% after nonresection procedures in contrast to 17% after resection and no recurrences after resection with wide surgical margin. In addition, the recurrence rate of tumors in the extremities was 55%, and 25% of these patients eventually required amputation [16]. In an early Mayo clinic series of 19 patients with available information on treatment, local recurrence developed in all but 2 of 10 patients treated by lesional curettage, but no recurrences were reported after en-bloc resection with wide margins [4]. DFB does not metastasize no matter how many local recurrences occur, and can be eventually cured by multiple en-bloc resection in the majority of cases because the lesion is absolutely benign despite its local aggressiveness [1]. Because of the infiltrative pattern of growth and histologic resemblance, DFB has been considered the osseous counterpart of desmoid-type fibromatosis in soft tissue [1, 2, 17]. However, Hauben et al. reported that cytoplasmic overexpression of β-catenin was detected in half of the cases with accumulation in the nucleus only in one case, whereas desmoid-type fibromatosis of soft tissue notes both nuclear and cytoplasmic overexpression in most cases. The authors suggested that the β-catenin pathway does not seem to have the same essential role in the tumorigenesis of DFB as in the desmoid-type fibromatosis of soft tissue despite the morphological overlap with regard to epidemiology, histology, and immunohistochemical profile [18, 19].

References

1. Mirra JM. Desmoid tumor of bone. In: Mirra JM, editor. Bone tumors: clinical, radiologic, and pathologic correlations. 2nd ed. Philadelphia: Lea & Febiger; 1989. p. 735–47.
2. Czerniak B. Fibrous and fibrohistiocytic lesions. In: Dorfman HD, Czerniak B, editors. Dorfman and Czerniak's bone tumors. 2nd ed. (eBook): Elsevier; 2016. p. 617–91.
3. Evans S, Ramasamy A, Jeys L, Grimer R. Desmoplastic fibroma of bone: a rare bone tumour. J Bone Oncol. 2014;3(3–4):77–9.
4. Inwards CY, Krishnan Unni K, Beabout JW, Sim FH. Desmoplastic fibroma of bone. Cancer. 1991;68(9):1978–83.
5. Unni KK, Inwards CY. Desmoplastic fibroma. In: Unni KK, Inwards CY, editors. Dahlin's bone tumors: general aspects and data on 10,165 cases. 6th ed. Philadelphia: Lippincott William & Wilkins; 2010. p. 175–8.
6. Crim J, Gold RH, Mirra JM, Eckardt J, Bassett L. Desmoplastic fibroma of bone: radiographic analysis. Radiology. 1989;172(3):827–32.
7. Campanacci M. Desmoid fibroma. In: Campanacci M, editor. Bone and soft tissue tumors. Wien New York: Springer-Verlag; 1999. p. 143–8.
8. Sundaram M, McGuire M, Schajowicz F. Soft-tissue masses: histologic basis for decreased signal (short T2) on T2-weighted MR images. Am J Roentgenol. 1987;148(6):1247–50.
9. Yu JS, Lawrence S, Pathria M, Resnick D, Haghighi P. Desmoplastic fibroma of the calcaneus. Skeletal Radiol. 1995;24:451–4.
10. Bahk WJ, Kang YK, Lee AH, Mirra JM. Desmoid tumor of bone with enchondromatous nodules, mistaken for chondrosarcoma. Skeletal Radiol. 2003;32:223–6.
11. Callahan KS, Eberhardt SC, Fechner RE, Cerilli LA. Desmoplastic fibroma of bone with extensive cartilaginous metaplasia. Ann Diagn Pathol. 2006;10(6):343–6.
12. Mirra JM. Fibrous tumors of bone with enchondroma-like nodules. In: Mirra JM, editor. Bone tumors: clinical, radiologic, and pathologic correlations. 2nd ed. Philadelphia: Lea & Febiger; 1989. p. 674–90.
13. Nag H, Kumar R, Bhan S, Awasthy B, Julka P, Ray R. Radiotherapy for desmoplastic fibroma of bone: a case report. J Orthop Surg. 2003;11(1):90–3.
14. Sanfilippo NJ, Wang GJ, Larner JM. Desmoplastic fibroma: a role for radiotherapy? South Med J. 1995;88(12):1267–9.
15. Seidensaal K, Harrabi S, Weykamp F, Herfarth K, Welzel T, Mechtersheimer G, et al. Radiotherapy in the treatment of aggressive fibromatosis: experience from a single institution. Radiat Oncol. 2020;15(1):1–9.
16. Böhm P, Kröber S, Greschniok A, Laniado M, Kaiserling E. Desmoplastic fibroma of the bone: a report of two patients, review of the literature, and therapeutic implications. Cancer. 1996;78(5):1011–23.
17. Jaffe HL. Desrnoplastic fibroma and fibrosarcoma. In: Jaffe HL, editor. Tumors and tumorous conditions of the bones and joints. Phildelphia: Lea & Febiger; 1958. p. 298–303.
18. Hauben EI, Jundt G, Cleton-Jansen AM, Yavas A, Hrron HM, Van Mark E, et al. Desmoplastic fibroma of bone: an immunohistochemical study including β-catenin expression and mutational analysis for β-catenin. Hum Pathol. 2005;36(9):1025–30.
19. Hauben E, Cleton-Jansen AM. In: Fletcher CDM, Bridge JA, Hogendoorn PCW, Mertens F, editors. Desmoplastic fibroma of bone. In WHO classification of tumors of soft tissue and bone. IARC Lyon; 2013. p. 298. https://hdl.handle.net/2066/132068.

Fibrosarcoma

33

33.1 Definition

Fibrosarcoma (FSA) of bone is a rare malignant spindle cell tumor exhibiting a fibroblastic differentiation, consisting of relatively monomorphic fibroblastic cells with variable amount of collagen production but no osteoid or cartilage production. It may occur as a primary, de novo, lesion and secondarily after irradiation or through malignant transformation from various preexisting benign conditions such as fibrous dysplasia, giant cell tumor, Paget disease, bone infarction, diaphyseal medullary stenosis, or chronic osteomyelitis [1, 2]. The majority cases of FSAB are solitary lesions, but a few cases of multifocal FSA have been reported sporadically [3–6]. Only 3 out of 286 cases (1%) were multifocal skeletal disease at presentation in the Mayo Clinic series [2].

33.2 Incidence

FRA of bone is rare, representing approximately 3–5% of primary malignant bone tumors [1, 2, 7, 8]. Secondary FSA accounted for 22% of all FSA (64 of 286 cases) in the Mayo Clinic files [2].

33.3 Age

The lesion can occur in all age groups with an even distribution from the second through seventh decades [2, 9], but most commonly affects middle-aged and elderly individuals, with an average in the fourth decade of life [1, 8] and a peak in the fifth decade [9].

33.4 Location

The common skeletal distribution is similar to that of osteosarcoma (OSA) [1]. The metaphysea region extending to the diaphyseal of the long bone is involved in more than half of the patients. The lesion can be medullary (70%) or periosteal (30%) in location [8]. The most frequent location is the distal and proximal tibia, followed by the proximal humerus, proximal femur, pelvis, and jaw. Over 40% of the cases occur around the knee joint (distal femur and proximal tibia) [1, 9, 10].

W.-J. Bahk, *Diagnosis and Management of Primary Bone Tumors*,
https://doi.org/10.1007/978-981-96-3484-2_33

33.5 Clinical Features

The most common symptom is pain in medullary presentation and mass or swelling with or without pain/tenderness in periosteal presentation [8]. The pain is usually milder and of long duration in lower-grade tumors, or more severe and of short duration in higher-grade tumors. Swelling, limitation of joint motion, stress or pathologic fracture can be more frequently associated in higher-grade FSA.

33.6 Radiologic Findings

Plain radiograph FSA of bone presents with nonspecific features, usually indicating local aggressiveness such as cortical destruction and soft tissue extension as in other malignant bone tumors. FSA is usually centered within the metaphysis or meta-diaphysis of long bones (Figs. 33.1 and 33.2). Typically, the lesion is eccentric, purely osteolytic, and expansile without internal cartilage or bone production. *Lower-grade* lesions usually exhibit a geographic destruction pattern with cortical thinning or breakthrough. The lesion margin is usually well-defined, with no discernible sclerotic rim. Cortical ridging and multiple septations by irregular, lobulated destruction of the cortex produce a more prominent "*soap-bubble*" appearance. The cortex can be breached or focally destructed, but periosteal reaction is usually minimal (Fig. 33.1a). *Higher-grade* lesions show an ill-defined extensive geographic destruction with more locally aggressive, moth-eaten to permeative pattern. The multilobulated or "*soap-bubble*" appearance becomes less prominent due to severe medullary destruction, and residual bony trabeculae are rare. However, the cortex is more extensively destructed and extends into soft tissue, forming a large mass in most cases [1] (Fig. 33.2a). A periosteal reaction is also rarely observed, and it is usually laminated, spiculate, or Codman triangle if presents. **Bone scan** The lesion usually presents homogeneously or heterogeneously strong uptake in the lesion (Figs. 33.1b and 33.2b). It can easily detect the exceedingly rare multifocal FSA. **CT scan** is useful to evaluate the amount of bone destruction and the amount and quality of intact bone remaining. CT may substitute for MRI if a patient cannot undergoes for various reasons. **PET/CT scan** shows heterogeneous intense FDG uptake in the lesion (Fig. 33.2d) corresponding to the destruction noted on CT scan, and is also useful to detect exceptionally rare multifocal lesions or distant metastasis. **MR images** can more clearly define the degree of intraosseous spread and the extent of soft tissue invasion (Figs. 33.1c and 33.2c). The SI is intermediate on T1-weighted image and heterogeneous intermediate and high on T2-weighted image. The lesion is avidly enhanced by contrast medium.

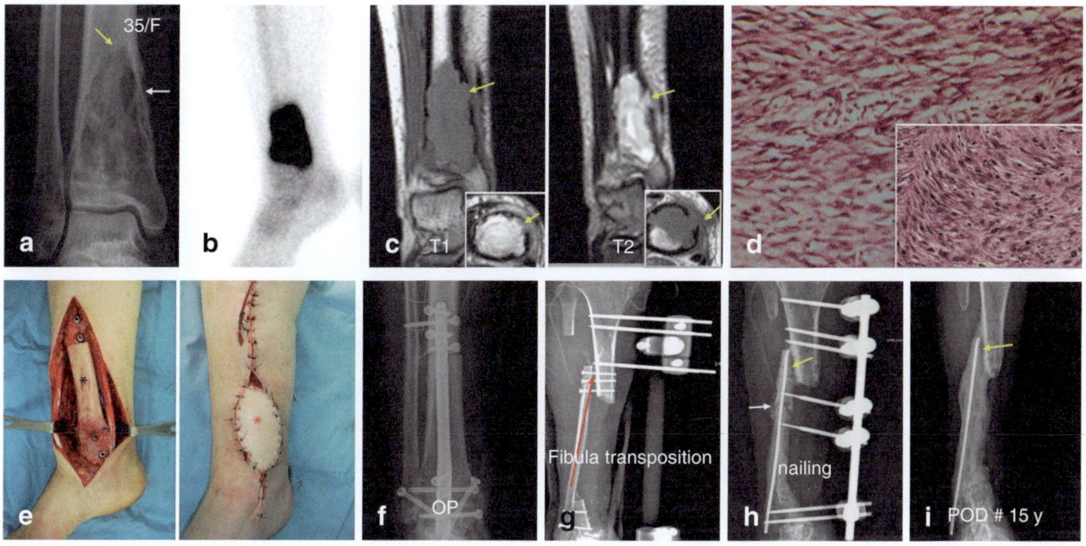

Fig. 33.1 ***Low-grade FSA with a focal higher-grade tumor.*** (**a**) Radiograph taken for right ankle pain of 4–5 months' duration in a 35-year-old lady shows an ill-defined, multilobulated geographic destruction with a wide zone of transition (yellow arrow). There are cortical ridges and multiple septations by irregular, lobulated destruction of the cortex with a prominent "*soap-bubble*" appearance in the meta-diaphysis of the distal tibia. The cortex is undulate and irregularly thinned and possibly perforated, but no definite periosteal reaction (white arrow). (**b**) Bone scan reveals a homogeneous strong uptake only in the distal tibia, indicating a solitary lesion. (**c**) MR images demonstrate a relatively well-defined, intramedullary mass-like lesion with intermediate SI on T1-weighted image and heterogeneous intermediate and high SI on T2-weighted image. The cortices are irregularly eroded and markedly thinned. There is a focal cortical perforation with minimal soft tissue extension (arrows). (**d**) Microscopic examination notes mostly bland-looking, monotonous spindle cells arranged in the same way as a school of fishes, focally interlacing at an acute angle, a typical "*herring-bone*" arrangement, suggesting low-grade FSA. There is another focal area of higher cellularity with more striking anaplasia including brisk mitotic activity, indicating higher-grade (Grade 3) FSA (inset). (**e**) (Left) Wide resection followed by reconstruction using allogenic tibia graft (black asterisk) was performed. (Right) The soft tissue defect was covered by a sural artery local flap (red asterisk). (**f**) Immediate postoperative radiograph shows well-matched tibia graft fixed by retrograde intramedullary nail. The ankle is fused with additional screw fixation. (**g**) Postoperative infection with skin necrosis was complicated at 1 year after initial surgery. After infection control by several procedures, the ipsilateral fibula was transposed (arrow) and fixed by external fixator and screws with autogenous bone graft at the junction of fibula and tibia. (**h**) Two years later, closed reduction and internal fixation with Nancy nail was done for fracture of the transposed fibula (white arrow). The external fixator was changed to a bigger and stronger one, and autogenous chip bone graft was performed for nonunion at the junction site (yellow arrow). (**i**) Follow-up radiograph at 15 years after initial surgery reveals no evidence of local recurrence with complete union of the transposed fibula (arrow)

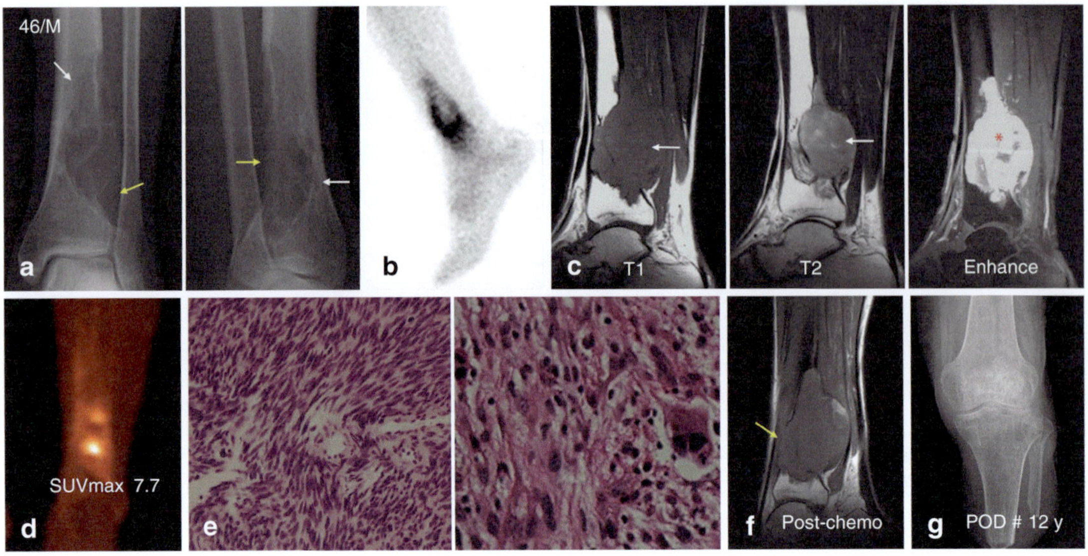

Fig. 33.2 ***High-grade FSA***. (**a**) Radiograph taken for left ankle pain of 2 months' duration in a 46-year-old man shows an ill-defined, eccentric, multilobulated geographic destruction with a less prominent "*soap-bubble*" pattern and rare residual bony trabeculae in the meta-diaphysis of the distal tibia. A moth-eaten type of destruction is also observed along the peripheral margin of the lesion, producing a wide margin of transition (white arrows). The cortex is significantly destructed but with no discernible periosteal reaction (yellow arrows). (**b**) Bone scan reveals heterogenous strong uptake with a focal void area only in the distal tibia, suggesting a solitary lesion. (**c**) MR images demonstrate an eccentric mass-like lesion with intermediate SI on T1-weighted image and heterogeneous intermediate SI withfocal areas of high signal on T2-weighted image. The cortex is significantly destructed with a large soft tissue mass formation (arrows). The lesion is strongly enhanced by contrast medium (asterisk). (**d**) PET/CT scan demonstrates heterogeneous intense FDG uptake (SUVmax 7.7) in the tibial lesion accompanied by severe cortical destruction on CT scan (not shown here). (**e**) Microscopic examination: (Left) Medium-power magnification shows exuberant monotonous fibroblastic spindle cells arranged in a characteristic "*herringbone*" pattern. There is no osteoid or chondroid deposition. Collagen production is relatively minimal, and chronic inflammatory cells are also seen in the right lower field. (Right) Higher-magnification shows individual cells with markedly bizarre nuclei, large nucleoli, hyperchromatism, and brisk mitotic activity including atypical mitoses, indicating Grade 4 FSA. (**f**) Follow-up MR image after neoadjuvant chemotherapy reveals newly developed anterior cortical destruction with soft tissue extension (arrow), without reduction of the tumor size, indicating further progression of the tumor. (**g**) Below-knee amputation was performed. Fortunately, the patient is still alive without local recurrence at 12 years after amputation

33.7 Histologic Findings

FSA typically consists of spindle cells (fibroblasts) and collagen fibers but lacks bone or cartilage matrix production. The lesion is typified by uniform proliferation of spindle-shaped cells arranged in parallel bundles with variable amounts of collagen production. All individual cells are uniformly oriented like a school of fishes, focally interlacing at an acute angle, so-called "*herringbone*" pattern (Figs. 33.1d, and 33.2e). Reactive multinucleated giant cells and chronic inflammatory cells may occasional be found. Based on differentiation, number of cells, mitotic activity, collagen production, nuclear pleomorphism, and overall histologic pattern, FSA of bone can be divided into 4 grades. The cellularity is inversely proportional to the amount of collagen production by the tumor cells. The histologic pattern varies from a better-differentiated, not highly cellular lesion with heavy collagen production (grade 1–2/low-grade), to poorly differentiated highly cellular lesion with obvious nuclear pleomorphism, high mitotic rate, and minimal collagen production (grade 3–4/high-grade) [1, 2]. *Low-grade FSA* is rarer and characterized by monotonous fibroblastic cells with abundant collagen fibers arranged in fascicles or streams. The cells are not very numerous but mildly hyperchromatic and pleomorphic with some mitotic figures. The amount of collagen is usually prominent. *Grade 1* is often difficult to differentiate from locally aggressive desmoplastic fibroma or benign lesion such as nonossifying fibroma because of the overlapping range of mild cytologic atypia. Thus, a clinic-pathologic-radiologic correlation is mandatory to distinguish such cases. *Grade 2* is more cellular with plumper nuclei, more frequent mitotic figures, but less collagen. *High-grade FSA* (Grade 3, 4) is typified by areas with low-grade FSA and other areas of very high cellularity with striking anaplasia, including bizarre plump nuclei, large nucleoli with hyperchromatism, brisk mitotic activity, or even atypical mitoses. However, the typical "*herringbone*" pattern is less prominent and collagen production is rather minimal. In a Rizzoli Institute series of 80 patients, Bertoni et al. reported two cases (2.5%) of grade 1, 11 cases (14%) of grade 2, 42 (53%) cases of grade 3, and 25 cases (31%) of grade 4 [11].

33.8 Management

Wide resection with reconstruction is the treatment of choice if feasible (Fig. 33.1). However, amputation can be considered if it is difficult to obtain an adequate margin, especially in high-grade lesions (Fig. 33.2). Perioperative adjuvant chemotherapy should be considered for high-grade FSA because of a high probability of metastases (>70%) [10], although the lesion respond poorly to chemotherapy. Unfortunately, FSA is also resistant to radiotherapy.

33.9 Prognosis

The prognosis is much worse than that of OSA because of resistance to chemotherapy and radiotherapy, as well as higher incidence of metastasis. However, the 5-year survival rate has gradually improved, from 37% in the 1970s to 54% during the past decade [9]. In 1975, Huvos et al. [8] reported that the overall 5-, 10-, 15-, and 20-year survival rates were 34%, 28%, 27%, and 25% respectively, which were much poorer than those of OSA in their large series including 130 patients. The authors reported 5-year and 10-year survival rates of 27% and 20% in medullary FSA, and 52% and 48% in periosteal FSA. They also reported metastases in 45% of the patients, with the most common site being the lung (81%), followed by other bones (34%). In 1984, an analysis of Rizzoli Institute series including 80 patients reported the 10-year survival rate of 83% for low-grade lesions but 34% for high-grade tumors. The authors also found that local recurrence was a poor prognostic factor [11]. In 1985, a study of 102 patients reported that there was no significant difference in behavior in FSA with or without areas of malignant fibrous histiocytoma, but the prognosis correlated closely with the histologic grade of the tumors. The 5-year survival were 64% in Grade 1 tumors, 41% in Grade 2 tumors, and 23% in Grade 3 tumors, with an overall survival of 34% [12]. Later in 2000, a multivariate analysis of the Mayo Clinic data including 92 patients suggested that high-grade tumor, age more than 40 years, and tumor location in the axial skeleton were the most significant risk factors affecting overall survival. The overall 5-year survival was 33.4%, with the rate of 50% for patients with a low-grade tumor compare to 29% for those with a high-grade lesion. Despite the low rate of local recurrence (15%), the disease-free survival was low mainly due to high incidence of development of metastatic disease in over 60% of the patients. The most common site for metastasis was lung (about 80%), followed by skeleton (7%). The 5-year disease-specific survival rate was only 29% for patients who had surgery before 1980, but it improved to 45% for those having surgery in 1980 or later due to adjuvant chemotherapy and radiation therapy as well as the advent of new imaging modalities and instrumentation [10]. Secondary FSA shows significantly worse prognosis, with 10-year survival rate less than 10% [1].

References

1. Picci P, Mirra JM. Fibrosarcoma. In: Mirra JM, editor. Bone tumors: clinical, radiologic, and pathologic correlations. 2nd ed. Philadelphia: Lea & Febiger; 1989. p. 747–59.
2. Unni KK, Inwards CY. Fibrosarcoma and desmoplastic fibroma. In: Unni KK, Inwards CY, editors. Dahlin's bone tumors: general aspects and data on 10,165 cases. 6th ed. Philadelphia: Lippincott William & Wilkins; 2010. p. 169–78.
3. Hernandez FJ, Fernandez BB. Multiple diffuse fibrosarcoma of bone. Cancer. 1976;37(2):939–45.
4. Kabukcuoglu Y, Kabukcuoglu F, Carter S, Oztürk I, Erseven G, Kuzgun U. Multiple diffuse fibrosarcoma of bone. Am J Orthop. 1999;28(12):715–7.
5. Nielsen AR, Poulsen H. Multiple diffuse fibrosarcomata of the bones. Acta Pathol Microbiol Scand. 1962;55(3):265–72.
6. Steiner PE. Multiple diffuse fibrosarcoma of bone. Am J Pathol. 1944;20(5):877.
7. Dorfman HD, Czerniak B. Bone cancers. Cancer. 1995;75(S1):203–10.
8. Huvos AG, Higinbotham NL. Primary fibrosarcoma of bone. A clinicopathologic study of 130 patients. Cancer. 1975;35(3):837–47.
9. Czerniak B. Fibrous and fibrohistiocytic lesions. In: Dorfman HD, Czerniak B, editors. Dorfman and Czerniak's bone tumors. 2nd ed. eBook: Elsevier; 2016. p. 617–91.
10. Papagelopoulos PJ, Galanis E, Frassica FJ, Sim FH, Larson DR, Wold LE. Primary fibrosarcoma of bone: outcome after primary surgical treatment. Clin Orthop Relat Res. 2000;373:88–103.
11. Bertoni F, Capanna R, Calderoni P, Patrizia B, Campanacci M. Primary central (medullary) fibrosarcoma of bone. Semin Diagn Pathol. 1984;1:185–98.
12. Taconis W, Van Rijssel T, Fibrosarcoma of long bones. A study of the significance of areas of malignant fibrous histiocytoma. J Bone Joint Surg Br. 1985;67(1):111–6.

MIX
Papier aus verantwortungsvollen Quellen
Paper from responsible sources
FSC® C105338

If you have any concerns about our products,
you can contact us on
ProductSafety@springernature.com

In case Publisher is established outside the EU,
the EU authorized representative is:
Springer Nature Customer Service Center GmbH
Europaplatz 3, 69115 Heidelberg, Germany

Printed by Libri Plureos GmbH
in Hamburg, Germany